Clinical Anesthesiology Board Review

A Test Simulation and Self-Assessment Tool

Larry Chu, MD, MS

Assistant Professor of Anesthesia
Department of Anesthesiology and Critical Care Medicine
Stanford University School of Medicine
Stanford, California

McGraw-Hill

MEDICAL PUBLISHING DIVISION

New York / Chicago / San Francisco / Lisbon / London / Madrid
Mexico City / New Delhi / San Juan / Seoul / Singapore / Sydney / Toronto

Clinical Anesthesiology Board Review:
A Test Simulation and Self-Assessment Tool

5 6 7 8 9 0   DIG/DIG   10

ISBN: 0-07-143778-9

Notice

Medicine is an ever-changing science. As new research and clinical experience broaden our knowledge, changes in treatment and drug therapy are required. The authors and the publisher of this work have checked with sources believed to be reliable in their efforts to provide information that is complete and generally in accord with the standards accepted at the time of publication. However, in view of the possibility of human error or changes in medical science, neither the editors nor the publisher nor any other party who has been involved in the preparation or publication of this work warrants that the information contained herein is in every respect accurate or complete, and they disclaim all responsibility for any errors or omissions or for the results obtained from use of the information contained in this work. Readers are encouraged to confirm the information contained herein with other sources. For example and in particular, readers are advised to check the product information sheet included in the package of each drug they plan to administer to be certain that the information contained in this work is accurate and that changes have not been made in the recommended dose or in the contraindications for administration. This recommendation is of particular importance in connection with new or infrequently used drugs.

This book was set in Times Roman by Matrix Publishing.
The editors were Marc Strauss, Marsha Loeb, and Patrick Carr.
The production supervisor was Catherine Saggese.
The cover designer was Aimee Nordin.
The text designer was Marsha Cohen, Parallelogram Graphics.
Quebecor World was printer and binder.

This book is printed on acid-free paper.

Library of Congress Cataloging-in-Publication Data
Chu, Larry F.
    Clinical anesthesiology board review : a test simulation and self-assessment tool / [edited by] Larry F. Chu
        p.   ; cm.
    Includes index.
    ISBN 0-07-143778-9 (alk. paper)
    1. Anesthesiology—Examinations, questions, etc.   2. Anesthesiologists—Licenses—United States—Examinations—Study Guides.   I. Chu, Larry F.   II. Title
    [DNLM: 1. Anesthesia—Examination Questions.   2. Anesthetics—Examination Questions.
WO 18.2 C559c 2005]
    RD82.3.C49 2005
617.9′6′0076—dc22
                                                            2004065570

Contents

Contributing Authors

Aileen Marie Adriano, MD
Clinical Instructor
Department of Anesthesia
Stanford University School of Medicine
Stanford, California

Ian Richard Carroll, MD
Clinical Assistant Professor, Division of Pain Management
Department of Anesthesia
Stanford University School of Medicine
Stanford, California

Andrea Fuller, MD
Clinical Instructor, Division of Obstetric Anesthesia
Department of Anesthesia
Stanford University School of Medicine
Stanford, California

Thomas Kyle Harrison, MD
Clinical Instructor
Department of Anesthesia
Palo Alto Veterans Affairs Hospital
Palo Alto, California

James E. Janik, MD
Anesthesia Resident
Department of Anesthesia
Stanford University School of Medicine
Stanford, California

Shanthala Keshavacharya, MD
Anesthesia Fellow, Cardiac Anesthesia
Department of Anesthesia
Stanford University School of Medicine
Stanford, California

Calvin C. Kuan, MD
Clinical Assistant Professor, Division of Pediatric Anesthesia
Department of Anesthesia
Stanford University School of Medicine
Stanford, California

Edward R. Mariano, MD
Assistant Clinical Professor
Department of Anesthesiology
University of California at San Diego
San Diego, California

Bridget M. Phillip, MD
Anesthesia Fellow, Pediatric Anesthesia
Department of Anesthesia
Stanford University School of Medicine
Stanford, California

Jeannie L. Seybold, MD
Anesthesia Resident
Department of Anesthesia
Stanford University School of Medicine
Stanford, California

Chris R. Stasny, MD
Anesthesia Resident
Department of Anesthesia
Stanford University School of Medicine
Stanford, California

Elizabeth Steele, MD
Clinical Instructor
Case Western Reserve Medical School
Metrohealth Medical Center
Cleveland, Ohio

Kathleen Vuong, MD
Staff Anesthesiologist
Kaiser Permanente Hospital
Redwood City, California

Heidi L. Witherell, MD, MA
Anesthesia Resident
Department of Anesthesia
Stanford University School of Medicine
Stanford, California

REVIEWERS

Timothy Angelotti, MD, PhD

Assistant Professor of Anesthesia
Department of Anesthesia
Stanford University School of Medicine
Stanford, California

Martin Angst, MD

Assistant Professor of Anesthesia
Department of Anesthesia
Stanford University School of Medicine
Stanford, California

Gail Boltz, MD

Assistant Professor of Anesthesia, Division of Pediatric Anesthesia
Department of Anesthesia
Stanford University School of Medicine
Stanford, California

John Brock-Utne, MD, PhD, FFA(SA)

Professor of Anesthesia
Department of Anesthesia
Stanford University School of Medicine
Stanford, California

Jay Brodsky, MD

Professor of Anesthesia
Department of Anesthesia
Stanford University School of Medicine
Stanford, California

Brendan Carvalho, MBBCh(SA), FRCA(UK)

Assistant Professor of Anesthesia, Division of Obstetric Anesthesia
Department of Anesthesia
Stanford University School of Medicine
Stanford, California

John L. Chow, MD

Assistant Professor of Anesthesia
Department of Anesthesia
Stanford University School of Medicine
Stanford, California

J. David Clark, MD, PhD

Assistant Professor of Anesthesia
Department of Anesthesia, Division of Pain Management
Stanford University School of Medicine
Stanford, California
Staff Physician
Veterans Affairs Palo Alto Health Care System
Palo Alto, California

Kristin Lynn Cobb, PhD

Instructor
Department of Health Research and Policy, Division of Epidemiology
Stanford University School of Medicine
Stanford, California

David Drover, MD

Assistant Professor of Anesthesia
Department of Anesthesia
Stanford University School of Medicine
Stanford, California

Gregory Engel, MD

Chief Fellow, Cardiovascular Medicine
Department of Medicine, Division of Cardiovascular Medicine
Stanford University School of Medicine
Stanford, California

Pamela Fish, MB, ChB

Associate Professor of Anesthesia
Department of Anesthesia
Stanford University School of Medicine
Stanford, California
Staff Physician
Veterans Affairs Palo Alto Health Care System
Palo Alto, California

J. Kent Garman, MD, MS

Associate Professor of Anesthesia, Division of Cardiac Anesthesia
Department of Anesthesia
Stanford University School of Medicine
Stanford, California

Brenda Golianu, MD

Assistant Professor of Anesthesia, Division of Pediatric Anesthesia
Department of Anesthesia
Stanford University School of Medicine
Stanford, California

Leland Hanowell, MD

Associate Professor of Anesthesia, Division of Cardiac Anesthesia
Department of Anesthesia
Stanford University School of Medicine
Stanford, California

Ethan Jackson, MD

Clinical Instructor
Department of Anesthesia, Division of Cardiac Anesthesia
Stanford University School of Medicine
Stanford, California

Richard A. Jaffe, MD, PhD

Professor of Anesthesia and Neurosurgery, Chief of Neurosurgical
Anesthesia
Department of Anesthesia
Stanford University School of Medicine
Stanford, California

Steve Lipman, MD

Clinical Assistant Professor of Anesthesia, Division of Obstetric
Anesthesia
Department of Anesthesia
Stanford University School of Medicine
Stanford, California

Alex Macario, MD, MBA

Associate Professor of Anesthesia
Department of Anesthesia
Stanford University School of Medicine
Stanford, California

Frederick G. Mihm, MD

Professor of Anesthesia, Division of Critical Care Medicine
Department of Anesthesia
Stanford University School of Medicine
Stanford, California

Christina Mora-Mangano, MD

Professor of Anesthesia, Chief of Cardiac Anesthesia
Department of Anesthesia
Stanford University School of Medicine
Stanford, California

Chandra Ramamoorthy, MD

Associate Professor of Anesthesia, Chief of Pediatric Anesthesia
Department of Anesthesia
Stanford University School of Medicine
Stanford, California

Stephen J. Ruoss, MD

Associate Professor of Medicine, Division of Pulmonary
    and Critical Care
Department of Medicine
Stanford University School of Medicine
Stanford, California

Steve Shafer, MD

Professor of Anesthesia
Department of Anesthesia
Stanford University School of Medicine
Stanford, California
Staff Physician
Veterans Affairs Palo Alto Health Care System
Palo Alto, California

Pieter van der Starre, MD

Associate Professor of Anesthesia, Division of Cardiac Anesthesia
Department of Anesthesia
Stanford University School of Medicine
Stanford, California

Preface

This is a new type of anesthesia review book. It does not present a comprehensive topical review of anesthesiology. What this book does provide—for the first time—are detailed and thoroughly researched answers to actual examination questions used in a previous American Board of Anesthesiology (ABA) examination. We believe that it provides an authentic test-simulation experience that is an important self-assessment tool for candidates preparing for board certification in anesthesia.

My colleagues at Stanford, both faculty and residents, have worked diligently to produce the answers you are about to read. In addition to factual information, we also have included a "reasoning" section for each answer. Simply put, this is how experienced test takers would have answered the question and why they chose their answers. We also have provided indexed answer sheets so that the reader can conveniently locate and review examination questions by topic.

It is important to emphasize to the reader that the answers you are about to read are simply that: our best attempt to derive the best possible answer for each question. The ABA has not published an answer key to the examination. We anticipate that there may be controversy and debate surrounding some of our answers. Our goal is to provide a framework to use retired questions as a self-assessment tool and to stimulate discussion and debate about controversies in anesthesia. Indeed, we invite you to participate in the discussion by visiting our Web site *http://ether.stanford.edu*. We have designed it to help connect you with colleagues who are also preparing for the ABA examination. Errata and updates also will be posted to the Web site.

We hope that you will find our approach to board preparation a useful adjunct to your study plans. Nothing can replace a comprehensive topical review of the field of anesthesia as a foundation for your board preparation and future career in anesthesiology. However, putting knowledge into practice is equally important for success. The ABA's retired board questions are an important resource to let you flex your anesthesia muscles, to help you identify areas of weakness, and to get into the test-taking frame of mind. We believe that *Clinical Anesthesiology Board Review: A Test Simulation and Self-Assessment Tool* is the ideal review companion that will provide you with high-yield, relevant review information to help you achieve your goal: passing the written ABA board examination.

I would like to thank the numerous contributors and faculty reviewers who have made this book possible. I would like to express special gratitude to John Brock-Utne, MD, PhD, Richard Jaffe, MD, PhD, and Steve Shafer, MD, for valuable advice and suggestions that have improved the quality of this book substantially. My editors at McGraw-Hill, Janet Foltin, Marsha Loeb, Patrick Carr, and Marc Strauss, have each played an important role in the success of this publication.

Finally, I would like to especially thank and acknowledge Francis and Krystal Wong for their invaluable assistance in the preparation of this book.

Larry Chu, MD, MS
Stanford, California

Acknowledgments

I would like to thank and acknowledge the important work of the American Board of Anesthesiology (ABA) and the American Society of Anesthesiologists (ASA) and their members. The ABA-written board examination, oral board examination, and maintenance of certification in anesthesiology (MOCA) are important components of high-quality anesthesia education and clinical practice. They serve a vital role in advancing the specialty of anesthesiology. We are indebted to these organizations for the use of their examination material in this publication.

A career development award to the author from the National Institutes of General Medical Sciences of the National Institutes of Health (1K23GM071400-01) provided scholarly time necessary for completion of this work and is gratefully acknowledged. A portion of this manuscript was completed during a research fellowship grant to the author from the Foundation for Anesthesia Education and Research. Their support is also gratefully acknowledged.

The American Board of Anesthesiology/American Society of Anesthesiologists In-Training Examination 1993 is reprinted with permission of the American Society of Anesthesiologists, 520 N. Northwest Highway, Park Ridge, Illinois 60068-2573.

How to Use This Book

This text is designed as a test simulation and self-assessment tool. It is not intended to replace a comprehensive topical review of anesthesia that is the foundation of high-quality anesthesia education and clinical practice. Readers who have already completed a rigorous topical review may wish to use this text as a simulation of an actual American Board of Anesthesiology (ABA) examination. The actual ABA test booklets are reprinted in this text and should be completed sequentially by the reader. Time restrictions should be followed strictly to assist the reader in assessing the pacing of an actual examination. Readers who have not yet completed a complete review or feel that they require assessment of specific areas of knowledge may choose to use the topical answer sheets that are provided.

OPTIONAL QUESTIONS

The ABA occasionally tests knowledge of controversial topics in anesthesia. In addition, some aspects of clinical knowledge and the practice of anesthesiology have changed significantly since this examination was first administered. New knowledge advances the specialty of anesthesia but also can affect the structure of the K-type logic of this examination. Accordingly, some questions that were written in 1993 cannot be answered in 2005. In addition, certain drugs (e.g., pipecuronium and enflurane) are no longer used commonly by anesthesiologists in the United States. We have prepared detailed answers and explanations for all these questions and encourage the reader to review them. We have indicated these questions as "optional" on the examination answer sheets for readers who wish to omit them from their test simulation or self-assessment exercises. Our answers provide useful information that can be reviewed after these exercises have been completed. Readers who wish to preserve the pacing of the test simulation should limit the examination time to 3 hours and 17 minutes (Book A) and 3 hours and 15 minutes (Book B) if optional questions are ommitted.

HOW TO ACCESS THE WEB SITE

A companion Web site for this book can be accessed at *http://ether.stanford.edu*.

The Web site contains additional supplementary information not available in this text. In addition, errata and updates will be posted regularly. A computerized analysis of your completed examination is also available. It may assist the reader in identifying areas requiring further study.

Discussion forums are available for readers to interact with other candidates preparing for the anesthesia board examination. Authors of this book will be available periodically to respond to questions and discussions that are posted to the Web site.

Readers will need to register a unique login in order to post messages to the Web site and access the test analysis software. The passcode needed to complete the registration process is provided below.

Passcode: copperkettle

AMERICAN BOARD OF ANESTHESIOLOGY

AMERICAN SOCIETY OF ANESTHESIOLOGISTS

IN-TRAINING EXAMINATION

Book A

$3^1/_2$ hours

Do not break the seal until you are told to do so.

Read the directions on the back cover.

PREPARED IN COOPERATION WITH NATIONAL BOARD OF MEDICAL EXAMINERS©

ABA/ASA 93SA
pp 40, qtn 175

Printed in
U.S.A.

DIRECTIONS For each of the questions or incomplete statements below, ONE or MORE of the answers or completions given is correct. On the answer sheet fill in the circle containing

A if only *1, 2, and 3* are correct,
B if only *1 and 3* are correct,
C if only *2 and 4* are correct,
D if only *4* is correct,
E if all are correct.

FOR EACH QUESTION FILL IN ONLY ONE CIRCLE ON YOUR ANSWER SHEET

DIRECTIONS SUMMARIZED				
A	B	C	D	E
1, 2, 3	1, 3	2, 4	4	All are
only	only	only	only	correct

1. During mechanical ventilation, factors that influence the correlation between set tidal volume and exhaled tidal volume include

   (1) inspiratory time
   (2) fresh gas flow
   (3) compliance of the breathing circuit
   (4) addition of positive end-expiratory pressure to the circuit

2. In a 45-year-old man with adult respiratory distress syndrome, which of the following will result from institution of mechanical ventilation with positive end-expiratory pressure?

   (1) Decreased intrapulmonary shunt
   (2) Increased pulmonary compliance
   (3) Increased ventilation-perfusion ratio in the dependent portion of lung
   (4) Decreased dead space to tidal volume ratio

3. A 58-year-old man with suspected carcinoma of the lung requires postoperative ventilation following general anesthesia for mediastinoscopy. Preoperatively, his shoulder muscles are weak bilaterally, but strength improves with exercise. This patient will show

   (1) inadequate reversal of neuromuscular block with an anticholinesterase drug
   (2) increased sensitivity to both depolarizing and nondepolarizing muscle relaxants
   (3) increased muscle strength following plasmapheresis
   (4) resolution of symptoms following administration of hydrocortisone

	DIRECTIONS SUMMARIZED			
A	B	C	D	E
1, 2, 3	1, 3	2, 4	4	All are
only	only	only	only	correct

4. Which of the following statements concerning postoperative shivering is true?

    (1) It increases carbon dioxide production
    (2) It is suppressed by intravenous meperidine
    (3) It accentuates halothane-related tremors
    (4) It increases heat loss

5. The elimination half-life of an amide local anesthetic is prolonged in which of the following conditions?

    (1) Liver disease
    (2) Term pregnancy
    (3) Heart failure
    (4) Kidney disease

6. A 10-year-old child with asthma is undergoing anesthesia with nitrous oxide, oxygen, and halothane. Effects of the accidental injection of atropine 2 mg in this patient would include

    (1) postoperative delirium
    (2) ventricular dysrhythmias
    (3) increased body temperature
    (4) bronchospasm

7. True statements concerning the oculocardiac reflex include:

    (1) It is more likely to occur in a patient with hypercarbia than in a patient with normocarbia
    (2) It is not seen during operative procedures on an empty orbit
    (3) Its afferent limb is the trigeminal nerve
    (4) It does not occur in the awake patient

8. Phase II succinylcholine block is characterized by

    (1) a train-of-four ratio less than 0.7
    (2) nonsustained response to tetanic stimulation
    (3) post-tetanic facilitation
    (4) improvement by edrophonium

9. Advantages of closed circuit anesthesia over a semiclosed anesthesia system include the ability to

    (1) more quickly alter the inspired anesthetic concentration
    (2) decrease the total amount of inhalational anesthetic used
    (3) more easily increase $PaCO_2$ during emergence
    (4) decrease heat loss to a greater extent

DIRECTIONS SUMMARIZED				
A	**B**	**C**	**D**	**E**
1, 2, 3	1, 3	2, 4	4	All are
only	only	only	only	correct

10. Chronic hyperglycemia from excessive glucose administration during parenteral hyperalimentation causes

    (1) retinal degeneration
    (2) depression of granulocyte function
    (3) inhibition of platelet aggregation
    (4) hypercarbia

11. Which of the following produces effective transtracheal jet ventilation through a 14-gauge intravenous catheter?

    (1) Oxygen through a 50 psi pressure regulator
    (2) An Ambu bag with oxygen flow at 15 L/min
    (3) Oxygen flush from the fresh gas outlet from the anesthesia machine
    (4) The reservoir bag from the anesthesia circle system

12. During intraoperative mapping of a seizure focus under general anesthesia, EEG activation may be enhanced or seizures induced by the use of

    (1) ketamine
    (2) methohexital
    (3) enflurane
    (4) thiopental

13. Transthoracic resistance to DC defibrillation is decreased by

    (1) use of conductive gel
    (2) multiple attempts at defibrillation
    (3) defibrillation during expiration
    (4) larger electrodes

14. Compared with a healthy 20-year-old, respiratory function in a healthy 1-year-old is characterized by

    (1) greater chest wall compliance
    (2) lesser lung compliance
    (3) greater small airway resistance
    (4) similar functional residual capacity/total lung volume (FRC/TLC) ratio

15. True statements concerning insertion of a total hip prosthesis with methylmethacrylate cement include:

    (1) Hypotension is more likely with placement in the acetabulum than with insertion in the femoral shaft
    (2) Absorbed volatile monomer causes vasodilation
    (3) A deliberate hypotensive technique is contraindicated
    (4) Arterial hemoglobin desaturation may result from fat embolization

16. True statements concerning <u>direct</u> ventricular defibrillation during cardiopulmonary bypass include:

    (1) Shocks greater than 30 joules are associated with myocardial damage
    (2) Hypokalemia increases the chance of defibrillation
    (3) Myocardial impedance decreases after a single shock
    (4) Thin-walled ventricles defibrillate more easily than hypertrophied ventricles

17. The indications for administration of fresh frozen plasma include

    (1) acute volume expansion in a hypovolemic patient
    (2) bleeding in a patient with a normal activated clotting time after cardiopulmonary bypass
    (3) transfusion of 6 units of red blood cells in a 70-kg patient
    (4) bleeding in a patient with a prolonged bleeding time and abnormal factor VIII

18. Immediately after sustaining a traumatic cord transection with a T4 level, a patient requires emergency laparotomy. Disease-related factors affecting anesthetic management include

    (1) venous pooling
    (2) hypothermia
    (3) decreased peripheral vascular resistance
    (4) decreased alveolar ventilation

19. Trigeminal neuralgia is characterized by

    (1) unilateral, intense, paroxysmal pain of sudden onset
    (2) diminished sensation in the distribution of the maxillary division of the trigeminal nerve
    (3) normal function of the glossopharyngeal nerve
    (4) resolution of symptoms by injection of local anesthetic at trigger points

20. During general anesthesia in a healthy patient, hypothermia to 33°C results in

    (1) prolongation of vecuronium action
    (2) protection against cerebral ischemia
    (3) potentiation of isoflurane
    (4) increased risk for ventricular dysrhythmias

21. Factors that decrease the incidence of deep vein thrombosis following total hip replacement include

    (1) external compression of the lower extremities
    (2) epidural anesthesia intraoperatively
    (3) prophylactic aspirin
    (4) deliberate hypotension intraoperatively

		DIRECTIONS SUMMARIZED		
A	B	C	D	E
1, 2, 3	1, 3	2, 4	4	All are
only	only	only	only	correct

22. Ketamine administered in anesthetic doses

   (1) increases intracranial pressure
   (2) does not cause respiratory depression
   (3) is eliminated by hepatic metabolism
   (4) increases bronchomotor tone

23. During laser excision of a sublaryngeal tumor, the risk of airway ignition would be decreased by using

   (1) water-based lubricants
   (2) jet ventilation without an endotracheal tube
   (3) saline solution in the endotracheal tube cuff
   (4) nitrous oxide

24. A 24-year-old patient with hypertension and hypercalcemia is scheduled for a parathyroidectomy. Serum calcium concentration may be decreased by the administration of

   (1) a calcium channel blocker
   (2) magnesium sulfate
   (3) sodium bicarbonate
   (4) vigorous volume expansion

25. Effects of open cholecystectomy under general anesthesia with mechanical ventilation include

   (1) increased intrapulmonary shunting
   (2) decreased lung volumes up to 48 hours postoperatively
   (3) decreased functional residual capacity
   (4) decreased dead space

26. Features of the neonate's prompt adjustment to extrauterine life include

   (1) lung expansion resulting in increased pulmonary vascular resistance
   (2) nonshivering thermogenesis as a response to cold stress
   (3) anatomic closure of the ductus arteriosus
   (4) initial expansion of airless collapsed lungs by creation of negative pressures of 40 to 80 cmH_2O

27. Landmarks used in performing a superior laryngeal nerve block include the

   (1) transverse process of C6
   (2) cricoid cartilage
   (3) angle of the mandible
   (4) greater cornu of the hyoid cartilage

FOR EACH ITEM FILL IN ONLY ONE CIRCLE ON YOUR ANSWER SHEET

DIRECTIONS SUMMARIZED				
A	**B**	**C**	**D**	**E**
1, 2, 3	1, 3	2, 4	4	All are
only	only	only	only	correct

28. Blood products that transmit viruses include

    (1) factor IX concentrate
    (2) plasma protein fraction
    (3) cryoprecipitate
    (4) albumin

29. Compared with heated cascade-type humidifiers, heated nebulizers used for humidification are associated with a greater risk for

    (1) bacterial transmission
    (2) increased airway resistance
    (3) water intoxication
    (4) inspissated secretions in large airways

30. Landmarks for caudal block include the

    (1) sciatic notch
    (2) posterior-superior iliac spines
    (3) iliac crests
    (4) sacral cornu

31. Changes in pulmonary function associated with advanced age include

    (1) decreased lung compliance
    (2) increased alveolar dead space
    (3) decreased functional residual capacity
    (4) decreased maximum voluntary ventilation

32. The MAC of isoflurane is decreased by

    (1) ethanol-induced enzyme induction
    (2) hyperventilation to a $PaCO_2$ of 25 mmHg
    (3) chronic anemia to a hematocrit of 20%
    (4) decreased body temperature to 34°C

33. Compared with fentanyl, characteristics of alfentanil include

    (1) greater protein binding
    (2) more rapid clearance
    (3) shorter elimination half-life
    (4) greater volume of distribution

DIRECTIONS SUMMARIZED				
A	B	C	D	E
1, 2, 3	1, 3	2, 4	4	All are
only	only	only	only	correct

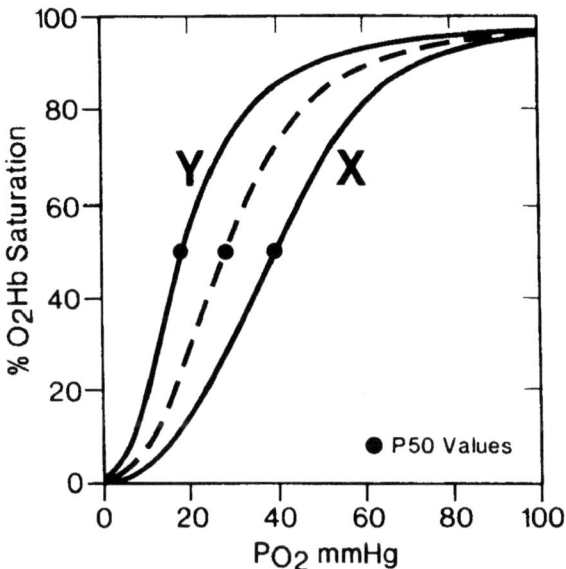

34. The oxygen-dissociation curve in the center of the graph represents normal adult hemoglobin. True statements concerning curves X and Y include:

    (1) Curve Y represents hemoglobin characteristic of a normal neonate
    (2) Curve X represents hemoglobin characteristic of 3-week-old banked blood
    (3) Curve Y represents hemoglobin characteristic of an alkalotic patient
    (4) Curve X represents hemoglobin characteristic of a hypothermic patient

35. A 45-year-old man who is scheduled for coronary artery bypass grafting is receiving heparin and nitroglycerin infusions for preinfarction angina. True statements concerning use of heparin during coronary revascularization in this patient include:

    (1) The anticoagulant effect is enhanced by the nitroglycerin
    (2) Platelet count should be determined prior to the operation
    (3) Activated coagulation time is unreliable after prolonged administration of heparin
    (4) The dose of heparin necessary to provide adequate systemic anticoagulation is likely to be increased

36. True statements concerning negative pressure pulmonary edema include:

    (1) It is associated with airway obstruction
    (2) It responds to diuretic therapy
    (3) Resolution occurs within 24 hours
    (4) Debilitated adults are predisposed to it

DIRECTIONS SUMMARIZED				
A	B	C	D	E
1, 2, 3	1, 3	2, 4	4	All are
only	only	only	only	correct

37. Landmarks for the sciatic nerve via a posterior approach include the

    (1) posterior superior iliac spine
    (2) coccyx
    (3) greater trochanter of the femur
    (4) iliac crest

38. Epidural anesthesia for cesarean delivery is planned for a 30-year-old woman in labor. She has preeclampsia and takes propranolol for mitral valve prolapse. A test dose of 3 ml of 2% lidocaine containing 15 μg of epinephrine is administered, and no change in heart rate is noted by palpation of the pulse. Prior to injection of more local anesthetic, blood is freely aspirated from the catheter.

    Explanations for failure of the intravenous test dose include:

    (1) The pain of labor masked the change usually seen with the test dose
    (2) Pre-existing beta-adrenergic blockade blunted the tachycardia from the intravenous epinephrine
    (3) Changes in pulse rate were too brief to be noted by palpation of the pulse
    (4) Preeclampsia decreased the sensitivity to exogenously administered catecholamines

39. A 76-year-old man with a history of angina, dyspnea on exertion, and syncope attributable to aortic stenosis is brought to the operating room for open reduction of an ankle fracture. An ECG shows sinus rhythm. Anesthetic considerations include:

    (1) Nitroglycerin is contraindicated
    (2) Atrial fibrillation should be treated with synchronized cardioversion
    (3) The risk for cardiac complications is the same as that of patients with coronary artery stenosis
    (4) Spinal anesthesia is relatively contraindicated

40. Use of hyperventilation to decrease brain swelling also decreases

    (1) P_{50} of hemoglobin
    (2) serum ionized calcium concentration
    (3) serum potassium concentration
    (4) cerebral metabolic rate

41. A neonate born at 32 weeks' gestation has cyanosis, tachypnea, a scaphoid abdomen, and a cardiac impulse on the right. Immediate management of this child should include

    (1) insertion of a chest tube
    (2) limiting inspired oxygen concentration to 50%
    (3) administration of rapid positive pressure ventilation by mask
    (4) insertion of a nasogastric tube

		DIRECTIONS SUMMARIZED		
A	B	C	D	E
1, 2, 3	1, 3	2, 4	4	All are
only	only	only	only	correct

42. The principle underlying diffusion hypoxia also explains

    (1) apneic oxygenation
    (2) the concentration effect
    (3) the solubility effect
    (4) the second gas effect

43. True statements concerning carbon dioxide absorption in breathing-system canisters include:

    (1) The major reactant of baralyme is barium hydroxide
    (2) Baralyme contains silica to minimize dust
    (3) The major component of soda lime is sodium hydroxide
    (4) Both baralyme and soda lime contain calcium hydroxide

44. Factors that decrease local anesthetic concentration in the fetus include

    (1) maternal hypotension
    (2) maternal acidemia
    (3) maternal serum alpha acid glycoprotein concentration
    (4) fetal acidosis

45. An oxygen analyzer sensor placed in the inspiratory limb of a circle system

    (1) is useful as a disconnect alarm if placed near the patient
    (2) will increase dead space
    (3) will be more pressure sensitive than one placed in the expiratory limb
    (4) should not be placed distal to an in-circuit humidifier

46. Agents that produce an acute withdrawal response in patients addicted to heroin include

    (1) pentazocine
    (2) nalbuphine
    (3) buprenorphine
    (4) naloxone

47. A 68-year-old man has had severe, constant burning and aching in the right forehead and anterior scalp for six weeks after an episode of herpes zoster. True statements concerning this patient's condition include:

    (1) It is more common in elderly patients
    (2) The neuralgia involves the supraorbital branches of the ophthalmic division of the facial nerve
    (3) Tricyclic antidepressants often provide effective pain relief
    (4) Opioid analgesics are the first-line treatment

11

DIRECTIONS SUMMARIZED				
A	B	C	D	E
1, 2, 3	1, 3	2, 4	4	All are
only	only	only	only	correct

48. Three weeks after exposure to toxic levels of an organophosphate insecticide, a farm worker is scheduled for inguinal herniorrhaphy. Which of the following should be avoided?

    (1) Spinal anesthesia with tetracaine
    (2) Epidural anesthesia with 2-chloroprocaine
    (3) Atracurium neuromuscular block
    (4) Succinylcholine infusion

49. The addition of halothane 0.5% to nitrous oxide and oxygen 50% each for cesarean delivery

    (1) increases the incidence of low Apgar scores
    (2) increases operative blood loss
    (3) increases the incidence of maternal hypotension
    (4) decreases the incidence of maternal awareness

50. Stellate ganglion block is associated with ipsilateral

    (1) mydriasis
    (2) diaphoresis
    (3) exophthalmos
    (4) scleral hyperemia

51. A 22-year-old man is unconscious after free-basing "crack." Likely findings include

    (1) depressed ST segments
    (2) hyperthermia
    (3) premature ventricular contractions
    (4) pinpoint pupils

52. Administration of halothane to a healthy patient causes

    (1) decreased myocardial contractility
    (2) depressed baroreceptor response
    (3) increased venous capacitance
    (4) decreased systemic vascular resistance

53. Indications for administration of calcium chloride during cardiopulmonary resuscitation include

    (1) acute hyperkalemia
    (2) electromechanical dissociation
    (3) verapamil toxicity
    (4) digoxin toxicity

DIRECTIONS SUMMARIZED				
A	B	C	D	E
1, 2, 3	1, 3	2, 4	4	All are
only	only	only	only	correct

54. A 27-year-old man is undergoing emergency bronchoscopy with propofol-vecuronium anesthesia after aspirating a peanut. Intervals of apneic oxygenation are used to facilitate the procedure. Initial blood gas values while breathing pure oxygen are PaO_2 400 mmHg and $PaCO_2$ 30 mmHg. Effects of 10 minutes of apneic oxygenation at a flow rate of 10 L/min include

   (1) decreased heart rate
   (2) decreased PaO_2 to 50 mmHg
   (3) cutaneous vasoconstriction
   (4) increased $PaCO_2$ to 60 mmHg

55. In a patient with normal hemodynamics, systemic blood pressure is measured using a radial artery catheter and a noninvasive oscillometric blood pressure (NIBP) monitor on the same arm. Compared with the readings from the NIBP monitor, the indwelling catheter would show

   (1) the same or higher systolic blood pressure
   (2) lower diastolic pressure if the transducer is damped
   (3) the same mean blood pressure
   (4) lower blood pressure values if the catheter is replaced by one with a larger diameter

56. A 20-kg, 4-year-old boy receives atropine 0.3 mg intramuscularly one hour prior to inguinal herniorrhaphy under general anesthesia. Forty minutes later while still in the preoperative preparation room, his temperature is 38.6°C. Likely causes of the temperature elevation include

   (1) malignant hyperthermia
   (2) alteration of central temperature regulation
   (3) release of catecholamines
   (4) suppression of sweating

57. If ketorolac 30 mg were substituted for meperidine 100 mg after an outpatient inguinal herniorrhaphy, the patient would experience less

   (1) respiratory depression
   (2) analgesia
   (3) nausea
   (4) bleeding

58. An asymptomatic 32-year-old man with asthma undergoes herniorrhaphy under 1.5% lidocaine epidural anesthesia to a sensory level of T2-3. Which of the following will occur with this level of anesthesia?

   (1) The ability to cough will be normal
   (2) Vital capacity will be unchanged
   (3) Intraoperative bronchospasm will be prevented
   (4) Tidal volume will be unchanged

DIRECTIONS SUMMARIZED				
A	B	C	D	E
1, 2, 3	1, 3	2, 4	4	All are
only	only	only	only	correct

59. True statements concerning epidurally administered morphine include:

    (1) The long duration of analgesia results from high lipid solubility
    (2) Pruritus is completely reversed by naloxone
    (3) Plasma morphine levels are lower than those seen after intramuscular administration
    (4) Analgesia is inadequate for the pain of labor

60. A 36-year-old woman is scheduled for cholecystectomy. She is 65 inches tall and weighs 180 kg. Compared with a patient of the same height who weighs 60 kg, this patient is at increased risk for

    (1) hypoxemia in the supine position
    (2) fasting hypoglycemia
    (3) acid aspiration syndrome
    (4) difficult reversal of neuromuscular block

61. Radiologic findings in advanced emphysema include

    (1) ground-glass appearance of lung fields
    (2) increased cardiothoracic ratio
    (3) increased bronchial markings
    (4) flattening of the hemidiaphragms

62. Anesthetic agents that are safe for use in a patient with acute intermittent porphyria include

    (1) ketamine
    (2) isoflurane
    (3) pancuronium
    (4) etomidate

63. Recurrent laryngeal nerve paralysis is a recognized complication of which of the following procedures?

    (1) Ligation of a patent ductus arteriosus
    (2) Stellate ganglion block
    (3) Mediastinoscopy
    (4) Use of a topical ice slush during heart surgery

64. Clinical situations associated with an increase in parasympathetic activity include

    (1) manipulation of the carotid sinus
    (2) intestinal insufflation during colonoscopy
    (3) traction on the superior oblique muscle during strabismus surgery
    (4) caudal anesthesia for excision of a pilonidal cyst

DIRECTIONS SUMMARIZED				
A	**B**	**C**	**D**	**E**
1, 2, 3	1, 3	2, 4	4	All are
only	only	only	only	correct

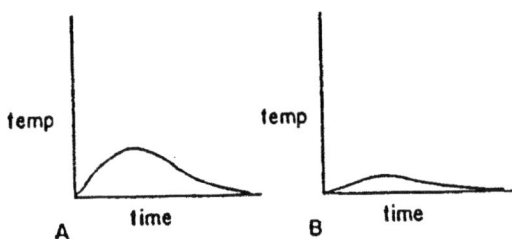

65. Curve A shown above is an accurate thermodilution curve from a patient with a cardiac output of 4 L/min. Curve B was obtained at the same time from the same patient. Curve B is consistent with

    (1) an opening at the syringe-catheter junction that allows some injectate to leak out of the system
    (2) use of room temperature injectate when the computer is programmed for iced injectate
    (3) injection of cold indicator solution through a long extension tube rather than directly into the correct catheter lumen
    (4) use of 10 ml of cold indicator solution when the cardiac output computer is programmed for 5 ml of injectate

66. While evaluating oliguria following operative repair of an aortic aneurysm, large "V" waves are noted in a pulmonary artery occlusion pressure trace. This finding is consistent with which of the following disorders?

    (1) Tricuspid regurgitation
    (2) Mitral regurgitation
    (3) Aortic regurgitation
    (4) Coronary artery disease

67. The output of an agent-specific vaporizer is higher than the dial setting under which of the following conditions?

    (1) The vaporizer is filled with an agent of higher vapor pressure
    (2) Ambient temperature increases from 20°C to 24°C
    (3) The vaporizer is used at an elevation of 5000 feet
    (4) The inspiratory valve is incompetent

68. The advantages of colloid over crystalloid for massive volume replacement include

    (1) lower incidence of pulmonary edema
    (2) greater urine output
    (3) less disruption of hemostasis
    (4) greater potency in restoring circulatory homeostasis

DIRECTIONS SUMMARIZED				
A	B	C	D	E
1, 2, 3	1, 3	2, 4	4	All are
only	only	only	only	correct

69. A 24-year-old man has constant burning pain three months after sustaining a crush injury to the arm. The injured muscles and joints are healed. Findings consistent with a diagnosis of causalgia include

    (1) beads of perspiration on the skin
    (2) skin discoloration
    (3) hypersensitivity to touch
    (4) warm extremity

70. A 45-year-old patient who takes tranylcypromine (Parnate), an MAO inhibitor, is scheduled for elective surgery under general anesthesia. True statements include:

    (1) Meperidine can produce hyperthermia
    (2) Surgery must be delayed for two weeks after discontinuation of MAO inhibitor therapy
    (3) An exaggerated response to ephedrine should be expected
    (4) A decrease in pressor response to phenylephrine should be expected

71. A 52-year-old man with a chronic cough associated with a long history of smoking is scheduled for elective cholecystectomy. Cessation of smoking for 48 hours will result in

    (1) decreased bronchial secretions
    (2) shift of the oxyhemoglobin dissociation curve to the right
    (3) decreased airway irritability
    (4) decreased carboxyhemoglobin level

72. A 55-year-old woman has a urine output of 15 ml during the first two hours following a radical hysterectomy. Findings consistent with a prerenal cause include

    (1) urine osmolality 590 mOsm/L
    (2) plasma creatinine concentration 1.1 mg/dl
    (3) urine specific gravity 1.025
    (4) urine sodium concentration 40 mEq/L

73. An 8-kg, 1-year-old child has a measured blood loss of 50 ml during the first two hours of a rectal pull-through operation. Preoperative hematocrit was 31%. Balanced saline solution 150 ml has been administered for replacement. Urine output has been 2 ml for the last hour, heart rate is 160 bpm, and blood pressure is 40/15 mmHg.

The most appropriate fluid therapy is

   (A) 25% albumin
   (B) balanced salt solution
   (C) balanced salt solution and mannitol
   (D) 5% dextrose in 0.45% saline solution
   (E) packed red blood cells

74. An increased initial dose and a decreased maintenance dose of pancuronium are required in patients with

   (A) advanced age
   (B) burns
   (C) cirrhosis
   (D) chronic renal failure
   (E) fever

75. Which of the following statements concerning banked blood is true?

   (A) Red blood cells preserved with CPDA-1 have a shelf life of approximately 21 days
   (B) Packed red blood cells deliver oxygen normally immediately after administration
   (C) Packed red blood cells contain most of the leukocytes present in the donated unit
   (D) Citrate is used as a source of energy for whole blood
   (E) Stored whole blood contains all coagulation factors except II and VIII

76. A 73-year-old woman with a preoperative serum creatinine concentration of 2.1 mg/dl develops oliguria during enflurane anesthesia. Urine sodium concentration is 10 mEq/L and urine osmolality is 450 mOsm/L. The most likely cause of these findings is

   (A) acute renal failure
   (B) chronic renal insufficiency
   (C) decreased renal perfusion
   (D) fluoride nephrotoxicity
   (E) intraoperative administration of furosemide

77. During active labor, 10 ml of bupivacaine 0.5% with epinephrine 1:200,000 is administered epidurally. Fifteen minutes later, maternal blood pressure is 70/50 mmHg and heart rate is 70 bpm; fetal heart rate is 90 bpm for 45 seconds, with loss of beat-to-beat variability. The most likely explanation for the fetal vital signs is

   (A) fetal bupivacaine cardiotoxicity
   (B) maternal bupivacaine cardiotoxicity
   (C) maternal hypotension
   (D) uterine artery vasoconstriction
   (E) umbilical cord compression

78. Compared with diazepam, midazolam

    (A) is more lipid soluble
    (B) has a longer elimination half-life
    (C) has a larger volume of distribution
    (D) has a greater clearance
    (E) undergoes slower hepatic metabolism

79. A 30-year-old woman has difficulty talking 15 minutes after initiation of interscalene block for closed reduction of a dislocated shoulder. The most likely cause is

    (A) cervical sympathetic block
    (B) delayed systemic toxic reaction
    (C) phrenic nerve paralysis
    (D) pneumothorax
    (E) recurrent laryngeal nerve block

80. An acutely ill 65-year-old man with sepsis has severe hypophosphatemia. Which of the following is most likely to result from this electrolyte disorder?

    (A) Bronchospasm
    (B) Diarrhea
    (C) Muscle weakness
    (D) Seizures
    (E) Ventricular ectopy

81. During a right lower lobe resection, SpO_2 decreases from 99% to 70% after institution of one-lung ventilation. FIO_2 is 1.0. The most appropriate management is to

    (A) administer an inhaled bronchodilator
    (B) apply continuous positive airway pressure to the right lung
    (C) apply positive end-expiratory pressure to the left lung
    (D) increase tidal volume
    (E) reinflate the right lung

82. Carbon dioxide retention first occurs when the ratio of forced expiratory volume in 1 second to vital capacity (FEV_1/VC) decreases below

    (A) 15%
    (B) 35%
    (C) 50%
    (D) 65%
    (E) 75%

83. During recovery from halothane anesthesia, an alveolar concentration of 0.1% will have the greatest effect on

    (A) myocardial contractility
    (B) ventilatory response to hypercarbia
    (C) atrioventricular conduction
    (D) ventilatory response to hypoxia
    (E) neuromuscular transmission

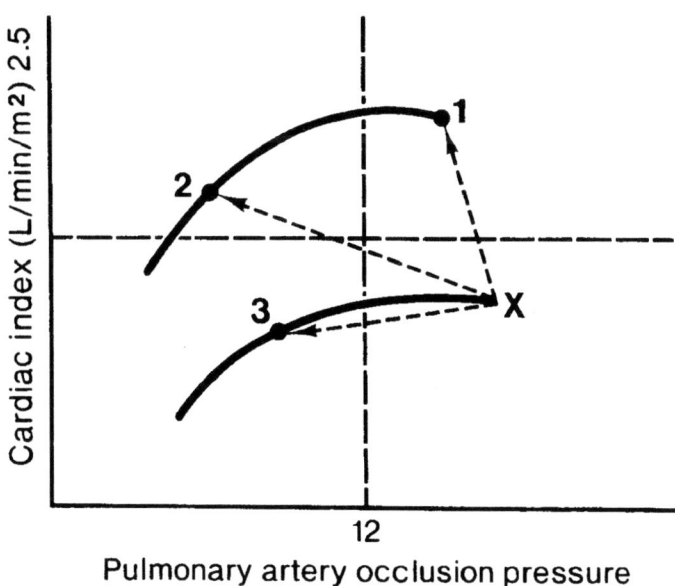

Pulmonary artery occlusion pressure
(mmHg)

84. In the diagram above, point "X" represents a patient with severe left ventricular dysfunction. The points labeled 1, 2, and 3 each represent the results of a different therapeutic intervention. Which of the following represents the most likely intervention at each point?

	Point 1	Point 2	Point 3
(A)	Dopamine	Furosemide	Nitroprusside
(B)	Dopamine	Nitroprusside	Furosemide
(C)	Furosemide	Dopamine	Nitroprusside
(D)	Nitroprusside	Dopamine	Furosemide
(E)	Nitroprusside	Furosemide	Dopamine

85. With long-term administration, which of the following drugs produces the most prolonged sedative effect of diazepam?

(A) Cimetidine
(B) Famotidine
(C) Metoclopramide
(D) Ranitidine
(E) Warfarin

86. During uncomplicated mask induction with halothane and 50% nitrous oxide in oxygen in a 6-month-old infant with a large ventricular septal defect and valvular pulmonic stenosis, SpO_2 decreases from 85% (room air) to 60%; heart rate is 100 bpm and blood pressure is 62/40 mmHg. The most appropriate management is to

(A) administer atropine
(B) administer phenylephrine
(C) administer propranolol
(D) increase anesthetic depth
(E) intubate the trachea

87. Which of the following statements concerning variable decelerations of fetal heart rate is true?

    (A) It indicates compression of the umbilical cord
    (B) It indicates compression of the fetal head
    (C) It indicates prematurity
    (D) It is obliterated by atropine
    (E) It occurs normally following epidural anesthesia

88. During enflurane anesthesia for colectomy in a 75-year-old man with sepsis, urine output decreases to 10 ml/hr. Heart rate is 120 bpm, blood pressure is 100/50 mmHg, central venous pressure is 10 mmHg, and pulmonary artery occlusion pressure is 15 mmHg. The most appropriate management at this time is to

    (A) measure cardiac output
    (B) increase fluid administration
    (C) infuse dopamine
    (D) administer propranolol
    (E) switch from enflurane to isoflurane

89. The effect of neomycin at the neuromuscular junction is

    (A) decreased by depolarizing relaxants
    (B) partially reversed by calcium
    (C) potentiated by anticholinesterases
    (D) prevented by pretreatment with magnesium
    (E) primarily prejunctional

90. A patient is bleeding excessively after routine transurethral resection of the prostate. Re-exploration discloses diffuse oozing. The most appropriate management is administration of

    (A) platelets
    (B) fresh frozen plasma
    (C) desmopressin
    (D) epsilon-aminocaproic acid
    (E) cryoprecipitate

91. Which of the following statements concerning functional residual capacity is true?

    (A) It decreases linearly during a three-hour anesthetic
    (B) It decreases in pregnancy primarily because of a decrease in the expiratory reserve volume
    (C) It increases in patients with a history of heavy smoking
    (D) It increases with pulmonary contusions
    (E) It is smaller (ml/kg) in children than in adults

92. After two hours of anesthesia with halothane 1.2% and oxygen, nitrous oxide 75% is added to the inspired gas mixture. This addition would

    (A) increase the alveolar halothane and oxygen concentrations above inspired
    (B) increase the alveolar halothane concentration only
    (C) cause no change in alveolar gas concentrations compared with inspired
    (D) decrease alveolar oxygen concentration compared with inspired
    (E) decrease alveolar oxygen and halothane concentrations below inspired

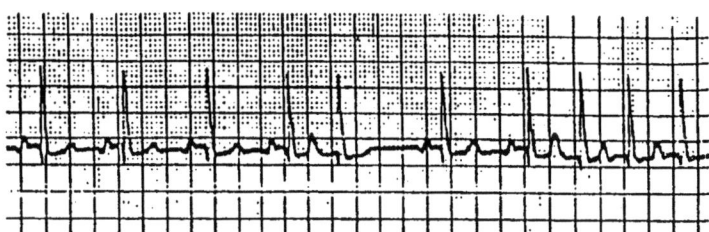

93. The ECG tracing above shows

   (A) aberrant intraventricular conduction
   (B) acceleration of phase 4 depolarization of the sinus node
   (C) a compensatory pause
   (D) initiation of re-entrant supraventricular tachycardia
   (E) paroxysmal atrial fibrillation

94. One hour after an open cholecystectomy, a 42-year-old patient is hemodynamically stable and breathing spontaneously (rate 10/min and regular) at an FIO$_2$ of 0.4. Fentanyl, isoflurane, nitrous oxide, and pancuronium were used during the procedure. Analysis of arterial blood gases is most likely to show:

	pH	PCO$_2$ (mmHg)	PO$_2$ (mmHg)
(A)	7.18	40	100
(B)	7.18	60	140
(C)	7.28	50	85
(D)	7.40	26	220
(E)	7.40	40	40

95. A 6-year-old child with asthma begins wheezing during anesthesia with halothane and nitrous oxide in oxygen. A loading dose of aminophylline is administered followed by continuous infusion. Premature ventricular contractions appear on the ECG. The most appropriate management is to

   (A) administer fentanyl
   (B) discontinue aminophylline
   (C) increase exhalation time
   (D) increase the inspired concentration of halothane
   (E) switch the inhalational agent to isoflurane

96. Oxygen 100 ml/min is bubbled through a vaporizer containing an anesthetic with a vapor pressure of 150 mmHg, and this mixture is added to a fresh gas flow of 5 L/min. The delivered anesthetic concentration is

   (A) 0.25%
   (B) 0.5%
   (C) 1%
   (D) 2.5%
   (E) 5%

97. A 50-year-old man who takes aspirin and nifedipine is scheduled for thoracotomy with one-lung ventilation. Which of the following is associated with the greatest risk for intraoperative hypoxemia?

   (A) Preoperative withdrawal of nifedipine therapy
   (B) Intraoperative mild respiratory acidosis
   (C) Intraoperative administration of isoflurane
   (D) Intraoperative administration of nitroglycerin
   (E) Intraoperative thoracic epidural morphine

98. A 35-year-old woman with severe myasthenia gravis is scheduled for thymectomy. Which of the following preoperative pulmonary function tests is most likely to be normal?

   (A) Forced expiratory volume in 1 second (FEV_1)
   (B) Forced vital capacity (FVC)
   (C) FEV_1/FVC
   (D) Maximum voluntary ventilation
   (E) Peak inspiratory force

99. A 66-year-old man with aortic regurgitation is brought to the operating room for aortic valve replacement after having received morphine, scopolamine premedication. PO_2 is 40 mmHg in a sample of pulmonary artery blood drawn 10 minutes after the patient started breathing pure oxygen. This finding is compatible with

   (A) wedging of the catheter tip
   (B) left-to-right intracardiac shunting
   (C) increased intrapulmonary shunting
   (D) excessively depressed ventilation
   (E) normal cardiac output

100. Which of the following statements concerning metoclopramide is true?

   (A) It is antagonized by concomitant administration of atropine
   (B) It decreases gastrointestinal motility
   (C) It decreases gastric secretion
   (D) It lacks antiemetic properties
   (E) It stimulates dopamine receptors

101. During halothane anesthesia with spontaneous ventilation, the most reliable sign of malignant hyperthermia is

   (A) hypertension
   (B) increased temperature
   (C) increased minute ventilation
   (D) muscle rigidity
   (E) tachycardia

102. Which of the following is the most appropriate action after an anesthetic vaporizer is tipped?

   (A) Return to the manufacturer for recalibration
   (B) Flush the vaporizer with oxygen at 5 L/min for 24 hours
   (C) Store the vaporizer for 24 hours at room temperature
   (D) Set the vaporizer at low concentration and flush with oxygen at 10 L/min for 30 minutes
   (E) Verify the vaporizer output with mass spectrography

103. Following pneumonectomy, a paralyzed patient being mechanically ventilated has the following arterial blood gas values: PaO_2 71 mmHg, $PaCO_2$ 55 mmHg, pH 7.29. SvO_2 is 45%. The most likely explanation for this SvO_2 is

    (A) decreased red cell mass
    (B) high cardiac output
    (C) hypothermia
    (D) peripheral left-to-right arteriovenous shunt
    (E) ventilation/perfusion mismatch

104. Which of the following is a sign of cyclosporine toxicity?

    (A) Abnormal hepatic enzyme activity
    (B) Decreased hemoglobin concentration
    (C) Increased serum creatinine concentration
    (D) Nodular density on radiograph of the chest
    (E) ST-T wave changes on ECG

105. Myofascial pain is an example of

    (A) a central pain state
    (B) neuropathic pain
    (C) psychogenic pain
    (D) somatic pain
    (E) visceral pain

106. In children with preoperative upper respiratory tract infection, which of the following is associated with the greatest risk for postoperative airway obstruction?

    (A) Age less than 1 year
    (B) Endotracheal intubation
    (C) Head and neck surgery
    (D) Inadequate airway humidification
    (E) Surgery for more than two hours

107. In an anesthetized patient being mechanically ventilated, end-expired carbon dioxide is 58 mmHg and peak inspiratory airway pressure is 15 cmH$_2$O. Ventilator settings indicate a delivered tidal volume of 800 ml, but the expiratory flow-meter shows a tidal volume of 360 ml. Which of the following is the most likely cause of this discrepancy?

    (A) Fresh gas flow of 0.5 L/min
    (B) Incompetence of the pressure-relief valve
    (C) Low ventilatory rate
    (D) Presence of a hole in the ventilator bellows
    (E) Prolongation of the inspiratory phase

108. Which of the following statements concerning pipecuronium is true?

    (A) It has a faster onset than pancuronium
    (B) It increases systemic vascular resistance
    (C) It induces tachycardia
    (D) It is eliminated by the kidney
    (E) It induces histamine release

109. Left ventricular end-diastolic volume is most likely to be underestimated by pulmonary artery occlusion pressure in patients with

    (A) acute myocardial ischemia
    (B) aortic insufficiency
    (C) mitral stenosis
    (D) primary pulmonary hypertension
    (E) tricuspid stenosis

110. Which of the following statements concerning the cardiovascular effects of intravenous bupivacaine is true?

    (A) Bretylium is effective in treating bupivacaine-induced ventricular arrhythmias
    (B) Cardiovascular toxicity is decreased during pregnancy
    (C) Cardiovascular toxicity occurs at lower blood levels than central nervous system toxicity
    (D) Systemic vascular resistance is unchanged
    (E) The rate of impulse conduction through the heart is increased

111. Which of the following is indicated by an alarm condition in the line-isolation monitor?

    (A) An electrical shock to the patient
    (B) A power surge in the main hospital power supply
    (C) Disconnection of the patient from an electrocautery grounding pad
    (D) Overload of the operating room circuits
    (E) The presence of a current leak between an operating room electrical device and ground

112. Which of the following statements concerning ketorolac is true?

    (A) It binds to opioid receptors
    (B) It causes dose-related thrombocytopenia
    (C) It decreases heart rate during isoflurane anesthesia
    (D) It is eliminated unchanged in urine
    (E) It reversibly inhibits cyclooxygenase

113. Postoperatively, a patient is being mechanically ventilated by a constant-flow, pressure-cycled ventilator with the following initial settings: inspiratory/expiratory (I/E) ratio of 1:2, peak inspiratory pressure (PIP) of 25 cmH_2O, and rate of 10/min. One hour later, the I/E ratio is 1:4. Which of the following would ensure that the minute ventilation is the same as that initially set?

    (A) Inflate the endotracheal tube cuff to prevent leakage
    (B) Double the respiratory rate
    (C) Decrease the expiratory pause until the I/E ratio is 1.0
    (D) Increase the PIP until the I/E ratio is 1:2
    (E) Increase the PIP to 50 cmH_2O

114. Left ventricular subendocardial perfusion pressure is best estimated by the difference between

    (A) mean arterial and central venous pressures
    (B) diastolic arterial and pulmonary artery occlusion pressures
    (C) mean arterial and pulmonary artery occlusion pressures
    (D) systolic arterial and pulmonary artery occlusion pressures
    (E) diastolic arterial and central venous pressures

115. A 29-year-old man who has been nasotracheally intubated for two weeks following a motor vehicle accident has a fever (39°C) and a constant headache. Leukocyte count is 18,000/mm³. The most likely cause is

    (A) fractured nasal septum
    (B) retropharyngeal abscess
    (C) maxillary sinusitis
    (D) meningitis
    (E) rhinovirus infection

116. Surgery is cancelled 10 minutes after initiation of intravenous regional anesthesia with 50 ml of lidocaine 0.5%. To terminate anesthesia safely, what is the most appropriate timing for deflating the tourniquet?

    (A) Immediately if benzodiazepines have been administered
    (B) Immediately after intravenous administration of ephedrine 10 mg
    (C) Immediately, followed by repeated reinflation and deflation
    (D) In no less than 20 minutes after initial injection
    (E) In no less than 45 minutes after initial injection

117. A 2500-g, 12-hour-old infant is tracheally intubated and mechanically ventilated at a rate of 20/min with an FIO_2 of 0.4 and peak inspiratory pressure of 25 cmH₂O. At birth, amniotic fluid was meconium stained and Apgar scores were 2 and 7. The most recent arterial blood gas levels are PaO_2 50 mmHg, $PaCO_2$ 55 mmHg, and pH 7.20. The most appropriate management is to

    (A) administer sodium bicarbonate
    (B) begin intravenous infusion of prostaglandin E_1
    (C) increase FIO_2
    (D) increase ventilation
    (E) perform bronchial lavage

118. A 60-year-old woman who is taking propranolol for hypertension and is allergic to penicillin is anesthetized with thiopental and halothane for resection of an abdominal aortic aneurysm. Shortly after intubation she is given vancomycin 500 mg intravenously, after which her blood pressure decreases from 140/80 to 70/50 mmHg while her heart rate remains steady at 64 bpm.

The most likely explanation for the decrease in blood pressure is

    (A) cross-sensitivity of penicillin and vancomycin
    (B) interaction of vancomycin and propranolol
    (C) vancomycin-induced anaphylactoid reaction
    (D) interaction of halothane and propranolol
    (E) interaction of halothane and vancomycin

119. During a reoperative total hip arthroplasty requiring transfusion of 8 units of packed red blood cells, blood begins to ooze from the operative field and intravenous catheter sites. Urine is pink. The most likely cause is

    (A) citrate intoxication
    (B) factor V and VIII deficiencies
    (C) rhabdomyolysis
    (D) thrombocytopenia
    (E) transfusion reaction

120. Eight hours after abdominal surgery, a 51-year-old patient becomes increasingly somnolent. Epidural morphine 5 mg was administered immediately following the procedure. Postoperatively, respiratory rate has not decreased below 12/min and SpO_2 has remained greater than 92%. Arterial blood gas analysis shows PaO_2 80 mmHg, $PaCO_2$ 82 mmHg, and pH 7.1.

Which of the following is the most appropriate conclusion?

(A) Analysis of the blood sample was delayed
(B) The blood sample was venous rather than arterial
(C) The patient is receiving supplemental oxygen
(D) The pulse oximeter readings are falsely high
(E) No treatment is required at this time

121. A 76-year-old patient is restless and hallucinating in the preoperative holding area. He received morphine 5 mg and scopolamine 0.4 mg intramuscularly as premedication and is now breathing oxygen 2 L/min through nasal prongs. SpO_2 is 98%. Which of the following is the most appropriate next step?

(A) Administration of naloxone
(B) Administration of physostigmine
(C) Induction of general anesthesia
(D) Determination of serum electrolyte concentrations
(E) CT scan of the head

122. For any given FIO_2 and $PaCO_2$, the PaO_2 is lower in a healthy paralyzed patient anesthetized with isoflurane than in the same patient unanesthetized and breathing spontaneously. The primary cause of this difference is

(A) controlled ventilation
(B) increased airway resistance
(C) inhibition of hypoxic pulmonary vasoconstriction
(D) intraoperative hypothermia
(E) preferential ventilation of nondependent lung

123. Normal pseudocholinesterase

(A) is highly concentrated at the motor end-plate
(B) hydrolyzes succinylcholine by Hofmann elimination
(C) is produced primarily at nerve terminals
(D) is antagonized by acetylcholinesterase inhibitors
(E) resists dibucaine inhibition more than its atypical variant

124. Thirty-six hours after primary repair of meningomyelocele, a term newborn has frequent periods of apnea lasting 25 seconds and associated with oxygen desaturation to 80%. The most likely explanation is

(A) hyperglycemia
(B) loss of cerebrospinal fluid
(C) obstructive hydrocephalus
(D) residual anesthetic effect
(E) normal postoperative events

125. Inhalation induction of anesthesia is more rapid in a 6-month-old infant than in an adult because infants have

    (A) greater ratio of alveolar ventilation to functional residual capacity
    (B) greater ratio of blood volume to body weight
    (C) greater solubility of anesthetic in blood
    (D) lower anesthetic requirement
    (E) lower distribution of cardiac output to vessel-rich organs

126. Which the following findings is most hazardous in premature infants?

    (A) Hematocrit of 55%
    (B) Rectal temperature of 35°C
    (C) Umbilical arterial blood PO_2 of 50 mmHg
    (D) Umbilical arterial blood PCO_2 of 45 mmHg
    (E) Umbilical arterial systolic pressure of 60 mmHg

127. A 40-year-old patient has pain following injection of 8 ml of thiopental 2.5% through a right radial artery catheter. His hand remains pink. Which of the following is the most appropriate next step?

    (A) Injection of lidocaine through the catheter
    (B) Injection of nitroglycerin through the catheter
    (C) Injection of papaverine through the catheter
    (D) Right stellate ganglion block
    (E) No intervention

128. During nitrous oxide anesthesia, which of the following expands most rapidly?

    (A) Air bubble in the blood
    (B) Air in the intestine
    (C) Endotracheal tube cuff
    (D) Pneumothorax
    (E) Sulfahexafluoride bubble in the vitreal cavity

129. While checking an anesthesia machine, opening the oxygen flow-control valve yields no oxygen flow, although the wall-mounted oxygen pipeline supply gauge reads 50 psig. Opening the backup oxygen cylinder results in normal oxygen flow. The most likely cause is

    (A) failure of the oxygen pipeline supply
    (B) failure of the second-stage oxygen pressure regulator
    (C) a malfunctioning check valve in the oxygen pipeline supply inlet
    (D) a malfunctioning fail-safe valve
    (E) a malfunctioning oxygen flow-control valve

130. Which of the following statements concerning pulmonary function in patients with pulmonary fibrosis is true?

    (A) Diffusion capacity is decreased
    (B) Pulmonary artery diastolic-to-occlusion pressure gradients are normal
    (C) Ventilation-perfusion relationships are normal
    (D) Static pulmonary compliance is unchanged
    (E) Mechanical ventilation with slow rate and large tidal volume is optimal

131. Mismatching of ventilation to perfusion in the lung is greatest in which of the following situations?

    (A) Awake patient, spontaneous ventilation, lateral decubitus position
    (B) Anesthetized patient, controlled ventilation, supine position
    (C) Anesthetized patient, controlled ventilation, lateral decubitus position
    (D) Anesthetized patient, controlled ventilation, sitting position
    (E) Anesthetized patient, spontaneous ventilation, prone position

132. The hemodynamic profile below is from a 62-year-old man in the ICU after coronary artery bypass grafting.

	Entering ICU	+30 Minutes
Heart rate (bpm)	90	120
Blood pressure (mmHg)	125/75	80/30
PADP (mmHg)	12	25
PAOP (mmHg)	10	25
CVP (mmHg)	6	8

Which of the following is the most likely cause of the changes occurring after 30 minutes?

    (A) Anaphylactic reaction
    (B) Left ventricular ischemia
    (C) Pericardial tamponade
    (D) Pulmonary embolism
    (E) Septic shock

133. The odor of isoflurane is noted during isoflurane anesthesia with an endotracheal tube and mechanical ventilation. Mean airway pressure is unchanged. A scavenging system with an open interface and an active disposal system is being used. The most likely cause of the isoflurane odor is

    (A) a leak in the inspiratory limb of the anesthesia circuit
    (B) application of excessive negative pressure to the scavenging interface
    (C) malfunction of the pop-off valve of the anesthesia machine
    (D) obstruction of the gas disposal tubing leading from the scavenging interface
    (E) obstruction of the transfer tubing to the scavenging interface

134. Which of the following statements concerning the volume of distribution of a drug is true?

    (A) It is equal to the sum of the volumes of the tissue spaces into which it diffuses
    (B) It is equal to the volume to which it is distributed outside the plasma volume
    (C) It is unaltered by the amount bound to red blood cells and plasma proteins
    (D) It depends on elimination from plasma
    (E) It relates the total amount of the drug in the body to the plasma concentration

135. Which of the following statements concerning propofol is true?

    (A) Active metabolites can produce residual postoperative sedation
    (B) It causes less cardiovascular depression than an equivalent induction dose of thiopental
    (C) It causes less respiratory depression than an equivalent induction dose of thiopental
    (D) It has analgesic properties
    (E) The vehicle emulsion is associated with hypersensitivity reactions

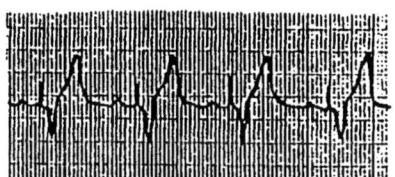

136. The ECG strip shown above is recorded as a patient with a permanent transvenous DDD pacemaker enters the operating room. These changes indicate that the pacemaker is

    (A) sensing the T waves
    (B) sensing the retrograde P waves
    (C) triggering off the intrinsic atrial activity
    (D) malfunctioning in the atrial pacing mechanism
    (E) prematurely stimulating the ventricle

137. Acute epiglottitis usually

    (A) requires a lateral radiograph of the neck for diagnosis
    (B) occurs in children 2 to 4 years of age
    (C) is treated effectively with racemic epinephrine
    (D) has a viral etiology
    (E) requires immediate awake intubation by direct laryngoscopy in the emergency department

138. Characteristics of postdural puncture headache include

    (A) incidence unrelated to the timing of ambulation
    (B) increased severity with addition of vasoconstrictors to the anesthetic
    (C) less frequent occurrence if the needle bevel is perpendicular to the direction of dural fibers
    (D) more frequent occurrence in men
    (E) prevention by prophylactic epidural blood patch

139. Which of the following statements concerning the superior laryngeal nerve is true?

    (A) It provides sensory innervation to the subglottic surface of the vocal cord
    (B) It provides sensory innervation to the inferior surface of the epiglottis
    (C) It is a branch of the glossopharyngeal nerve
    (D) It is blocked by injection of anesthetic near the lateral portion of the cricothyroid membrane
    (E) It is the most commonly injured nerve during thyroid surgery

140. Which of the following is a complication of glycine used for irrigation during transurethral resection of the prostate?

    (A) Epileptiform activity on EEG
    (B) Peripheral neuropathy
    (C) Tachycardia
    (D) Transient blindness
    (E) Transient deafness

141. In the event of a leak in the air flowmeter, which flowmeter arrangement produces the lowest risk for delivering hypoxic gas mixtures?

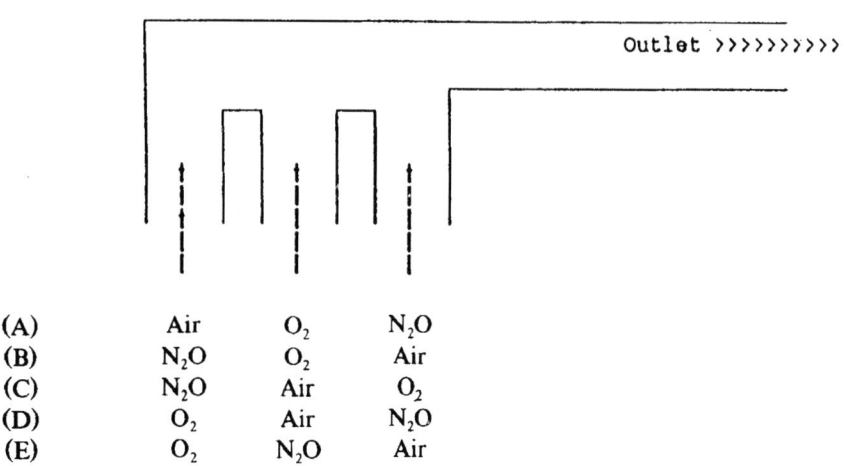

(A)	Air	O_2	N_2O
(B)	N_2O	O_2	Air
(C)	N_2O	Air	O_2
(D)	O_2	Air	N_2O
(E)	O_2	N_2O	Air

142. A 100-kg, 42-year-old woman received enflurane and oxygen for clipping of an intracranial aneurysm lasting eight hours. In the first two postoperative hours, urine output is 2 liters. Serum sodium concentration is 152 mEq/L. Urine osmolarity and central venous pressure are low. Which of the following is best used to establish the diagnosis?

(A) Pulmonary artery occlusion pressure
(B) Serum fluoride concentration
(C) Serum osmolarity
(D) Response to antidiuretic hormone
(E) Response to fluid restriction

143. The drug that causes dose-dependent EEG evidence of both central nervous system excitation and depression is

(A) lidocaine
(B) halothane
(C) thiopental
(D) nitrous oxide
(E) midazolam

144. Which of the following findings differentiates the pickwickian syndrome from morbid obesity?

(A) Carbon dioxide retention
(B) Upper airway obstruction
(C) Decreased forced expiratory volume
(D) Increased shunt fraction
(E) Increased functional residual capacity

145. Which of the following is the most likely sequela of interscalene brachial plexus block?

   (A) Cervical epidural block
   (B) Hemidiaphragmatic paralysis
   (C) Pneumothorax
   (D) Seizure
   (E) Vocal cord paralysis

146. Which of the following is the most reliable indicator of adequate reversal of neuromuscular block?

   (A) Inspiratory force equal to -30 cmH$_2$O
   (B) Sustained head lift for 5 seconds
   (C) Train-of-four ratio of 0.7
   (D) Twitch height at 100% of control
   (E) Vital capacity of 15 ml/kg

147. A 25-year-old man requires exploratory laparotomy following a motor vehicle accident. He is acutely intoxicated with alcohol. Which of the following is the most likely result of the alcohol ingestion?

   (A) Hyperdynamic circulation
   (B) Hyperglycemia
   (C) Hyperthermia
   (D) Increased respiratory depression from opioids
   (E) Increased sensitivity to neuromuscular blocking drugs

148. The decreased duration of action of an intravenous dose of fentanyl compared with an intravenous dose of morphine is best explained by

   (A) greater lipid solubility
   (B) increased hepatic metabolism
   (C) less protein binding
   (D) shorter elimination half-life
   (E) smaller volume of distribution

149. Which of the following complications of caudal anesthesia with 0.25% bupivacaine is more likely in children than in adults?

   (A) Intravascular injection
   (B) Neurotoxicity
   (C) Profound motor block
   (D) Systemic toxicity
   (E) Total spinal block

150. After an axillary brachial plexus block, the patient feels pain when the surgeon clips the skin over the thenar eminence. The most likely cause is inadequate anesthesia in the distribution of the

   (A) intercostobrachial nerve
   (B) median nerve
   (C) musculocutaneous nerve
   (D) radial nerve
   (E) ulnar nerve

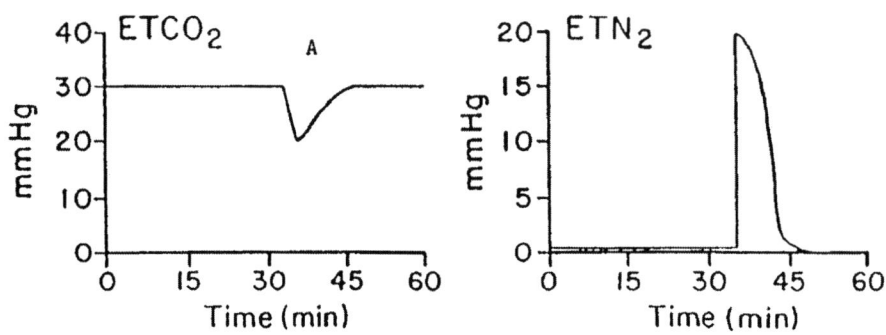

151. The trend plot above shows end-tidal gases measured during a radical neck dissection. The event occurring at A is most likely

    (A) acute hypotension
    (B) endobronchial intubation
    (C) kinking of the endotracheal tube
    (D) rupture of the endotracheal tube cuff
    (E) venous air embolism

---

152. A 36-year-old woman develops acute airway obstruction 24 hours after total thyroidectomy. The most likely cause is

    (A) bilateral recurrent laryngeal nerve injury
    (B) unilateral recurrent laryngeal nerve injury
    (C) hypocalcemia
    (D) subglottic edema
    (E) tracheomalacia

153. Arterial pressure in the radial artery is 155/70 mmHg measured by a correctly calibrated catheter-transducer system. At the same time, aortic pressure is 140/75 mmHg using a high-fidelity catheter tip transducer. The most likely cause of this discrepancy is

    (A) a large amount of air in the dome of the radial artery transducer
    (B) coarctation of the aorta
    (C) peripheral vascular constriction produced by sympathetic stimulation
    (D) physiologic amplification of the waveform from the aorta to the radial artery
    (E) too high a frequency response in the catheter-transducer system

154. During insertion of a Harrington rod with deliberate hypotension for correction of spinal scoliosis, accurate interpretation of somatosensory evoked potentials requires

    (A) core temperature greater than 35°C
    (B) hematocrit of at least 25%
    (C) mean arterial pressure greater than 70 mmHg
    (D) PO_2 of at least 80 mmHg
    (E) reversal of neuromuscular block

155. During insufflation of the peritoneal cavity with carbon dioxide at the start of laparoscopy, heart rate increases to 140 bpm, blood pressure decreases to 70/40 mmHg, and a loud murmur is heard through the esophageal stethoscope. The most appropriate immediate step is to

    (A) administer a vasoconstrictor
    (B) infuse crystalloid solution rapidly
    (C) discontinue the inhaled anesthetic
    (D) insert a central venous catheter
    (E) deflate the abdomen

156. A 35-year-old man has acute onset of low back pain, lower extremity weakness, and bladder dysfunction. He had a lumbar laminectomy two years ago. A myelogram shows disk herniation at L4-5. The most appropriate management is

    (A) bed rest
    (B) administration of a nonsteroidal anti-inflammatory agent
    (C) epidural administration of a corticosteroid
    (D) epidural administration of a local anesthetic
    (E) surgical decompression

157. A patient with chronic obstructive pulmonary disease is undergoing spinal anesthesia to a T6 sensory level. The most pronounced effect on pulmonary function will be a decrease in

    (A) minute ventilation
    (B) peak expiratory flow
    (C) physiologic dead space
    (D) tidal volume
    (E) vital capacity

158. A 70-year-old patient is shivering and has chest pain in the PACU following a cholecystectomy. Heart rate is 120 bpm, and blood pressure is 220/120 mmHg. SpO_2 is 97% at an FIO_2 of 0.4. An ECG shows ST-T wave changes, which are not affected by intravenous administration of nitroglycerin. Which of the following is the most appropriate next step?

    (A) Administration of esmolol
    (B) Administration of hydralazine
    (C) Administration of nitroprusside
    (D) Application of a warming blanket
    (E) Increasing FIO_2

159. A 24-year-old man who sustained multiple rib fractures in a motor vehicle accident has air leaks through bilateral chest tubes. Which of the following is most likely following initiation of high-frequency jet ventilation?

    (A) Airway pressure will be measured most reliably at the proximal (external) end of the endotracheal tube
    (B) Atelectatic areas of the lungs will re-expand
    (C) Changes in end-tidal carbon dioxide tension measured at the tip of the endotracheal tube will match changes in $PaCO_2$
    (D) Hypercarbia will develop
    (E) The air leaks will be proportional to peak airway pressure

160. Which of the following statements concerning the risk of acquiring hepatitis from a blood transfusion is true?

    (A) Most patients with post-transfusion hepatitis become clinically jaundiced
    (B) Most cases of post-transfusion hepatitis are caused by the hepatitis B virus
    (C) The risk for hepatitis is less than the risk for AIDS
    (D) The risk for post-transfusion hepatitis is less than 1% per unit transfused
    (E) The incidence of post-transfusion hepatitis has remained unchanged over the past decade

161. Which of the following is more likely to occur with use of trimethaphan to induce hypotension than with use of nitroprusside?

    (A) A predictable decrease in mean arterial pressure
    (B) Increased mixed venous PO_2
    (C) Increased serum lactate concentration
    (D) Mydriasis
    (E) Reflex tachycardia

162. Local anesthetics block nerve conduction by

    (A) closing calcium channels
    (B) decreasing intracellular calcium concentration
    (C) decreasing potassium conductance
    (D) causing extrusion of intracellular potassium
    (E) inhibiting cellular influx of sodium

163. Which of the following drugs decreases lower esophageal sphincter tone?

    (A) Edrophonium
    (B) Glycopyrrolate
    (C) Metoclopramide
    (D) Prochlorperazine
    (E) Succinylcholine

164. In patients homozygous for atypical pseudocholinesterase, which of the following best explains the prolonged action of succinylcholine?

    (A) An increased proportion of the dose reaches the neuromuscular junction
    (B) Diffusion away from the neuromuscular junction is slowed
    (C) Hepatic clearance of succinylcholine is decreased
    (D) Prejunctional activity is unopposed
    (E) Succinylmonocholine induces neuromuscular block

165. Recognized side effects of magnesium sulfate used for the treatment of preeclampsia that would be of anesthetic concern include each of the following EXCEPT

    (A) maternal pulmonary edema
    (B) neonatal hypotonia
    (C) increased maternal sensitivity to succinylcholine
    (D) increased maternal sensitivity to vecuronium
    (E) maternal hypokalemia

166. A comatose 40-year-old man is to undergo evacuation of an acute subdural hematoma. His left pupil is dilated and blood is present behind the left tympanic membrane. Each of the following is an acceptable intervention EXCEPT

    (A) application of 5 cmH$_2$O positive end-expiratory pressure
    (B) blind nasotracheal intubation
    (C) use of isoflurane
    (D) use of nitrous oxide
    (E) use of succinylcholine

167. A jaundiced patient requires general anesthesia for portocaval shunt. He has a long history of alcohol abuse and is cirrhotic with ascites. Special considerations relevant to induction of anesthesia for this patient include each of the following EXCEPT:

    (A) Denitrogenation by mask may be more rapid than expected
    (B) The risk of aspiration is increased
    (C) The dose of thiopental necessary for induction will be predictably reduced
    (D) The duration of succinylcholine action may be prolonged
    (E) Alfentanil would be an appropriate supplement

168. A patient being mechanically ventilated in the ICU requires wound debridement twice daily. Each of the following agents would be appropriate for induction of brief general anesthesia EXCEPT

    (A) nitrous oxide
    (B) etomidate
    (C) ketamine
    (D) methohexital
    (E) midazolam

169. A computer program for hemodynamic calculations has the following input values: body surface area, arterial blood pressure, heart rate, pulmonary artery occlusion pressure, pulmonary artery pressure, and cardiac output. Each of the following values can be derived with this program EXCEPT

    (A) cardiac index
    (B) stroke volume index
    (C) systemic vascular resistance
    (D) pulmonary vascular resistance
    (E) left ventricular stroke work index

170. A successful ankle block for transmetatarsal amputation of the first and second toes should include each of the following nerves EXCEPT the

    (A) saphenous
    (B) deep peroneal
    (C) superficial peroneal
    (D) sural
    (E) tibial

171. Each of the following contributes to hypotension following induction of anesthesia with propofol EXCEPT

(A) central vagal stimulation
(B) decreased central sympathetic tone
(C) direct myocardial depression
(D) resetting of arterial baroreceptors
(E) systemic vasodilation

172. Inhibition of labor by terbutaline causes each of the following maternal side effects EXCEPT

(A) hyperkalemia
(B) hypotension
(C) ventricular dysrhythmias
(D) hyperglycemia
(E) pulmonary edema

173. A 66-year-old man with chronic obstructive pulmonary disease who underwent colectomy 12 hours ago has been receiving an epidural infusion of fentanyl at a rate of 100 μg/hr. Which of the following is LEAST likely to develop?

(A) Hypotension
(B) Nausea
(C) Pruritus
(D) Respiratory depression
(E) Urinary retention

174. A 65-year-old man is disoriented and has a headache and nausea in the recovery room 30 minutes after transurethral resection of the prostate with glycine irrigation performed under spinal anesthesia. Heart rate is 50 bpm and blood pressure is 180/110 mmHg. Which of the following is LEAST likely?

(A) Decreased serum osmolality
(B) Serum sodium concentration 132 mEq/L
(C) Increased serum ammonia concentration
(D) Bibasilar rales
(E) Jugular venous distention

175. A 70-year-old man sustains injuries to both carotid bodies during bilateral carotid endarterectomies performed four days apart. Two hours after the second procedure, the patient is breathing room air in the PACU. Which of the following sets of arterial blood gas values is LEAST likely?

	pH	PCO$_2$ (mmHg)	PO$_2$ (mmHg)
(A)	7.3	50	58
(B)	7.3	50	86
(C)	7.4	40	86
(D)	7.4	42	58
(E)	7.5	32	58

GENERAL INSTRUCTIONS

1. Please write your name and identification number in the space provided on the front of this test book. If you are taking the examination for Board Certification, your identification number is printed on your notification card. If you are an In-Training Resident, use your U.S. Social Security Number. If you do not have a U.S. Social Security Number, use your Canadian Social Insurance Number.

2. Your name and identification number and all of your answers must be recorded on the separate answer sheet enclosed in this booklet.

   The sample on the right shows how to record your identification number on the answer sheet. Be sure to enter your number in the boxes provided and also to mark it in the appropriate spaces as illustrated.

3. Credit will be given only for answers marked on the answer sheet. You may make any preliminary notes or calculations in the test books, but be sure that all of your answers are marked on the answer sheet. Only one choice should be marked for each question. Multiple answers for the same question are treated as wrong answers. In marking your answer sheet use only a soft (#2) lead pencil. Do NOT use a pen or pencil with hard lead. Make each mark heavy and black enough to obliterate completely the letter within the circle. Marks should fill the circle; if marks are light or outside the circle, you may not receive credit for your answers. Make no stray marks on the answer sheet, as these could lower your score. If you wish to change an answer, be sure to erase your first mark completely.

4. This test book contains two different types of questions, each of which is preceded by special directions. You are advised to study the directions carefully. Even though you may be in doubt about the correct answer, select the choice that you consider to be the best. Your score is the number of questions you answered correctly.

5. You will have 3¹/₂ hours to work on this section of the test which contains 175 questions.

RULES OF CONDUCT FOR EXAMINEES DURING ABA/ASA IN-TRAINING EXAMINATION

1. Do not falsify information required for admission to the examination or impersonate another ABA/ASA examinee.

2. Do not bring calculators, watches with memory capability, books, papers, or memoranda of any kind into the examination room.

3. Do not break the seal on your test books until you are instructed to do so by the proctor.

4. Do not tear any pages or portions of pages from the test books or tear your answer sheet.

5. Do not disturb the examination process by talking, smoking, or interfering with others who are taking the examination.

6. Do not attempt to observe the test books or answer sheets of other examinees. Do not copy the answers of another examinee, permit answers to be copied, or in any way provide or receive unauthorized information about the content of the examination while it is in progress.

7. Terminate the examination immediately upon instruction by the proctor to do so.

8. Do not take the test books, answer sheets, or any documents, examination material, or memoranda from the room.

Failure to abide by these rules of conduct during this examination may result in disciplinary actions by the ABA/ASA In-Training Council or by the American Board of Anesthesiology. Statistical analyses may be used to verify observations and/or reports of suspected irregularities in conduct.

AMERICAN BOARD OF ANESTHESIOLOGY

AMERICAN SOCIETY OF ANESTHESIOLOGISTS

IN-TRAINING EXAMINATION

Book B

$3^1/_2$ hours

Do not break the seal until you are told to do so.

Read the directions on the back cover.

PREPARED IN COOPERATION WITH NATIONAL BOARD OF MEDICAL EXAMINERS®

ABA/ASA 93TB
pp 40, qtn 174

Printed in
U.S.A.

DIRECTIONS : Each of the numbered items or incomplete statements in this section is followed by answers or by completions of the statement. Select the ONE lettered answer or completion that is BEST in each case and fill in the circle containing the corresponding letter on the answer sheet.

1. The need for increased doses of nondepolarizing muscle relaxants in patients with extensive burns is best explained by

(A) increased protein binding
(B) hypermetabolism
(C) increased glomerular filtration rate
(D) proliferation of receptors on burned muscle
(E) decreased volume of distribution

2. Which of the following parts of the infant's airway determines the appropriate diameter of a nasotracheal tube?

(A) Nares
(B) Glottis
(C) Vocal cords
(D) Cricoid cartilage
(E) Third tracheal ring

3. Administration of 200 mEq of sodium bicarbonate during cardiopulmonary resuscitation is associated with

(A) CSF alkalosis
(B) hypercalcemia
(C) hypercarbia
(D) hyperkalemia
(E) shift of the oxyhemoglobin dissociation curve to the right

4. When compared with diazepam, midazolam

(A) metabolites contribute more significantly to the sedative effect
(B) elimination is less dependent on hepatic metabolism
(C) has more predictable action after intramuscular administration
(D) produces less respiratory depression
(E) produces less hypotension during induction of anesthesia with opioids

5. Which of the following statements concerning a patient who has been receiving nitroprusside for several days is true?

(A) Biotransformation of cyanide requires a sulfur donor
(B) Formation of methemoglobin increases cyanide toxicity
(C) Increased serum thiocyanate concentrations are innocuous
(D) Mixed venous PO_2 decreases as cyanide toxicity develops
(E) Serum thiocyanate concentrations reflect the degree of cyanide toxicity

6. Which of the following increases the cephalad spread of hyperbaric intrathecal local anesthetics?

(A) Cephalad-directed needle bevel
(B) Coughing
(C) Lithotomy position
(D) Obesity
(E) Rapid injection

7. Compared with a patient without liver disease, a patient with cirrhosis will have

(A) greater accumulation of vecuronium with infusion
(B) increased unbound plasma vecuronium concentration
(C) more frequent occurrence of phase II block after succinylcholine administration
(D) prolonged elimination half-life of atracurium
(E) unchanged volume of distribution for pancuronium

8. Intrathecally administered opioids exert their analgesic effects primarily in the

(A) brain stem
(B) fourth ventricle
(C) spinal nerve roots
(D) spinothalamic tracts
(E) substantia gelatinosa

9. During laser excision of vocal cord polyps in a 5-year-old boy, dark smoke suddenly appears in the surgical field. The trachea is intubated and anesthesia is being maintained with halothane, nitrous oxide, and oxygen. The most appropriate initial step is to

(A) change from oxygen and nitrous oxide to air
(B) fill the oropharynx with water
(C) instill water into the endotracheal tube
(D) remove the endotracheal tube
(E) ventilate with carbon dioxide

10. During craniotomy in the sitting position, end-tidal carbon dioxide tension suddenly decreases. Ventilatory excursion of the chest is normal. Further evaluation is most likely to show a decrease in

(A) alveolar-to-arterial oxygen tension difference
(B) alveolar-to-arterial carbon dioxide tension difference
(C) dead space ventilation
(D) pulmonary artery pressure
(E) pulmonary artery occlusion pressure

11. Which of the following is a cardiorespiratory effect of epidural block to a T4 sensory level?

(A) Decreased expiratory reserve volume
(B) Decreased tidal volume
(C) Increased circulating catecholamine concentrations
(D) Increased heart rate
(E) Unchanged vital capacity

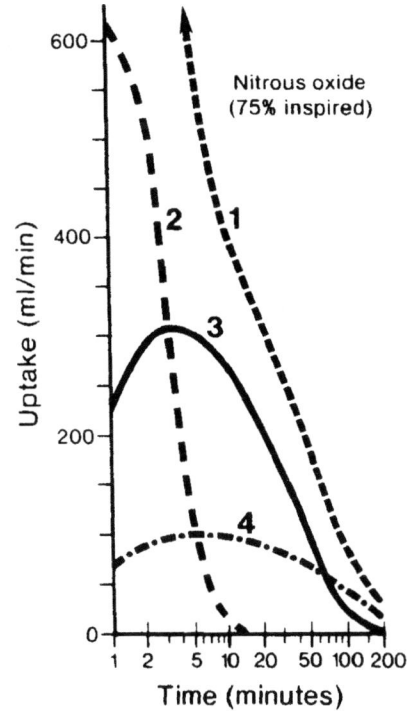

12. The figure above describes the uptake of nitrous oxide 75% by individual tissue groups (VRG=vessel-rich group, MG=muscle group, FG=fat group) and their sum (total uptake, TU). Which set of labels accurately describes the curves?

	1	2	3	4
(A)	MG	FG	VRG	TU
(B)	VRG	MG	FG	TU
(C)	FG	MG	TU	VRG
(D)	TU	FG	MG	VRG
(E)	TU	VRG	MG	FG

13. A 67-year-old man undergoes spinal anesthesia with hyperbaric tetracaine 10 mg for transurethral resection of the prostate. At the end of the 50-minute procedure, the level of anesthesia is T6 and blood pressure is 120/70 mmHg. Within two minutes after transfer to a stretcher, the patient has nausea and blood pressure decreases to 76/42 mmHg. Which of the following is the most likely cause of the acute hypotension?

(A) Acute congestive heart failure
(B) Decreased venous return
(C) Dilutional hyponatremia
(D) Progression of sympathetic block
(E) Unrecognized bladder perforation

14. A 26-year-old woman has persistent uterine bleeding following a normal spontaneous delivery without anesthesia. The uterus is firm on manual examination. Which of the following anesthetics is most appropriate for manual extraction of the placenta?

(A) Halothane
(B) Pudendal block with lidocaine
(C) Subarachnoid tetracaine
(D) Thiopental
(E) Vecuronium

15. Compared with intermittent positive pressure ventilation (IPPV), intermittent mandatory ventilation (IMV)

(A) better maintains cardiac output
(B) provides less than full mechanical ventilatory support
(C) requires a greater level of sedation
(D) requires a higher FiO_2
(E) requires a lower inspiratory flow rate

16. Which of the following findings would be considered normal in the EEG of an adult?

(A) Decreased frequency during induction with halogenated anesthetics
(B) Decreased frequency in frontal areas with administration of nitrous oxide 50%
(C) Dominance of beta rhythm at 20 to 30 Hz during the awake relaxed state
(D) Electrical silence with administration of isoflurane 2.5 MAC
(E) The presence of burst-suppression during natural sleep

17. Proper zeroing of an arterial pressure transducer attached to a supine anesthetized patient is best accomplished by

(A) continuous flow of fluid through the intravascular catheter
(B) opening the system to air at heart level
(C) placement of the transducer diaphragm at heart level
(D) proper damping of the transducer system
(E) zeroing the transducer during the expiration phase of mechanical ventilation

18. A 1-month-old infant becomes hypoxemic faster during apnea than an adult. Which of the following is the primary cause of this difference?

(A) Functional residual capacity in an infant is half that of an adult
(B) Metabolic rate in an infant is twice that of an adult
(C) Resting PaO_2 in an infant is lower than that in an adult
(D) The number of alveoli in an infant is 12% the number in an adult
(E) The hemoglobin dissociation curve in an infant is shifted to the right

19. During extracorporeal shock wave lithotripsy, the shock wave should be synchronized with

(A) the P wave of the ECG
(B) the R wave of the ECG
(C) the T wave of the ECG
(D) peak inspiration
(E) end-expiration

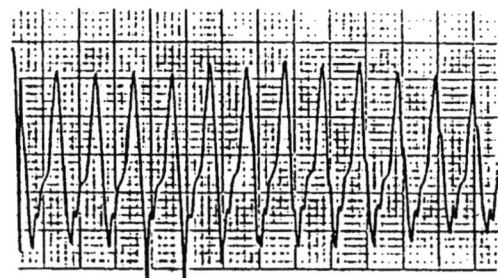

20. The cardiac rhythm illustrated above appeared suddenly in an anesthetized patient. The most appropriate management is

    (A) administration of adenosine
    (B) administration of digoxin
    (C) administration of epinephrine
    (D) overdrive pacing
    (E) synchronous cardioversion

---

21. Which of the following statements concerning hyperkalemia after succinylcholine administration to a patient with a spinal cord injury is true?

    (A) It is unlikely to occur if the lesion is located below T6
    (B) It is unlikely to occur within 24 hours of the injury
    (C) It is unlikely to occur more than 60 days after the initial injury
    (D) It is prevented by pretreatment with small doses of a nondepolarizing agent
    (E) It is decreased in magnitude by pretreatment with calcium chloride

22. The severity of chronic bronchitis is best assessed by measuring

    (A) tidal volume
    (B) carbon dioxide diffusion capacity
    (C) sputum production over 24 hours
    (D) forced vital capacity
    (E) arterial blood gases

23. An 8-kg, 1-year-old boy is scheduled for a bilateral inguinal hernia repair. If regional anesthesia is to be used for postoperative analgesia, which of the following statements is true?

    (A) Caudal administration of 0.25% bupivacaine will provide analgesia without evidence of motor block
    (B) Caudal administration of 0.125% bupivacaine is as effective as caudal administration of 0.25% bupivacaine
    (C) Caudal analgesia is more difficult to achieve in young children than in adults
    (D) The recommended volume of local anesthetic used for caudal analgesia in children is 3 ml per year of age
    (E) The volume of 0.25% bupivacaine required for bilateral ilioinguinal and iliohypogastric nerve blocks would be too large

24. After inserting a left-sided double-lumen endotracheal tube, both cuffs are inflated. When the right (tracheal) lumen is clamped, breath sounds are heard only in the lower right lung field. When the left (bronchial) lumen is clamped, breath sounds are heard over the entire left lung field. Where is the tube positioned?

(A) Tracheal orifice above the carina and bronchial limb in the right bronchus
(B) Tracheal orifice above the carina and bronchial limb in the left bronchus
(C) Tracheal orifice and bronchial limb both above the carina
(D) Tracheal cuff and bronchial limb both in the right bronchus
(E) Tracheal orifice and bronchial limb both in the left bronchus

25. A 27-year-old man with type I von Willebrand's disease requires internal fixation of an open fracture of the femur. Prothrombin time, partial thromboplastin time, and platelet count are normal. During surgery, there is significant oozing from the wound and the surgeon notes poor clot quality. The most appropriate therapy at this time is administration of

(A) cryoprecipitate
(B) desmopressin
(C) fresh frozen plasma
(D) lyophilized factor VII concentrate
(E) platelets

26. A 30-year-old man is brought to the emergency department after being rescued from a house fire. With the trachea intubated and FIO_2 at 1.0, arterial blood gas values are PaO_2 495 mmHg, $PaCO_2$ 28 mmHg, and pH 7.28. Hemoglobin saturation measured by co-oximeter is 50%. The most appropriate next step is to

(A) add positive end-expiratory pressure
(B) add n-acetylcysteine to the inhaled gases
(C) administer sodium bicarbonate intravenously
(D) transfuse 2 units of packed red blood cells
(E) transfer to a hyperbaric chamber

27. A 60-kg, 45-year-old woman who takes digoxin for atrial fibrillation receives furosemide 40 mg and mannitol 60 g during resection of a supratentorial meningioma. After initiation of hyperventilation to decrease $PaCO_2$ from 35 to 20 mmHg, multifocal premature ventricular contractions are noted on the ECG. The most likely cause is

(A) acute hypokalemia
(B) cerebral ischemia
(C) impending herniation of the brain stem
(D) paradoxical air embolism
(E) surgical manipulation of the meningioma

28. A 50-year-old woman with subarachnoid hemorrhage and left hemiparesis undergoes clipping of a right cerebral aneurysm. On the second postoperative day, mental status deteriorates. Blood pressure is 110/70 mmHg. A cerebral angiogram shows vasospasm. The most appropriate management is to

(A) administer dexamethasone
(B) administer mannitol
(C) administer phentolamine
(D) expand intravascular volume
(E) intubate and hyperventilate to a $PaCO_2$ of 28 mmHg

29. Which of the following statements concerning cerebral blood flow (CBF) during anesthesia is true?

    (A) CBF changes minimally when $PaCO_2$ increases from 30 to 40 mmHg
    (B) CBF changes minimally when PO_2 decreases from 160 to 100 mmHg
    (C) CBF is autoregulated when mean arterial pressure is 40 mmHg
    (D) CBF is coupled to cerebral metabolism during isoflurane anesthesia
    (E) CBF is unaffected by 1.2% isoflurane at a $PaCO_2$ of 40 mmHg

30. Which of the following drugs is contraindicated in patients with Parkinson's disease?

    (A) Atropine
    (B) Dopamine
    (C) Droperidol
    (D) Fentanyl
    (E) Isoflurane

31. A 70-kg patient with no acute bleeding has a preoperative platelet count of $40,000/mm^3$. Following preoperative transfusion of platelets 10 units, the predicted platelet count would be

    (A)   50,000/mm^3
    (B)   80,000/mm^3
    (C)   90,000/mm^3
    (D) 140,000/mm^3
    (E) 190,000/mm^3

32. Two hours after coronary artery bypass grafting, a 60-year-old man has a heart rate of 140 bpm and blood pressure of 80/60 mmHg. Cardiac index is 1.5 L/min/m^2. Central venous pressure is 23 mmHg with large a-waves in the right atrial pressure tracing. A pulsus paradoxus of 6 mmHg is noted. Which of the following is the most likely diagnosis?

    (A) Atrial flutter
    (B) Cardiac tamponade
    (C) Hypovolemia
    (D) Junctional tachycardia
    (E) Tension pneumothorax

33. Which of the following is the strongest indication for one-lung ventilation?

    (A) Descending thoracic aortic aneurysm
    (B) Esophageal resection
    (C) Lobectomy for lung abscess
    (D) Lobectomy for tumor
    (E) Pneumonectomy for tumor

34. In a 65-year-old man, which of the following findings on preoperative pulmonary function testing is associated with the highest risk for respiratory insufficiency following pneumonectomy?

    (A) Maximum voluntary ventilation at 65% of predicted
    (B) Mean pulmonary artery pressure of 28 mmHg
    (C) Predicted postoperative forced expiratory volume in one second (FEV_1) of 800 ml
    (D) Residual volume to total lung capacity (RV/TLC) ratio of 0.35
    (E) Vital capacity of 3 liters

35. During transurethral resection of the prostate, intravascular absorption of glycine irrigant most commonly produces

   (A) alkalosis
   (B) hemolysis
   (C) hypertension
   (D) tachycardia
   (E) wheezing

36. A 2.2-kg, 6-hour-old neonate is to undergo gastrostomy followed by repair of a tracheoesophageal fistula. During induction with halothane, air, and oxygen, the abdomen becomes distended. Appropriate management is to

   (A) intubate and assist spontaneous ventilation
   (B) intubate and control ventilation
   (C) insert an orogastric tube
   (D) allow the patient to breathe spontaneously by mask until gastrostomy
   (E) control ventilation by mask until gastrostomy

37. Which of the following is an advantage of a circle system over a Mapleson D system?

   (A) Better anesthetic conservation
   (B) Lower dead space
   (C) Lower circuit resistance
   (D) More efficient scavenging
   (E) More rapid changes in inspired gas concentration

38. A 27-year-old man with a one-month history of quadriplegia at a C6 level is given general anesthesia for cystoscopy. During the cystoscopy, blood pressure suddenly increases to 220/120 mmHg. Further evaluation is most likely to show

   (A) atrial fibrillation (ventricular rate 100 bpm)
   (B) paroxysmal atrial tachycardia (150 bpm)
   (C) sinus bradycardia
   (D) piloerection above the level of C6
   (E) sweating above the level of C6

39. Which of the following is the primary factor regulating normal coronary blood flow?

   (A) Aortic diastolic pressure
   (B) Coronary perfusion pressure
   (C) Heart rate
   (D) Myocardial oxygen consumption
   (E) Systolic wall tension

40. Which of the following statements concerning pressure support ventilation is true?

   (A) Continuous positive airway pressure is provided during inspiration and expiration
   (B) Delivered tidal volume remains the same with decreasing lung compliance
   (C) Inspiratory effort less than -2 cmH$_2$O is not assisted
   (D) The overall work of breathing decreases when weaning from mechanical ventilation
   (E) The patient will need more sedation than during intermittent mandatory ventilation

41. If administered epidurally in equipotent doses, which of the following opioids will produce analgesia over the greatest number of dermatomes?

    (A) Fentanyl
    (B) Hydromorphone
    (C) Meperidine
    (D) Morphine
    (E) Sufentanil

42. Which of the following is decreased by alkalinization of a 1.5% lidocaine solution?

    (A) Concentration of free base
    (B) Dose required for anesthesia
    (C) Duration of anesthesia
    (D) Intracellular concentration of ionized lidocaine
    (E) Time to onset of anesthesia

43. Cyanide toxicity from nitroprusside is unlikely in patients with renal dysfunction because

    (A) renal excretion of thiosulfate is decreased
    (B) metabolic acidosis inactivates cyanide
    (C) anemia inhibits breakdown of nitroprusside by oxyhemoglobin
    (D) thiocyanate is formed in the liver
    (E) the dose of nitroprusside necessary to lower blood pressure is greatly decreased

44. Twelve hours after an uneventful hysterectomy with lidocaine epidural anesthesia, a 70-year-old woman has partial paralysis of the lower extremities. She is receiving morphine 0.5 mg/hr through an epidural catheter and is pain free. On examination, definite motor loss is noted in the lower extremities, but no other deficits are apparent. The most appropriate action at this time is to

    (A) administer naloxone
    (B) substitute fentanyl for morphine infusion
    (C) remove the epidural catheter
    (D) obtain an MRI of the lumbar spine
    (E) reassure the patient

45. Equipment that is attached to a patient should have leakage current no greater than

    (A)   10 microamps
    (B) 100 microamps
    (C)   1 milliamp
    (D)   10 milliamps
    (E) 100 milliamps

46. When the inspired gas is changed from air to 20% oxygen and 80% nitrous oxide, PaO_2 increases because

    (A) increased pulmonary artery pressure perfuses alveoli that previously enhanced dead space
    (B) nitrous oxide stimulates the respiratory center
    (C) rapid absorption of nitrous oxide increases alveolar oxygen concentration
    (D) replacement of nitrogen by nitrous oxide expands atelectatic alveoli
    (E) respiratory depression from nitrous oxide shifts the oxyhemoglobin dissociation curve

47. Which of the following characteristics of local anesthetics is associated with long duration of action?

    (A) High degree of lipid solubility
    (B) High degree of protein binding
    (C) High molecular weight
    (D) High pK,
    (E) Presence of ester linkage

48. Which of the following drugs used to produce or reverse muscle relaxation has the greatest prolongation of action in a patient with end-stage renal disease?

    (A) Atracurium
    (B) Neostigmine
    (C) Pancuronium
    (D) Succinylcholine
    (E) Vecuronium

49. In a patient with chronic congestive heart failure, the safest pharmacologic approach to brain swelling during a craniotomy is

    (A) dexamethasone
    (B) furosemide
    (C) mannitol
    (D) thiopental
    (E) urea

50. In clinical anesthesia practice, the term "informed consent" is best described as a legal concept in which patients

    (A) agree to anesthesia care based on full disclosure of facts needed to make the decision intelligently
    (B) are told of all possible risks of anesthesia and anesthetic procedures
    (C) delegate all decisions regarding anesthesia care to the anesthesiologist
    (D) release the physicians from liability
    (E) sign global consent forms for surgical procedures that cover the administration of anesthesia care

51. The low fetal/maternal plasma ratio of bupivacaine compared with lidocaine is due to

    (A) fetal tissue binding
    (B) fetal plasma protein binding
    (C) maternal plasma protein binding
    (D) ionization in maternal blood
    (E) ionization in fetal blood

52. A previously healthy 28-year-old man is admitted to the emergency department with a probable opioid overdose. Arterial blood gas values are: PaO_2 49 mmHg, $PaCO_2$ 76 mmHg, and pH 7.12 while breathing room air. Which of the following statements is true?

    (A) Aspiration of gastric contents must have occurred
    (B) Hypoventilation alone can explain the acidosis and hypoxemia
    (C) The hypoxemia is probably due to noncardiogenic pulmonary edema
    (D) Naloxone should be administered only if the patient is normothermic
    (E) Pure oxygen is contraindicated

53. In which of the following clinical circumstances does down-regulation of beta-adrenergic receptors occur?

   (A) Chronic congestive heart failure
   (B) Hypothyroidism
   (C) Long-term clonidine administration
   (D) Long-term metoprolol administration
   (E) Stable angina

54. Which of the following is the most likely cause of apnea occurring after a retrobulbar block?

   (A) Epidural injection
   (B) Increased intracranial pressure
   (C) Oculopontine reflex
   (D) Ophthalmic artery injection
   (E) Subarachnoid injection

55. A 40-year-old man is undergoing open reduction and internal fixation of a fractured femur. During anesthesia with fentanyl, enflurane, and oxygen, heart rate decreases to 20 bpm and 6 premature ventricular contractions per minute are noted. No pulse is detected. The most appropriate next step is to

   (A) administer atropine
   (B) administer epinephrine
   (C) administer lidocaine
   (D) apply a transthoracic pacemaker
   (E) start cardiopulmonary resuscitation

56. A 35-year-old woman with systemic lupus erythematosus is admitted to the critical care unit following sudden onset of severe chest pain. Examination shows tachycardia, hypotension, pulmonary edema, and a blowing systolic murmur in the left parasternal region. The most appropriate management is

   (A) aerosol administration of terbutaline
   (B) intravenous infusion of phenylephrine and nitroglycerin
   (C) intravenous infusion of esmolol
   (D) intravenous infusion of epinephrine and nitroprusside
   (E) volume loading with lactated Ringer's solution

57. The table below shows the pharmacokinetic effects of a new neuromuscular blocker.

	Normal	Renal Failure
Volume of distribution	15 L	21 L
Clearance	200 ml/min	100 ml/min

In a patient with renal failure, which of the following will result in a response to this drug most similar to that of a normal individual?

   (A) Increased loading dose
   (B) The same maintenance dose
   (C) Decreased maintenance dose interval
   (D) Avoidance of continuous infusion
   (E) Increased dose of anticholinesterase for reversal

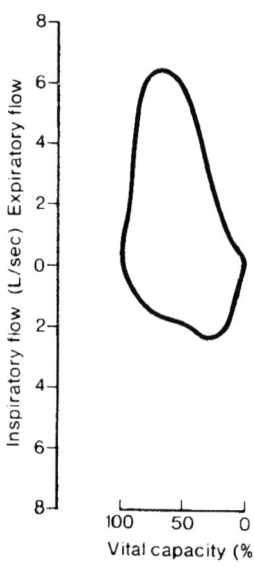

58. The flow-volume loop shown above is most likely from a patient with which of the following?

   (A) Bilateral vocal cord paralysis
   (B) Chronic bronchitis
   (C) Tracheal stenosis six months after a previous tracheostomy
   (D) Tumor of the lower trachea
   (E) Normal respiratory status

---

59. A 66-year-old patient with aortic stenosis is scheduled for aortic valve replacement. Examination shows blood pressure of 110/60 mmHg and sinus rhythm at a rate of 75 bpm. Pulmonary artery occlusion pressure (PAOP) is 20 mmHg with a prominent a-wave on the tracing. Which of the following is the most appropriate management?

   (A) Increasing myocardial contractility
   (B) Maintaining PAOP below 20 mmHg
   (C) Maintaining sinus rhythm
   (D) Promoting mild tachycardia
   (E) Decreasing peripheral resistance

60. During rapid-sequence induction prior to an emergency surgical procedure, a 20-year-old patient vomits gastric contents containing particulate matter. An endotracheal tube is easily inserted and ventilation with pure oxygen is initiated. Despite the presence of bilateral breath sounds, SpO$_2$ is 90%. Which of the following is the most appropriate next step?

   (A) Administration of broad-spectrum antibiotics
   (B) Intravenous administration of high-dose methylprednisolone
   (C) Bronchial lavage with normal saline solution
   (D) Bronchoscopy to remove particulate matter
   (E) Cancellation of the surgical procedure

61. A radial artery catheter is to be used for blood pressure measurement during a sitting craniotomy. When zeroing the transducer, which of the following describes the best levels for placement of the transducer and opening of the system to air?

	Transducer	Opening to Air
(A)	Head	Wrist
(B)	Head	Head
(C)	Head	Heart
(D)	Heart	Heart
(E)	Heart	Wrist

62. The gauge pressure on a cylinder of nitrous oxide

    (A) varies with the size of the cylinder
    (B) is the same for full and half-full cylinders
    (C) is the same as that of a full cylinder of oxygen if both are full
    (D) is independent of the temperature of the cylinder
    (E) reliably indicates the amount of nitrous oxide in the cylinder

63. Immediately after sustaining severe head injury, a 20-year-old man has a blood pressure of 150/90 mmHg and an intracranial pressure of 35 mmHg. After one hour of thiopental infusion, blood pressure is 105/60 mmHg, intracranial pressure is 20 mmHg, central venous pressure is 5 mmHg, and temperature is 36°C. The EEG shows slow-wave activity. The most appropriate next step is administration of

    (A) additional thiopental
    (B) a corticosteroid
    (C) furosemide
    (D) nimodipine
    (E) phenylephrine

64. Following induction of anesthesia with sufentanil and pancuronium, a patient with left main coronary artery disease has a decrease in blood pressure from 110/70 to 60/40 mmHg. There is no change in heart rate or ECG. The most appropriate management of the hypotension is administration of

    (A) calcium chloride
    (B) ephedrine
    (C) epinephrine
    (D) isoproterenol
    (E) phenylephrine

65. In a 35-year-old patient, which of the following is associated with an increased duration of clinical narcosis following infusion of a total dose of 10 mg/kg thiopental over three hours?

    (A) Alcoholism in remission
    (B) Asthma
    (C) Fever
    (D) Obesity
    (E) Use of appetite suppressants

66. A previously healthy, 60-kg, 17-year-old boy is undergoing emergency surgery for a gunshot wound involving the iliac vein. Ventilation is controlled with a tidal volume of 700 ml/breath, rate of 10/min, and peak inspiratory pressure of 30 cmH_2O. Body temperature is normal. The most likely cause of an end-tidal carbon dioxide partial pressure of 16 mmHg is

   (A) endobronchial intubation
   (B) excessive expiratory time
   (C) excessive tidal volume
   (D) low cardiac output
   (E) pulmonary aspiration

67. Which of the following statements concerning anesthetic management for MRIs is true?

   (A) ECG wires are associated with patient burns
   (B) Mechanical ventilation of the lungs is not feasible
   (C) Monitors with ferromagnetic components may be used
   (D) Oxygen analysis of inspired gas is inaccurate
   (E) Pulse oximetry is not reliable near the MR scanner

68. Intraocular pressure is

   (A) decreased by glycopyrrolate
   (B) increased by hyperventilation
   (C) decreased by halothane
   (D) increased by nondepolarizing muscle relaxants
   (E) increased by phenylephrine eye drops

69. Compared with adult hemoglobin, which of the following is a characteristic of fetal hemoglobin?

   (A) It has a greater oxygen-carrying capacity
   (B) It has a lower P_{50}
   (C) It is more likely to cause an artifactual increase in SpO_2
   (D) It is more likely to sickle
   (E) It unloads oxygen more readily at the tissues

70. Which of the following is most effective in decontaminating an anesthesia machine that was splattered with HIV-contaminated blood?

   (A) Bleach
   (B) De-ionized water
   (C) Ethylene oxide
   (D) Hydrogen peroxide
   (E) Isopropyl alcohol

71. Which of the following is greater in an obese patient than in a nonobese patient of equal height?

   (A) Milliliters of local anesthetic required for epidural block
   (B) Milligrams of succinylcholine required for intubation
   (C) Clearance of diazepam
   (D) Clearance of fentanyl
   (E) Oxygen consumption per body surface area

72. The best premedication regimen for a known active narcotic addict would include

    (A) secobarbital
    (B) diazepam
    (C) nalbuphine
    (D) morphine
    (E) droperidol

73. During cardiopulmonary bypass at a nasopharyngeal temperature of 28°C and a hematocrit of 20%, temperature-corrected $PaCO_2$ is 50 mmHg and uncorrected $PaCO_2$ is 60 mmHg. The most appropriate management is to

    (A) administer additional opioid
    (B) administer packed red blood cells to increase hematocrit to 25%
    (C) further decrease the patient's temperature
    (D) increase fresh gas flow to the oxygenator
    (E) institute mechanical ventilation

74. Two days after coronary artery bypass grafting, a 62-year-old man remains sedated, tracheally intubated, and mechanically ventilated with full neuromuscular block. Over the next three hours, PaO_2 decreases from 90 to 70 mmHg at an FIO_2 of 0.7, peak inspiratory pressure measured proximally in the ventilatory circuit increases from 40 to 66 cmH$_2$O, and plateau pressure remains unchanged at 30 cmH$_2$O.

    Which of the following is the most likely cause of these changes?

    (A) Adult respiratory distress syndrome
    (B) Bronchial mucus plugging
    (C) Left ventricular failure
    (D) Lobar pneumonia
    (E) Tension pneumothorax

75. A combined epidural and general anesthetic is used for aortofemoral bypass surgery. Just prior to extubation, the patient received morphine 5 mg through the epidural catheter. Eleven hours later, he is unresponsive while breathing 40% oxygen from a face mask. Respiratory rate is 6/min and SpO_2 is 92%. Arterial blood gas analysis shows PaO_2 80 mmHg, $PaCO_2$ 84 mmHg, and pH 7.16.

    Which of the following statements concerning this patient is true?

    (A) Hypercarbia is contributing to the decreased level of consciousness
    (B) Naloxone is ineffective for reversing the respiratory depression
    (C) The oxygen saturation is higher than expected because of the pH
    (D) The risk for respiratory depression would have been lower with subarachnoid administration of 0.5 mg morphine
    (E) Residual local anesthetic is contributing to the respiratory depression

76. A rapid shallow ventilatory pattern is most energy efficient for a patient who

    (A) has a low ratio of forced expiratory volume in one second to vital capacity (FEV_1/VC)
    (B) has a high ratio of tidal volume to vital capacity, and diminished vital capacity
    (C) has increased pulmonary compliance
    (D) is using the accessory muscles of respiration
    (E) has increased airway resistance

77. A 70-year-old patient has absence of the left radial pulse one month after repair of an aortic aneurysm. Arterial pressure was monitored perioperatively with a 20-gauge left radial artery catheter. Which of the following statements concerning this complication is true?

(A) A preoperative Allen's test would have predicted this complication
(B) Stellate ganglion block should be performed
(C) This complication would have been less likely with an 18-gauge catheter
(D) This patient has poor collateral circulation in the hand
(E) The pulse will likely return

78. Five minutes after intrathecal administration of tetracaine 12 mg in hyperbaric solution, a 60-year-old man has a weak hand grasp. Respirations are normal, heart rate has decreased from 80 to 45 bpm, and blood pressure has decreased from 150/80 to 90/50 mmHg. The most appropriate management at this time is

(A) administration of atropine
(B) administration of ephedrine
(C) administration of phenylephrine
(D) placement of the patient in the head-down position
(E) observation

79. A burn is found at the site of the electrocautery pad. Which of the following is most likely?

(A) The electrosurgical unit was in the bipolar mode
(B) The electrocautery pad became partially detached
(C) The electrosurgical unit ground wire was severed
(D) The line-isolation monitor alarmed
(E) The patient became grounded

80. Which property of oxygen is detected by the fail-safe device on the anesthesia machine?

(A) Concentration
(B) Flow
(C) Pressure
(D) Partial pressure
(E) Reserve volume

81. Which of the following nerves should be blocked for an operation at the medial aspect of the lower leg?

(A) Femoral
(B) Sciatic
(C) Obturator
(D) Common peroneal
(E) Tibial

82. Which of the following is most effective in preventing intraoperative hypothermia in adults?

(A) Heating and humidifying inspired gases
(B) Maintaining a warm operating room
(C) Using a circulating warm-water mattress
(D) Using reflective coverings
(E) Warming intravenous fluids

83. Which of the following shaded areas most accurately represents the dead space of a properly functioning circle system?

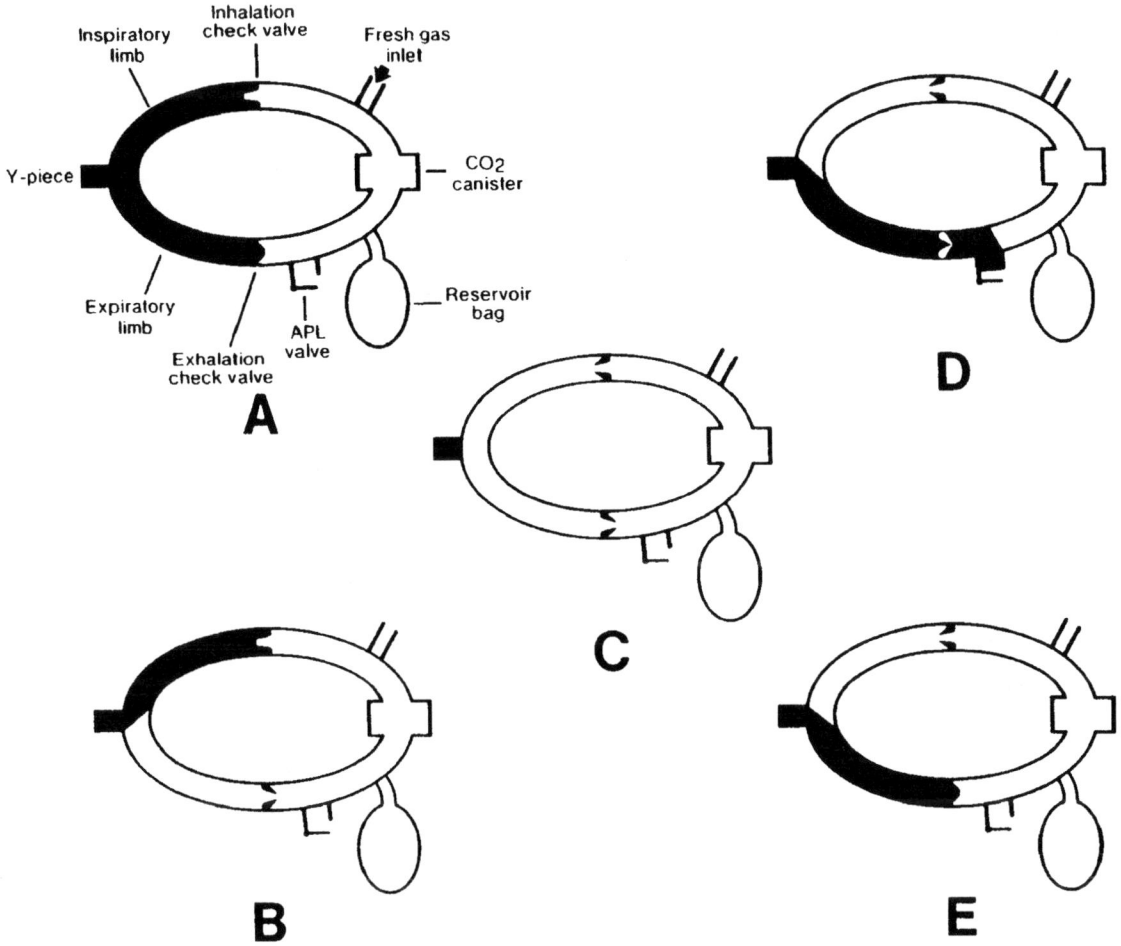

84. The effect of succinylcholine is terminated at postsynaptic effector cells by

   (A) binding and uptake by effector cells
   (B) diffusion into capillaries
   (C) hydrolysis by junctional cholinesterase
   (D) hydrolysis by pseudocholinesterase
   (E) spontaneous degradation to succinylmonocholine

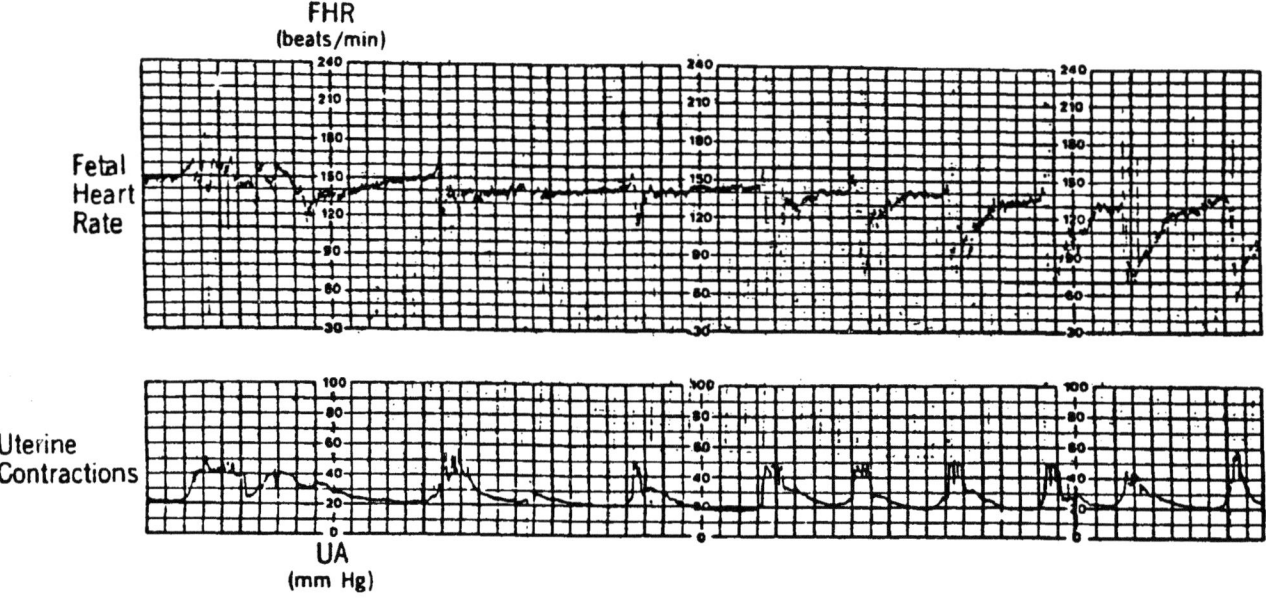

FHR
(beats/min)

Fetal Heart Rate

Uterine Contractions

UA
(mm Hg)

85. The fetal heart rate and uterine contraction tracings shown above are most consistent with

(A) fetal acidosis
(B) fetal cerebral hemorrhage
(C) fetal head compression
(D) fetal hypoxia
(E) uteroplacental insufficiency

86. The cardiovascular effects of an inhalational anesthetic are evaluated in 10 normal volunteers in the awake resting state and after 15 minutes of constant inspired concentration. Results were analyzed by t-test for paired data and are presented below as mean $\pm$ standard deviation.

	Mean Arterial Pressure (mmHg)	Heart Rate (bpm)	Cardiac Output (L/min)
Awake	94 ± 5	82 ± 2	4.2 ± 0.5
Anesthetized	83 ± 9	$90 \pm 2^*$	3.9 ± 0.7

$^*p < 0.05$

Based on these data, which of the following conclusions is most valid?

(A) A decrease in cardiac output would have been evident if more subjects were included in the study
(B) The anesthetic decreases mean arterial pressure
(C) The anesthetic does not cause cardiac depression
(D) The anesthetic is unsafe for patients with coronary artery disease
(E) There is a 95% to 100% chance that the anesthetic increases heart rate

87. A patient with alcoholic cirrhosis, ascites, and gastrointestinal bleeding receives 4 units of red blood cells prior to anesthesia with isoflurane in oxygen for emergency exploratory laparotomy. After the peritoneum is opened and the fluid is drained, blood pressure decreases to 60/40 mmHg and SpO_2 decreases to 90%. The most likely cause of the hypoxemia is

(A) acute myocardial ischemia
(B) decreased 2,3-diphosphoglycerate in transfused blood
(C) increased intrapulmonary shunting
(D) relative hypovolemia
(E) venous air embolism

88. Which of the following statements concerning barbiturate protection from cerebral ischemia is true?

(A) It may be achieved with dosages low enough to avoid cardiovascular effects
(B) It is linearly dose-related
(C) It improves neurologic outcome following cardiac arrest
(D) It is most useful in patients with focal ischemia
(E) It is unrelated to EEG activity

89. A 77-year-old woman is still intubated and breathing spontaneously following a total hip replacement. The muscle relaxant has been reversed. Tidal volume is 400 ml, end-tidal carbon dioxide tension is 45 mmHg, and SpO_2 is 98% at an FIO_2 of 1.0. On transfer from the operating table to the gurney, heart rate increases from 65 to 100 bpm and blood pressure decreases from 130/80 to 80/50 mmHg. End-tidal carbon dioxide tension is 30 mmHg and SpO_2 is 94%.

The most likely diagnosis is

(A) anaphylactic reaction
(B) bronchospasm
(C) myocardial infarction
(D) pulmonary embolism
(E) unreplaced blood loss

90. A 40-year-old woman has continuous nondermatomal burning pain of the distal foot four weeks after sustaining a metatarsal fracture. On examination, the foot is mildly swollen, tender, and cool. Which of the following statements concerning this condition is true?

(A) A radiograph of the distal bones of the painful foot will show severe osteoporosis
(B) A technetium scan of the distal joints of the painful foot will show decreased uptake
(C) Early use of opioid analgesia will prevent progression of the symptoms
(D) Intravenous phentolamine will relieve the pain
(E) The chance of spontaneous recovery within eight weeks is greater than 80%

91. Evaluation of a postoperative neurologic deficit discloses inability to oppose the thumb and little finger, weakness of abduction of the thumb, and loss of flexion of the distal phalanx of the index finger. This problem is most likely related to

(A) paresthesia occurring during an interscalene brachial plexus block
(B) attempted radial artery cannulation at the wrist
(C) inadequate padding under the elbow
(D) attempted venipuncture in the antecubital fossa
(E) abduction of the upper humerus against an "ether screen"

92. Arterial oxyhemoglobin desaturation develops more rapidly following apnea in a pregnant patient at term than in a nonpregnant patient with a large intra-abdominal tumor. Which of the following findings in pregnancy is the most likely cause?

   (A) Higher cardiac output
   (B) Higher oxygen consumption
   (C) Larger anatomic dead space
   (D) Smaller blood volume
   (E) Smaller functional residual capacity

93. Which of the following best describes the relationship between cerebral perfusion pressure and cerebral blood flow in a patient with untreated chronic hypertension?

   (A) It is constant at mean blood pressures between 50 and 150 mmHg
   (B) It is linear for all blood pressures
   (C) Flow versus pressure curve is hyperbolic
   (D) Flow versus pressure curve is shifted to the right
   (E) Flow versus pressure curve is shifted to the left

94. The accuracy of oxyhemoglobin saturation determined by digital pulse oximetry is affected significantly by each of the following EXCEPT

   (A) movement of the patient
   (B) isovolemic hemodilution to a hematocrit of 23%
   (C) position of the operating room light
   (D) intravenous administration of methylene blue
   (E) infusion of phenylephrine

95. The use of droperidol as a preanesthetic medication has been associated with each of the following EXCEPT

   (A) acute anxiety
   (B) anterograde amnesia
   (C) hypotension
   (D) extrapyramidal signs
   (E) catalepsy

96. Each of the following changes is expected with deliberate hypothermia EXCEPT

   (A) decreased unloading of oxygen from hemoglobin
   (B) a 5% decrease in MAC for each 1°C decrease in temperature
   (C) increased arterial oxygen and carbon dioxide contents
   (D) a 50% decrease in cerebral metabolic rate at 28°C
   (E) spike and dome EEG activity at temperatures below 30°C

97. Each of the following drugs is a cause of central anticholinergic syndrome EXCEPT

   (A) amitriptyline
   (B) atropine
   (C) diphenhydramine
   (D) promethazine
   (E) ranitidine

98. A 24-year-old woman requires anesthesia for emergency repair of open fractures of the tibia and fibula. She used cocaine two hours ago. Blood pressure is 170/110 mmHg. Each of the following is useful in managing the hypertension EXCEPT

   (A) hydralazine
   (B) labetalol
   (C) nitroprusside
   (D) phentolamine
   (E) propranolol

99. Carbon monoxide poisoning with a carboxyhemoglobin concentration of 20% is characterized by each of the following EXCEPT

   (A) decreased oxygen-carrying capacity of hemoglobin
   (B) decreased PaO_2
   (C) shift of the oxyhemoglobin dissociation curve to the left
   (D) normal minute volume of ventilation
   (E) headache and nausea

100. A 40-year-old woman receives alfentanil 75 μg/kg followed by an infusion of 1.5 μg/kg/min for a one-hour cholecystectomy and cholangiogram. This regimen could be associated with each of the following EXCEPT

   (A) muscle rigidity
   (B) increased biliary tract pressure
   (C) inadequate anesthesia
   (D) postoperative respiratory depression
   (E) two to four hours of postoperative analgesia

101. Monitoring sensory evoked potentials may be useful in detecting functional derangement of each of the following EXCEPT

   (A) cranial nerve pathways during posterior fossa operations
   (B) motor pathways during anterior cervical diskectomy
   (C) dorsal column pathways during operations for spinal tumors
   (D) visual pathways during operations on the sphenoid wing
   (E) cortical pathways during carotid artery operations

102. Which of the following drugs is LEAST likely to cross the placenta?

   (A) Lidocaine
   (B) Meperidine
   (C) Midazolam
   (D) Thiopental
   (E) Vecuronium

DIRECTIONS For each of the questions or incomplete statements below, ONE or MORE of the answers or completions given is correct. On the answer sheet fill in the circle containing

A if only *1, 2, and 3* are correct,
B if only *1 and 3* are correct,
C if only *2 and 4* are correct,
D if only *4* is correct,
E if all are correct.

FOR EACH QUESTION FILL IN ONLY ONE CIRCLE ON YOUR ANSWER SHEET

DIRECTIONS SUMMARIZED				
A	B	C	D	E
1, 2, 3	1, 3	2, 4	4	All are
only	only	only	only	correct

103. Characteristics of a depolarizing neuromuscular block include

    (1) tetanic fade at 50 Hz for 5 seconds
    (2) decreased train-of-four ratio
    (3) post-tetanic facilitation
    (4) decreased twitch height

104. Before awake nasal intubation in a patient who has been NPO, areas to be anesthetized are supplied by which of the following nerves?

    (1) Glossopharyngeal
    (2) Superior laryngeal
    (3) Recurrent laryngeal
    (4) Hypoglossal

105. A 40-year-old patient is referred to a pain clinic for evaluation of right upper quadrant pain six months after cholecystectomy performed through a subcostal incision. Which of the following procedures would provide diagnostic information?

    (1) Intercostal nerve blocks
    (2) Celiac plexus block
    (3) Differential spinal block
    (4) Lumbar sympathetic block

106. Compared with intermittent injections of intramuscular opioids for postoperative pain relief, patient-controlled analgesia is associated with

    (1) lower incidence of nausea and vomiting
    (2) increased risk for ventilatory depression
    (3) greater variability in opioid pharmacokinetics
    (4) lower total opioid requirement

DIRECTIONS SUMMARIZED				
A	**B**	**C**	**D**	**E**
1, 2, 3	1, 3	2, 4	4	All are
only	only	only	only	correct

107. Adverse reactions to protamine include

    (1) markedly increased pulmonary vascular resistance
    (2) anaphylaxis
    (3) decreased systemic vascular resistance
    (4) noncardiogenic pulmonary edema

108. Causes of the hypoxemia that occurs in patients with advanced cirrhosis include

    (1) decreased total lung capacity
    (2) decreased cardiac output
    (3) right-to-left pulmonary shunting
    (4) decreased 2,3-diphosphoglycerate concentration in erythrocytes

109. In a patient who is spontaneously breathing room air at the conclusion of a nitrous oxide (70%)-opioid anesthetic, causes of hypoxemia include

    (1) decreased functional residual capacity
    (2) dilution of alveolar oxygen by outpouring of nitrous oxide
    (3) opioid-induced respiratory depression
    (4) increased physiologic dead space

110. Compared with an induction dose of midazolam, an induction dose of thiopental causes a greater decrease in

    (1) blood pressure
    (2) cerebral blood flow
    (3) cerebral metabolic rate
    (4) cortical EEG activity

111. The FIO_2 achieved by nasal prongs with oxygen flowing at 8 L/min depends on

    (1) tidal volume
    (2) respiratory frequency
    (3) inspiratory flow rate
    (4) volume of the nasopharynx

112. The administration of mannitol 1 g/kg over 15 minutes produces an acute increase in

    (1) serum potassium concentration
    (2) central venous pressure
    (3) systemic vascular resistance
    (4) serum osmolality

DIRECTIONS SUMMARIZED				
A	B	C	D	E
1, 2, 3	1, 3	2, 4	4	All are
only	only	only	only	correct

113. Compared with a term infant, an infant born at 32 weeks' gestation who receives anesthesia at 2 months of age is at increased risk for

    (1) pulmonary oxygen toxicity
    (2) postoperative apnea
    (3) renal failure
    (4) retrolental fibroplasia

114. Advantages of performing spinal anesthesia via the lateral approach include

    (1) larger opening for needle insertion than for the midline approach
    (2) avoidance of the calcified interspinous ligament in the elderly
    (3) less flexion of the spine required than for the midline approach
    (4) less likelihood of peridural vein puncture than for the midline approach

115. In meralgia paresthetica

    (1) there is pain in the anterolateral aspect of the thigh
    (2) the obturator nerve is involved
    (3) obesity is an associated factor
    (4) neurolytic alcohol block is the treatment of choice

116. In patients undergoing transsphenoidal hypophysectomy for acromegaly, anesthesia is complicated by

    (1) decreased subglottic diameter
    (2) temporomandibular joint dysfunction
    (3) glucose intolerance
    (4) diabetes insipidus

117. The infant airway differs from that of the adult in which of the following ways?

    (1) The larynx is more cephalad
    (2) The vocal cords are perpendicular to the plane of the trachea
    (3) The cricoid cartilage is the narrowest part of the airway
    (4) The larynx is more anterior

118. The duration of an epidural block can be increased clinically by

    (1) use of a local anesthetic with low protein binding
    (2) use of a local anesthetic with low pK_a
    (3) addition of sodium bicarbonate to the local anesthetic
    (4) increasing the total dose of the local anesthetic

119. Prior to vaginal delivery at term, a primiparous woman receives epidural anesthesia administered through a catheter inserted at L2-3. The following day she has left footdrop and sensory loss over the left outer calf. Causes of these complications include

    (1) compression of the obturator nerve by excessive thigh flexion
    (2) compression of the lumbosacral trunk by the fetal head
    (3) nerve root injury by the epidural needle
    (4) compression of the common peroneal nerve by the stirrup

120. A 2-year-old boy with tetralogy of Fallot is scheduled for repair of bilateral inguinal hernias. True statements concerning this child include:

    (1) Oxygen saturation will improve with crying
    (2) Cyanosis will increase with use of halothane
    (3) Resistance to pulmonary outflow will be fixed
    (4) An increased red cell mass will compensate for right-to-left shunt

121. A previously healthy 28-year-old woman who had a subarachnoid hemorrhage two days ago is scheduled for a craniotomy and clipping of an anterior communicating artery aneurysm. She is awake, oriented, and neurologically intact. True statements concerning anesthetic management include:

    (1) The arterial pressure should be maintained above the preoperative values during induction
    (2) Hyperventilation to a $PaCO_2$ of 25 to 30 mmHg should be initiated prior to endotracheal intubation
    (3) Mannitol should be given immediately following induction
    (4) The mean arterial pressure should be decreased to 50 mmHg if necessary for surgical exposure

122. A 45-year-old man is scheduled for elective antrectomy and vagotomy. He has drunk a 6-pack of beer daily for 20 years. Laboratory evaluation shows the following findings.

	Patient	Normal
AST (SGOT) (U/L)	75	0-45
ALT (SGPT) (U/L)	56	0-45
LDH (U/L)	300	50-250
Alkaline phosphatase (U/L)	120	25-115
Bilirubin (mg/dl)	1.2	0.1-1.2

Based on these laboratory findings, anticipated problems in anesthetic management include

    (1) increased risk for halothane hepatotoxicity
    (2) coagulation disorders
    (3) large peripheral arteriovenous shunts
    (4) increased anesthetic requirements

FOR EACH ITEM FILL IN ONLY ONE CIRCLE ON YOUR ANSWER SHEET

		DIRECTIONS SUMMARIZED		
A	B	C	D	E
1, 2, 3	1, 3	2, 4	4	All are
only	only	only	only	correct

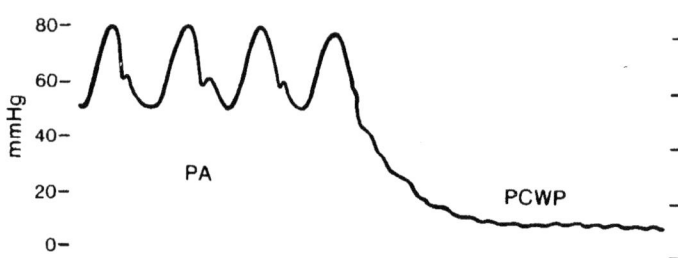

123. Causes of the pulmonary artery pressure and pulmonary artery occlusion pressure waveforms shown above include

(1) catheter overwedging
(2) protamine reaction
(3) acute mitral regurgitation
(4) primary pulmonary hypertension

124. Electrolyte profiles consistent with pyloric stenosis in a 6-week-old infant include:

	Na$^+$ (mEq/L)	K$^+$ (mEq/L)	Cl$^-$ (mEq/L)	HCO$_3^-$ (mEq/L)
(1)	145	3.5	108	24
(2)	145	2.5	85	15
(3)	160	5.5	120	36
(4)	128	2.5	85	32

125. True statements concerning regional anesthesia with peripheral nerve blocks for an operation on the knee using a tourniquet include:

(1) The inguinal perivascular block includes the obturator nerve
(2) Paresthesias are required during sciatic block
(3) The lateral femoral cutaneous nerve must be blocked
(4) Block of the lumbar plexus in the psoas compartment provides adequate anesthesia

126. Proximal spread of a local anesthetic solution placed in the axillary perivascular space is promoted by

(1) increased volume of the local anesthetic agent
(2) digital pressure distal to the injection site
(3) cephalad direction of the needle
(4) adduction of the shoulder after the injection

		DIRECTIONS SUMMARIZED		
A	**B**	**C**	**D**	**E**
1, 2, 3	1, 3	2, 4	4	All are
only	only	only	only	correct

127. Indications for neurolytic celiac plexus ablation include pain due to carcinoma of the

    (1) sigmoid colon
    (2) kidney
    (3) ovary
    (4) pancreas

128. Compared with a 20-year-old patient, an 80-year-old patient will

    (1) have similar EEG sensitivity to the same blood concentrations of thiopental
    (2) require lower induction doses (mg/kg) of thiopental
    (3) have increased sensitivity to volatile anesthetics
    (4) require lower doses (mg/kg) of succinylcholine

129. Induction of anesthesia with usual drug dosages and concentrations may lead to cardiovascular signs of overdose in patients with hypothyroidism because of expected decreases in

    (1) respiratory quotient
    (2) minute volume of breathing
    (3) circulating blood volume
    (4) cardiac output

130. The duration of the anticoagulant effect of heparin is

    (1) independent of body temperature
    (2) determined primarily by renal excretion
    (3) prolonged two to three times with hypoalbuminemia
    (4) dose dependent

131. During general endotracheal anesthesia, early signs of an acute asthma attack include

    (1) alteration of the expiratory plateau on capnography
    (2) increased $PaCO_2$
    (3) increased peak airway pressure
    (4) hypoxemia

132. At the placental interface, the efficiency of oxygen transport to the fetus is enhanced by

    (1) movement of the maternal oxyhemoglobin dissociation curve to the right
    (2) diffusion of carbon dioxide from fetal blood
    (3) movement of the fetal oxyhemoglobin dissociation curve to the left
    (4) maternal hyperventilation

133. During a carbon dioxide challenge test in a healthy patient, the $PaCO_2$ increases to 60 mmHg. Expected effects include

    (1) decreased pulmonary vascular resistance
    (2) increased cardiac output
    (3) renovascular dilation
    (4) sympathetic stimulation

134. Which of the following peripheral nerves must be blocked for removal of a glass splinter from the plantar surface of the heel?

    (1) Tibial
    (2) Saphenous
    (3) Sural
    (4) Superficial peroneal

135. A 26-year-old woman is to undergo emergency laparotomy for a ruptured appendix. She has been taking propylthiouracil and an oral beta-adrenergic blocker for two days for acute hyperthyroidism. Appropriate perioperative therapy includes administration of

    (1) potassium iodide
    (2) hydrocortisone
    (3) propranolol
    (4) propylthiouracil

136. A previously healthy 55-year-old patient is spontaneously breathing oxygen, nitrous oxide, and halothane during a minor surgical procedure. The end-tidal halothane concentration measured by mass spectrometry is 0.7%, end-tidal nitrous oxide concentration is 50%, and end-tidal carbon dioxide concentration is 9%. Findings consistent with these concentrations include

    (1) tachycardia
    (2) decreased requirement for halothane
    (3) premature ventricular contractions
    (4) serum bicarbonate concentration of 35 mEq/L

137. A 48-year-old man who is undergoing a right upper lobectomy for cancer has a PaO_2 of 67 mmHg while his left lung is being ventilated at 10 ml/kg at a rate of 10 breaths/min. Measures to increase PaO_2 include

    (1) hyperventilation to a $PaCO_2$ of 30 mmHg
    (2) insufflation of the right lung with continuous positive airway pressure
    (3) application of positive end-expiratory pressure 15 cmH_2O to the left lung
    (4) partial occlusion of right pulmonary blood flow

DIRECTIONS SUMMARIZED				
A	B	C	D	E
1, 2, 3	1, 3	2, 4	4	All are
only	only	only	only	correct

138. Uterine contractility is decreased by

    (1) epidural lidocaine
    (2) terbutaline
    (3) ketamine anesthesia
    (4) halothane

139. During induction of anesthesia for removal of a large intracranial tumor, effects of adding 1 MAC of isoflurane at normocarbia include

    (1) decreased cerebral metabolic rate
    (2) attenuated cerebrovascular response to $PaCO_2$
    (3) increased intracranial pressure
    (4) abolished cerebral autoregulation

140. Intraoperative events that may cause an increased arterial to end-tidal carbon dioxide tension difference include

    (1) pulmonary embolus
    (2) induced hypotension
    (3) application of positive end-expiratory pressure
    (4) atelectasis

141. Factors that decrease beat-to-beat variability of the fetal heart rate include

    (1) epidural administration of lidocaine
    (2) maternal hypotension
    (3) intravenous administration of ephedrine
    (4) intravenous administration of glycopyrrolate

142. Neural fibers that transmit pain include

    (1) B fibers
    (2) C fibers
    (3) A-alpha fibers
    (4) A-delta fibers

143. Gas flow through an endotracheal tube is

    (1) directly related to the change in pressure along the length of the tube
    (2) inversely related to the viscosity of the gas
    (3) inversely related to the length of the tube
    (4) directly related to the square of the radius of the tube

DIRECTIONS SUMMARIZED				
A	B	C	D	E
1, 2, 3	1, 3	2, 4	4	All are
only	only	only	only	correct

144. Hetastarch

   (1) produces a hypercoagulable state
   (2) complicates blood crossmatching
   (3) is contraindicated in patients with diabetes mellitus
   (4) is metabolized by amylase

145. During pelvic laparoscopy under epidural anesthesia, the patient is placed in the Trendelenburg position and the abdomen is distended by insufflation of carbon dioxide. Anticipated responses include

   (1) hyperpnea to maintain normal minute ventilation
   (2) pain despite sensory block to T4
   (3) decreased venous return and cardiac output
   (4) metabolic acidosis from absorption of carbon dioxide

146. When triggered by the R wave, the intra-aortic balloon pump is likely to be ineffective with

   (1) prolonged use of electrocautery
   (2) development of rapid atrial fibrillation
   (3) sudden onset of aortic regurgitation
   (4) sudden onset of mitral regurgitation

147. An asymptomatic 40-year-old woman with a systolic click and a late systolic murmur is scheduled for total abdominal hysterectomy. Anesthetic considerations include:

   (1) Prophylactic antibiotics are recommended
   (2) Intraoperative fluid restriction is indicated
   (3) The patient is predisposed to tachyarrhythmias
   (4) Myocardial depressant inhalational agents are contraindicated

148. A 24-year-old woman who is receiving magnesium sulfate for severe preeclampsia requires emergency cesarean delivery. True statements concerning succinylcholine-induced muscle relaxation in this patient include:

   (1) It will be potentiated by the magnesium sulfate
   (2) Fasciculations will be absent following succinylcholine administration
   (3) It will be prolonged
   (4) It can be antagonized by calcium chloride

DIRECTIONS SUMMARIZED				
A	B	C	D	E
1, 2, 3	1, 3	2, 4	4	All are
only	only	only	only	correct

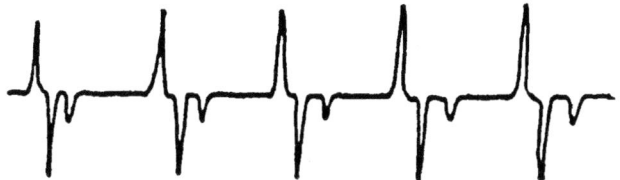

149. During posterior fossa surgery in the sitting position

(1) a single-lumen central venous catheter should display the ECG shown above
(2) pulmonary artery occlusion pressures greater than 10 mmHg prevent paradoxical air embolism
(3) if venous air embolism occurs, pulmonary artery pressure increases before precordial Doppler sounds change
(4) if venous air embolism occurs, aspiration of air from the distal lumen of a pulmonary artery catheter is less effective than aspiration from a multi-orificed central venous catheter

150. A patient undergoing strabismus repair develops acute bradycardia during traction on an eye muscle. This response is

(1) mediated by a facial nerve afferent
(2) also manifested by ventricular ectopy
(3) prevented by preanesthetic intramuscular administration of atropine
(4) treated by stopping the surgical stimulus

151. In a patient treated with propranolol and phenoxybenzamine prior to resection of a solitary pheochromocytoma, factors contributing to postoperative hypotension include

(1) residual alpha-adrenergic block
(2) heart failure
(3) residual beta-adrenergic block
(4) adrenal insufficiency

152. Anesthesia is induced with isoflurane and nitrous oxide in a patient with low cardiac output. Compared with a patient with normal cardiac function, which of the following will occur?

(1) Alveolar isoflurane concentration will approach the inspired concentration more rapidly
(2) Total uptake of isoflurane will be higher during the first 11 minutes
(3) The rate of rise of the alveolar concentration of isoflurane will be affected more than that of nitrous oxide
(4) Induction will be slower

DIRECTIONS SUMMARIZED				
A	B	C	D	E
1, 2, 3	1, 3	2, 4	4	All are
only	only	only	only	correct

153. Factors associated with post-intubation croup in children include

    (1) age less than 3 months
    (2) history of recent upper respiratory infection
    (3) use of a nasotracheal tube
    (4) surgery of the head and neck

154. True statements concerning the effects of amrinone include:

    (1) Systemic vascular resistance is decreased
    (2) Intracellular levels of cyclic AMP are increased
    (3) It acts independently of $beta_1$-adrenergic receptors
    (4) Simultaneous administration of norepinephrine enhances ventricular dysrhythmias

155. Deflation of a leg tourniquet after two hours of inflation decreases

    (1) mixed venous oxygen saturation
    (2) core temperature
    (3) systemic vascular resistance
    (4) end-tidal carbon dioxide tension

156. Compared with those of isoflurane, the respiratory effects of enflurane include

    (1) similar decrease in airway resistance
    (2) greater attenuation of hypoxic pulmonary vasoconstriction
    (3) greater increase in $PaCO_2$ during spontaneous ventilation at 1 MAC
    (4) less inhibition of hypoxic ventilatory drive at "MAC awake" concentrations

157. Intravenous drugs that produce central nervous system effects by modulating gamma-aminobutyric acid receptor activity include

    (1) midazolam
    (2) thiopental
    (3) flumazenil
    (4) ketamine

158. Findings consistent with heparin-induced thrombocytopenia include

    (1) platelet count of $25,000/mm^3$
    (2) subcutaneous route of heparin administration
    (3) thrombosis
    (4) onset within four hours of initiating heparin therapy

DIRECTIONS SUMMARIZED				
A	B	C	D	E
1, 2, 3	1, 3	2, 4	4	All are
only	only	only	only	correct

159. An anephric 12-year-old patient with a large pericardial effusion is to have pericardiocentesis under general anesthesia. Appropriate anesthetic management includes

    (1) maintenance of a high venous pressure
    (2) prevention of tachycardia
    (3) avoidance of positive end-expiratory pressure
    (4) reduction of systemic vascular resistance

160. Reliable indicators of left ventricular function in a patient with severe chronic obstructive pulmonary disease include

    (1) left ventricular end-diastolic volume
    (2) pulmonary artery diastolic pressure
    (3) left atrial pressure
    (4) cardiac index

161. A 38-year-old woman who takes verapamil for idiopathic hypertrophic subaortic stenosis is anesthetized with enflurane, nitrous oxide, oxygen, and fentanyl for laparoscopic cholecystectomy. After inflation of the abdomen with carbon dioxide, heart rate increases to 140 bpm, blood pressure decreases to 85/60 mmHg, and ST-segment depression occurs. End-tidal carbon dioxide concentration is unchanged. Appropriate pharmacologic management includes intravenous administration of

    (1) phenylephrine
    (2) nitroglycerin
    (3) esmolol
    (4) calcium chloride

162. Compared with intermittent bolus administration, effects of continuous infusion of a short-acting anesthetic include

    (1) increased therapeutic index
    (2) decreased serum concentration required
    (3) prolonged recovery time
    (4) decreased total amount of anesthetic required

163. During abdominal closure for gastroschisis in a 1-day-old infant, airway pressure increases and oxygen saturation decreases. Breath sounds are bilateral, and endotracheal suctioning does not improve ventilation. After increasing FIO_2, appropriate management includes

    (1) deepening volatile anesthesia
    (2) administering additional muscle relaxant
    (3) adding positive end-expiratory pressure
    (4) foregoing primary abdominal closure

DIRECTIONS SUMMARIZED				
A 1, 2, 3 only	B 1, 3 only	C 2, 4 only	D 4 only	E All are correct

164. True statements concerning airway management in a patient with suspected injury to the cervical spine following head and chest trauma include:

 (1) Cricothyroidotomy is the preferred method of securing the airway
 (2) Injuries at C1 or C2 place the patient at greatest risk for neurologic injury during laryngoscopy
 (3) Cricoid pressure is contraindicated
 (4) A normal lateral, AP, and open-mouth view of the cervical spine rules out spinal cord injury

165. A 30-year-old man with gunshot wounds receives an emergency transfusion of 4 units of uncrossmatched O, Rh-negative blood. His blood type is AB, Rh-positive. For further intraoperative transfusion he should receive

 (1) O, Rh-negative red cells
 (2) AB, Rh-positive red cells
 (3) AB, Rh-positive plasma
 (4) O, Rh-negative plasma

166. A 46-year-old man who takes clonidine for essential hypertension undergoes a 12-hour limb reimplantation under general anesthesia. Which of the following should be anticipated during the perioperative course?

 (1) Decreased anesthetic requirements
 (2) Postoperative hypertension
 (3) Blunting of tachycardia with tracheal intubation
 (4) Excessive postoperative drowsiness

167. Defective expiratory unidirectional valves in a circle system result in

 (1) increased dead space
 (2) decreased FIO_2
 (3) prolonged anesthetic induction
 (4) transformation to a nonrebreathing system

168. In the absence of a change in the ventilator settings, the measured exhaled tidal volume on the machine spirometer decreases when

 (1) the endotracheal tube migrates into the right main stem bronchus
 (2) fresh gas flow is decreased
 (3) a heated humidifier is added
 (4) the endotracheal tube cuff begins to leak

DIRECTIONS SUMMARIZED				
A	B	C	D	E
1, 2, 3	1, 3	2, 4	4	All are
only	only	only	only	correct

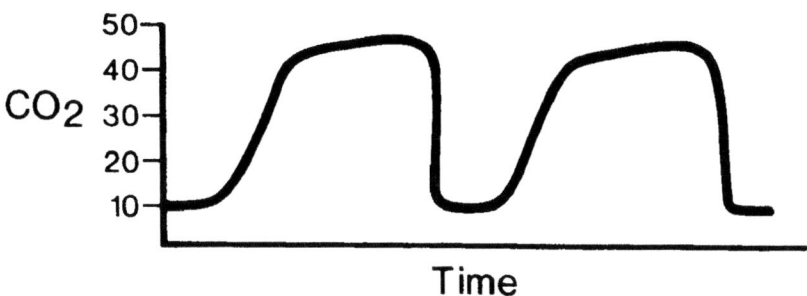

169. The capnographic waveform shown above was obtained during anesthesia using a semiclosed circle system and mechanical ventilation. This waveform is consistent with

    (1) increased body temperature to 40°C
    (2) kinking of the endotracheal tube
    (3) inadequate minute ventilation
    (4) an incompetent expiratory valve

170. A 45-year-old woman is scheduled for a cholecystectomy following an episode of acute cholecystitis. Thirty minutes after premedication with morphine and midazolam, she has nausea and acute right upper quadrant pain. Drugs that alleviate these symptoms include

    (1) glucagon
    (2) nitroglycerin
    (3) naloxone
    (4) flumazenil

171. During a blood transfusion, a patient develops sudden hypotension and oozing from the puncture sites. Laboratory studies useful in establishing the diagnosis include

    (1) serum free hemoglobin concentration
    (2) direct antiglobulin (Coombs') test
    (3) urine hemoglobin concentration
    (4) serum haptoglobin concentration

172. A continuous infusion of atracurium for 60 hours has been associated with

    (1) seizure activity
    (2) histamine release
    (3) increased anesthetic requirements
    (4) adrenal suppression

DIRECTIONS SUMMARIZED				
A	B	C	D	E
1, 2, 3	1, 3	2, 4	4	All are
only	only	only	only	correct

173. The anesthetic recovery of a newborn infant is complicated by the slow return of neuromuscular function. Factors that would cause this complication include

    (1) an inadequate dose of anticholinesterase
    (2) active maternal myasthenia gravis
    (3) a core temperature of 35°C
    (4) intraoperative administration of cefamandole

174. Complications of stellate ganglion block include

    (1) elevation of the ipsilateral hemidiaphragm
    (2) total spinal anesthesia
    (3) seizures
    (4) hoarseness

GENERAL INSTRUCTIONS

1. Please write your name and identification number in the space provided on the front of this test book. If you are taking the examination for Board Certification, your identification number is printed on your notification card. If you are an In-Training Resident, use your U.S. Social Security Number. If you do not have a U.S. Social Security Number, use your Canadian Social Insurance Number.

2. Your name and identification number and all of your answers must be recorded on the separate answer sheet enclosed in this booklet.

   The sample on the right shows how to record your identification number on the answer sheet. Be sure to enter your number in the boxes provided and also to mark it in the appropriate spaces as illustrated.

3. Credit will be given only for answers marked on the answer sheet. You may make any preliminary notes or calculations in the test books, but be sure that all of your answers are marked on the answer sheet. Only one choice should be marked for each question. Multiple answers for the same question are treated as wrong answers. In marking your answer sheet use only a soft (#2) lead pencil. Do NOT use a pen or pencil with hard lead. Make each mark heavy and black enough to obliterate completely the letter within the circle. Marks should fill the circle; if marks are light or outside the circle, you may not receive credit for your answers. Make no stray marks on the answer sheet, as these could lower your score. If you wish to change an answer, be sure to erase your first mark completely.

4. This test book contains two different types of questions, each of which is preceded by special directions. You are advised to study the directions carefully. Even though you may be in doubt about the correct answer, select the choice that you consider to be the best. Your score is the number of questions you answered correctly.

5. You will have 3½ hours to work on this section of the test which contains 174 questions.

RULES OF CONDUCT FOR EXAMINEES DURING ABA/ASA IN-TRAINING EXAMINATION

1. Do not falsify information required for admission to the examination or impersonate another ABA/ASA examinee.

2. Do not bring calculators, watches with computer capability, books, papers, or memoranda of any kind into the examination room.

3. Do not break the seal on your test books until you are instructed to do so by the proctor.

4. Do not tear any pages or portions of pages from the test books or tear your answer sheet.

5. Do not disturb the examination process by talking, smoking, or interfering with others who are taking the examination.

6. Do not attempt to observe the test books or answer sheets of other examinees. Do not copy the answers of another examinee, permit answers to be copied, or in any way provide or receive unauthorized information about the content of the examination while it is in progress.

7. Terminate the examination immediately upon instruction by the proctor to do so.

8. Do not take the test books, answer sheets, or any documents, examination material, or memoranda from the room.

Failure to abide by these rules of conduct during this examination may result in disciplinary actions by the ABA/ASA In-Training Council or by the American Board of Anesthesiology. Statistical analyses may be used to verify observations and/or reports of suspected irregularities in conduct.

Book A Answer Sheet

1)	1	2	3	4	45)	1	2	3	4	89)	A	B	C	D	E
2)	1	2	3	4	46)	1	2	3	4	90)	A	B	C	D	E
3)	1	2	3	4	47)	1	2	3	4	91)	A	B	C	D	E
4)	1	2	3	4	48)	1	2	3	4	92)	A	B	C	D	E
5)	1	2	3	4	49)	1	2	3	4	93)	A	B	C	D	E
6)	1	2	3	4	50)	1	2	3	4	94)	A	B	C	D	E
7)	1	2	3	4	51)	1	2	3	4	95)	A	B	C	D	E
8)	1	2	3	4	52)	1	2	3	4	96)	A	B	C	D	E
9)	1	2	3	4	53)	1	2	3	4	97)	A	B	C	D	E
10)	1	2	3	4	54)	1	2	3	4	98)	A	B	C	D	E
11)	1	2	3	4	55)	1	2	3	4	99)	A	B	C	D	E
12)	1	2	3	4	56)	1	2	3	4	100)	A	B	C	D	E
13)	1	2	3	4	57)	1	2	3	4	101)	A	B	C	D	E
14)	1	2	3	4	58)	1	2	3	4	102)	A	B	C	D	E
15)	1	2	3	4	59)	1	2	3	4	103)	A	B	C	D	E
16)	1	2	3	4	60)	1	2	3	4	104)	A	B	C	D	E
17)	1	2	3	4	61)	1	2	3	4	105)	A	B	C	D	E
18)	1	2	3	4	62)	1	2	3	4	106)	A	B	C	D	E
19)	1	2	3	4	63)	1	2	3	4	107)	A	B	C	D	E
20)	1	2	3	4	64)	1	2	3	4	108)	A	B	C	D	E
21)	1	2	3	4	65)	1	2	3	4	109)	A	B	C	D	E
22)	1	2	3	4	66)	1	2	3	4	110)	A	B	C	D	E
23)	1	2	3	4	67)	1	2	3	4	111)	A	B	C	D	E
24)	1	2	3	4	68)	1	2	3	4	112)	A	B	C	D	E
25)	1	2	3	4	69)	1	2	3	4	113)	A	B	C	D	E
26)	1	2	3	4	70)	1	2	3	4	114)	A	B	C	D	E
27)	1	2	3	4	71)	1	2	3	4	115)	A	B	C	D	E
28)	1	2	3	4	72)	1	2	3	4	116)	A	B	C	D	E
29)	1	2	3	4	73)	A	B	C	D	E	117)	A	B	C	D	E
30)	1	2	3	4	74)	A	B	C	D	E	118)	A	B	C	D	E
31)	1	2	3	4	75)	A	B	C	D	E	119)	A	B	C	D	E
32)	1	2	3	4	76)	A	B	C	D	E	120)	A	B	C	D	E
33)	1	2	3	4	77)	A	B	C	D	E	121)	A	B	C	D	E
34)	1	2	3	4	78)	A	B	C	D	E	122)	A	B	C	D	E
35)	1	2	3	4	79)	A	B	C	D	E	123)	A	B	C	D	E
36)	1	2	3	4	80)	A	B	C	D	E	124)	A	B	C	D	E
37)	1	2	3	4	81)	A	B	C	D	E	125)	A	B	C	D	E
38)	1	2	3	4	82)	A	B	C	D	E	126)	A	B	C	D	E
39)	1	2	3	4	83)	A	B	C	D	E	127)	A	B	C	D	E
40)	1	2	3	4	84)	A	B	C	D	E	128)	A	B	C	D	E
41)	1	2	3	4	85)	A	B	C	D	E	129)	A	B	C	D	E
42)	1	2	3	4	86)	A	B	C	D	E	130)	A	B	C	D	E
43)	1	2	3	4	87)	A	B	C	D	E	131)	A	B	C	D	E
44)	1	2	3	4	88)	A	B	C	D	E	132)	A	B	C	D	E

133)	A	B	C	D	E
134)	A	B	C	D	E
135)	A	B	C	D	E
136)	A	B	C	D	E
137)	A	B	C	D	E
138)	A	B	C	D	E
139)	A	B	C	D	E
140)	A	B	C	D	E
141)	A	B	C	D	E
142)	A	B	C	D	E
143)	A	B	C	D	E
144)	A	B	C	D	E
145)	A	B	C	D	E
146)	A	B	C	D	E
147)	A	B	C	D	E
148)	A	B	C	D	E
149)	A	B	C	D	E
150)	A	B	C	D	E
151)	A	B	C	D	E
152)	A	B	C	D	E
153)	A	B	C	D	E
154)	A	B	C	D	E
155)	A	B	C	D	E
156)	A	B	C	D	E
157)	A	B	C	D	E
158)	A	B	C	D	E
159)	A	B	C	D	E
160)	A	B	C	D	E
161)	A	B	C	D	E
162)	A	B	C	D	E
163)	A	B	C	D	E
164)	A	B	C	D	E
165)	A	B	C	D	E
166)	A	B	C	D	E
167)	A	B	C	D	E
168)	A	B	C	D	E
169)	A	B	C	D	E
170)	A	B	C	D	E
171)	A	B	C	D	E
172)	A	B	C	D	E
173)	A	B	C	D	E
174)	A	B	C	D	E
175)	A	B	C	D	E

Book B Answer Sheet

1)	A	B	C	D	E	45)	A	B	C	D	E	89)	A	B	C	D	E
2)	A	B	C	D	E	46)	A	B	C	D	E	90)	A	B	C	D	E
3)	A	B	C	D	E	47)	A	B	C	D	E	91)	A	B	C	D	E
4)	A	B	C	D	E	48)	A	B	C	D	E	92)	A	B	C	D	E
5)	A	B	C	D	E	49)	A	B	C	D	E	93)	A	B	C	D	E
6)	A	B	C	D	E	50)	A	B	C	D	E	94)	A	B	C	D	E
7)	A	B	C	D	E	51)	A	B	C	D	E	95)	A	B	C	D	E
8)	A	B	C	D	E	52)	A	B	C	D	E	96)	A	B	C	D	E
9)	A	B	C	D	E	53)	A	B	C	D	E	97)	A	B	C	D	E
10)	A	B	C	D	E	54)	A	B	C	D	E	98)	A	B	C	D	E
11)	A	B	C	D	E	55)	A	B	C	D	E	99)	A	B	C	D	E
12)	A	B	C	D	E	56)	A	B	C	D	E	100)	A	B	C	D	E
13)	A	B	C	D	E	57)	A	B	C	D	E	101)	A	B	C	D	E
14)	A	B	C	D	E	58)	A	B	C	D	E	102)	A	B	C	D	E
15)	A	B	C	D	E	59)	A	B	C	D	E	103)	1	2	3	4	
16)	A	B	C	D	E	60)	A	B	C	D	E	104)	1	2	3	4	
17)	A	B	C	D	E	61)	A	B	C	D	E	105)	1	2	3	4	
18)	A	B	C	D	E	62)	A	B	C	D	E	106)	1	2	3	4	
19)	A	B	C	D	E	63)	A	B	C	D	E	107)	1	2	3	4	
20)	A	B	C	D	E	64)	A	B	C	D	E	108)	1	2	3	4	
21)	A	B	C	D	E	65)	A	B	C	D	E	109)	1	2	3	4	
22)	A	B	C	D	E	66)	A	B	C	D	E	110)	1	2	3	4	
23)	A	B	C	D	E	67)	A	B	C	D	E	111)	1	2	3	4	
24)	A	B	C	D	E	68)	A	B	C	D	E	112)	1	2	3	4	
25)	A	B	C	D	E	69)	A	B	C	D	E	113)	1	2	3	4	
26)	A	B	C	D	E	70)	A	B	C	D	E	114)	1	2	3	4	
27)	A	B	C	D	E	71)	A	B	C	D	E	115)	1	2	3	4	
28)	A	B	C	D	E	72)	A	B	C	D	E	116)	1	2	3	4	
29)	A	B	C	D	E	73)	A	B	C	D	E	117)	1	2	3	4	
30)	A	B	C	D	E	74)	A	B	C	D	E	118)	1	2	3	4	
31)	A	B	C	D	E	75)	A	B	C	D	E	119)	1	2	3	4	
32)	A	B	C	D	E	76)	A	B	C	D	E	120)	1	2	3	4	
33)	A	B	C	D	E	77)	A	B	C	D	E	121)	1	2	3	4	
34)	A	B	C	D	E	78)	A	B	C	D	E	122)	1	2	3	4	
35)	A	B	C	D	E	79)	A	B	C	D	E	123)	1	2	3	4	
36)	A	B	C	D	E	80)	A	B	C	D	E	124)	1	2	3	4	
37)	A	B	C	D	E	81)	A	B	C	D	E	125)	1	2	3	4	
38)	A	B	C	D	E	82)	A	B	C	D	E	126)	1	2	3	4	
39)	A	B	C	D	E	83)	A	B	C	D	E	127)	1	2	3	4	
40)	A	B	C	D	E	84)	A	B	C	D	E	128)	1	2	3	4	
41)	A	B	C	D	E	85)	A	B	C	D	E	129)	1	2	3	4	
42)	A	B	C	D	E	86)	A	B	C	D	E	130)	1	2	3	4	
43)	A	B	C	D	E	87)	A	B	C	D	E	131)	1	2	3	4	
44)	A	B	C	D	E	88)	A	B	C	D	E	132)	1	2	3	4	

133)　1　2　3　4
134)　1　2　3　4
135)　1　2　3　4
136)　1　2　3　4
137)　1　2　3　4
138)　1　2　3　4
139)　1　2　3　4
140)　1　2　3　4
141)　1　2　3　4
142)　1　2　3　4
143)　1　2　3　4
144)　1　2　3　4
145)　1　2　3　4
146)　1　2　3　4
147)　1　2　3　4
148)　1　2　3　4
149)　1　2　3　4
150)　1　2　3　4
151)　1　2　3　4
152)　1　2　3　4
153)　1　2　3　4
154)　1　2　3　4
155)　1　2　3　4
156)　1　2　3　4
157)　1　2　3　4
158)　1　2　3　4
159)　1　2　3　4
160)　1　2　3　4
161)　1　2　3　4
162)　1　2　3　4
163)　1　2　3　4
164)　1　2　3　4
165)　1　2　3　4
166)　1　2　3　4
167)　1　2　3　4
168)　1　2　3　4
169)　1　2　3　4
170)　1　2　3　4
171)　1　2　3　4
172)　1　2　3　4
173)　1　2　3　4
174)　1　2　3　4
175)　1　2　3　4

Topic Indexed Answer Sheet

≡ BASIC SCIENCE ≡

BOOK A

89)	A	B	C	D	E
123)	A	B	C	D	E
162)	A	B	C	D	E
164)	A	B	C	D	E
169)	A	B	C	D	E

BOOK B

12)	A	B	C	D	E
46)	A	B	C	D	E
82)	A	B	C	D	E
84)	A	B	C	D	E
86)	A	B	C	D	E
157)	1	2	3	4	

≡ EQUIPMENT/PHYSICS ≡

BOOK A

1)	1	2	3	4	
9)	1	2	3	4	
11)	1	2	3	4	
13)	1	2	3	4	
29)	1	2	3	4	
43)	1	2	3	4	
45)	1	2	3	4	
55)	1	2	3	4	
65)	1	2	3	4	
67)	1	2	3	4	
96)	A	B	C	D	E
102)	A	B	C	D	E
107)	A	B	C	D	E
111)	A	B	C	D	E
113)	A	B	C	D	E
128)	A	B	C	D	E
129)	A	B	C	D	E
133)	A	B	C	D	E
141)	A	B	C	D	E
151)	A	B	C	D	E
153)	A	B	C	D	E

BOOK B

15)	A	B	C	D	E
17)	A	B	C	D	E
37)	A	B	C	D	E
40)	A	B	C	D	E
45)	A	B	C	D	E
61)	A	B	C	D	E
62)	A	B	C	D	E
67)	A	B	C	D	E
70)	A	B	C	D	E
79)	A	B	C	D	E
80)	A	B	C	D	E
83)	A	B	C	D	E
94)	A	B	C	D	E
111)	1	2	3	4	
143)	1	2	3	4	
146)	1	2	3	4	
167)	1	2	3	4	
168)	1	2	3	4	
169)	1	2	3	4	

≡ CARDIOVASCULAR ≡

BOOK A

16)	1	2	3	4	
35)	1	2	3	4	
39)	1	2	3	4	
53)	1	2	3	4	
66)	1	2	3	4	
84)	A	B	C	D	E
93)	A	B	C	D	E
95)	A	B	C	D	E
99)	A	B	C	D	E
109)	A	B	C	D	E
110)	A	B	C	D	E
114)	A	B	C	D	E
132)	A	B	C	D	E
136)	A	B	C	D	E
158)	A	B	C	D	E

BOOK B

20)	A	B	C	D	E
27)	A	B	C	D	E
32)	A	B	C	D	E
39)	A	B	C	D	E
53)	A	B	C	D	E
55)	A	B	C	D	E
59)	A	B	C	D	E
64)	A	B	C	D	E
73)	A	B	C	D	E
74)	A	B	C	D	E
123)	1	2	3	4	
147)	1	2	3	4	
161)	1	2	3	4	

≡ CLINICAL ANESTHESIA ≡

BOOK A

10)	1	2	3	4	
15)	1	2	3	4	
17)	1	2	3	4	
18)	1	2	3	4	
21)	1	2	3	4	
23)	1	2	3	4	
24)	1	2	3	4	
28)	1	2	3	4	
48)	1	2	3	4	
63)	1	2	3	4	
64)	1	2	3	4	
68)	1	2	3	4	
71)	1	2	3	4	
75)	A	B	C	D	E
81)	A	B	C	D	E
88)	A	B	C	D	E
90)	A	B	C	D	E
94)	A	B	C	D	E
97)	A	B	C	D	E
115)	A	B	C	D	E
118)	A	B	C	D	E
119)	A	B	C	D	E
120)	A	B	C	D	E
121)	A	B	C	D	E

127) A B C D E
152) A B C D E
155) A B C D E
159) A B C D E
160) A B C D E
166) A B C D E
167) A B C D E
168) A B C D E
174) A B C D E

BOOK B

3) A B C D E
7) A B C D E
19) A B C D E
21) A B C D E
24) A B C D E
25) A B C D E
26) A B C D E
31) A B C D E
33) A B C D E
50) A B C D E
52) A B C D E
54) A B C D E
56) A B C D E
60) A B C D E
72) A B C D E
77) A B C D E
87) A B C D E
89) A B C D E
91) A B C D E
98) 1 2 3 4
116) 1 2 3 4
122) 1 2 3 4
129) 1 2 3 4
135) 1 2 3 4
137) 1 2 3 4
150) 1 2 3 4
151) 1 2 3 4
159) 1 2 3 4
164) 1 2 3 4
165) 1 2 3 4
170) 1 2 3 4

NEUROANESTHESIA

BOOK A

12) 1 2 3 4
40) 1 2 3 4
142) A B C D E
143) A B C D E
154) A B C D E

BOOK B

10) A B C D E
16) A B C D E
28) A B C D E
29) A B C D E
38) A B C D E
49) A B C D E
63) A B C D E
88) A B C D E
93) A B C D E
101) A B C D E
121) 1 2 3 4
139) 1 2 3 4
149) 1 2 3 4

OBSTETRIC AND REGIONAL ANESTHESIA

BOOK A

27) 1 2 3 4
30) 1 2 3 4
37) 1 2 3 4
38) 1 2 3 4
44) 1 2 3 4
49) 1 2 3 4
58) 1 2 3 4
59) 1 2 3 4
77) A B C D E
79) A B C D E
87) A B C D E
116) A B C D E
138) A B C D E
145) A B C D E
149) A B C D E

150) A B C D E
157) A B C D E
170) A B C D E
172) A B C D E
173) A B C D E

BOOK B

6) A B C D E
11) A B C D E
13) A B C D E
14) A B C D E
44) A B C D E
51) A B C D E
75) A B C D E
78) A B C D E
81) A B C D E
85) A B C D E
92) A B C D E
102) A B C D E
104) 1 2 3 4
114) 1 2 3 4
118) 1 2 3 4
119) 1 2 3 4
125) 1 2 3 4
126) 1 2 3 4
132) 1 2 3 4
134) 1 2 3 4
138) 1 2 3 4
141) 1 2 3 4
148) 1 2 3 4

PAIN

BOOK A

19) 1 2 3 4
47) 1 2 3 4
50) 1 2 3 4
69) 1 2 3 4
105) A B C D E

Topic Indexed Answer Sheet

BOOK B					
90)	A	B	C	D	E
105)	1	2	3	4	
106)	1	2	3	4	
115)	1	2	3	4	
127)	1	2	3	4	
142)	1	2	3	4	
174)	1	2	3	4	

═══ PEDIATRICS ═══

BOOK A

6)	1	2	3	4	
14)	1	2	3	4	
26)	1	2	3	4	
41)	1	2	3	4	
56)	1	2	3	4	
73)	A	B	C	D	E
86)	A	B	C	D	E
106)	A	B	C	D	E
117)	A	B	C	D	E
124)	A	B	C	D	E
125)	A	B	C	D	E
126)	A	B	C	D	E
137)	A	B	C	D	E

BOOK B

2)	A	B	C	D	E
9)	A	B	C	D	E
18)	A	B	C	D	E
23)	A	B	C	D	E
36)	A	B	C	D	E
69)	A	B	C	D	E
113)	1	2	3	4	
117)	1	2	3	4	
120)	1	2	3	4	
124)	1	2	3	4	
153)	1	2	3	4	
163)	1	2	3	4	

173)	1	2	3	4	

═══ PHARMACOLOGY ═══

BOOK A

5)	1	2	3	4	
22)	1	2	3	4	
32)	1	2	3	4	
33)	1	2	3	4	
46)	1	2	3	4	
52)	1	2	3	4	
57)	1	2	3	4	
62)	1	2	3	4	
70)	1	2	3	4	
74)	A	B	C	D	E
78)	A	B	C	D	E
83)	A	B	C	D	E
85)	A	B	C	D	E
92)	A	B	C	D	E
100)	A	B	C	D	E
104)	A	B	C	D	E
108)	A	B	C	D	E
112)	A	B	C	D	E
134)	A	B	C	D	E
135)	A	B	C	D	E
140)	A	B	C	D	E
148)	A	B	C	D	E
161)	A	B	C	D	E
163)	A	B	C	D	E
165)	A	B	C	D	E
171)	A	B	C	D	E

BOOK B

1)	A	B	C	D	E
4)	A	B	C	D	E
5)	A	B	C	D	E
8)	A	B	C	D	E
30)	A	B	C	D	E
35)	A	B	C	D	E
41)	A	B	C	D	E
42)	A	B	C	D	E

43)	A	B	C	D	E
47)	A	B	C	D	E
48)	A	B	C	D	E
57)	A	B	C	D	E
65)	A	B	C	D	E
68)	A	B	C	D	E
95)	A	B	C	D	E
97)	A	B	C	D	E
100)	A	B	C	D	E
107)	1	2	3	4	
110)	1	2	3	4	
112)	1	2	3	4	
130)	1	2	3	4	
144)	1	2	3	4	
154)	1	2	3	4	
156)	1	2	3	4	
162)	1	2	3	4	
166)	1	2	3	4	
172)	1	2	3	4	

═══ PHYSIOLOGY ═══

BOOK A

2)	1	2	3	4	
3)	1	2	3	4	
4)	1	2	3	4	
7)	1	2	3	4	
8)	1	2	3	4	
20)	1	2	3	4	
25)	1	2	3	4	
31)	1	2	3	4	
34)	1	2	3	4	
36)	1	2	3	4	
51)	1	2	3	4	
54)	1	2	3	4	
60)	1	2	3	4	
61)	1	2	3	4	
72)	1	2	3	4	
76)	A	B	C	D	E
80)	A	B	C	D	E
82)	A	B	C	D	E
91)	A	B	C	D	E

98)	A	B	C	D	E
101)	A	B	C	D	E
103)	A	B	C	D	E
122)	A	B	C	D	E
130)	A	B	C	D	E
131)	A	B	C	D	E
139)	A	B	C	D	E
144)	A	B	C	D	E
146)	A	B	C	D	E
147)	A	B	C	D	E
175)	A	B	C	D	E

BOOK B

22)	A	B	C	D	E
34)	A	B	C	D	E
58)	A	B	C	D	E
66)	A	B	C	D	E
71)	A	B	C	D	E
76)	A	B	C	D	E
96)	A	B	C	D	E
99)	A	B	C	D	E
103)	1	2	3	4	
108)	1	2	3	4	
109)	1	2	3	4	
128)	1	2	3	4	
131)	1	2	3	4	
133)	1	2	3	4	
136)	1	2	3	4	
140)	1	2	3	4	
145)	1	2	3	4	
152)	1	2	3	4	
155)	1	2	3	4	
158)	1	2	3	4	
160)	1	2	3	4	
171)	1	2	3	4	

ANSWERS TO
BOOK A EXAMINATION

BOOK A:

QUESTION 1

Answer A

Equipment/
Physics

QUESTION (K-type):

During mechanical ventilation, factors that influence the correlation between set tidal volume and exhaled tidal volume include

(1) Inspiratory time.
(2) Fresh gas flow.
(3) Compliance of the breathing circuit.
(4) Addition of positive end-expiratory pressure to the circuit.

CORRECT ANSWER: A (1, 2, and 3 are correct.)

SUMMARY:

Often a difference exists between the set tidal volume of an anesthesia machine and the actual delivered tidal volume. This difference can be explained by several factors. One of these is the fresh gas flow rate. High flow rates can add additional volume to each inspired breath that results in increased delivered tidal volume. Prolonged inspiratory time also provides an opportunity for more gas to enter the lungs for a given breath. This translates into an increase in the delivered tidal volume to the patient. Also, the breathing circuit of an anesthesia machine can absorb some of the set tidal volume and result in a decreased delivered tidal volume. PEEP does not alter the delivered tidal volume from the ventilator.

EXPLANATION:

(1) **Correct.** Changing the I:E ratio such that the inspiratory time is prolonged will result in added volume for each breath delivered by the ventilator.
(2) **Correct.** High fresh gas flows can increase the delivered tidal volume to the patient's lungs from the ventilator.
(3) **Correct.** Compliance of the anesthesia breathing circuit can absorb tidal volume and result in a decrease in the delivered tidal volume.
(4) **Incorrect.** PEEP is not considered to be an influencing factor in the correlation of set versus delivered tidal volume.

REASONING:

This question tests knowledge of the anesthesia machine ventilator and factors that influence delivered tidal volumes. The first three options (especially choices 2 and 3) usually are recognized as influencing factors. This knowledge makes the first option correct by default. The last option is not correct. Although there may be some evidence that PEEP influences the delivered tidal volume (in certain anesthesia machines), it generally is not regarded as a correlating factor.

REFERENCE:

Ehrenwerth, J. Anesthesia Equipment: Principles and Applications. St. Louis, Mosby, 1993, p. 554. Morgan GE, Mikhail MS, Murray MJ. Clinical Anesthesiology, 3d ed. New York, McGraw-Hill, 2002, pp. 50–53.

Answer E

Physiology

QUESTION (K-type):

In a 45-year-old man with adult respiratory distress syndrome, which of the following will result from institution of mechanical ventilation with positive end-expiratory pressure?

(1) Decreased intrapulmonary shunt.
(2) Increased pulmonary compliance.
(3) Increased ventilation-perfusion ratio in the dependent portion of lung.
(4) Decreased dead-space-to-tidal-volume ratio.

CORRECT ANSWER: E (All are correct.)

SUMMARY:

Positive end-expiratory pressure (PEEP) is the elevation of transpulmonary pressure at the end of expiration. The main effect of PEEP is to increase functional residual capacity by preventing collapse of alveoli and recruiting atelectactic alveoli. This results in decreased intrapulmonary shunting that improves arterial oxygenation. Excessive PEEP can overdistend the alveoli, resulting in decreased lung compliance and increased dead space. Complications of PEEP therapy include barotrauma (e.g., pneumothorax, subcutaneous emphysema) and decreased cardiac output owing to decreased venous return. Care must be taken to adjust the amount of PEEP to an "optimal" level at which oxygen delivery to tissues is increased and the dead-space-to-tidal-volume ratio is lowest.[1] This is especially important in patients with acute respiratory distress syndrome (ARDS), in whom lung disease is heterogeneous, and PEEP may not be evenly distributed.[1]

EXPLANATION:

(1) *Correct.* Addition of PEEP decreases intrapulmonary shunting and improves arterial oxygenation by increasing FRC and tidal ventilation above closing capacity, improving lung compliance, and correcting ventilation-perfusion abnormalities. This is accomplished by stabilization and recruitment of partially collapsed alveoli.
(2) *Correct.* PEEP improves or increases lung compliance by increasing transpulmonary distending pressure.
(3) *Correct.* Alveoli in dependent portions of lung are at increased risk of atelectasis owing to accumulation of interstitial edema fluid. PEEP can recruit these alveoli and improve the ventilation-perfusion ratio.[1]
(4) *Correct.* Optimal PEEP is the amount that provides maximal oxygen delivery and the lowest dead-space-to-tidal-volume ratio.[1] Excessive PEEP can *increase* dead space by overdistending alveoli and lower cardiac output by decreasing venous return.

REASONING:

This question tests knowledge of respiratory physiology and the effects of PEEP. Choice 1 is correct because recruited alveoli can participate in oxygen exchange, thereby decreasing intrapulmonary shunt. The same effect of PEEP also increases the ventilation-perfusion ratio in dependent portions of lung, making choice 3 also correct. Choices 2 and 4 are correct if we assume that an *optimal* amount of PEEP is being used, in which case pulmonary compliance is increased and dead space is decreased. If *excessive* levels of PEEP are used, pulmonary compliance can decrease, and dead space can increase. Giving the question writer the benefit of the doubt, the reader can assume that an appropriate amount of PEEP is being used. Choices 1, 2, 3, and 4 are all correct; therefore, the best answer is E.

REFERENCE:

1. Miller RD, Miller ED, Reves JG, et al. Anesthesia, 5th ed. New York, Churchill Livingstone, 2000, pp. 2425–2426, Figs. 72-20 and 72-21, p. 2429.
2. Morgan GE, Mikhail MS, Murray MJ. Clinical Anesthesiology, 3d ed. New York, McGraw-Hill, 2002, pp. 968–970, 972–973.

BOOK A:

QUESTION 3

Answer A

Physiology

QUESTION (K-type):

A 58-year-old man with suspected carcinoma of the lung requires postoperative ventilation following general anesthesia for mediastinoscopy. Preoperatively, his shoulder muscles are weak bilaterally, but strength improves with exercise. This patient will show

(1) Inadequate reversal of neuromuscular block with an anticholinesterase drug.
(2) Increased sensitivity to both depolarizing and nondepolarizing muscle relaxants.
(3) Increased muscle strength following plasmapheresis.
(4) Resolution of symptoms following administration of hydrocortisone.

CORRECT ANSWER: A (1, 2, and 3 are correct.)

SUMMARY:

Muscle weakness that improves with exercise and is associated with carcinoma of the lung is a hallmark of Lambert-Eaton myasthenic syndrome (LEMS). Antibodies to presynaptic voltage-gated calcium channels cause decreased release of acetylcholine into the neuromuscular junction. Both myasthenia gravis and LEMS are diseases of the neuromuscular junction. Treatment of LEMS includes immunosupression and plasmapheresis. Anticholinesterases are less helpful in LEMS than in myasthenia gravis. Curative procedures are directed toward the carcinoma. Patients with LEMS are sensitive to both depolarizing and nondepolarizing muscle relaxants. Guanidine hydrochloride and 3,4-diaminopyridine (DAP) increase the release of acetylcholine and can improve the symptoms of LEMS.[1]

EXPLANATION:

(1) *Correct.* Anticholinesterases do not appreciably increase the amount of acetylcholine at the neuromuscular junction (NMJ) because it is not released in the first place in LEMS.
(2) *Correct.* Decreased release of acetylcholine at the neuromuscular junction makes these patients sensitive to all types of muscle relaxants.
(3) *Correct.* Plasmapheresis will reduce the amount of circulating antibodies and reduce the symptoms of LEMS.
(4) *Incorrect.* Symptoms will improve but are not likely to resolve with immune suppression. The underlying malignancy needs to be treated.

REASONING:

This question tests knowledge of the pathophysiology of Lambert-Eaton myasthenic syndrome (LEMS). Choice 4 is the easiest to eliminate with the knowledge that immune suppression is not curative. However, it does improve symptoms, so choice 3 is correct. Patients with LEMS are very sensitive to all types of muscle relaxants (choice 2) owing to decreased acetylcholine release into the NMJ. Anticholinesterases increase acetylcholine by inhibiting the enzymes that degrade acetylcholine. However, with very little acetylcholine to begin with, patients with LEMS do not respond to the administration of anticholinesterases (choice 1).[2] Choices 1, 2, and 3 are correct; therefore, the best answer is A.

REFERENCES:

1. Barash PG, Cullen BF, Stoelting RK. Clinical Anesthesia, 4th ed. Philadelphia, Lippincott Williams & Wilkins, 2001, p. 846.
2. Ibid., p. 825.
3. Darnell RB, Posner JB. Paraneoplastic syndromes involving the nervous system. N Engl J Med 349(16):1543–1554, 2003.
4. Morgan GE, Mikhail MS, Murray MJ. Clinical Anesthesiology, 3d ed. New York, McGraw-Hill, 2002, p. 754.

BOOK A:

Answer A

Physiology

QUESTION 4

QUESTION (K-type):

Which of the following statements concerning postoperative shivering is true?

(1) It increases carbon dioxide production.
(2) It is suppressed by intravenous meperidine.
(3) It accentuates halothane-related tremors.
(4) It increases heat loss.

CORRECT ANSWER: A (1, 2, and 3 are correct.)

SUMMARY:

Postoperative shivering is often more of a problem for patients than pain. The adult hypothermic patient shivers to generate heat. Unfortunately, shivering is an undesirable stress on the body. Shivering increases oxygen demand and carbon dioxide production by up to 800 percent.[1] Shivering is poorly tolerated in patients with marginal cardiac and pulmonary reserve and should be treated with active warming and medications. Meperidine is the agent used most commonly in the recovery room to treat postoperative shivering. Volatile agents decrease the vasoconstrictive response to hypothermia but also lower the threshold for shivering.

EXPLANATION:

(1) **Correct.** Shivering increases $\dot{V}O_2$ and $\dot{V}CO_2$ owing to the increased metabolic activity from skeletal muscle contraction.
(2) **Correct.** Meperidine is a first-line agent for the treatment of shivering. Other opioids can be used but generally are not as effective as meperidine.
(3) **Correct.** Shivering is common after general anesthesia.
(4) **Incorrect.** Shivering generates heat. In some instances, enough heat is generated that the patient becomes hyperthermic.

REASONING:

This question tests knowledge of the pathophysiology of postoperative shivering. It is somewhat challenging because each choice has some plausibility of being correct. Choices 3 and 4 are probably the more difficult choices to differentiate. Halothane is used rarely in clinical practice in North America, and experience with this agent among anesthesia residents is limited. Because of our confidence in choices 1 and 2, we can infer that choice 3 is also correct. In considering choice 4, one might reason that since shivering increases core body temperature, compensatory mechanisms such as peripheral vasoconstriction may be abolished, leading to increased heat loss. However, the reader is encouraged to avoid such circuitous reasoning.

REFERENCE:

1. Barash PG, Cullen BF, Stoelting RK. Clinical Anesthesia, 4th ed. Philadelphia, Lippincott Williams & Wilkins, 2001, p. 1397.
2. Morgan GE, Mikhail MS, Murray MJ. Clinical Anesthesiology, 3d ed. New York, McGraw-Hill, 2002, pp. 705–505, 940–941.

Answer B

Pharmacology

QUESTION (K-type):

The elimination half-life of an amide local anesthetic is prolonged in which of the following conditions?

(1) Liver disease.
(2) Term pregnancy.
(3) Heart failure.
(4) Kidney disease.

CORRECT ANSWER: B (1 and 3 are correct.)

SUMMARY:

The elimination half-life of amide local anesthetics is determined by liver function. Microsomal enzymes within the liver are responsible for their metabolism; therefore, decreases in liver function or liver blood flow increase their elimination half-life. Changes in kidney function do not appreciably alter excretion of amide local anesthetics because very little is excreted unchanged.

EXPLANATION:

(1) *Correct.* Liver disease decreases the metabolism of amide local anesthetics, prolonging their elimination.
(2) *Incorrect.* Liver function and blood flow to the liver do not change during pregnancy.
(3) *Correct.* Blood flow to the liver is decreased in patients with CHF. This decreases the delivery of amide local anesthetics to their site of metabolism, prolonging their elimination.
(4) *Incorrect.* The kidneys do not play a major role in the elimination of amide local anesthetics because little unchanged drug is present in urine.

REASONING:

This question tests knowledge of amide local anesthetics and their mechanism of elimination. Choices 1 and 3 obviously are correct because amide local anesthetics are metabolized in the liver. Since the kidney plays a small role in the elimination of amides, choice 4 can be eliminated. Only choice 2 remains. Choice 2 is incorrect because liver function is not affected by pregnancy, leaving answer B as the best answer.

REFERENCE:

Morgan GE, Mikhail MS, Murray MJ. Clinical Anesthesiology, 3d ed. New York, McGraw-Hill, 2002, pp. 238, 807.
Stoelting RK, Miller RD. Basics of Anesthesia, 4th ed. New York, Churchill Livingstone, 2000, pp. 83–84.

Answer B

Pharmacology

QUESTION (K-type):

A 10-year-old child with asthma is undergoing anesthesia with nitrous oxide, oxygen, and halothane. Effects of the accidental injection of atropine 2 mg in this patient would include

(1) Postoperative delirium.
(2) Ventricular dysrhythmias.
(3) Increased body temperature.
(4) Bronchospasm.

CORRECT ANSWER: B (1 and 3 are correct.)

SUMMARY:

Atropine belongs to the class of drugs that are commonly referred to as anticholinergic agents. More accurately, they are drugs that block muscarinic acetylcholine receptors. These are to be differentiated from neuromuscular blocking agents that act at nicotinic acetylcholine receptors. Anticholinergic agents competitively block acetylcholine from activating the acetylcholine receptor. They can affect several organ systems, including cardiovascular, respiratory, central nervous system (CNS), gastrointestinal, ophthalmic, genitourinary, and thermoregulatory. Other anticholinergics (scopolamine and glycopyrrolate) have varying effects on the different systems. An overdose of an anticholinergic agent may result in CNS effects, tachycardia, dry mouth, hyperthermia, mydriasis, and cycloplegia. Treatment includes acetylcholinesterase inhibitors (physostigmine is the only one that crosses the blood–brain barrier) and supportive care.

EXPLANATION:

(1) **Correct.** Atropine, a tertiary amine, can cross the blood–brain barrier and can cause memory deficits and excitatory reactions, including hallucinations, agitation, delirium, and even loss of consciousness. This is the central anticholinergic syndrome.

(2) **Incorrect.** Effects of muscarinic blockade on the heart can result in tachycardia, shortening of the PR interval, and atrial and nodal dysrhythmias. However, it has little effect on the ventricles.

(3) **Correct.** Blockade of sweat glands may lead to an inability to dissapate heat. This is also known as *atropine fever.*

(4) **Incorrect.** Anticholinergic agents inhibit secretions of respiratory tract mucosa and cause relaxation of bronchial smooth muscle. Ipratropium bromide, an atropine derivative, is used as a metered-dose inhaler or nebulized solution for treatment of asthma.

REASONING:

This question tests knowledge of the pharmacology of atropine. Clearly, anticholinergic toxicity may cause delirium and hyperthermia. Ventricular dysrhythmias may result from tachycardia in patients with coronary artery disease, but healthy patients, including most children, will get only a transient sinus tachycardia. A case report of three children aged 7 to 9 years who were accidentally given massive doses of atropine (16 to 21 mg/kg orally) indicated that they suffered CNS symptoms and tachycardia, both of which resolved within 48 hours. Mydriasis, however, lasted for a week.[1]

REFERENCE:

1. Arthurs GJ, Davies R. Atropine–a safe drug. Anaesthesia 35(11):1077–1079, 1980.
2. Morgan GE, Mikhail MS, Murray MJ. Clinical Anesthesiology, 3d ed. New York, McGraw-Hill, 2002, pp. 207–211.

BOOK A: **QUESTION 7**

Answer B

Physiology

QUESTION (K-type):

True statements concerning the oculocardiac reflex include

(1) It is more likely to occur in a patient with hypercarbia than in a patient with normocarbia.

(2) It is not seen during operative procedures on an empty orbit.

(3) Its afferent limb is the trigeminal nerve.

(4) It does not occur in the awake patient.

CORRECT ANSWER: B (1 and 3 are correct.)

SUMMARY:

The oculocardiac reflex can be triggered by manipulation, pressure, or pain of the eyeball or extraocular muscles and results in bradycardia and/or other dysrhythmias, including ventricular tachycardia and asystole.[1] It also can be elicited by eye trauma, hematoma, and performing a retrobulbar block on an awake or anesthetized patient of any age, but it is seen most commonly in pediatric patients during strabismus surgery. Hypercarbia can increase the incidence of bradycardia during strabismus surgery.[2] Thus it is important to maintain normocarbia to help prevent the reflex. Treatment includes discontinuing the inciting stimulus, ensuring adequate anesthetic depth and oxygenation, Trendelenburg positioning, and possibly atropine, although routine use for prophylaxis is controversial.[2] With repeated stimulation, the oculocardiac reflex fatigues.

EXPLANATION:

(1) **Correct.** Bradycardia is more likely to occur with hypercarbia during strabismus surgery. Maintaining normocarbia can help to reduce the incidence and severity of the oculocardiac reflex.[2]

(2) **Incorrect.** The oculocardiac reflex can be elicited by direct pressure on the tissue in the orbit after enucleation.[1]

(3) **Correct.** Afferent impulses travel along the short and long ciliary nerves to the ciliary ganglion and then to the gasserian ganglion via the ophthalmic division (V_1) of the trigeminal nerve. The efferent limb is the vagus nerve.[2,3]

(4) **Incorrect.** The oculocardiac reflex can be elicited by pressure on the eyeball, traction on extraocular muscles, orbital hematomas, eye trauma or pain, and retrobulbar blockade.[1] All may occur in the awake patient, who may experience somnolence and nausea instead of or in addition to bradycardia and dysrhythmias.

REASONING:

This question tests knowledge of the physiology of the oculocardiac reflex. The reader should be able to rule out choices 2 and 4 by knowing the various stimuli that can cause the oculocardiac reflex and knowing that they can occur in the awake patient and in an enucleated patient. The reader is then left with answer B (choices 1 and 3) because all the choices cannot be incorrect. The reader also should know that the afferent limb is the trigeminal nerve or that increased P_{CO_2} increases the incidence of the oculocardiac reflex, making the correct answers choices 1 and 3.

REFERENCES:

1. Barash PG, Cullen BF, Stoelting RK. Clinical Anesthesia, 4th ed. Philadelphia, Lippincott Williams & Wilkins, 2001, pp. 973–974.

2. Miller RD, Miller ED, Reves JG, et al. Anesthesia, 5th ed. New York, Churchill Livingstone, 2000, p. 2181.

3. Ibid., p. 642.

4. Morgan GE, Mikhail MS, Murray MJ. Clinical Anesthesiology, 3d ed. New York, McGraw-Hill, 2002, p. 763.

BOOK A:

Answer E

Physiology

QUESTION 8

QUESTION (K-type):

Phase II succinylcholine block is characterized by

(1) A train-of-four ratio less than 0.7.
(2) Nonsustained response to tetanic stimulation.
(3) Post-tetanic facilitation.
(4) Improvement by edrophonium.

SUMMARY:

Succinylcholine is a depolarizing muscle relaxant that can cause both phase I and II blocks. Phase I is the commonly recognized effect of succinylcholine: an acetylcholine receptor agonist causing motor end plate depolarization (equally diminished train-of-four stimulation without fade). However, if enough succinylcholine is administered, a block that resembles a nondepolarizing block will develop (train-of-four stimulation with fade). This is thought to relate to conformational changes that accompany prolonged muscle membrane depolarization. Characteristics of phase II block include train-of-four fade, prolonged recovery, anticholinesterase antagonism, and fade with repeated tetanic stimulation.

EXPLANATION:

(1) *Correct.* Monitoring a patient receiving succinylcholine will show a decrease in the train of four to a ratio of less than 0.7 as the patient transitions from phase I to phase II block. Once the ratio is less than 0.4, the patient has a phase II block.

(2) *Correct.* Repeated tetanic stimulation has no effect on the patient with a normal phase I block, but phase II shows a reduced response with successive stimulations.

(3) *Correct.* A single tetanus will increase the ratio on train of four in phase II block.

(4) *Correct.* Phase II block can be improved with anticholinesterases. Phase I block is prolonged after administration of anticholinesterases.

REASONING:

This question tests knowledge of type I and type II neuromuscular blockade. Knowing that phase II block of succinylcholine has similar characteristics to nondepolarizing muscle relaxation makes answering this question much easier. Choices 2, 3, and 4 are clearly characteristics of phase II block. The first choice is a bit challenging because phase II is not formally established before a train-of-four ratio of less than 0.4. But if choices 2, 3, and 4 are true, choice 1 must be as well. All choices are correct, and E is the best answer.

REFERENCE:

Miller RD, Miller ED, Reves JG, et al. Anesthesia, 5th ed. New York, Churchill Livingstone, 2000, pp. 425–426.

Morgan GE, Mikhail MS, Murray MJ. Clinical Anesthesiology, 3d ed. New York, McGraw-Hill, 2002, p.182.

BOOK A:	QUESTION 9

Answer C

Equipment/Physics

QUESTION (K-type):

Advantages of closed-circuit anesthesia over a semiclosed anesthesia system include the ability to

(1) More quickly alter the inspired anesthetic concentration.
(2) Decrease the total amount of inhalational anesthetic used.
(3) More easily increase $PaCO_2$ during emergence.
(4) Decrease heat loss to a greater extent.

CORRECT ANSWER: C (2 and 4 are correct.)

SUMMARY:

Closed-circuit anesthesia differs from semi-closed-circuit anesthesia in the following way: All exhaled gases, except CO_2, are rebreathed in closed-circuit breathing systems, whereas the pressure-release valve in semi-closed-circuit anesthesia evacuates some of the exhaled gases. Advantages of closed-circuit breathing systems include maximal humidification and warming of inhaled gases, less pollution of gases into the environment, and less use of volatile anesthetics. Disadvantages of closed-circuit anesthesia are the inability to rapidly change concentrations of gases, including oxygen and volatile anesthetics, because of the low fresh gas flows.

EXPLANATION:

(1) **Incorrect.** Closed-circuit anesthesia uses low gas flows, making it difficult to quickly alter inspired anesthetic concentration.
(2) **Correct.** Closed-circuit anesthesia minimizes the amount of anesthetic used.
(3) **Incorrect.** There is no difference between closed- and semi-closed-circuit anesthesia with respect to the rate of rise of $Paco_2$ during emergence. This is so because CO_2 is not rebreathed during closed-circuit anesthesia; it is removed from the circuit by the CO_2 absorber.
(4) **Correct.** Closed-circuit anesthesia conserves the maximum amount of heat and humidification.

REASONING:

This is question tests knowledge of the differences between closed-circuit and semi-closed-anesthesia systems. Choices 2 and 4 are clearly correct because closed-circuit anesthesia conserves heat and minimizes use of anesthetics through low flows. This allows answers A, B, and D to be eliminated. Choices 1 and 3 are either both correct or incorrect based on the answer choices. Both answers 1 and 3 are incorrect because closed-circuit anesthesia slows the rate of rise of inspired anesthetic concentration and does not affect the rise of $Paco_2$ during emergence. Choice C is the best answer.

REFERENCE:

Morgan GE, Mikhail MS, Murray MJ. Clinical Anesthesiology, 3d ed. New York, McGraw-Hill, 2002, pp.146–150.
Stoelting RK, Miller RD. Basics of Anesthesia, 4th ed. New York, Churchill Livingstone, 2000, pp. 139–141.

BOOK A: QUESTION 10

Answer C

Clinical Anesthesia

QUESTION (K-type):

Chronic hyperglycemia from excessive glucose administration during parenteral hyperalimentation causes

(1) Retinal degeneration.
(2) Depression of granulocyte function.
(3) Inhibition of platelet aggregation.
(4) Hypercarbia.

CORRECT ANSWER: C (2 and 4 are correct.)

SUMMARY:

Hyperalimentation frequently leads to hyperglycemia, which has a number of deleterious effects. Among these effects are an inhibition of granulocyte function and an increase in CO_2 production. Hyperglycemia has been reported to either have no effect or actually in-

crease platelet aggregation. Retinal degeneration is not a typical problem associated with total parenteral nutrition (TPN)–induced hyperglycemia. TPN is linked to the retinopathy of prematurity in the newborn.

EXPLANATION:

(1) **Incorrect.** Retinal degeneration is not a complication of excessive glucose administration during TPN.

(2) **Correct.** Granulocyte function is depressed from chronic hyperglycemia during TPN.

(3) **Incorrect.** Platelet aggregation is not diminished in patients receiving hyperalimentation.

(4) **Correct.** Hypercarbia can occur owing to excessive glucose administration during hyperalimentation.

REASONING:

Retinal degeneration has not been linked to the chronic hyperglycemia that can be seen with TPN. TPN is a risk factor for the retinopathy of prematurity. Granulocyte function is clearly depressed by hyperglycemia, and it has been postulated that this may account for the increased risk of infection in diabetic patients on TPN. Several studies have examined platelet function and hemostasis during TPN administration. Platelet aggregation is not depressed by TPN. The respiratory quotient (RQ) is the ratio of CO_2 production to O_2 consumption and normally is approximately 0.8. Excess glucose administration during hyperalimentation increases the RQ to approximately 1 and results in excess CO_2 production. This can be severe enough to precipitate respiratory failure in the patient with severe obstructive pulmonary disease. Choice C is the best answer.

REFERENCES:

Miller RD, Miller ED, Reves JG, et al. Anesthesia, 5th ed. New York, Churchill Livingstone, 2000, pp. 907, 2520–2523.

Porta I, Planas M, Padro JB, et al. Effect of two lipid emulsions on platelet function. Infusionsther Transfusionsmed 21:316–321, 1994.

Skibowska A, Raszeja-Specht A, Szutowicz A. Platelet function and acetyl-coenzyme A metabolism in type 1 diabetes mellitus. Clin Chem Lab Med 41:1136–1143, 2003.

BOOK A:

QUESTION 11

Answer B

Clinical Anesthesia

QUESTION (K-type):

Which of the following produces effective transtracheal jet ventilation through a 14-gauge intravenous catheter?

(1) Oxygen through a 50 psi pressure regulator
(2) An Ambu bag with oxygen flow at 15 L/min
(3) Oxygen flush from the fresh gas outlet of the anesthesia machine
(4) The reservoir bag from the anesthesia circle system

CORRECT ANSWER: B (1 and 3 are correct.)

SUMMARY:

Transtracheal jet ventilation is a lifesaving maneuver that generally is reserved for patients who cannot be ventilated or intubated by other means. Its purpose is to temporarily restore oxygenation until a more definitive airway can be established. A high-pressure oxygen source must be attached via noncompliant tubing to a 14-gauge intravenous catheter placed through the cricothyroid membrane. Oxygen through a 50 psi regulator or from the oxygen flush valve are both adequate sources. Unfortunately, an Ambu bag and the reservoir bag from the circle system are likely to be too compliant to reliably generate the pressures necessary for transtracheal ventilation.

EXPLANATION:

(1) **Correct.** A 14-gauge catheter requires a driving force of 50 psi for effective ventilation. The small, high-pressure jet of gas generates a negative pressure gradient via the Venturi effect to entrain additional gas for ventilation. This jet can be provided both by an oxygen source (cylinder, etc.) connected to a regulator to drop the pressure to 50 psi and by the anesthesia machine through the oxygen flush valve.

(2) **Incorrect.** An Ambu bag cannot generate the driving force needed for effective ventilation through a 14-gauge catheter.

(3) **Correct.** See above.

(4) **Incorrect.** The reservoir bag cannot generate the driving force needed for effective ventilation through a 14-gauge catheter.

REASONING:

This question tests knowledge of transtracheal jet ventilation. As outlined earlier, choices 1 and 3 are correct: Oxygen must be provided at 50 psi either through the oxygen flush valve or another source connected to a regulator. Choices 2 and 4 are incorrect: An Ambu bag and the reservoir bag are too compliant for effective transtracheal ventilation. Therefore, the best answer is B.

REFERENCE:

Barash PG, Cullen BF, Stoelting RK. Clinical Anesthesia, 4th ed. Philadelphia, Lippincott Williams & Wilkins, 2001, p. 835.
Morgan GE, Mikhail MS, Murray MJ. Clinical Anesthesiology, 3d ed. New York, McGraw-Hill, 2002, pp. 769–771.

BOOK A:

Answer A

Neuroanesthesia

QUESTION 12

QUESTION (K-type):

During intraoperative mapping of a seizure focus under general anesthesia, electroencephalograph (EEG) activation may be enhanced or seizures induced by the use of

(1) Ketamine.
(2) Methohexital.
(3) Enflurane.
(4) Thiopental.

CORRECT ANSWER: A (1, 2, and 3 are correct.)

SUMMARY:

Several commonly used anesthetics can induce seizures either directly or through their metabolites in susceptible individuals. These include enflurane, methohexital, ketamine, etomidate, meperidine, atracurium, and cis-atracurium. Both thiopental and propofol suppress seizure activity and would not help elicit seizure foci during mapping.

EXPLANATION:

(1) **Correct.** Ketamine has been shown to induce subcortical seizure activity in patients with epilepsy.
(2) **Correct.** Methohexital is used to elicit seizure foci during cortical mapping, with a propensity to elicit seizures in patients with foci in the temporal lobe.
(3) **Correct.** Enflurane increases both EEG voltage and frequency, which can progress to spike-and-wave patterns and then tonic-clonic seizures.
(4) **Incorrect.** Thiopental suppresses seizure activity and would not be desirable during epileptic foci mapping.

REASONING:

This question tests knowledge of central nervous system (CNS) effects of several anesthetics, some of which are now used rarely (e.g., enflurane). Choice 4 is clearly incorrect because thiopental is used to induce anesthesia in patients with seizures, suppressing the seizure activity. This means that answers C, D, and E are incorrect and choices 1 and 3 are correct. There is only a question as to whether choice 2 is correct or incorrect. The use of methohexital during ECT may help the reader determine that choice 2 is correct. A is the best answer.

REFERENCE:

Miller RD, Miller ED, Reves JG, et al Anesthesia, 5th ed. New York, Churchill Livingstone, 2000, pp. 713–714.
Morgan GE, Mikhail MS, Murray MJ. Clinical Anesthesiology, 3d ed. New York, McGraw-Hill, 2002, pp. 585–586.

BOOK A:

Answer E

Equipment/Physics

QUESTION 13

QUESTION (K-type):

Transthoracic resistance to direct-current (DE) defibrillation is decreased by

(1) Use of conductive gel.
(2) Multiple attempts at defibrillation.
(3) Defibrillation during expiration.
(4) Larger electrodes.

CORRECT ANSWER: E (All are correct.)

SUMMARY:

Proper defibrillation during cardiac arrest depends on appropriate flow of current through the heart. Based on Ohm's law, current flow (amperes) equals potential (volts) divided by impedence or resistance (ohms). Therefore, during defibrillation, current flow depends on the resistance or transthoracic impedence. Several factors can decrease transthoracic impedence and improve the current delivered to the heart. These include larger electrode size, use of electrode-skin coupling material, increased number of shocks, decreased time interval between shocks, end-expiratory phase of ventilation, proper placement of electrodes, and firm electrode-to-chest contact pressure.

EXPLANATION:

(1) **Correct.** Conductive gel or paste used between the defibrillators and skin decrease transthoracic impedence. In addition, use of gel or paste can prevent burning the skin with the paddles. Care must be taken to ensure that the gel does not connect the electrodes because the current will preferentially flow through the gel on the surface of the chest between the two electrodes.

(2) **Correct.** Transthoracic impedence decreases with repeated shocks, increasing current flow to the heart.

(3) **Correct.** Defibrillation during end expiration results in the least resistance to flow. This is so because the chest diameter and therefore distance the current must flow to the heart are at a minimum.

(4) **Correct.** The larger the electrodes, the greater is the area of contact for current flow, and the less is the impedence.

REASONING:

This question tests knowledge of electric current flow during defibrillation. Choice 1 is correct because conductive gel always should be used to decrease resistance during defibrillation. Since choice 1 is correct, both C and D are incorrect. Common sense shows that choice 4 is correct because a larger electrode decreases resistance to flow. Since choices 1 and 4 are correct, the only possible answer is E. Knowledge of choices 2 and 3, although important to review, is not required to determine the correct answer.

REFERENCES:

Cummens RO. Advanced Cardiac Life Support. Dallas, American Heart Association, 1997, Secs. 4.3–4.6.

Miller RD, Miller ED, Reves JG, et al. Anesthesia, 5th ed. New York, Churchill Livingstone, 2000, p. 2545.

Morgan GE, Mikhail MS, Murray MJ. Clinical Anesthesiology, 3d ed. New York, McGraw-Hill, 2002, p. 922.

BOOK A:	**QUESTION 14**

Answer A

Pediatrics

QUESTION (K-type):

Compared with a healthy 20-year-old, respiratory function in a healthy 1-year-old is characterized by

(1) Greater chest wall compliance.
(2) Lesser lung compliance.
(3) Greater small airway resistance.
(4) Similar functional residual capacity/total lung volume (FRC/TLC) ratio.

CORRECT ANSWER: A (1, 2, and 3 are correct.)

SUMMARY:

The anatomy and physiology of the lungs and chest wall are different and evolving in a neonate and infant compared with an older child and adult. The ribs of the neonate are horizontally oriented from the vertebral column such that they have very little cephalad-caudad movement with inspiration. Accessory respiratory muscles are less effective owing to the rib orientation. This improves when the ribs gradually slant downward after the child learns to stand and walk.[1] The chest wall commonly displays paradoxical movement with inspiration owing to rib orientation, poor muscular development, incomplete calcification, and higher cartilage content.[1] Prior to 37 weeks gestational age, diaphragmatic muscles have less than 10 percent of type I (slow twitch, high oxidative capacity) muscle fibers compared with about 50 percent in an adult.[1] Along with a higher rate of oxygen consumption, this leads to earlier fatigue.

EXPLANATION:

(1) **Correct.** Neonates and infants have greater chest wall compliance owing to weaker intercostal and diaphragmatic muscles, more horizontal rib orientation, pliable ribs, and greater proportion of cartilage versus bone in the ribs.

(2) **Correct.** Neonates and infants have fewer and smaller alveoli that result in decreased lung compliance. For the first 3 years of life, alveoli increase in number but not size. After that, the increase is greatest until 5 years of age.[2] At about 8 years of age, alveolar maturation is complete.

(3) **Correct.** Neonates and infants have less developed small airways that lead to greater small airways resistance. Resistance in the larger "central airways" is constant in all age groups, but resistance in the smaller airways is decreased with age.

(4) **Incorrect.** FRC per kilogram, about 30 mL/kg, is similar for all ages. The healthy adult has a TLC of 82 mL/kg, whereas the healthy infant has a TLC of 63 mL/kg. Thus, because adults have a greater TLC, the ratio of FRC/TLC is not similar between a 20-year-old and 1-year-old.[3]

REASONING:

Key concepts for answering this question include understanding respiratory physiology and how it changes with age. Choices 1, 2, and 3 are clearly true because of the anatomy and physiology of the infant lung. Choice 4 then can be eliminated by understanding that adults have a greater volume per kilogram of lung capacity. All the preceding reasons explain why children desaturate and tire more quickly and have less tolerance for upper and lower respiratory illnesses.

REFERENCES:

1. Cote CJ. A Practice of Anesthesia for Infants and Children, 3d ed. Philadelphia, Saunders, 2001, p. 11.
2. Ibid., p. 13.
3. Ibid., p. 12.
4. Morgan GE, Mikhail MS, Murray MJ. Clinical Anesthesiology, 3d ed. New York, McGraw-Hill, 2002, p. 850.

BOOK A:

Answer C

Clinical Anesthesia

QUESTION 15

QUESTION (K-type):

True statements concerning insertion of a total hip prosthesis with methylmethacrylate cement include

(1) Hypotension is more likely with placement in the acetabulum than with insertion in the femoral shaft.
(2) Absorbed volatile monomer causes vasodilation.
(3) A deliberate hypotensive technique is contraindicated.
(4) Arterial hemoglobin desaturation may result from fat embolization.

CORRECT ANSWER: C (2 and 4 are correct.)

SUMMARY:

Methylmethacrylate cement is used to bind prosthetic devices to bone. Mixing the liquid and powder methylmethacrylate together causes an exothermic reaction that results in cement hardening. As it hardens, the cement expands against the prosthesis and within the bone, resulting in intramedullary hypertension (>500 mm Hg) that may cause embolization of fat, bone marrow, cement, or air into the venous system. This bone cement implantation syndrome manifests clinically as hypoxemia, dysrhythmias, pulmonary hypertension, or decreased cardiac output. The monomer also can cause vasodilation and hypotension. Despite the aforementioned risks, a deliberate or controlled hypotensive technique is recommended for total hip replacement because of the advantages of reduced blood loss, improved cementing, and shorter surgical time.

EXPLANATION:

(1) *Incorrect.* Hypotension due to fat or bone marrow embolization is more likely with insertion in the femoral shaft than the acetabulum presumably because there is more marrow in the former.

(2) *Correct.* Residual methylmethacrylate monomer can cause vasodilation and decreased systemic vascular resistance.

(3) *Incorrect.* Deliberate hypotensive anesthetic technique is *indicated* because it reduces blood loss by 30 to 50 percent,[1] improves prosthetic cementing, and decreases the duration of surgery.

(4) *Correct.* Arterial desaturation can result from fat or bone marrow embolization at the time of cementing and has been reported up to 5 days postoperatively.[1]

REASONING:

Key concepts for answering this question are understanding the surgical issues with total hip arthroplasty and the potential problems using methylmethacrylate. An understanding of the bone cement implantation syndrome should allow the reader to determine that choices 2 and 4 are correct. Understanding the indications and advantages of a deliberate hypotensive anesthetic technique should allow the reader to eliminate choice 3. Choice 1 therefore can be eliminated along with choice 3 even if the reader does not know whether hypotension is more likely with acetabulum placement or femoral shaft insertion. C is the best answer.

REFERENCE:

1. Miller RD, Miller ED, Reves JG, et al. Anesthesia, 5th ed. New York, Churchill Livingstone, 2000, pp. 2123–2124.
2. Morgan GE, Mikhail MS, Murray MJ. Clinical Anesthesiology, 3d ed. New York, McGraw-Hill, 2002, pp. 784–787.

BOOK A:

Answer B

Cardiovascular

QUESTION 16 (OPTIONAL)

QUESTION (K-type):

True statements concerning <u>direct</u> ventricular defibrillation during cardiopulmonary bypass include

(1) Shocks greater than 30 joules are associated with myocardial damage.
(2) Hypokalemia increases the chance of defibrillation.
(3) Myocardial impedance decreases after a single shock.
(4) Thin-walled ventricles defibrillate more easily than hypertrophied ventricles.

CORRECT ANSWER: B (1 and 3 are correct.)

SUMMARY:

Direct ventricular defibrillation usually can be achieved with 5 to 10 J. Up to 60 J can be used, but higher and repeated defibrillations can be associated with myocardial injury. Success with defibrillation can be improved by correcting any pH, blood gas, or electrolyte abnormalities and ensuring adequate myocardial rewarming. Potassium at a high-normal level favors defibrillation.

EXPLANATION:

(1) *Correct.* The higher energy levels used for direct defibrillation can lead to myocardial injury.

(2) *Incorrect.* Hypokalemia decreases the likelihood of defibrillation.

(3) *Correct.* Resistance to the electric current flow is decreased after the initial shock.

(4) *Incorrect.* Lake and colleagues studied energy dose and other variables that affect direct ventricular fibrillation during open heart surgery in a cohort of 150 adult cardiac patients. They found that heart weight and thickness of ventricular myocardium appeared to be less important factors in direct defibrillation. The only exception was during low (1 J) shocks, where thinner-walled ventricles appeared to defibrillate more easily.[1] Given that most delivered shocks are greater than 1 J and that choices 1 and 3 are correct, this statement must be incorrect.

REASONING:

This is a somewhat challenging question that tests knowledge of direct ventricular defibrillation. It may not be entirely clear to the reader that thin-walled ventricles do not defibrillate more easily than hypertrophied ventricles. Indeed, there are some data in the literature to suggest that thin-walled ventricles defibrillate more easily when 1-J shocks are delivered.[1] However, choice 1 is correct, and choice 2 is clearly incorrect. By the process of elimination, B (choices 1 and 3) is the best answer.

REFERENCES:

1. Lake CL, Sellers TD, Nolan SP, et al. Energy dose and other variables possibly affecting ventricular defibrillation during cardiac surgery. Anesth Analg 63:743–751, 1984.
2. Kaplan, JA, Reich DL, Konstadt SN. Cardiac Anesthesia, 4th ed. Philadelphia, Saunders, 1999, pp. 1086–1087.

BOOK A:

QUESTION 17

Answer C

Clinical Anesthesia

QUESTION (K-type):

The indications for administration of fresh frozen plasma include

(1) Acute volume expansion in a hypovolemic patient.
(2) Bleeding in a patient with a normal activated clotting time after cardiopulmonary bypass.
(3) Transfusion of 6 units of red blood cells in a 70-kg patient.
(4) Bleeding in a patient with a prolonged bleeding time and abnormal factor VIII.

CORRECT ANSWER: C (2 and 4 are correct.)

SUMMARY:

Fresh frozen plasma (FFP) contains all plasma proteins, which include all the clotting factors. FFP is used for the following: (1) treatment of isolated clotting factor deficiencies, (2) reversal of warfarin anticoagulation, (3) correction of coagulopathies secondary to liver disease, (4) bleeding in patients with normal activated clotting times after cardiopulmonary bypass, (5) patients with antithrombin III deficiencies, and (6) patients who undergo massive transfusions (roughly one to two times a patients blood volume). FFP is not used for volume expansion because it carries the same infectious risk as a unit of whole blood and can cause transfusion reactions.

EXPLANATION:

(1) *Incorrect.* FFP is not used for volume expansion.
(2) *Correct.* FFP is indicated for patients with normal activated clotting times who are bleeding after cardiopulmonary bypass.
(3) *Incorrect.* Transfusion of 6 units in a 70-kg patient would not be considered a massive transfusion because the blood volume is approximately 5 L, and a massive transfusion would be roughly 5 L or more.

(4) **Correct.** Administration of FFP corrects a factor VIII deficiency because all clotting factors are contained within FFP. Therefore, it is indicated in a patient with a factor VIII deficiency and prolonged bleeding time.

REASONING:

This question tests knowledge of the criteria for transfusion of fresh frozen plasma. Choice 1 is clearly incorrect because FFP is not used for volume expansion. This eliminates answers A, B, and E. Choice 4 is correct because both remaining answers contain choice 4. Choice 2 is the only remaining question, and it is correct because FFP is indicated in persistent bleeding after cardiopulmonary bypass with a normal activated clotting time.

REFERENCE:

Morgan GE, Mikhail MS, Murray MJ. Clinical Anesthesiology, 3d ed. New York, McGraw-Hill, 2002, pp. 458, 635, 638.
Stoelting RK, Miller RD. Basics of Anesthesia, 4th ed. New York, Churchill Livingstone, 2000, pp. 139–141.

BOOK A:

Answer E

Neuroanesthesia

QUESTION 18

QUESTION (K-type):

Immediately after sustaining a traumatic cord transection with a T4 level, a patient requires emergency laparotomy. Disease-related factors affecting anesthetic management include

(1) Venous pooling.
(2) Hypothermia.
(3) Decreased peripheral vascular resistance.
(4) Decreased alveolar ventilation.

CORRECT ANSWER: E (All are correct.)

SUMMARY:

Spinal cord injury has significant bearing on the acute and chronic anesthetic management of patients. Acute injury at the T4 level can influence the respiratory, cardiovascular, and thermoregulatory systems markedly. Many of the hemodynamic changes that result from spinal cord injury can be explained by damage in the T1–L2 region of the sympathetic nervous system. Loss of sympathetic tone from this area of the cord results in loss of vascular tone with venous pooling, loss of peripheral vascular resistance, and hypotension. Lesions at or above the T7 level often cause hypoventilation and hypoxia secondary to reduction in vital capacity (VC), FEV_1, expiratory reserve volume, and paralysis or impairment of intercostal muscle function. Thermoregulatory function is also impaired because of injured sympathetic pathways to the hypothalamic center.

EXPLANATION:

(1) **Correct.** Venous pooling is a likely result of injury to segments between T1–L2. This is secondary to loss of sympathetic tone and vasodilation.
(2) **Correct.** Hypothermia results secondary to loss of sympathetic relay to the hypothalamic regulatory center.
(3) **Correct.** Loss of sympathetic tone to the vasculature results in loss of peripheral vascular resistance and orthostatic hypotension.
(4) **Correct.** A lesion at T7 or higher can cause significant alteration in respiratory function with decreased alveolar ventilation.

REASONING:

Knowledge of physiologic changes that occur during acute spinal cord injury is required to answer this question correctly. Knowing that loss of sympathetic outflow to the vasculature occurs with a lesion at this level makes choices 1 and 3 correct. Also, remembering that these patients become hypothermic in the operating room and that we must take measures to prevent this makes choice 2 correct. Significant respiratory compromise occurs at lesions above T7 that can lead to alveolar hypoventilation and hypoxia.

REFERENCE:

Miller RD, Miller ED, Reves JG, et al. Anesthesia, 5th ed. New York, Churchill Livingstone, 2000, pp. 568–569, 925.

Morgan GE, Mikhail MS, Murray MJ. Clinical Anesthesiology, 3d ed. New York, McGraw-Hill, 2002, pp. 589–590.

BOOK A: **QUESTION 19**

Answer B

Pain

QUESTION (K-type):

Trigeminal neuralgia is characterized by

(1) Unilateral, intense, paroxysmal pain of sudden onset.
(2) Diminished sensation in the distribution of the maxillary division of the trigeminal nerve.
(3) Normal function of the glossopharyngeal nerve.
(4) Resolution of symptoms by injection of local anesthetic at trigger points.

CORRECT ANSWER: B (1 and 3 are correct.)

SUMMARY:

Trigeminal neuralgia (tic douloureux) is a chronic disorder characterized by severe, unilateral, paroxysmal, recurrent lancinating pain in the trigeminal nerve distribution. Glossopharyngeal nerve function typically is normal. Diminished sensation can occur in any trigeminal distribution, but typically, minimal or no sensory deficits are present. Trigger point injections are not used for trigeminal neuralgia.

EXPLANATION:

(1) **Correct.** Trigeminal neuralgia is characterized by unilateral, intense, paroxysmal pain of sudden onset.
(2) **Incorrect.** Diminished sensation in the distribution of the maxillary division can occur but certainly does not characterize trigeminal neuralgia.
(3) **Correct.** Glossopharyngeal function is characteristically normal in trigeminal neuralgia.
(4) **Incorrect.** "Trigger point injection" typically refers to injection of local anesthetic into muscle to treat myofascial pain. Injection of trigger points is not done for trigeminal neuralgia, although some patients have defined "trigger zones." These are areas that are not painful but when touched will trigger the patient's typical pain. Short-term reduction of symptoms sometimes is seen when these "trigger zone" areas are injected with local anesthetic.

REASONING:

This question tests knowledge of the pathophysiology of trigeminal neuralgia. Patients with trigeminal neuralgia suffer from chronic recurrent paroxysmal unilateral lancinating pains. These are often the result of compression of the trigeminal nerve at the level of the pons by aberrant blood vessels, tumor, or bone. A minority of patients may have involvement of the nervus intermedius or glossopharyngeal nerve or have sensory deficits in the trigeminal nerve. However, these are the exceptions rather than the rule. Choice 1 is correct. Choice 2 is incorrect, and therefore, choice 3 is correct. Choice 4 is incorrect—trigger point injections are not used in trigeminal neuralgia. Therefore, B is the best answer.

REFERENCES:

Benzon R, Borsook M, Strichartz. Essentials of Pain Medicine and Regional Anesthesia. New York, Churchill Livingstone, 1999, pp. 194–196.
Love S, Coakham HB. Trigeminal neuralgia: Pathology and pathogenesis. Brain 124:2347–2360, 2001; erratum in Brain 125:687, 2002.

BOOK A:

Answer E

Physiology

QUESTION 20

QUESTION (K-type):

During general anesthesia in a healthy patient, hypothermia to 33°C results in

(1) Prolongation of vecuronium action.
(2) Protection against cerebral ischemia.
(3) Potentiation of isoflurane.
(4) Increased risk for ventricular dysrhythmias.

CORRECT ANSWER: E (All are correct.)

SUMMARY:

Mild hypothermia is associated with many adverse and few positive effects. Hypothermia causes (1) coagulopathy, increasing the need for transfusions, (2) increased susceptibility to surgical wound infections, (3) prolonged recovery from anesthesia, (4) increased incidence of ventricular dysrhythmias and cardiac events, and (5) decreased metabolism of most drugs, including anesthetic agents and muscle relaxants. On the positive side, hypothermia provides a measure of protection against cerebral and cardiac ischemia and may help in recovery from ARDS.

EXPLANATION:

(1) *Correct.* Hypothermia prolongs the action of muscle relaxants by decreasing metabolism and excretion.
(2) *Correct.* Hypothermia protects against cerebral ischemia by lowering $CMRO_2$.
(3) *Correct.* Hypothermia decreases MAC requirements for all potent inhalational agents.
(4) *Correct.* Even mild hypothermia triples the incidence of ventricular dysrhythmias and cardiac events.

REASONING:

This question tests knowledge of the physiologic effects of hypothermia. Hypothermia can cause multisystem physiologic derangements and contribute to perioperative morbidity. The reader should review these effects carefully.[1] All the choices are well-known effects of hypothermia; therefore, E is the correct answer.

REFERENCE:

1. Sessler DI. Mild perioperative hypothermia. N Engl J Med 24:1730–1737, 1997.
2. Morgan GE, Mikhail MS, Murray MJ. Clinical Anesthesiology, 3d ed. New York, McGraw-Hill, 2002, pp. 117, 136, 189.

Answer B

OB/Regional

QUESTION (K-type):

Factors that decrease the incidence of deep vein thrombosis (DVT) following total hip replacement include

(1) External compression of the lower extremities.
(2) Epidural anesthesia intraoperatively.
(3) Prophylactic aspirin.
(4) Deliberate hypotension intraoperatively.

CORRECT ANSWER: B (1 and 3 are correct.)

SUMMARY:

Several studies comparing intraoperative epidural with general anesthesia for hip surgery have found no significant decrease in the rate of postoperative DVT formation. Hoek and colleagues found a postoperative DVT rate of 37 percent for the epidural group and 36 percent for general anesthesia.[1] Another prospective, randomized trial also confirmed their observation.[2] A recent meta-analysis by the Pulmonary Embolism Prevention (PEP) trial found that aspirin prophylaxis reduced the risk of pulmonary embolism (PE) and DVT by almost a third in patients undergoing hip replacement surgery.[3]

EXPLANATION:

(1) *Correct.* External compression devices of the lower extremities have been shown to reduce the incidence of DVT following total hip replacement surgery.
(2) *Incorrect.* A prospective, randomized trial comparing general anesthesia with general anesthesia plus intraoperative epidural found no statistical difference in the rate of postoperative DVT following hip replacement surgery.[2] These results corroborate previous findings.[1]
(3) *Correct.* The Sixth ACCP Consensus Conference on Anticoagulation did not recommend aspirin as the *sole* therapy for DVT prophylaxis following hip replacement surgery (grade 1A recommendation). However, a recent meta-analysis of over 17,000 patients found that patients who received perioperative aspirin prophylaxis (160 mg for up to 35 days postoperatively) had at least one-third reduction in risk of PE and DVT.
(4) *Incorrect.* A prospective, randomized trial comparing intraoperative hypotension versus normotensive anesthesia showed no difference in the incidence of DVT following hip replacement surgery.[4]

REASONING:

This question is challenging because there are conflicting data in the literature regarding the effects of prophylactic aspirin and incidence of DVT. Most people would have confidence in choice 1, and thus choice 3 also must be correct, regardless of the conflicting data. The best answer is B.

REFERENCES:

1. Hoek JA, Henny CP, Knipscheer HC, et al. The effect of different anaesthetic techniques on the incidence of thrombosis following total hip replacement. Thromb Haemost 65(2):122–125, 1991.
2. Dauphin A, Raymer KE, Stanton EB, Fuller HD. Comparison of general anesthesia with and without lumbar epidural for total hip arthroplasty: Effects of epidural block on hip arthroplasty. J Clin Anesth 9:200–203, 1997.

3. Prevention of pulmonary embolism and deep vein thrombosis with low dose aspirin: Pulmonary Embolism Prevention (PEP) trial. Lancet 355:1295–1302, 2000.

4. Fredin H, Gustafson C, Rosberg B. Hypotensive anesthesia, thromboprophylaxis and postoperative thromboembolism in total hip arthroplasty. Acta Anaesthesiol Scand 28:503–507, 1984.

BOOK A:

Answer A

Pharmacology

QUESTION 22

QUESTION (K-type):

Ketamine administered in anesthetic doses

(1) Increases intracranial pressure.
(2) Does not cause respiratory depression.
(3) Is eliminated by hepatic metabolism.
(4) Increases bronchomotor tone.

CORRECT ANSWER: A (1, 2, and 3 are correct.)

SUMMARY:

Ketamine is a unique nonopioid analgesic/hypnotic/amnestic agent. It induces a state of dissociative anesthesia and is unique because of its minimal effects on respiration. It is also the only intravenous induction agent that has stimulatory effects on the cardiovascular system.

EXPLANATION:

(1) *Correct.* Ketamine is well known to increase cerebral blood flow and subsequently increase intracranial and cerebrospinal fluid pressures. There are conflicting reports on the effect of ketamine on intraocular pressure, but it generally should be avoided for penetrating eye injuries.

(2) *Correct.* Ketamine has very few respiratory effects and does not cause significant respiratory depression.

(3) *Correct.* Ketamine is converted to norketamine through hydroxylation and demethylation by the liver. Factors that reduce hepatic blood flow, such as halothane, also prolong the effects of ketamine by imparing elimination.

(4) *Incorrect.* Ketamine has well documented bronchodilatory properties and has been used to induce anesthesia in patients with reactive airways diseases such as asthma. Bronchodilatory effects of ketamine reflect a decrease in bronchomotor tone.

REASONING:

This question tests knowledge of the pharmacology of ketamine. Most readers will recognize immediately that choices 1 and 2 are true, leading them to conclude that choice 3 is also true even if the reader is unsure of the elimination mechanism. Choice 4 is obviously true if the reader is familiar with the meaning of *bronchomotor tone.*

REFERENCE:

Barash PG, Cullen BF, Stoelting RK. Clinical Anesthesia, 4th ed. Philadelphia, Lippincott Williams & Wilkins, 2001, pp. 327–328.

Answer A

Clinical Anesthesia

QUESTION (K-type):

During laser excision of a sublaryngeal tumor, the risk of airway ignition would be decreased by using

(1) Water-based lubricants.
(2) Jet ventilation without an endotracheal tube.
(3) Saline solution in the endotracheal tube cuff.
(4) Nitrous oxide.

CORRECT ANSWER: A (1, 2, and 3 are correct.)

SUMMARY:

A major hazard of laser airway surgery is fire. Endotracheal tubes can burn, particularly in the oxygen-enriched environment of the operating field. Nitrous oxide also supports combustion. Thus it is imperative to reduce the amount of oxygen as much as possible, ideally to under 30 percent, and to avoid the use of N_2O. Other methods to reduce the risk of airway fire are (1) nonintubation techniques such as jet ventilation, (2) periods of apnea and spontaneous breathing, (3) conventional tubes with protection such as metallic tape wrapping and saline in the cuff, and (4) laser-resistant tubes. Other measures include using saline-soaked pledgets and limiting laser use and power.

EXPLANATION:

(1) **Correct.** Lubricants should be water-based to reduce the risk of ignition.
(2) **Correct.** Jet ventilation avoids placement of an endotracheal tube that could support combustion.
(3) **Correct.** If laser or fire should break the cuff, the water will help to douse the flames.
(4) **Incorrect.** Nitrous oxide supports combustion and should not be used.

REASONING:

This question tests knowledge of airway fires. Choice 4 is clearly incorrect because nitrous oxide is a flammable gas that increases the risk of airway fire. Choice 2 is one of several techniques that can be used to ventilate the patient having laser airway surgery. If choice 2 is true and choice 4 has been eliminated, then choices 1 and 3 also must be true. The addition of water to the field helps reduce the risk of ignition.

REFERENCE:

Morgan GE, Mikhail MS, Murray MJ. Clinical Anesthesiology, 3d ed. New York, McGraw-Hill, 2002, pp. 773–774.
Upper airway management guide provided for laser airway surgery. Anesthesia Patient Safety Foundation Newsletter 8(2), 1993.

Answer D

Physiology

QUESTION (K-type):

A 24-year-old patient with hypertension and hypercalcemia is scheduled for a parathyroidectomy. Serum calcium concentration may be decreased by the administration of

(1) A calcium channel blocker.
(2) Magnesium sulfate.
(3) Sodium bicarbonate.
(4) Vigorous volume expansion.

SUMMARY:

Hyperparathyroidism from parathyroid tumor usually is due to parathyroid adenoma (90 percent) or hyperplasia (9 percent) and can cause hypercalcemia.[1] The effects of hypercalcemia can be broad and include polyuria/dipsia, nephrolithiasis, skeletal muscle weakness, gastrointestinal symptoms, and psychiatric sequelae such as depression, memory loss, confusion, or psychosis.[1] Hypertension occurs in 20 to 50 percent of patients and usually resolves with treatment of the hyperparathyroidism. Treatment of hypercalcemia consists of establishing a diuresis with volume expansion and a loop diuretic, bisphosphonate (pyrophosphate analogues that inhibit bone resorption), calcitonin (inhibits bone resorption), and in certain cases plicamycin or corticosteroids.

EXPLANATION:

(1) *Incorrect.* The addition of a calcium channel blocker is not only not advocated for hypercalcemia but also would do nothing to lower the serum calcium concentration.

(2) *Incorrect.* Magnesium would not reduce the serum calcium concentration. This is a distracter based on the antagonistic effects of calcium and magnesium. For example, hypermagnesemia can be treated temporarily with intravenous calcium.

(3) *Incorrect.* Hyperventilation will cause a respiratory alkalosis. This may result in a decrease in ionized calcium as serum proteins bind more calcium. However, the total serum calcium remains unchanged. Only the fraction of calcium that is bound changes.

(4) *Correct.* Vigorous volume expansion with saline dilutes calcium, and the sodium inhibits renal tubular calcium absorption.

REASONING:

This is an example of a question with a variety of distracter choices. Calcium channel blockers and magnesium administration do nothing to lower serum calcium. However, they sound like they might have some vague "anticalcium effect." Similarly, hyperventilation can induce signs of hypocalcemia such as tetany by lowering ionized calcium but does not affect total serum calcium. The only choice that reduces calcium levels is vigorous volume expansion. D is the best answer.

REFERENCES:

1. Barash PG, Cullen BF, Stoelting RK. Clinical Anesthesia, 4th ed. Philadelphia, Lippincott Williams & Wilkins, 2001. p. 1124.

2. Stoelting RK, Dierdorf SF. Anesthesia and Co-existing Disease, 3d ed. New York, Churchill Livingstone, 1993, pp. 330–332.

3. Morgan GE, Mikhail MS, Murray MJ. Clinical Anesthesiology, 3d ed. New York, McGraw-Hill, 2002, p. 537.

BOOK A:

QUESTION 25

Answer A

Physiology

QUESTION (K-type):

Effects of open cholecystectomy under general anesthesia with mechanical ventilation include

(1) Increased intrapulmonary shunting.
(2) Decreased lung volumes up to 48 hours postoperatively.
(3) Decreased functional residual capacity.
(4) Decreased dead space.

SUMMARY:

Positive-pressure ventilation and general anesthesia have a number of adverse effects on pulmonary mechanics. These effects include increased shunting, decreased vital capacity, decreased functional residual capacity, and increased dead space. These changes are exacerbated by upper abdominal surgery and may persist for several days postoperatively. These changes are offset intraoperatively by increasing the delivered FIO_2 and minute ventilation.

EXPLANATION:

(1) *Correct.* General anesthesia consistently produces a decrease in functional residual capacity of 15 to 20 percent that results in increased intrapulmonary shunting as blood continues to perfuse unventilated regions. This effect is augmented by the impairment of hypoxic pulmonary vasoconstriction that accompanies general anesthesia.

(2) *Correct.* Decreased lung volumes including vital capacity and functional residual capacity remain depressed for 10 to 14 days following upper abdominal surgery with general anesthesia.

(3) *Correct.* See above.

(4) *Incorrect.* Positive-pressure ventilation increases dead space as alveolar dead space increases. This occurs as superior alveoli are ventilated but not perfused while the patient is under general anesthesia.

REASONING:

This question tests knowledge of changes in respiratory physiology associated with anesthesia. Choices 1 and 3 are common effects of mechanical ventilation under general anesthesia. Choice 4 is incorrect because positive-pressure ventilation is well known to increase dead space. Therefore, A is the best answer.

REFERENCE:

Morgan GE, Mikhail MS, Murray MJ. Clinical Anesthesiology, 3d ed. New York, McGraw-Hill, 2002, pp. 421–425.
Stoelting RK, Dierdorf SF. Anesthesia and Coexisting Disease, 3d ed. New York, Churchill Livingstone, 1993, p. 142.

BOOK A:

Answer C

Pediatrics

QUESTION 26

QUESTION (K-type):

Features of the neonate's prompt adjustment to extrauterine life include

(1) Lung expansion resulting in increased pulmonary vascular resistance.
(2) Nonshivering thermogenesis as a response to cold stress.
(3) Anatomic closure of the ductus arteriosus.
(4) Initial expansion of airless collapsed lungs by creation of negative pressures of 40 to 80 cm H_2O.

CORRECT ANSWER: C (2 and 4 are correct.)

SUMMARY:

Many physiologic changes occur at birth to allow the neonate to adapt to extrauterine life. In utero, the fetal lungs contain fluid that is normally expelled during vaginal birth. This is not absolutely necessary for normal respirations after birth, as evidenced by successful births after cesarean deliveries.[1] The fluid that remains is normally absorbed by the pulmonary capillaries and lymphatics. Transient tachypnea of the newborn is the self-limiting condition in which there is residual fluid in the lungs for 24 to 72 hours. This is manifested by tachypnea and chest x-ray findings (i.e., perihilar markings, fluid in the fissures, and streaky linear opacities in the parenchyma).[1] Increased arterial oxygen content from expanded lungs decreases pulmonary vascular resistance and leads to increased pulmonary blood flow and increased blood return to the left atrium. Elevated left atrial pressures help to close the foramen ovale. Decreased pulmonary vascular resistance, along with increased oxygen tensions, functionally closes the ductus arteriosus, resulting in adult circulation.

EXPLANATION:

(1) **Incorrect.** Lung expansion at birth results in *decreased* pulmonary vascular resistance (PVR). Also, initiation of breathing, increased pH, and increased alveolar oxygen tension contribute to the rapid drop in PVR that begins from the first 5 minutes of life and continues over the next few weeks.[2]

(2) **Correct.** The neonate has a large body-surface-area-to-weight ratio and is at risk for significant heat loss. During the first 3 months of life, the infant is unable to shiver. Nonshivering thermogenesis (metabolism of brown fat) is the primary mechanism of heat production.[3]

(3) **Incorrect.** The ductus arteriosus closes *functionally* when pulmonary arterial pressure decreases to less than systemic arterial pressure, and there is increased arterial oxygen content. The ductus may not close *anatomically* until the full-term neonate is 10 to 14 days old.[2]

(4) **Correct.** The initial expansion of airless collapsed lungs requires a gasp that generates negative pressures of 40 to 80 cm H_2O. This amount of transpulmonary pressure is required to distend the lungs that have until then been filled with lung fluid.

REASONING:

Key concepts for answering this question include understanding the physiologic and anatomic changes in the fetus during and after birth. One should be able to recognize that choices 1 and 3 are incorrect. Both attempt to deceive, but the reader should know that pulmonary vascular resistance *decreases* at birth. The reader may be deceived by the term *anatomic closure* versus *functional closure* but should remember that sometimes patients require surgery to ligate a patent ductus arteriosus. Choices 2 and 4 are reasonable and logical. Therefore, C is the best answer.

REFERENCES:

1. Cote CJ. A Practice of Anesthesia for Infants and Children, 3d ed. Philadelphia, Saunders, 2001, pp. 10–11.
2. Miller RD, Miller ED, Reves JG, et al. Anesthesia, 5th ed. New York, Churchill Livingstone, 2000, p. 2070.
3. Ibid., p. 2092.
4. Morgan GE, Mikhail MS, Murray MJ. Clinical Anesthesiology, 3d ed. New York, McGraw-Hill, 2002, p. 816.

BOOK A:

QUESTION 27

Answer D

OB/Regional

QUESTION (K-type):

Landmarks used in performing a superior laryngeal nerve block include the

(1) Transverse process of C6.
(2) Cricoid cartilage.
(3) Angle of the mandible.
(4) Greater cornu of the hyoid cartilage.

CORRECT ANSWER: D (4 only is correct.)

SUMMARY:

The superior laryngeal nerve is a branch of the vagus nerve, which, in turn, branches into the internal laryngeal nerve (sensory branch) and external laryngeal nerve (motor branch), providing sensory innervation between the epiglottis and vocal cords and motor innervation to the cricothyroid muscle. The superior laryngeal nerve block is used to anesthetize the airway for awake fiberoptic intubations. The block is performed by infiltrating local anesthetic 1 cm below the greater cornu of the hyoid bone. This is where the superior laryngeal nerve divides into its external and internal branches prior to the internal branch entering the thyrohyoid membrane.

EXPLANATION:

(1) *Incorrect.* The transverse process of C6, the cricoid cartilage, and the angle of the mandible are not used as landmarks for the superior laryngeal nerve block.
(2) *Incorrect.* See above.
(3) *Incorrect.* See above.
(4) *Correct.* The greater cornu of the hyoid bone is the only landmark used for the superior laryngeal nerve block.

REASONING:

Either knowledge of the anatomy of the upper airway nerves or having performed the block enables the reader to correctly answer this question. Knowing that the superior laryngeal nerve branches off the vagus nerve and supplies sensory innervation to the area between the epiglottis and the vocal cords allows choices 1 and 2 to be eliminated because the cricoid cartilage and transverse process of C6 are caudal to the sensory innervation. Only D is a possibility.

REFERENCE:

Brown DL. Atlas of Regional Anesthesia, 2d ed. Philadelphia, Saunders, 1999, pp. 211–212.
Morgan GE, Mikhail MS, Murray MJ. Clinical Anesthesiology, 3d ed. New York, McGraw-Hill, 2002, pp. 60, 83–84.

BOOK A: **QUESTION 28**

Answer E

Clinical Anesthesia

QUESTION (K-type):

Blood products that transmit viruses include

(1) Factor IX concentrate.
(2) Plasma protein fraction.
(3) Cryoprecipitate.
(4) Albumin.

CORRECT ANSWER: E (All are correct.)

SUMMARY:

Despite routine testing and pasteurization of certain blood products, transfusion of blood products from one human to another carries the risk of transmitting infectious diseases such as viruses or prions. All the products listed are being transferred from one person to another and carry the risk of transmitting infection.

EXPLANATION:

(1) **Correct.** Factor IX concentrate is used to treat hemophilia B (an X-linked recessive disorder causing factor IX deficiency). Factor IX is derived from human plasma and has potential for infection.[1] Virus-inactivated factor IX is now available.[2]

(2) **Correct.** Plasma protein fraction is derived from human plasma and is comprised of albumin plus α and β globulins.

(3) **Correct.** Cryoprecipitate is derived from plasma and contains factor VIII, fibrinogen, von Willebrand factor, and fibronectin.

(4) **Correct.** Both albumin and plasma protein fraction are heat treated at 60°C for 10 hours to minimize the risk of transmission of viruses. In fact, in the United States, only one case of hepatitis B virus (HBV) and no cases of hepatitis C (HCV) or human immunodeficiency virus (HIV) infection have been noted from transfusion of albumin or fibrinogen.[3] Since these are the most concerning viruses, the risk is very low, but other viruses such as parvovirus B19 have been shown to be present in clotting factors and albumin.[4]

REASONING:

The key to answering this question is in knowing that anything that comes from one person and goes into another can transmit infectious processes despite testing and treatment. All the answers come from human blood and therefore pose some risk of transmitting infectious diseases, however miniscule, as in the case of albumin and plasma protein fraction. The best answer is E, all the above.

REFERENCES:

1. Barash PG, Cullen BF, Stoelting RK. Clinical Anesthesia, 4th ed. Philadelphia, Lippincott Williams & Wilkins, 2001, p. 226.
2. McLoughlin TM, Greilich PE. Preexisting hemostatic defects and bleeding disorders. In Lake CL, Moore RA (eds): Blood: Hemostasis, Transfusion and Alternatives in the Perioperative Period. New York, Raven Press, 1995, p. 25.
3. Tabor E. The epidemiology of virus transmission by plasma derivatives: Clinical studies verifying the lack of transmission of hepatitis B and C viruses and HIV type I. Transfusion 39:1160–1168, 1999.
4. Laub R, Strengers P. Parvoviruses and blood products. Pathol Biol 50:339–348, 2002.
5. Miller RD, Miller ED, Reves JG, et al. Anesthesia, 5th ed. New York, Churchill Livingstone, 2000, pp. 1637–1639.
6. Morgan GE, Mikhail MS, Murray MJ. Clinical Anesthesiology, 3d ed. New York, McGraw-Hill, 2002, pp. 630, 638.

BOOK A:

QUESTION 29

Answer A

Clinical Anesthesia

QUESTION (K-type):

Compared with heated cascade-type humidifiers, heated nebulizers used for humidification are associated with a greater risk for

(1) Bacterial transmission.
(2) Increased airway resistance.
(3) Water intoxication.
(4) Inspissated secretions in large airways.

CORRECT ANSWER: A (1, 2, and 3 are correct.)

SUMMARY:

Heated nebulizers work by passing a jet of gas over water that subsequently entrains some water droplets via the Bernoulli effect. The gas subsequently contains both water vapor and, unlike cascade-type humidifiers, small droplets. This may result in large quantities of water being delivered with a subsequent increased airway resistance (as secretion volume increases), water intoxication, and atelectasis. In addition, these droplets can deliver bacteria to the lungs quite efficiently because the units themselves are difficult to sterilize. Inspissation of secretions is not a significant problem because the devices transfer large amounts of water to the secretion. Heated cascade-type nebulizers have been criticized for some of the same failings but appear to have fewer problems.

EXPLANATION:

(1) **Correct.** Bacterial transmission (particularly *Pseudomonas*), while a problem with both, is considered more serious for nebulizers.
(2) **Correct.** Increased airway resistance can be a problem with nebulizers through increasing secretion volume.
(3) **Correct.** The nebulizers are so efficient that water overload has been reported, and the large volume of water delivered can increase secretion volume beyond the ability of the mucociliary clearance system to clear.
(4) **Incorrect.** Inspissation of secretions is not a problem with the nebulizers.

REASONING:

This is a moderately difficult K-type question that requires detailed knowledge to differentiate cascade-type humidifiers from heated nebulizers. Without specific knowledge, one might guess that nebulizers would not cause inspissation of secretions because they are used commonly in respiratory therapy. Having excluded choice 4, one should focus on choice 2 because that will determine if the answer is A or B. Since choice 2 is most likely correct, the best answer would be A.

REFERENCES:

Ballard K, Cheeseman W, Ripiner T, Wells S. Humidification for ventilated patients. Intens Crit Care Nurs 8:2–9, 1992.

Barash PG, Cullen BF, Stoelting RK. Clinical Anesthesia, 3d ed. Philadelphia, Lippincott-Raven Publishers, 1997, p. 563.

Chamney AR. Humidification requirements and techniques: Including a review of the performance of equipment in current use. Anaesthesia 24:602–617, 1969.

Morgan GE, Mikhail MS, Murray MJ. Clinical Anesthesiology, 3d ed. New York, McGraw-Hill, 2002, pp. 45–46.

Shelly MP, Lloyd GM, Park GR. A review of the mechanisms and methods of humidification of inspired gases. Intens Care Med 14:1–9, 1988.

BOOK A:

Answer C

OB/Regional

QUESTION 30

QUESTION (K-type):

Landmarks for caudal block include the

(1) Sciatic notch.
(2) Posterior-superior iliac spines.
(3) Iliac crests.
(4) Sacral cornu.

CORRECT ANSWER: C (2 and 4 are correct.)

SUMMARY:

Caudal anesthesia is a commonly used regional technique for pediatric surgery, especially urologic, rectal, and inguinal procedures. It also can be performed in adults and has historical significance in obstetric anesthesia, where it can be especially useful in the second stage of labor. The caudal space is the sacral portion of the epidural space. The procedure is performed with the patient in the prone or lateral position by inserting a needle through the sacral hiatus at a 45-degree angle. A characteristic "pop" is felt as the needle punctures the sacrococcygeal ligament (a distal extension of the ligamentum flavum), and the angle of the needle is flattened and then advanced. Aspiration for cerebrospinal fluid (CSF) and blood is mandatory. Local anesthetic is injected as a single shot, or a catheter is placed. The technique overall is very safe, but complications can include arrhythmias or seizures from inadvertent intravascular injection, total spinal intraosseous injection, or damage to the fetal head or maternal rectum when used for obstetrics. The risk of dural puncture is highest in infants because the dural sac extends to S3 in this population and to S1 in adults.

EXPLANATION:

(1) *Incorrect.* The greater and lesser sciatic notches are located on the ileum and ischium, respectively. The sciatic nerve exits the pelvis through the greater sciatic notch. Both these notches are located below the gluteus maximus muscle and are not identified easily from the surface because of their depth in the pelvis.[1]

(2) *Correct.* The sacral hiatus can best be identified by palpating the posterior-superior iliac spines, drawing a line between these two points, and forming an equilateral triangle. The tip of the triangle will rest on the sacral hiatus.[2] The midpoint between the posterior-superior iliac spines is a useful way to identify the midline of the sacral hiatus.

(3) *Incorrect.* The iliac crests are too superior to be useful landmarks for a caudal block.

(4) *Correct.* The sacral cornua are the lateral borders of the sacral hiatus.[3]

REASONING:

Determining the correct answer to this question requires knowledge of how a caudal block is performed and the anatomy of the sacrum. The major landmark for this block is the sacral hiatus, so choice 4 is correct. Choice 3 can be eliminated because the iliac crests are too high in the pelvis to serve as effective landmarks for a caudal block. Choice 1 is eliminated because the sciatic notch is not an easily palpable landmark. Choice 2 is correct because identifying the posterosuperior iliac spines can be useful in finding the sacral hiatus. Therefore, C is the best answer.

REFERENCES:

1. Netter FH. Atlas of Human Anatomy. Summit, NJ, Ciba-Geigy Corporation, 1994, Plates 457 and 465.
2. Brown DL. Atlas of Regional Anesthesia. Philadelphia, Saunders, 1999, pp. 347–355.
3. Netter FH. Atlas of Human Anatomy. Summit, NJ, Ciba-Geigy Corporation, 1994, Plate 145.
4. Morgan GE, Mikhail MS, Murray MJ. Clinical Anesthesiology, 3d ed. New York, McGraw-Hill, 2002, pp. 273–275.

BOOK A:

QUESTION 31

Answer C

Physiology

QUESTION (K-type):

Changes in pulmonary function associated with advanced age include

(1) Decreased lung compliance.
(2) Increased alveolar dead space.
(3) Decreased functional residual capacity.
(4) Decreased maximum voluntary ventilation.

SUMMARY:

Reduced lung elasticity and recoil secondary to a decrease of elastin in lung tissue is the most profound effect of age on lung physiology, causing premature closure of small airways on expiration.[1] Elderly lung tissue is more compliant (stretches more easily with volume expansion) yet exhibits decreased alveolar surface area available for effective gas exchange. These changes result in an increase in alveolar dead space, as well as functional residual capacity. Maximum voluntary ventilation or forced vital capacity are decreased in patients owing to the loss of elastic recoil.[2]

EXPLANATION:

(1) **Incorrect.** Elderly patients exhibit calcific chest walls leading to decreased thoracic (not lung) compliance.

(2) **Correct.** Lung parenchyma in elderly patients exhibit decreased alveolar surface area available for effective gas exchange, leading to increased alveolar dead space.

(3) **Incorrect.** Functional residual capacity is slightly increased in elderly patients secondary to the loss of elastic recoil that results in increased residual volume (FRC = ERV + RV).

(4) **Correct.** Maximum voluntary ventilation or forced vital capacity is decreased in patients owing to the loss of elastic recoil.

REASONING:

This is a difficult K-type question that challenges inherent assumptions concerning changes in respiratory physiology with age. They key to this question lies with the understanding that elastic recoil and alveolar surface area are most affected by age. The choices can be reasonably differentiated with this basic understanding.

REFERENCES:

1. Miller RD, Miller ED, Reves JG, et al. Anesthesia, 5th ed. New York, Churchill Livingstone, 2000, p. 2149.
2. Ibid., p. 2151, Figs. 61-6 and 61-8.
3. Morgan GE, Mikhail MS, Murray MJ. Clinical Anesthesiology, 3d ed. New York, McGraw-Hill, 2002, pp. 876–878.

BOOK A: **QUESTION 32**

Answer D

Pharmacology

QUESTION (K-type):

The MAC of isoflurane is decreased by

(1) Ethanol-induced enzyme induction.
(2) Hyperventilation to a Pa_{CO_2} of 25 mm Hg.
(3) Chronic anemia to a hematocrit of 20 percent.
(4) Decreased body temperature to 34°C.

CORRECT ANSWER: D (4 only is correct.)

SUMMARY:

Minimum alveolar concentration (MAC) is defined as the alveolar concentration of volatile anesthetic that will prevent movement following surgical incision in 50 percent of patients. Factors that decrease MAC include hypothermia, additional sedative medications, pregnancy, acute alcohol intoxication, chronic amphetamine abuse, advanced age, *neonates, hyponatremia, hypercalcemia, hematocrit less than 10 percent, Pa_{CO_2} less than 15 mm Hg or greater than 95 mm Hg, Pa_{O_2} less than 40 mm Hg, and hypotension with a MAP less than 40 mm Hg.*

EXPLANATION:

(1) **Incorrect.** Ethanol-induced enzyme induction from chronic alcohol abuse most likely will increase MAC.[1] Acute alcohol intoxication tends to decrease MAC.

(2) **Incorrect.** Pa_{CO_2} in the range of 15 to 95 mm Hg has no effect on MAC.[1] Therefore, hyperventilation to a Pa_{CO_2} of 25 mm Hg will have no effect.

(3) **Incorrect.** Chronic anemia with a hematocrit of 20 percent will have no effect on MAC. Only anemia to a hematocrit of less than 10 percent will decrease MAC.

(4) **Correct.** Hypothermia will decrease MAC.

REASONING:

This commonly used question tests knowledge of factors that influence MAC. Choice 1 is incorrect because hepatic enzyme induction owing to ethanol should increase MAC. Since choice 1 is incorrect, choice 3 also must be incorrect. Hypothermia definitely decreases MAC, so choice 4 is correct. Choice 2 is not obvious, but the reader may recall that very high Pa_{CO_2} values can cause narcosis. The easiest way to answer this question correctly is to memorize a table of factors affecting MAC found in commonly used texts.

REFERENCE:

1. Stoelting RK, Miller RD. Basics of Anesthesia, 4th ed. New York, Churchill Livingstone, 2000, p. 32.
2. Morgan GE, Mikhail MS, Murray MJ. Clinical Anesthesiology, 3d ed. New York, McGraw-Hill, 2002, pp. 135–137, Table 7-4 (p. 136), Factors Affecting MAC.

BOOK A:

Answer B

Pharmacology

QUESTION 33

QUESTION (K-type):

Compared with fentanyl, characteristics of alfentanil include

(1) Greater protein binding.
(2) More rapid clearance.
(3) Shorter elimination half-life.
(4) Greater volume of distribution.

CORRECT ANSWER: B (1 and 3 are correct.)

SUMMARY:

Parenteral opioids differ greatly in their pharmacokinetic and pharmacodynamic profiles. Fentanyl and alfentanil differ in their extent of protein binding, their context-sensitive half-lives (based on a multicompartment model that includes two distribution half-lives and a terminal elimination half-life), their volume of distribution, their rate of clearance, and their extent of hepatic metabolism. Alfentanil is slightly more protein bound and has a shorter elimination half-life and a smaller volume of distribution compared with fentanyl. These properties cause alfentanil to have a relatively short duration of action compared with fentanyl despite its lower rate of clearance.[1] Alfentanil is used commonly in clinical settings in which rapid onset and short duration of action are desired (such as in placement of ocular blocks for ophthalmic surgery).

EXPLANATION:

(1) *Correct.* Alfentanil is more protein bound than fentanyl.
(2) *Incorrect.* Alfentanil has a slower rate of clearance than fentanyl.
(3) *Correct.* Alfentanil has a shorter elimination half-life (in terms of both terminal half life and distribution or central compartment half-life).
(4) *Incorrect.* Alfentanil has a lower volume of distribution than fentanyl.

REASONING:

This K-type question asks you to identify the pharmacokinetic properties of alfentanil compared with fentanyl. You should know that the volume of distribution of alfentanil is lower than that of fentanyl because this is one of the primary reasons alfentanil's clinical effect is so short. You can eliminate answers C and D based on this knowledge. The challenging part of this question is not being tempted to select answer A, which includes the item "more rapid clearance." It would seem rational that a drug with a shorter duration of action would have a more rapid rate of clearance, but this is not the case with respect to alfentanil. Alfentanil's clinical effect is so short because it has so little volume of distribution, not because of its clearance. B is the best answer.

REFERENCE:

1. Miller RD, Miller ED, Reves JG, et al. Anesthesia, 5th ed. New York, Churchill Livingstone, 2000, pp. 312–315.
2. Morgan GE, Mikhail MS, Murray MJ. Clinical Anesthesiology, 3d ed. New York, McGraw-Hill, 2002, pp. 152–155, 164–167.

BOOK A:　　　　**QUESTION 34**

Answer B

Physiology

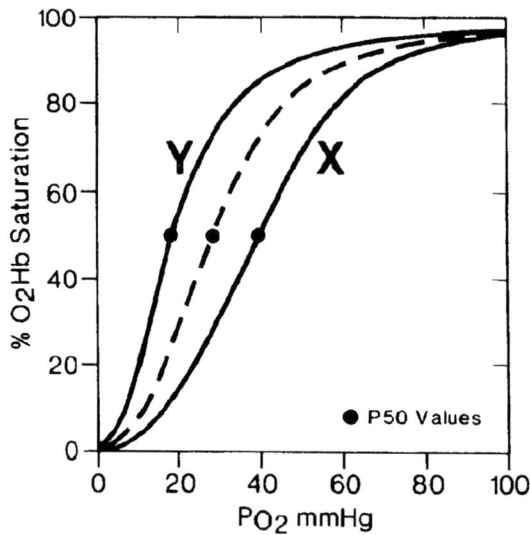

QUESTION (K-type):

The oxygen-dissociation curve in the center of the graph represents normal adult hemoglobin. True statements concerning curves *X* and *Y* include

(1) Curve *Y* represents hemoglobin characteristic of a normal neonate.
(2) Curve *X* represents hemoglobin characteristic of 3-week-old banked blood.

(3) Curve *Y* represents hemoglobin characteristic of an alkalotic patient.

(4) Curve *X* represents hemoglobin characteristic of a hypothermic patient.

CORRECT ANSWER: B (1 and 3 are correct.)

SUMMARY:

The hemoglobin-oxygen dissociation curve describes how avidly hemoglobin binds to oxygen as a function of P_{O_2}. Up to four oxygen molecules can bind one hemoglobin molecule. Many factors alter this curve, such as pH, body temperature, different forms of hemoglobin molecules, and levels of 2,3-DPG. When the curve shifts to the right, less oxygen is bound to hemoglobin at any given Pa_{O_2}, and the opposite is true when the curve is shifted to the left. Shifting to the right favors oxygen delivery to tissue, which occurs during hyperthermia, acidosis, and increased levels of 2,3-DPG. Increased oxygen delivery is important during tissue hypoxia, when acidosis and increased 2,3-DPG occur. Increased temperature can result in increased cellular metabolism, a situation that also demands increased oxygen delivery. Conversely, hypothermia, alkalosis, and decreased 2,3-DPG suggest decreased oxygen demand and shift the curve leftward.

EXPLANATION:

(1) *Correct.* Fetal hemoglobin has a higher affinity for oxygen because it relies on this to extract oxygen from their mother's adult hemoglobin. Neonatal hemoglobin is comprised primarily of fetal hemoglobin, which has a greater affinity for oxygen, demonstrated by a shift to the left in the oxygen-hemoglobin dissociation curve.

(2) *Incorrect.* The longer blood is stored, the lower are the levels of 2,3-DPG, which shifts the oxygen-hemoglobin curve to the left, not right.

(3) *Correct.* Alkalosis shifts the oxygen-hemoglobin curve to the left because hemoglobin binds oxygen more avidly.

(4) *Incorrect.* Hypothermia shifts the curve to the left because hemoglobin binds oxygen more avidly.

REASONING:

This commonly used question asks for knowledge of the oxyhemoglobin dissociation curve and factors that can affect oxygen loading and unloading from hemoglobin. Choice 4 is obviously incorrect because alkalosis shifts the curve to the left. This allows answers C, D, and E to be eliminated, leaving choices 1 and 3 as correct. The only question is whether choice 2 is correct or incorrect. It is actually incorrect because banked blood causes a shift in the oxyhemoglobin dissociation curve to the left. B is correct.

REFERENCE:

Miller RD, Miller ED, Reves JG, et al. Anesthesia, 5th ed. New York, Churchill Livingstone, 2000, pp. 1618–1621.

Morgan GE, Mikhail MS, Murray MJ. Clinical Anesthesiology, 3d ed. New York, McGraw-Hill, 2002, pp. 501–502.

Answer C

Cardiovascular

QUESTION (K-type):

A 45-year-old man who is scheduled for coronary artery bypass grafting is receiving heparin and nitroglycerin infusions for preinfarction angina. True statements concerning the use of heparin during coronary revascularization in this patient include

(1) The anticoagulant effect is enhanced by the nitroglycerin.
(2) Platelet count should be determined prior to the operation.
(3) Activated coagulation time is unreliable after prolonged administration of heparin.
(4) The dose of heparin necessary to provide adequate systemic anticoagulation is likely to be increased.

CORRECT ANSWER: C (2 and 4 are correct.)

SUMMARY:

This patient is at risk for heparin resistance. There are various clinical factors and drugs that can influence the anticoagulant effect of heparin. Both heparin and nitroglycerine can cause heparin resistance, necessitating higher doses of heparin to achieve the required level of anticoagulation during cardiopulmonary bypass.

EXPLANATION:

(1) *Incorrect.* Heparin's anticoagulant effect is decreased by nitroglycerine.
(2) *Correct.* A heparin infusion can affect platelet count. Heparin-induced thrombocytopenia (HIT) can cause a decrease in platelet count and hypercoagulable state. The time frame usually is within 2 to 5 days in type I HIT, which is characterized by mild thrombocytopenia without thrombosis (proaggregatory effect on platelets). Type II HIT is a more serious and severe immune-mediated effect seen on average after 7 to 9 days of heparin infusion. This disorder produces clots in various arteries with significant morbidity and mortality.
(3) *Incorrect.* The reliability of ACT is not affected.
(4) *Correct.* Heparin's anticoagulant effect is decreased by nitroglycerine and an increased dose may be necessary. Antithrombin III deficiency should also be considered in the setting of heparin resistence. Antithrombin III binds to and inactivates thrombin and other activated clotting factors. Antithrombin III–thrombin binding is accelerated severalfold by the presence of heparin, which binds to a separate binding site on antithrombin III.[1] Thus heparin's anticoagulation effect is mediated via antithrombin III. Antithrombin III deficiency can be treated with transfusion of fresh frozen plasma.

REASONING:

This is an often-seen board question requiring knowledge of heparin resistance. Since choice 1 is clearly incorrect, answers A, B, and E can be eliminated. That leaves answers C and D. The pharmacologic effect of a heparin infusion includes an aggregatory effect on platelets (type I HIT and the more severe and serious type II HIT). C is the best answer.

REFERENCES:

1. Barash PG, Cullen BF, Stoelting RK. Clinical Anesthesia, 4th ed. Philadelphia, Lippincott Williams & Wilkins, 2001, p. 204.
2. Hensley F, Martin DE, Gravlee FP. Practical Approach to Cardiac Anesthesia, 3d ed. Philadelphia, Lippincott Williams & Wilkins, 2002, pp. 498–499.
3. Morgan GE, Mikhail MS, Murray MJ. Clinical Anesthesiology, 3d ed. New York, McGraw-Hill, 2002, p. 450.

Answer B

Physiology

QUESTION (K-type):

True statements concerning negative-pressure pulmonary edema include

(1) It is associated with airway obstruction.
(2) It responds to diuretic therapy.
(3) Resolution occurs within 24 hours.
(4) Debilitated adults are predisposed to it.

CORRECT ANSWER: B (1 and 3 are correct.)

SUMMARY:

Postobstructive or negative-pressure pulmonary edema (NPPE) is the development of sudden pulmonary edema following upper airway obstruction such as laryngospasm or endotracheal tube obstruction. Starling forces govern the amount of fluid filtration across a capillary bed into the interstitium. Forceful inspiration against a closed airway creates negative intrathoracic pressure, increases pulmonary blood volume and capillary hydrostatic pressure, and causes fluid exudation into the interstitium. In addition, hypoxia associated with airway obstruction causes hypoxic pulmonary vasoconstriction, further increasing capillary hydrostatic pressure and causing more fluid exudation. The greater the negative pressure created, the worse is the pulmonary edema, explaining why young athletic men have an increased susceptibility to NPPE.

EXPLANATION:

(1) *Correct.* Forceful inspiration against a closed airway or airway obstruction causes NPPE.
(2) *Incorrect.* Current consensus therapy for NPPE involves oxygen and intubation. Diuretics have been used in some instances, but their role is unclear. Diuretics potentially could be harmful because they can further decrease the intravascular volume causing hypotension.
(3) *Correct.* Resolution of NPPE is rapid, typically occurring within 24 hours.
(4) *Incorrect.* Young athletic males are predisposed to NPPE because they can generate the largest negative intrathoracic pressure.

REASONING:

This question tests knowledge of negative-pressure pulmonary edema. Clearly, choice 1 is correct, and choice 4 is incorrect because high negative intrathoracic pressure needs to be created to cause NPPE that occurs with upper airway obstruction in young athletes. This leaves only a question as to whether or not choice 2 is correct. It is incorrect because diuretics potentially can be harmful to patients with NPPE. B is correct.

REFERENCE:

Van Kooy M, Gargiulo R. Postobstructive pulmonary edema. Am Fam Phys 62:401–404, 2000. Morgan GE, Mikhail MS, Murray MJ. Clinical Anesthesiology, 3d ed. New York, McGraw-Hill, 2002, pp. 942–943.

Answer B

OB/Regional

QUESTION (K-type):

Landmarks for the sciatic nerve via a posterior approach include the

(1) Posterior-superior iliac spine.
(2) Coccyx.
(3) Greater trochanter of the femur.
(4) Iliac crest.

CORRECT ANSWER: B (1 and 3 are correct.)

SUMMARY:

The sciatic nerve is composed of fibers from L4 to S3. It exits the pelvis below the piriformis muscle in the sciatic notch and passes distally dorsal to the lesser trochanter of the femur. At the superior portion of the popliteal fossa the sciatic nerve divides into the common peroneal and tibial nerves, which when combined with the saphenous nerve provide sensory and motor innervation to the lower leg and foot. A saphenous nerve block is appropriate for surgery on the lower leg, foot, and ankle but most often must be combined with femoral and other nerve blocks to provide complete anesthesia.

EXPLANATION:

(1) ***Correct.*** To perform a sciatic nerve block via the posterior approach, a line is drawn between the greater trochanter of the femur and the posterosuperior iliac spine with the patient in the lateral position with the hip flexed. A second line 4 to 5 cm in length is drawn perpendicular and caudomedially to the midpoint of the first. The sciatic nerve is located at the terminus of this second line.[1]
(2) ***Incorrect.*** The coccyx is the distal end of the vertebral column and is not a landmark for the sciatic nerve block.
(3) ***Correct.*** As discussed earlier, the greater trochanter of the femur is an important landmark for sciatic nerve block via the posterior approach.
(4) ***Incorrect.*** The iliac crest is not a landmark for the sciatic nerve block.

REASONING:

Knowledge of the anatomy of the lower extremity and course of the sciatic nerve is essential to perform an effective sciatic nerve block. This question is one of many commonly tested regional procedures the reader should memorize in preparation for the written examination. Other important blocks for the examination include the axillary, ankle, interscalene, caudal, and stellate ganglion blocks. Choices 1 and 3 are used consistently to locate the sciatic nerve from the posterior approach. Therefore, B is correct.

REFERENCE:

1. Brown DL. Atlas of Regional Anesthesia. Philadelphia, Saunders, 1999, pp. 95–101.
2. Morgan GE, Mikhail MS, Murray MJ. Clinical Anesthesiology, 3d ed. New York, McGraw-Hill, 2002, pp. 300–302.

Answer A

OB/Regional

QUESTION (K-type):

Epidural anesthesia for cesarean delivery is planned for a 30-year-old woman in labor. She has preeclampsia and takes propranolol for mitral valve prolapse. A test dose of 3 mL of 2% lidocaine containing 15 μg epinephrine is administered, and no change in heart rate is noted by palpation of the pulse. Prior to injection of more local anesthetic, blood is freely aspirated from the catheter.

Explanations for failure of the intravenous test dose include:

(1) The pain of labor masked the change usually seen with the test dose.
(2) Preexisting β-adrenergic blockade blunted the tachycardia from the intravenous epinephrine.
(3) Changes in pulse rate were too brief to be noted by palpation of the pulse.
(4) Preeclampsia decreased the sensitivity to exogenously administered catecholamines.

CORRECT ANSWER: A (1, 2, and 3 are correct.)

SUMMARY:

The administration of epinephrine containing epidural test doses in laboring women is controversial because detection of an intravascular catheter in parturients can be hindered by many factors. The heart rate increase associated with epinephrine administration may be masked by pain associated with uterine contractions or too brief to detect. Administration of β-antagonists for other medical conditions can mask heart rate increases. Because of these limitations, it is imperative to aspirate catheters prior to dosing and always give incremental doses in laboring women.

EXPLANATION:

(1) **Correct.** The patient in the question is in labor, and it is possible that the heart rate response from the clearly intravascular catheter was masked by pain associated with labor.
(2) **Correct.** Propranolol is a β-antagonist and can prevent the tachycardic response to intravascular epinephrine.[1]
(3) **Correct.** The average increased time to tachycardia with intravenous epinephrine is approximately 60 seconds, and the duration is approximately 60 seconds.[2] Experts recommend a pulse oximeter or electrocardiogram (ECG) to detect this response because palpitation of the pulse or measurement of blood pressure can be unreliable.[2]
(4) **Incorrect.** Preeclampsia increases sensitivity to exogenously administered catecholamines.

REASONING:

This question tests knowledge of epidural catheter management and test dose administration to parturients. Choice 2 is clearly correct because the patient is on β-blocking medication. The next step is to examine choice 4, which is clearly incorrect because preeclamptic patients are more sensitive to catecholamines. These two steps eliminate B, C, D, and E as answers and make the only possible correct answer A. However, it is best to check yourself and verify that choices 1 and 3 are indeed correct prior to choosing A as the answer. Since the patient is in labor and you know that this can mask the tachycardia associated with test doses, choice 1 is clearly correct. Choice 3 is slightly more difficult to prove but makes intuitive sense and is proven correct on further review of the literature.

REFERENCES:

1. Chestnut DH. Obstetric Anesthesia Principles and Practice, 2d ed. St. Louis, Mosby, 1999, pp. 364–368.
2. Hughes SC, Levinson G, Rosen MA. Shnider and Levinson's Anesthesia for Obstetrics, 4th ed. Philadelphia, Lippincott Williams & Wilkins, 2002, pp. 134–146.
3. Morgan GE, Mikhail MS, Murray MJ. Clinical Anesthesiology, 3d ed. New York, McGraw-Hill, 2002, pp. 825, 837–38.

BOOK A:

Answer E

Cardiovascular

QUESTION 39

QUESTION (K-type):

A 76-year-old man with a history of angina, dyspnea on exertion, and syncope attributable to aortic stenosis is brought to the operating room for open reduction of an ankle fracture. An ECG shows sinus rhythm. Anesthetic considerations include

(1) Nitroglycerin is contraindicated.
(2) Atrial fibrillation should be treated with synchronized cardioversion.
(3) The risk for cardiac complications is the same as that in patients with coronary artery stenosis.
(4) Spinal anesthesia is relatively contraindicated.

CORRECT ANSWER: E (All are correct.)

SUMMARY:

The patient's symptoms are indicative of severe aortic stenosis (AS). Anesthetic considerations include maintaining adequate preload, good myocardial contractility and perfusion pressure, sinus rhythm, and normal rate. Myocardial supply and demand are impaired. Myocardial O_2 demand is increased by a hypertrophic ventricle. Increased intraventricular pressure compromises oxygen supply while increasing the demand. For these reasons, these patients do not tolerate even mild vasodilation and hypotension.

EXPLANATION:

(1) **Correct.** Venodilation, decreased preload, and possible hypotension make nitroglycerine unsafe.
(2) **Correct.** The hypertrophic noncompliant ventricle in AS develops diastolic dysfunction, which increases left ventricular end-diastolic pressure, thus decreasing the LA-to-LV pressure gradient in diastole, compromising passive filling. Atrial contraction assumes a greater role in maintaining cardiac output.
(3) **Correct.** Pathophysiology in AS leads to increased left ventricular (LV) afterload, resulting in ventricular hypertrophy and increased myocardial oxygen requirements. Supply also can be impaired in AS because aortic diastolic pressure can be decreased and ventricular filling pressures are increased owing to the noncompliant ventricle. This supply-demand imbalance places these patients at increased risk for myocardial ischemia.[1]
(4) **Correct.** Spinal anesthesia can decrease afterload, leading to decreased coronary perfusion during diastole and possible myocardial ischemia.

REASONING:

Aortic stenosis is a cardiac lesion that is tested frequently on board examinations. The key to the anesthetic management of aortic stenosis is understanding that the pathophysiology stems from the fixed afterload increase of the stenotic valve. Normal aortic valve area is about 3 cm^2, and symptoms of AS appear when the valve narrows to less than 0.8 cm^2.[1] Patients with AS need well-timed atrial contractions to augment left ventricular filling. These contractions can account for up to 30 to 40 percent of left ventricular end-diastolic volume.[1] Adequate preload is also important to help offset decreased LV compliance from LV hypertrophy. Decreases in afterload should be avoided because they do not significantly offset the fixed afterload increase from the stenotic valve. Heart rates should be kept normal (60 to 70 beats per minute) to allow adequate time for coronary perfusion during diastole while avoiding bradycardia (decreased cardiac output) and tachycardia (myocardial O_2 supply-demand imbalance and ischemia).[1] The fact that choices 1, 2, and 4 are correct makes E the only possibility.

REFERENCE:

1. Barash PG, Cullen BF, Stoelting RK. Clinical Anesthesia, 4th ed. Philadelphia, Lippincott Williams & Wilkins, 2001, p. 894.
2. Morgan GE, Mikhail MS, Murray MJ. Clinical Anesthesiology, 3d ed. New York, McGraw-Hill, 2002, pp. 416–418.

BOOK A:

QUESTION 40

Answer A

Physiology

QUESTION (K-type):

Use of hyperventilation to decrease brain swelling also decreases

(1) P_{50} of hemoglobin.
(2) Serum ionized calcium concentration.
(3) Serum potassium concentration.
(4) Cerebral metabolic rate.

CORRECT ANSWER: A (1, 2, and 3 are correct.)

SUMMARY:

Hyperventilation causes a variety of physiologic changes. Because of the respiratory alkalosis created by hyperventilation, there is a leftward shift in the oxyhemoglobin curve, which lowers the P_{50}. Also, the alkalosis will cause a decrease in ionized serum calcium and potassium (secondary to an intracellular shift). Hyperventilation does not decrease the cerebral metabolic rate, although it will decrease regional and global cerebral blood flow.

EXPLANATION:

(1) **Correct.** The alkalosis resulting from hyperventilation will shift the oxyhemoglobin curve to the left, causing a decreased hemoglobin P_{50}.
(2) **Correct.** Hyperventilation decreases the ionized serum calcium by promoting serum protein binding.
(3) **Correct.** Hyperventilation decreases serum potassium by causing an intracellular shift in exchange for hydrogen ions.
(4) **Incorrect.** Hyperventilation does not decrease the cerebral metabolic rate.

REASONING:

This question tests knowledge of the physiologic effects of hyperventilation. Circulating calcium is normally 40 percent bound to protein, 50 percent ionized, and 10 percent in chelated forms.[1] Respiratory alkalosis increases the protein-bound fraction and reduces ionized calcium levels. Hyperventilation and the resulting respiratory alkalosis also can decrease serum potassium levels and may lead to hypokalemia. Hyperventilation to a Pa_{CO_2} of 20 mm Hg also can reduce serum phosphate levels by 2 to 3 mg/dL.[2] It is also important to understand how physiologic changes affect the oxyhemoglobin curve and that it shifts leftward with alkalosis. The best answer is A.

REFERENCES:

1. Barash PG, Cullen BF, Stoelting RK. Clinical Anesthesia, 4th ed. Philadelphia, Lippincott Williams & Wilkins, 2001, p. 189.
2. Ibid., p. 193.
3. Morgan GE, Mikhail MS, Murray MJ. Clinical Anesthesiology, 3d ed. New York, McGraw-Hill, 2002, pp. 50–503.

BOOK A:

Answer D

Pediatrics

QUESTION 41

QUESTION (K-type):

A neonate born at 32 weeks' gestation has cyanosis, tachypnea, a scaphoid abdomen, and a cardiac impulse on the right. Immediate management of this child should include

(1) Insertion of a chest tube.
(2) Limiting inspired oxygen concentration to 50%.
(3) Administration of rapid positive-pressure ventilation by mask.
(4) Insertion of a nasogastric tube.

CORRECT ANSWER: D (4 only is correct.)

SUMMARY:

Congenital diaphragmatic hernia (CDH) occurs in about 1 in 5000 live births. Around the eighth week of gestation, portions of bowel, stomach, and abdominal viscera can herniate into the thorax through either the left or right posterolateral foramen of Bachdalek or the anterior foramen of Morgagni. Ninety percent of herniations are through the left foramen of Bachdalek.[1] Clinical signs include cyanosis, hypoxia, respiratory distress, scaphoid abdomen, bowel obstruction, and auscultation of bowel sounds in the chest. Radiographic studies will quickly reveal the diagnosis. The mass effect of the herniated abdominal contents leads to pulmonary hypoplasia and pulmonary hypertension. Despite modern therapies of ECMO, nitric oxide, surfactant, and high-frequency ventilation, morbidity and mortality remain relatively unchanged over the last few decades.[1]

EXPLANATION:

(1) *Incorrect.* Chest tube insertion may be necessary at some point because these patients are at risk for pneumothoraces. However, if there is no evidence that the patient has a pneumothorax, there is no need to insert a chest tube prophylactically.

(2) *Incorrect.* Limiting the concentration of inspired oxygen in a premature infant may prevent retinopathy of prematurity but is a low priority in a patient who is cyanotic and tachypneic. Patients with CDH are often hypoxic owing to pulmonary hypoplasia, and are at increased risk of pulmonary hypertension. Treatment of pulmonary hypertension can include oxygen, along with hyperventilation, alkalosis, sedation, paralysis, and other pharmacologic agents.[1]

(3) *Incorrect.* In extreme situations, the patient may require positive-pressure mask ventilation, but this must be administered carefully because increased airway pressures will insufflate air into the stomach and increase the size of the intrathoracic herniated bowel. Ideally, mask ventilation should be avoided, and the patient should be allowed to breath spontaneously, preoxygenated, and intubated awake.[1]

(4) *Correct.* Insertion of a nasogastric or orogastric tube serves to decompress the stomach of gas and fluids.[1]

REASONING:

This is a challenging question because all the options sound reasonable and, in fact, may be used at some point in the treatment. Choice 1 is not necessary for immediate management, so it can be ruled out. Choice 2 does not make good clinical sense, so it also can be ruled out. Choice 3, like choice 1, may be necessary in extreme situations, but this is not justified with the current clinical description. Choice 4 is the most reasonable immediate intervention.

REFERENCE:

1. Cote CJ. A Practice of Anesthesia for Infants and Children, 3d ed. Philadelphia, Saunders, 2001, pp. 304–305.
2. Morgan GE, Mikhail MS, Murray MJ. Clinical Anesthesiology, 3d ed. New York, McGraw-Hill, 2002, pp. 864–865.

BOOK A:

None of the Choices are Correct

Basic Science

QUESTION 42 (OPTIONAL)

QUESTION (K-type):

The principle underlying diffusion hypoxia also explains

(1) Apneic oxygenation.
(2) The concentration effect.
(3) The solubility effect.
(4) The second-gas effect.

CORRECT ANSWER: None of the choices are correct.

SUMMARY:

After extensive discussion and research regarding this question, we have concluded that none of the choices can be correct. Diffusion hypoxia occurs when a patient who has been receiving nitrous oxide is placed on room air at the conclusion of an anesthetic. The nitrous oxide diffuses rapidly from the blood into the lungs, decreasing the alveolar concentration of oxygen and carbon dioxide.[1] This is a dilutional effect on oxygen and carbon dioxide by nitrous oxide. The resulting hypocarbia can depress the respiratory drive, and the decreased alveolar oxygen concentration can lead to hypoxemia.[2] Administration of 100% oxygen can help to prevent this phenomenon.

EXPLANATION:

(1) *Incorrect.* Apneic oxygenation is based on the augmented gas inflow effect that is a component of the concentration effect.[3] With this technique, ventilation can be stopped for brief periods of time if 100% oxygen is insufflated—usually via a small catheter—into the airway. When oxygen is taken up from the alveoli into the blood, more gas (100% oxygen) is drawn in. Although adequate oxygenation often can be maintained effectively, development of hypercarbia and respiratory acidosis limits this technique. Arterial P_{CO_2} increases 6 mm Hg in the first minute of apnea and 3 to 4 mm Hg each minute thereafter. Diffusion hypoxia is a *dilutional* effect that is not explained by apneic oxygenation.

(2) *Incorrect.* The concentration effect is composed of two effects: (a) the augmented gas inflow effect (see choice 1) and (b) the concentrating effect.[3] The concentrating effect occurs when an anesthetic is taken up from the lungs into the bloodstream; the remaining anesthetic in the lungs is at a higher concentration than would be expected. For example, if an anesthetic is at 20 percent of total gas (20 parts per 100), and 10 are taken up into the bloodstream, then the remaining anesthetic is at a concentration of 11 percent (10 per 90 remaining parts), not 10 percent. As gas leaves the alveoli into the bloodstream, new gas (at 20 percent anesthetic concentration) enters the alveoli (augmented gas inflow effect). Diffusion hypoxia is a *dilutional* effect that is not explained by the concentration effect.

(3) *Incorrect.* A review of standard anesthesia texts and experts within our department failed to find a definition or description of the "solubility effect." This is unfortunate wording because the solubility of nitrous oxide does explain the phenomenon of diffusion hypoxia. The speed at which a gas diffuses across the alveolar capillary membrane down a concentration gradient (e.g., from areas of high gas concentration to low) is determined not only by the molecular weight of the gas but also by its solubility. Graham's law states that the rate at which gases diffuse is inversely proportional to the square root of their molecular weight, where

$$D_{N_2O} \alpha \ \frac{1}{\sqrt{MW_{N_2O}}} \quad D_{O_2} \alpha \ \frac{1}{\sqrt{MW_{O_2}}} \quad \frac{D_{N_2O}}{D_{O_2}} = 0.85 \quad \frac{D_{O_2}}{D_{N_2O}} = 1.2$$

By this measure, alveolar oxygen diffuses 1.2 times faster than nitrous oxide. However, solubility of gas in blood also plays a factor in determining the speed of diffusion across the alveolar capillary membrane.

$$\frac{\sqrt{MW_{O_2}}}{\sqrt{MW_{N_2O}}} \times \frac{Sol\ N_2O}{Sol\ O_2} = \frac{\sqrt{32}}{\sqrt{44}} \times \frac{0.47}{0.024} = 16.7$$

When the solubility of nitrous oxide is taken into consideration, we see that it diffuses 17 times more rapidly across the alveolar capillary membrane compared with oxygen. Thus the rapid washout of nitrous oxide at the end of an anesthetic that causes diffusion hypoxia is due to rapid diffusion across the alveolar concentration gradient, which is related to its solubility. However, there is no such thing as a "solubility effect," and thus this choice is incorrect.

(4) *Incorrect.* The second-gas effect occurs when one gas, nitrous oxide, speeds the uptake of a potent anesthetic.[4] For example, if a patient breathes 50% nitrous oxide (50 parts per 100) and 4% sevoflurane (4 parts per 100), and all the nitrous is taken up, the remaining 4 parts of sevoflurane is in only 50 parts of total gas. Its concentration is now 4/50 = 8%. The overall effect is concentration of the second gas, in this case sevoflurane. As we have already discussed, diffusion hypoxia is cause by a *dilutional* effect on alveolar oxygen and carbon dioxide.

REASONING:

This is a challenging question because none of the choices reflects a clearly correct answer. The likely intent of this question is to test knowledge of the concentration effect, the second-gas effect, and diffusion hypoxia. It is important to understand the determinants of diffusion rates across the alveolar-capillary membrane. Blood/gas solubility is a major determinant of diffusion rates across the alveolar-capillary membrane and is the best reason that explains why nitrous oxide diffuses rapidly from blood and can lead to dilution of alveolar oxygen and carbon dioxide at the end of an anesthetic. Unfortunately, the choice "solubility effect" is not a widely known or conventional anesthetic term. None of the choices is correct.

REFERENCES:

[1] Fink BR. Diffusion anoxia. Anesthesiology 16:511–519, 1955.

2. Barash PG, Cullen BF, Stoelting RK. Clinical Anesthesia, 4th ed. Philadelphia, Lippincott Williams & Wilkins, 2001, p. 387.

3. Ibid., p. 383.

4. Ibid., p. 384.

5. Stoelting RK, Miller RD. Basics of Anesthesia, 4th ed. New York, Churchill Livingstone, 2000, pp. 26–27.

6. Morgan GE, Mikhail MS, Murray MJ. Clinical Anesthesiology, 3d ed. New York, McGraw-Hill, 2002, pp. 132, 539.

Answer D

Equipment/Physics

QUESTION (K-type):

True statements concerning carbon dioxide absorption in breathing-system canisters include

(1) The major reactant of baralyme is barium hydroxide.
(2) Baralyme contains silica to minimize dust.
(3) The major component of soda lime is sodium hydroxide.
(4) Both baralyme and soda lime contain calcium hydroxide.

CORRECT ANSWER: D (4 only is correct.)

SUMMARY:

Carbon dioxide is eliminated from semiclosed and closed breathing circuits through the use of CO_2 absorbers that chemically neutralize CO_2, such as soda lime and baralyme. The CO_2 reacts with water and hydroxides to form carbonates, water, and heat. In soda lime, the hydroxides are sodium hydroxide, potassium hydroxide, and calcium hydroxide. In baralyme, the hydroxides are barium hydroxide and calcium hydroxide. With both soda lime and baralyme, the sodium hydroxide and barium hydroxide are present as activators for the reaction, and calcium hydroxide comprises the majority of the absorber. Soda lime has silica added to prevent dust formation, whereas baralyme has harder granules and does not need silica because of water bound to the octahydrate salt of barium hydroxide.

EXPLANATION:

(1) *Incorrect.* The major reactant of baralyme is calcium hydroxide.
(2) *Incorrect.* Baralyme does not contain silica to minimize dust, as does soda lime.
(3) *Incorrect.* The major component of soda lime is calcium hydroxide.
(4) *Correct.* The major reactant of both soda lime and baralyme is calcium hydroxide.

REASONING:

This question tests knowledge of similarities and differences in soda lime and baralyme components of CO_2-absorbing systems. Choice 4 is obviously correct, which allows answers A and B to be eliminated. Choice 2 is not correct because one of the differences between soda lime and baralyme is that soda lime contains silica, whereas baralyme does not. Answers C and E both contain choice 2 and can be eliminated. Only D remains, and it is the best answer.

REFERENCE:

Morgan GE, Mikhail MS, Murray MJ. Clinical Anesthesiology, 3d ed. New York, McGraw-Hill, 2002, pp. 33–34.
Stoelting RK, Miller RD. Basics of Anesthesia, 4th ed. New York, Churchill Livingstone, 2000, pp. 143–144.

Answer A

OB/Regional

QUESTION (K-type):

Factors that decrease local anesthetic concentration in the fetus include

(1) Maternal hypotension.
(2) Maternal acidemia.
(3) Maternal serum alpha acid glycoprotein concentration.
(4) Fetal acidosis.

CORRECT ANSWER: A (1, 2, and 3 are correct.)

SUMMARY:

Fetal plasma drug concentration depends on delivery of drug to the placenta via the uterine artery, transfer of drug across the placenta, and fetal uptake. If blood flow to the uterine artery is compromised, as in the case of maternal hypotension or other conditions associated with uterine hypoperfusion (supine hypotension syndrome, administration of vasoconstrictors), delivery of drug to the placenta will be decreased. Transfer of drug across the placenta depends on many factors, including the concentration of free drug (non–protein-bound) and lipid solublity. Local anesthetics such as lidocaine are weak bases (the pK_a of lidocaine is 7.8) and therefore are primarily in the nonionized form with higher pH and in the ionized form in conditions associated with low pH such as acidosis. If fetal acidosis is present, this can result in the drug crossing the placenta in the lipid-soluble form while circulating in maternal blood and then becoming ionized when exposed to the acidotic environment within the fetus. This can result in high fetal concentrations of local anesthetic and has been termed ion trapping.[1]

EXPLANATION:

(1) **Correct.** Maternal hypotension decreases drug delivery to the placenta, which decreases drug concentration in the fetus.

(2) **Correct.** Lidocaine is a weak base. When the pH is below the pK_a, more of the drug is in the ionized form, which will impede placental transfer.[2]

(3) **Correct.** Alpha acid glycoprotein binds basic drugs like local anesthetics. A higher serum alpha acid concentration will cause more protein binding and less placental transfer.

(4) **Incorrect.** Fetal pH has the same effect on a drug as maternal pH. If the pH is less than the pK_a of a drug with weakly basic properties such as lidocaine, most of the drug will be in the ionized form and will not cross the placenta. When the fetus is acidotic and there is a significant difference in the maternal and fetal pH, this can result in a much higher concentration of local anesthetic in the fetus and has been termed *ion trapping.*

REASONING:

This question requires knowledge that lidocaine and most other local anesthetics are weak bases and therefore are in the nonionized form at high pH and in the ionized form at low pH. One also must know the factors that favor placental transfer, keeping in mind that the ionized form of the drug will tend not to cross the placenta. With this knowledge, one can identify choice 2 as correct and choice 4 as incorrect. With the K-type question, this means that the answer must be A (1, 2, and 3 are correct).

REFERENCES:

1. Hughes SC, Levinson G, Rosen MA. Shnider and Levinson's Anesthesia for Obstetrics, 4th ed. Philadelphia, Lippincott Williams & Wilkins, 2002, p. 63.
2. Ibid., p. 63.
3. Morgan GE, Mikhail MS, Murray MJ. Clinical Anesthesiology, 3d ed. New York, McGraw-Hill, 2002, pp. 153, 233–241; 808–811, Table 14-1 (pp. 236–237), Physicochemical Properties of Local Anesthetics.

Answer D

Equipment/Physics

QUESTION (K-type):

An oxygen analyzer sensor placed in the inspiratory limb of a circle system

(1) Is useful as a disconnect alarm if placed near the patient.
(2) Will increase dead space.
(3) Will be more pressure sensitive than one placed in the expiratory limb.
(4) Should not be placed distal to an in-circuit humidifier.

CORRECT ANSWER: D (4 only is correct.)

SUMMARY:

The oxygen analyzer is the only device on the anesthesia machine that monitors the integrity of the low-pressure circuit.[1] Oxygen concentration in the circuit can be measured electrochemically, by paramagnetic analysis, or by mass spectrometry. The oxygen analyzer sensor can be placed in the inspiratory or expiratory limb of the circle system. It should not be placed in the fresh gas line because it would only measure concentration of oxygen entering the circuit and not what is actually delivered to the patient.[2] Placement of the sensor closest to the patient may help to detect a disconnection, but if it is placed distal to the Y connection, it may increase dead space.

EXPLANATION:

(1) *Incorrect.* The oxygen analyzer placed near the patient will *not* reliably detect all disconnections because they may occur at locations far from the analyzer, and high fresh gas flow rates may prevent the oxygen concentration from dropping low enough to set off the alarm.[2]
(2) *Incorrect.* Placement of the oxygen analyzer in the *inspiratory* limb of the circle system will *not* increase dead space. Placing the analyzer between the Y piece and the endotracheal tube *will* increase dead space.[2]
(3) *Incorrect.* The expiratory limb has a slightly lower partial pressure of oxygen compared with the inspiratory limb owing to the patient's oxygen consumption. However, it is equally sensitive on either side.
(4) *Correct.* While increased humidity does not affect most modern oxygen analyzers, it is advisable to minimize exposure to excessive humidity, which may affect the sensor.[2]

REASONING:

Key concepts for answering this question are understanding the circle system and the purpose of the oxygen analyzer. While the sensor can detect a disconnection under some circumstances, choice 1 can be ruled out because the sensor should not be relied on to do so. Choice 2 also can be eliminated because placement in the inspiratory limb does not affect dead space. Choice 3 is more confusing because location of the analyzer does not affect the sensitivity. Thus it also can be ruled out on this basis alone or can be eliminated along with choice 1. Finally, while most modern analyzers are not affected by humidity, it is still recommended to minimize exposure to humidity.

REFERENCES:

1. Barash PG, Cullen BF, Stoelting RK. Clinical Anesthesia, 4th ed. Philadelphia, Lippincott Williams & Wilkins, 2001, p. 589.
2. Dorsch JA, Dorsch SE. Understanding Anesthesia Equipment: Construction, Care and Complications, 3d ed. Baltimore, Williams & Wilkins, 1994. pp. 210–211.
3. Morgan GE, Mikhail MS, Murray MJ. Clinical Anesthesiology, 3d ed. New York, McGraw-Hill, 2002, p. 55.

Answer E

Physiology

QUESTION (K-type):

Agents that produce an acute withdrawal response in patients addicted to heroin include

(1) Pentazocine.
(2) Nalbuphine.
(3) Buprenorphine.
(4) Naloxone.

CORRECT ANSWER: E (All are correct.)

SUMMARY:

Withdrawal from opioid addiction can occur within 3 to 4 hours after the last dose. Patients initially may exhibit restlessness, diaphoresis, nausea, nasal congestion, lacrimation, stomach cramps, and drug-seeking behavior. Later symptoms include piloerection (hence the descriptor "cold turkey"), muscle spasms ("kicking the habit"), fever, chills, hypertension, and tachycardia.[1] Acute withdrawal can be produced by pure opioid antagonists such as naloxone or opioid agonist-antagonists such as pentazocine, nalbuphine, nalorphine, or butorphanol. The agonists-antagonists have opposing effects at different opiate receptors and are used for both analgesia and treating the side effects of opiate use.

EXPLANATION:

(1) **Correct.** Pentazocine is an opioid agonist-antagonist (primarily κ receptor stimulation) that is one-fourth to one-half as potent as morphine. It can cause an acute withdrawal response in addicts.[2]

(2) **Correct.** Nalbuphine is an opioid agonist-antagonist structurally related to oxymorphone and naloxone that acts as an agonist at κ receptors and as an antagonist at μ receptors. Nalbuphine can cause acute withdrawal symptoms in addicts.[3]

(3) **Correct.** Buprenorphine is an opioid agonist-antagonist that is a partial μ-receptor antagonist. Withdrawal symptoms can sometimes be seen acutely after administration to patients addicted to heroin owing to its μ-receptor antagonist properties. However, buprenorphine has minimal effects on methadone-maintained opioid abusers compared with other agonist-antagonists.[3]

(4) **Correct.** Naloxone is a pure opioid antagonist ($\mu \gg \delta$ or κ) that can produce an acute withdrawal response in patients addicted to heroin. Because naloxone has a relatively short duration of action (30 to 45 minutes) compared with longer-acting opioids, repeated doses or continuous infusion may be required to treat respiratory depression.

REASONING:

Key concepts for answering this question include understanding opioid and opioid antagonist pharmacology. Choices 1, 2, and 4 definitely can cause an acute withdrawal response in patients addicted to heroin. Choice 3, buprenorphine, is described as having minimal effects on opioid abusers. However, because of its opioid antagonist properties, it is conceivable for buprenorphine to precipitate withdrawal. Choices 1, 2, and 4 are clearly correct. The only possible answer is E, which includes choice 3.

REFERENCES:

1. Miller RD, Miller ED, Reves JG, et al. Anesthesia, 5th ed. New York, Churchill Livingstone, 2000, p. 305.
2. Ibid., p. 345.
3. Ibid., pp. 346–347.
4. Morgan GE, Mikhail MS, Murray MJ. Clinical Anesthesiology, 3d ed. New York, McGraw-Hill, 2002, pp. 164–169, 249.

Answer B

Pain

QUESTION (K-type):

A 68-year-old man has had severe, constant burning and aching in the right forehead and anterior scalp for 6 weeks after an episode of herpes zoster. True statements concerning this patient's condition include

(1) It is more common in elderly patients.
(2) The neuralgia involves the supraorbital branches of the ophthalmic division of the facial nerve.
(3) Tricyclic antidepressants often provide effective pain relief.
(4) Opioid analgesics are the first-line treatment.

CORRECT ANSWER: B (1 and 3 are correct.)

SUMMARY:

Postherpetic neuralgia (PHN) more often afflicts the elderly and follows the distribution of a particular sensory nerve. Motor nerves are not affected. Antineuropathic pain medicines such as tricyclic antidepressants and gabapentin may be quite effective. Opioid analgesics may be effective, but their use is considered controversial.

EXPLANATION:

(1) **Correct.** The elderly are more at risk for herpes zoster.
(2) **Incorrect.** The facial nerve (cranial nerve VII) is a motor nerve. The question describes an affliction of the supraorbital branch of the ophthalmic division of cranial nerve V (the trigeminal nerve).
(3) **Correct.** Tricyclic antidepressants are first-line treatment of PHN.
(4) **Incorrect.** Opioids may be helpful to some, but their use in PHN is controversial.

REASONING:

This question tests knowledge of the pathophysiology of postherpetic neuralgia (PHN). Patients older than age 60 who get acute herpes zoster have an incidence of PHN that is 30 to 50 percent, whereas those under age 50 have only a 5 percent incidence. Only sensory nerves are affected because the varicella virus reactivates in sensory ganglia either in the dorsal root ganglia or the gasserian ganglia of the trigeminal nerve. No dermatome is more often affected than another. Treatment often involves tricyclic antidepressants, gabapentin, Lidoderm patches, or capsaicin cream, but use of opioids has been controversial. The best choice is B.

REFERENCE:

Benzon R, Borsook M, Strichartz. Essentials of Pain Medicine and Regional Anesthesia. New York, Churchill Livingstone, 1999, pp. 267–270.
Morgan GE, Mikhail MS, Murray MJ. Clinical Anesthesiology, 3d ed. New York, McGraw-Hill, 2002, p. 314.

QUESTION (K-type):

Three weeks after exposure to toxic levels of an organophosphate insecticide, a farm worker is scheduled for inguinal herniorrhaphy. Which of the following should be avoided?

(1) Spinal anesthesia with tetracaine.
(2) Epidural anesthesia with 2-chloroprocaine.
(3) Atracurium neuromuscular block.
(4) Succinylcholine infusion.

CORRECT ANSWER: E (All are correct.)

SUMMARY:

Ester-linked local anesthetics such as 2-chloroprocaine and tetracaine are metabolized by pseudocholinesterase. Pseudocholinesterase also degrades acetylcholine released at the neuromuscular junction, as well as succinylcholine and mivacurium.[1] Atracurium is largely degraded through enzymatic action by nonspecific plasma esterases. Organophosphates inhibit a number of enzymes, including pseudocholinesterase, acetylcholinesterase, and other nonspecific plasma esterases. Drugs that are substrates for these enzymes may have prolonged elimination following exposure to organophosphates.

EXPLANATION:

(1) *Correct.* Organophosphate insecticides are irreversible inhibitors of cholinesterases affecting pseudocholinesterase, acetylcholinesterase, and nonspecific plasma cholinesterases. Their effects may last several weeks. Pseudocholinesterase is involved in the metabolism of succinylcholine and ester-linked local anesthetics such as tetracaine and 2-chloroprocaine. Nonetheless, delayed metabolism of these local anesthetics in people with pseudocholinesterase deficiency has been documented rarely.
(2) *Correct.* See above.
(3) *Correct.* Atracurium undergoes ester hydrolysis by both nonspecific plasma esterases and nonenzymatic degradation (Hofmann reaction). It has been estimated that two-thirds of the degradation of atracurium occurs via enzymatic ester hydrolysis. *cis*-Atracurium, on the other hand, does not undergo significant enzymatic hydrolysis.
(4) *Correct.* See above.

REASONING:

This question tests knowledge of organophosphate poisoning and the enzymes that are affected. It is also important to review the physical signs and symptoms of organophosphate poisoning. Initially, symptoms may resemble a flulike syndrome (abdominal pain, headache, dizziness) and progress to include coma, convulsions, confusion, muscle weakness, dyspnea, cyanosis, and sometimes pancreatitis.[2] All the choices are best avoided in a patient exposed to organophosphates; thus E is the correct answer.

REFERENCES:

1. Barash PG, Cullen BF, Stoelting RK. Clinical Anesthesia, 4th ed. Philadelphia, Lippincott Williams & Wilkins, 2001, p. 540.
2. Goldman L, Ausiello D (eds). Cecil Textbook of Medicine, 22d ed. Philadelphia, Saunders, 2003, pp. 520–521.
3. Morgan GE, Mikhail MS, Murray MJ. Clinical Anesthesiology, 3d ed. New York, McGraw-Hill, 2002, p. 165.

Answer D

OB/Regional

QUESTION (K-type):

The addition of halothane 0.5% to nitrous oxide and oxygen 50% each for cesarean delivery

(1) Increases the incidence of low Apgar scores.
(2) Increases operative blood loss.
(3) Increases the incidence of maternal hypotension.
(4) Decreases the incidence of maternal awareness.

CORRECT ANSWER: D (4 only is correct.)

SUMMARY:

The addition of a low-dose volatile agent such as halothane or isoflurane is common practice during general anesthesia for cesarean section. When compared with a technique using 50% nitrous oxide and 50% oxygen and no volatile agent, many clinically significant differences are observed. A deeper level of anesthesia is achieved, which results in decreased circulating catecholamine levels and a significantly reduced incidence of maternal awareness. High maternal catecholamine levels have been shown to cause uterine artery vasoconstriction and decreased uterine blood flow, which is ablated with the use of volatile agents.[1] While intraoperative blood loss is greater in patients who receive general anesthesia for cesarean section, it is not increased with the addition of a volatile agent in low doses (<1 MAC). Adverse neonatal effects have not been observed.

EXPLANATION:

(1) *Incorrect.* Volatile agents have not been shown to cause low Apgar scores. In fact, the addition of volatile agents allows the anesthesiologist to give the mother higher inhaled oxygen concentrations for a given level of anesthesia, which has been shown to improve the condition of the newborn.[1,2]

(2) *Incorrect.* Halogenated agents produce a dose-related decrease in uterine tone. However, addition of low doses of these agents during cesarean section has not been shown to increase operative blood loss when compared with a technique using 50% nitrous oxide and 50% oxygen and no volatile agent.[3]

(3) *Incorrect.* Patients given a volatile agent in addition to nitrous oxide and oxygen have lower blood pressures than those without volatile agents. However, in the *hemodynamically stable* patient, the incidence of true maternal hypotension is not increased significantly.[1]

(4) *Correct.* Cesarean section is associated with a high incidence of awareness, especially in emergency cases. Compared with a technique with no volatile agent, the incidence of awareness is virtually eliminated by using a volatile agent.[1]

REASONING:

For K-type questions, it is best to first determine which statements are true. Once this is done, some answers can be eliminated just because of their location on the list. In this question, choice 4 is definitely true, which eliminates A and B as possible answers. Then one must decide if all the statements are true. Choice 1 is definitely not true owing to the low dose of halothane given, which eliminates E as a possible answer. Then one must decide if choice 2 is true in order to choose between C and D as answers. While it is true that halogenated agents cause decreased uterine tone, low doses have not been associated with increased operative blood loss. The key here is the low dose, which eliminates choice 2 and makes D the correct answer.

REFERENCES:

1. Hughes SC, Levinson G, Rosen MA. Shnider and Levinson's Anesthesia for Obstetrics, 4th ed. Philadelphia, Lippincott Williams & Wilkins, 2002, pp. 220–222.
2. Chestnut DH. Obstetric Anesthesia Principles and Practice, 2d ed. St. Louis, Mosby, 1999, pp. 483–484.
3. Hughes SC, Levinson G, Rosen MA. Shnider and Levinson's Anesthesia for Obstetrics, 4th ed. Philadelphia, Lippincott Williams & Wilkins, 2002, p. 222, Table 11.16.
4. Morgan GE, Mikhail MS, Murray MJ. Clinical Anesthesiology, 3d ed. New York, McGraw-Hill, 2002, pp. 830–833.

BOOK A:

Answer D

Pain

QUESTION 50

QUESTION (K-type):

Stellate ganglion block is associated with ipsilateral

(1) Mydriasis.
(2) Diaphoresis.
(3) Exophthalmos.
(4) Scleral hyperemia.

CORRECT ANSWER: D (4 only is correct.)

SUMMARY:

Stellate ganglion block is performed by injection of local anesthetic in the neck to block the sympathetic innervation of the ipsilateral head, face, and arm. Interruption of the sympathetic tone leads to Horner's syndrome. Horner's syndrome is characterized by ptosis, miosis, anhydrosis, and enopthalmos. In addition, interruption of sympathetic tone results in vasodilation of the affected areas. This yields an increase in temperature of the skin, hyperemia of the ipsilateral sclera, and nasal congestion.

EXPLANATION:

(1) *Incorrect.* Mydriasis (pupil enlargement) is the opposite of what is seen following successful stellate block.
(2) *Incorrect.* Diaphoresis (sweating) is blocked by successful stellate block.
(3) *Incorrect.* Exophthalmos (protruding eye) is the opposite of what is seen following successful stellate.
(4) *Correct.* Scleral hyperemia owing to vasodilation is seen following successful stellate block.

REASONING:

The stellate ganglion is composed of the fusion of the inferior cervical ganglion and the first thoracic ganglion. However, the sympathetic innervation of the head, face, and upper extremity do not all pass through the stellate ganglion. Thus, when stellate ganglion block is performed, 15 to 20 mL of solution is used with the hope that it will spread along the prevertebral fascia superiorly and inferiorly down to T4. When this is accomplished, interruption of sympathetic tone will result in ipsilateral ptosis (lid droop) by blocking sympathetic innervation to the superior tarsal muscle (Mueller's third), anhydrosis (lack of facial sweating), miosis (small pupil), and enophthalmos (recession of the eyeball into the orbit). Slight enophthalmos results from interruption of sympathetic tone to the orbitalis muscle (Mueller's first), which spans the inferior orbital fissure. Release of vasoconstrictive tone results in nasal congestion, scleral hyperemia, facial flushing, and upper extremity temperature increase. The best answer is D.

REFERENCES:

Cousins M, Bridenbaugh P. Neural Blockade in Clinical Anesthesia and Management of Pain, 3d ed. Philadelphia: Lippincott Williams & Wilkins, 1998, pp. 428–429.

Morgan GE, Mikhail MS, Murray MJ. Clinical Anesthesiology, 3d ed. New York, McGraw-Hill, 2002, p. 294.

BOOK A:

Answer A

Pharmacology

QUESTION 51

QUESTION (K-type):

A 22-year-old man is unconscious after free-basing "crack." Likely findings include

(1) Depressed ST segments.
(2) Hyperthermia.
(3) Premature ventricular contractions.
(4) Pinpoint pupils.

CORRECT ANSWER: A (1, 2, and 3 are correct.)

SUMMARY:

Crack is cocaine. Signs of cocaine overdose relate to its actions both as a local anesthetic and its inhibition of norepinephrine reuptake. Complications include myocardial ischemia or infarction, serious and sudden arrhythmias, high-output congestive heart failure, rhabdomyolysis, acute renal failure, seizures, hyperpyrexia, and respiratory depression. The increased sympathetic tone associated with cocaine use leads to enlarged pupils.

EXPLANATION:

(1) *Correct.* Cocaine use through its sympathomimetic effects increases heart rate, blood pressure, and myocardial work. Myocardial ischemia is not infrequent and can manifest as ST-segment depression.
(2) *Correct.* Cocaine is associated with life-threatening hyperthermia.
(3) *Correct.* Premature ventricular contractions are seen often in cocaine overdose.
(4) *Incorrect.* The increased sympathetic tone leads to the look of "wide-eyed surprise" associated with increased sympathetic tone. Pupil size is increased. Pinpoint pupils are associated with opiate overdose rather than crack. When an opiate is mixed with cocaine or an amphetamine, this is referred to as "speedballing." The pupil size then may be hard to predict.

REASONING:

This question tests knowledge of the physical findings associated with acute cocaine intoxication. These effects can include hypertension, tachycardia, and other sequelae of increased sympathetic output. Importantly, propranolol was used widely in the past to control cocaine-induced hypertension but has been associated with lethal hypertensive exacerbation owing to unopposed α-adrenergic stimulation.[1] Labetalol is a better choice for controlling cocaine-induced hypertension because it has both α and β blockade.

REFERENCES:

1. Barash PG, Cullen BF, Stoelting RK. Clinical Anesthesia, 4th ed. Philadelphia, Lippincott Williams & Wilkins, 2001, p. 975.
2. Haim DY, Lippmann ML, Goldberg SK, Walkenstein MD. The pulmonary complications of crack cocaine: A comprehensive review. Chest 107:233–240, 1995.
3. Lange RA, Hillis LD. Medical progress: Cardiovascular complications of cocaine use. N Engl J Med 345:351–358, 2001.

4. Traub SJ, Hoffman RS, Nelson LS. Current concepts: Body packing—the internal concealment of illicit drugs. N Engl J Med 349:2519–2526, 2003.

BOOK A:

QUESTION 52

Answer A

Pharmacology

QUESTION (K-type):

Administration of halothane to a healthy patient causes

(1) Decreased myocardial contractility.
(2) Depressed baroreceptor response.
(3) Increased venous capacitance.
(4) Decreased systemic vascular resistance.

CORRECT ANSWER: A (1, 2, and 3 are correct.)

SUMMARY:

Halothane is a halogenated alkane volatile anesthetic that has many cardiovascular effects. It causes a decrease in mean arterial pressure (MAP) through direct myocardial depression. Halothane blunts the baroreceptor response because an elevated heart rate would be expected with a decreased MAP, but heart rate does not increase with halothane. Vasodilation does occur with halothane, but systemic vascular resistance does not change because cardiac output also decreases.

EXPLANATION:

(1) *Correct.* Halothane depresses the heart and cardiac output in a dose-dependent manner. This effect occurs because halothane interferes with intracellular calcium utilization.
(2) *Correct.* Halothane blunts the carotid and aortic arch baroreceptor response to decreases in MAP. Without halothane, a drop in blood pressure causes a decrease in parasympathetic output from the baroreceptors, and the heart rate rises. The heart rate does not rise with decreases in MAP caused by halothane.
(3) *Correct.* Halothane causes vasodilatation and increased venous capacitance.
(4) *Incorrect.* Although halothane causes vasodilatation and a drop in MAP, systemic vascular resistance (SVR) is unchanged because the drop in MAP caused by halothane parallels the drop in cardiac output (CO). This is illustrated by the equation

$$SVR = \frac{(MAP - CVP)}{CO}.$$

REASONING:

Choice 1 is clearly correct because one of the unique properties of halothane is its depression on myocardium. This allows answers C and D to be eliminated. Choice 2 is correct because an increase in heart rate is not seen when using halothane, leaving only answers A and E as possibilities. Answer A is correct because choice 4 is incorrect. When deciding whether or not choice 4 is correct, it is helpful to write out the equation for SVR. In examining the equation it becomes obvious that not only MAP affects SVR, but CO does as well, and since both decrease equally, SVR is unchanged. The best answer is A.

REFERENCES:

Stoelting RK, Miller RD. Basics of Anesthesia, 4th ed. New York, Churchill Livingstone, 2000, pp. 46–49.
Morgan GE, Mikhail MS, Murray MJ. Clinical Anesthesiology, 3d ed. New York, McGraw-Hill, 2002, pp. 139–140.

Answer A

Cardiovascular

QUESTION (K-type):

Indications for administration of calcium chloride during cardiopulmonary resuscitation (CPR) include

(1) Acute hyperkalemia.
(2) Electromechanical dissociation.
(3) Verapamil toxicity.
(4) Digoxin toxicity.

CORRECT ANSWER: A (1, 2, and 3 are correct.)

SUMMARY:

Calcium chloride is indicated during CPR under specific conditions such as hyperkalemia, hypocalcemia, calcium channel blocker toxicity, and hypermagnesemia. Electromechanical dissociation (EMD) or the newer term pulseless electrical activity (PEA) is a generic diagnosis where the patient has electrical cardiac activity without perfusion. It includes the above-mentioned conditions in addition to other causes such as hypoxia, hypovolemia, acidosis, hypothermia, drug overdose, tamponade, tension pneumothorax, and massive pulmonary embolus.

EXPLANATION:

(1) *Correct.* Calcium chloride is indicated in the treatment of hyperkalemia. It antagonizes the effect of high potassium levels on the heart.
(2) *Correct.* Pulseless electrical activity includes many conditions, among which are hyperkalemia, hypermagnesemia, and calcium channel blocker toxicity that can be treated with calcium chloride.
(3) *Correct.* Calcium chloride can be used to treat verapamil overdose.
(4) *Incorrect.* Hypercalemia and hypokalemia worsen the digoxin toxicity. Therefore, calcium chloride is contraindicated.

REASONING:

This question tests knowledge of the indications for calcium administration during CPR. Specific pathology such as hyperkalemia, hypermagnesemia, and calcium channel blocker toxicity all can be treated with administration of calcium chloride. Choices 1, 2, and 3 are correct. Therefore, A is the best answer.

REFERENCES:

Barash PG, Cullen BF, Stoelting RK. Clinical Anesthesia, 4th ed. Philadelphia, Lippincott Williams & Wilkins, 2001, pp. 1485–1501.
Morgan GE, Mikhail MS, Murray MJ. Clinical Anesthesiology, 3d ed. New York, McGraw-Hill, 2002, p. 924.

Answer D

Physiology

QUESTION (K-type):

A 27-year-old man is undergoing emergency bronchoscopy with propofol-vecuronium anesthesia after aspirating a peanut. Intervals of apneic oxygenation are used to facilitate the procedure. Initial blood gas values while breathing pure oxygen are Pa_{O_2} = 400 mm Hg and Pa_{CO_2} = 30 mm Hg. Effects of 10 minutes of apneic oxygenation at a flow rate of 10 L/min include

(1) Decreased heart rate.
(2) Decreased Pa_{O_2} to 50 mm Hg.
(3) Cutaneous vasoconstriction.
(4) Increased Pa_{CO_2} to 60 mm Hg.

CORRECT ANSWER: D (4 only is correct.)

SUMMARY:

Apneic oxygenation is a technique used to maintain oxygenation in the absence of ventilation. A catheter supplying oxygen is placed above the carina to replace oxygen absorbed by the lungs. This technique can provide adequate oxygenation for more than 30 minutes but is limited by the development of hypercapnia. Without ventilation, hypercapnia increases as a function of the duration of apnea. Hypercapnia leads to signs of increased sympathetic tone, including tachycardia, hypertension, and dilation of conjunctival and superficial facial vessels leading to flushing.

EXPLANATION:

(1) *Incorrect.* An increased heart rate rather than a decreased heart rate would be expected owing to the development of hypercapnia and its associated increase in sympathetic tone.
(2) *Incorrect.* Apneic oxygenation can maintain adequate levels of oxygen despite a lack of ventilation for up to a half hour, and the Pa_{O_2} would be expected to be significantly higher than 50 mm Hg after only 10 minutes.
(3) *Incorrect.* Hypercapnia also leads to facial flushing and cutaneous vasodilation rather than vasoconstriction despite the increase in sympathetic tone.
(4) *Correct.* During apnea, carbon dioxide is not eliminated, and the arterial partial pressure rises. The partial pressure of carbon dioxide typically rises by approximately 6 mm Hg in the first minute and by 3 mm Hg every minute thereafter. The expected rise after 10 minutes would be approximately $6 + (3 \times 9) = 33$. With a staring Pa_{CO_2} of 30 mm Hg, the total Pa_{CO_2} would be approximately 63 mm Hg. Therefore, an increase in Pa_{CO_2} to 60 mm Hg would be expected.

REASONING:

This question tests knowledge of apneic oxygenation. The most important aspects to understand include the ability of the technique to maintain oxygenation in the absence of ventilation for significant periods of time. It is also important to know that the technique is limited by the development of hypercarbia and respiratory acidosis. The sympathetic effects of hypercarbia are well known and include tachycardia, arrhythmias, hypertension, and cutaneous flushing. The best answer is choice D.

REFERENCE:

Barash PG, Cullen BF, Stoelting RK. Clinical Anesthesia, 4th ed. Philadelphia, Lippincott Williams & Wilkins, 2001, p. 834.
Morgan GE, Mikhail MS, Murray MJ. Clinical Anesthesiology, 3d ed. New York, McGraw-Hill, 2002, p. 465.

Answer B

Equipment/Physics

QUESTION (K-type):

In a patient with normal hemodynamics, systemic blood pressure is measured using a radial artery catheter and a noninvasive oscillometric blood pressure (NIBP) monitor on the same arm. Compared with the readings from the NIBP monitor, the indwelling catheter would show

(1) The same or higher systolic blood pressure.
(2) Lower diastolic pressure if the transducer is damped.
(3) The same mean blood pressure.
(4) Lower blood pressure values if the catheter is replaced by one with a larger diameter.

CORRECT ANSWER: B (1 and 3 are correct.)

SUMMARY:

The "gold standard" for blood pressure monitoring is intraarterial monitoring. Overdamping by lengthy tubing, extra stopcocks, air bubbles, and increased blood viscosity would reduce the arterial waveform and therefore systolic pressure. Underdamping by decreasing tubing size or increasing catheter size would raise the blood pressure artifactually. Compared with the noninvasive blood pressure cuff, the catheter-transducer system usually gives a higher blood pressure value owing to underdamping and resonance. (See also Question 153, Book A for an explanation of pulse-wave amplification.)

EXPLANATION:

(1) ***Correct.*** An old study comparing automated auscultatory and oscillometric pressure against direct invasive measurements of arterial pressure showed that indirect methods underestimated the systolic and overestimated diastolic pressure.[1] One way to remember this is that the catheter-transducer system includes extra components such as tubing and stopcocks that contribute to underdamping and resonance. This results in direct systolic arterial pressure often exceeding indirect noninvasive pressure.

(2) ***Incorrect.*** A dampened system would result in lowered systolic but not diastolic pressure. This occurs when the frequency of the system is too low to faithfully reproduce the arterial waveform, producing a more protracted or smaller wave.[2]

(3) ***Correct.*** Mean arterial pressure (MAP) is the most accurate value measured by oscillometry and is taken at the cuff pressure at which maximal oscillation of the arterial pulse occurs. In the catheter-transducer system, the MAP is calculated by integrating the area under the arterial waveform. Although studies have reported slight differences between the invasive and noninvasive MAP, this is questionably significant. Overthinking would lead one to eliminate this choice. However, simply understanding that the MAP is one of the more accurate values measured in oscillimetry and less subjected to a dampening or overshooting in the catheter-transducer system would make this choice correct.

(4) ***Incorrect.*** Larger catheters create greater ringing or resonance in the system. This would result in higher systolic pressure.

REASONING:

This is a challenging question that demands a thorough understanding of noninvasive and catheter-transducer methods for measuring arterial blood pressure. It is important for the reader to review the principles of oscillometric methods as well as factors that affect damping of catheter-transducer systems. Understanding the physics behind intraarterial monitoring helps eliminate choices 2 and 4. Whether or not one knows that choice 3 is correct, the only logical choice left is answer B (1 and 3).

REFERENCES:

1. Davis RF. Clinical comparison of automated auscultatory and oscillometric and catheter-transducer measurements of arterial pressure. J Clin Monit 1:114, 1985.
2. Miller RD, Miller ED, Reves JG, et al. Anesthesia, 5th ed. New York, Churchill Livingstone, 2000, pp. 1132–133, Fig. 30-12.
3. Morgan GE, Mikhail MS, Murray MJ. Clinical Anesthesiology, 3d ed. New York, McGraw-Hill, 2002, p. 93.

BOOK A:

QUESTION 56

Answer D

Pharmacology

QUESTION (K-type):

A 20-kg 4-year-old boy receives atropine 0.3 mg intramuscularly 1 hour prior to inguinal herniorrhaphy under general anesthesia. Forty minutes later while still in the preoperative preparation room, his temperature is 38.6°C. Likely causes of the temperature elevation include

(1) Malignant hyperthermia.
(2) Alteration of central temperature regulation.
(3) Release of catecholamines.
(4) Suppression of sweating.

CORRECT ANSWER: D (4 only is correct.)

SUMMARY:

Anticholinergic agents are used in anesthesia for various purposes. Understanding the pharmacology of these agents is important because there are many side effects, including atrial dysrhythmias, central nervous system (CNS) effects of both stimulation and depression, decreased peristalsis, mydriasis, cycloplegia, and urinary retention. Atropine is a tertiary amine that can be administered intravenously, intramuscularly, and into the trachea. It is particularly effective on the heart (treating bradycardia) and the bronchial smooth muscle (bronchodilation). Scopolamine is also a tertiary amine with greater antisialagogue properties than atropine. It also has greater CNS effects, as evidenced by use of this agent as a sedative, and for prevention of motion sickness. Glycopyrrolate is a quaternary agent that does not cross the blood–brain barrier. It causes a mild increase in heart rate, has antisialagogue effects, and has little or no CNS effects. Glycopyrrolate is often given to counter the bradycardia of neostigmine when reversing neuromuscular blockade. (Also see Question 6, Book A.)

EXPLANATION:

(1) *Incorrect.* While malignant hyperthermia (MH) always should be a concern in the presence of hyperthermia, there is no other clinical indication that the patient is at risk for MH or that the patient has signs of MH other than the elevated temperature.

(2) *Incorrect.* While atropine, a tertiary amine, does cross the blood-brain barrier, the CNS effects are behavioral, including memory deficits, restlessness, unconsciousness, and hallucinations. This is known as *central anticholinergic syndrome*. There is no known alteration of central temperature regulation.

(3) *Incorrect.* Anticholinergic agents block acetylcholine from binding to the muscarinic cholinergic receptor. Blockade of the receptors in the sinoatrial node results in tachycardia. This, however, is due to inhibition of vagal tone and not release of catecholamines.

(4) **Correct.** Suppression of sweating is a known effect of anticholinergic agents and is the likely mechanism of the patient's elevated temperature.

REASONING:

This question tests the reader's understanding of the pharmacology of anticholinergic agents. Choice 1 is possible, but without further information, it is not *likely*. If there is any uncertainty about choice 1, the reader should know that choice 3 is not the mechanism of anticholinergic agents. This should narrow the choices to 2 and 4. The reader should know that the mechanism of hyperthermia with anticholinergic agents is suppression of sweating and not central alterations. D is the best answer.

REFERENCE:

Barash PG, Cullen BF, Stoelting RK. Clinical Anesthesia, 4th ed. Philadelphia, Lippincott Williams & Wilkins, 2001, p. 561.

Morgan GE, Mikhail MS, Murray MJ. Clinical Anesthesiology, 3d ed. New York, McGraw-Hill, 2002, pp. 207–211.

BOOK A:

Answer B

Pharmacology

QUESTION 57

QUESTION (K-type):

If ketorolac 30 mg were substituted for meperidine 100 mg after an outpatient inguinal herniorrhaphy, the patient would experience less

(1) Respiratory depression.
(2) Analgesia.
(3) Nausea.
(4) Bleeding.

CORRECT ANSWER: B (1 and 3 are correct.)

SUMMARY:

Ketorolac is a nonsteroidal anti-inflammatory drug that is administered either intravenously or intramuscularly. It is used for short-term management of acute pain and works by blocking prostaglandin synthesis. Ketorolac is mainly a peripherally acting drug and causes minimal, if any, central side effects associated with opiates such as nausea and vomiting, sedation, and respiratory depression. Disadvantages of ketorolac include inhibition of platelet aggregation, renal toxicity, gastrointestinal ulcerations, and a ceiling effect to the amount of analgesia produced by increasing the dose of ketorolac. In addition, patients with asthma, nasal polyps, and aspirin allergies have a higher incidence of allergic reactions to ketorolac.

EXPLANATION:

(1) **Correct.** Ketorolac primarily acts peripherally, with no respiratory depressive effects and minimal nausea in comparison with opiates, which act centrally and can cause both side effects.
(2) **Incorrect.** Ketorolac 30 mg and meperedine 100 mg are equivalent analgesic doses.
(3) **Correct.** See above.
(4) **Incorrect.** Ketorolac produces more bleeding when compared with opiates because ketorolac inhibits platelet aggregation. This occurs because ketorolac inhibits cyclooxygenase, preventing thromboxane synthesis, which is necessary for platelet aggregation.

145

Clearly, choices 1 and 3 are correct because nausea and respiratory depression are well-known opiate side effects not usually associated with ketorolac. Choice 4 is incorrect because one of the principal concerns with using ketorolac is the increased bleeding postoperatively caused by platelet inhibition. This allows answers C, D, and E to be eliminated. Only choice 2 remains, which is incorrect because the doses listed provide roughly equivalent analgesia. B is the best answer.

REFERENCE:

Stoelting RK. Pharmacology and Physiology in Anesthetic Practice, 3d ed. Philadelphia, Lippincott Raven Publishers, 1999, pp. 255–256.

Morgan GE, Mikhail MS, Murray MJ. Clinical Anesthesiology, 3d ed. New York, McGraw-Hill, 2002, p. 248.

BOOK A: **QUESTION 58**

Answer D

OB/Regional

QUESTION (K-type):

An asymptomatic 32-year-old man with asthma undergoes herniorrhaphy under 1.5% lidocaine epidural anesthesia to a sensory level of T2–3. Which of the following will occur with this level of anesthesia?

(1) The ability to cough will be normal.
(2) Vital capacity will be unchanged.
(3) Intraoperative bronchospasm will be prevented.
(4) Tidal volume will be unchanged.

CORRECT ANSWER: D (4 only is correct.)

SUMMARY:

Epidural anesthesia with high sensory levels can cause paralysis of abdominal and intercostal muscles, leading to decreased expiratory reserve volume, peak expiratory flow, and maximum minute ventilation.[1] Vital capacity is reduced in these patients as a result of the decrease in expiratory reserve volume. Abdominal and intercostal muscle paralysis with high sensory levels is also associated with decreased ability to cough, which can be problematic in patients with lung disease and/or copious secretions. While the sympathectomy associated with high sensory epidural anesthesia theoretically could increase bronchomotor tone owing to unopposed parasympathetic innervation of the airways, this is not a clinically significant problem in asthmatic patients.[2]

EXPLANATION:

(1) *Incorrect.* The ability to cough in these patients is abnormal owing to paralysis of abdominal and intercostal muscles.
(2) *Incorrect.* Vital capacity is reduced owing to the reduction in expiratory reserve volume.
(3) *Incorrect.* Intraoperative bronchospasm will not be prevented in this patient because the airways will have primarily parasympathetic tone owing to the sympathectomy associated with a T2 epidural sensory level.
(4) *Correct.* Tidal volume is unchanged in patients with high sensory levels from neuraxial anesthesia.[1]

REASONING:

The question tests the reader's knowledge of the effects of a high sensory level of anesthesia associated with neuraxial blockade. Choice 1 is incorrect because cough is impaired in this situation. Since expiratory reserve volume is a component of vital capacity and is reduced, vital capacity must be reduced, making choice 2 incorrect. Choice 3 can be eliminated because choice 1 is incorrect. However, bronchospasm in an asthmatic patient will not be prevented by a sympathectomy because increased sympathetic tone favors bronchodilation. Choice 4 is correct because lung volumes do not change considerably with high sensory levels. This makes D the best answer.

REFERENCES:

1. Barash PG, Cullen BF, Stoelting RK. Clinical Anesthesia, 4th ed. Philadelphia, Lippincott Williams & Wilkins, 2001, p. 663.
2. Stoelting RK, Dierdorf SF. Anesthesia and Co-Existing Disease, 4th ed. New York, Churchill Livingstone, 2002, pp. 200–201.
3. Morgan GE, Mikhail MS, Murray MJ. Clinical Anesthesiology, 3d ed. New York, McGraw-Hill, 2002, p. 484, Fig. 22-5 (pp. 271–273), Spirogram Showing Static Lung Volumes.

BOOK A:

QUESTION 59

Answer D

OB/Regional

QUESTION (K-type):

True statements concerning epidurally administered morphine include

(1) The long duration of analgesia results from high lipid solubility.
(2) Pruritus is completely reversed by naloxone.
(3) Plasma morphine levels are lower than those seen after intramuscular administration.
(4) Analgesia is inadequate for the pain of labor.

CORRECT ANSWER: D (4 only is correct.)

SUMMARY:

Morphine is a hydrophilic opiate. With epidural administration, a small amount diffuses into the intrathecal space and acts on spinal opiate receptors. Its water solubility allows it to remain in the intrathecal space, resulting in a duration of action of approximately 12 to 16 hours.[1] Side effects of epidural morphine include pruritus, urinary retention, sedation, and respiratory depression. While epidural narcotics alone are inadequate for the pain of labor, they can be used to minimize local anesthetic concentration and the motor blockade associated with local anesthetics.[2]

EXPLANATION:

(1) **Incorrect.** Morphine is a water-soluble narcotic.
(2) **Incorrect.** The pruritus associated with epidural morphine is reduced significantly by naloxone but not completely eliminated.[3]
(3) **Incorrect.** When compared, plasma levels of morphine were similar when intravenous and epidural doses were given.[4] Plasma levels tend to fluctuate more with intramuscular bolus administration but have similar pharmacokinetics to intravenous dosing.[5] Therefore, plasma morphine levels are similar to those seen after intramuscular administration.
(4) **Correct.** Intrathecal morphine can provide adequate analgesia for labor.[6] When epidural morphine was studied, it had a slow onset and required high doses associated with unacceptable side effects to be used as a sole analgesic in labor.[7]

REASONING:

A good general rule when taking tests is that if an answer is absolute (such as choice 2), it is usually not true. Very few things are absolute in medicine. Naloxone is an effective agent for pruritus but will not completely reverse this side effect. This question requires knowledge that morphine is hydrophilic, which eliminates choice 1. Since choices 1 and 2 are wrong, the correct answer must be D.

REFERENCES:

1. Barash PG, Cullen BF, Stoelting RK. Clinical Anesthesia, 4th ed. Philadelphia, Lippincott Williams & Wilkins, 2001, p. 1321.
2. Hughes SC, Levinson G, Rosen MA: Shnider and Levinson's Anesthesia for Obstetrics, 4th ed. Philadelphia, Lippincott Williams & Wilkins, 2002, pp. 165–166.
3. Kendrick WD, Woods AM, Daly MY, et al. Naloxone versus nalbuphine infusion for prophylaxis of epidural morphine-induced pruritus. Anesth Analg 1996;82:641–647.
4. Barash PG, Cullen BF, Stoelting RK. Clinical Anesthesia, 4th ed. Philadelphia, Lippincott Williams & Wilkins, 2001, p. 1321, Fig. 54-7.
5. Ibid., p. 1319.
6. Hughes, SC, Levinson G, Rosen MA. Shnider and Levinson's Anesthesia for Obstetrics, 4th ed. Philadelphia, Lippincott Williams & Wilkins, 2002, pp. 155–156.
7. Ibid., pp. 162–163.
8. Morgan GE, Mikhail MS, Murray MJ. Clinical Anesthesiology, 3d ed. New York, McGraw-Hill, 2002, pp. 166–169, 823.

BOOK A:

Answer B

Clinical Anesthesia

QUESTION 60

QUESTION (K-type):

A 36-year-old woman is scheduled for cholecystectomy. She is 65 inches tall and weighs 180 kg. Compared with a patient of the same height who weighs 60 kg, this patient is at increased risk for

(1) Hypoxemia in the supine position.
(2) Fasting hypoglycemia.
(3) Acid aspiration syndrome.
(4) Difficult reversal of neuromuscular block.

CORRECT ANSWER: B (1 and 3 are correct.)

SUMMARY:

Obese patients have a higher incidence of many diseases, including type 2 diabetes, coronary artery disease, gastroesophageal reflux, and hypertension. In addition, increased abdominal mass leads to restrictive lung disease, reduced functional residual capacity (FRC), and arterial hypoxemia.[1] Morbid obesity is defined as a body mass index (BMI) of greater than 35 kg/m^2.[2] Lipid-soluble drugs have a higher volume of distribution and may require higher loading doses to achieve clinical effect, whereas water-soluble drugs such as neuromuscular blockers have a decreased volume of distribution and should be dosed according to ideal body weight.

EXPLANATION:

(1) **Correct.** Obese patients develop restrictive lung disease owing to compression of the diaphragm by abdominal adipose tissue. This results in decreased functional residual capacity (FRC) that may fall below closing capacity. The supine position further reduces FRC, leading to atelectasis and ventilation-perfusion mismatch.

(2) **Incorrect.** Obese patients are at risk for developing type 2 diabetes mellitus that is characterized by insulin resistance and hyperglycemia. These patients should not develop fasting hypoglycemia secondary to insulin resistance.

(3) **Correct.** Hiatal hernia and gastroesophageal reflux disease are more common in the obese. In addition, delayed gastric emptying and hyperacidic gastric fluid place obese patients at higher risk for acid aspiration syndrome.

(4) *Incorrect.* Water-soluble drugs such as neuromuscular blockers can have a decreased volume of distribution in obese patients. Following an appropriate dose of muscle relaxant based on ideal body weight, obese patients should respond to anticholinesterase reversal agents normally.

REASONING:

There are several challenging aspects to this question. Although choice 2 may sound good, obese patients with diabetes mellitus type 2 should not develop fasting hypoglycemia owing to their disease alone. Patients using exogenous insulin for glycemic control may be at risk for hypoglycemia when fasting. Choice 4 is incorrect because obese patients should respond to neuromuscular blocking drugs appropriately. B is the best answer.

REFERENCES:

1. Stoelting RK, Miller RD. Basics of Anesthesia, 4th ed. New York, Churchill Livingstone, 2000, pp. 316–318.
2. Barash PG, Cullen BF, Stoelting RK. Clinical Anesthesia, 4th ed. Philadelphia, Lippincott Williams & Wilkins, 2001, pp. 975, 1035–1041.
3. Morgan GE, Mikhail MS, Murray MJ. Clinical Anesthesiology, 3d ed. New York, McGraw-Hill, 2002, pp. 748–749.

BOOK A:

Answer D

Physiology

QUESTION 61

QUESTION (K-type):

Radiologic findings in advanced emphysema include

(1) Ground-glass appearance of lung fields.
(2) Increased cardiothoracic ratio.
(3) Increased bronchial markings.
(4) Flattening of the hemidiaphragms.

CORRECT ANSWER: D (4 only is correct.)

SUMMARY:

Emphysema is one of the chronic obstructive pulmonary diseases, characterized by loss of elasticity in lung tissue and disruption of alveolar septa creating large air sacs or bullae. This loss of elasticity that normally supports small airways causes premature airway collapse during exhalation. It also causes lung hyperinflation, leading to increased residual volume, increased functional residual capacity, and increased total lung capacity. Emphysema is characterized on chest x-ray as more radiolucent or darker, hyperinflated lungs with flattened hemidiaphragms and a long, narrow cardiac silhouette.

EXPLANATION:

(1) *Incorrect.* Ground-glass appearance of the lung fields is not associated with emphysema.
(2) *Incorrect.* Increased cardiothoracic ratio occurs with either an increase in heart size or decrease in lung size. Despite the fact that many patients with emphysema have cardiac disease and a potentially enlarged heart, cardiothoracic ratio is decreased in emphysematous patients as lung size increases significantly.
(3) *Incorrect.* Lungs are hyperinflated in emphysema, with less tissue density to absorb radiation, making bronchial markings less visible. Increased bronchial markings are seen in patients with chronic bronchitis because of increased secretions in the airways.
(4) *Correct.* The hemidiaphragms are flattened as the lungs are hyperinflated, pushing downward on the hemidiaphragms.

149

REASONING:

Knowing the physiology of emphysema, namely, destruction of the elasticity of the lungs causing hyperinflation, makes the correct answer obvious without much knowledge of radiology. Since the lungs are enlarged in emphysematous patients, the other structures will appear smaller or be pushed by the lungs. The heart will appear smaller, and the hemidiaphragms will be pushed downward. This eliminates choice 2 because the cardiothoracic ratio is smaller, and choice 4 is correct because the hemidiaphragms are pushed downward and flattened out. D is the best answer.

REFERENCE:

Goodman LR. Felson's Principles of Chest Roentgenology, 2d ed. Philadelphia, Saunders, 1999, pp. 159, 239–240.
Morgan GE, Mikhail MS, Murray MJ. Clinical Anesthesiology, 3d ed. New York, McGraw-Hill, 2002, pp. 516–517.

BOOK A:

Answer A

Pharmacology

QUESTION 62

QUESTION (K-type):

Anesthetic agents that are safe for use in a patient with acute intermittent porphyria include

(1) Ketamine.
(2) Isoflurane.
(3) Pancuronium.
(4) Etomidate.

CORRECT ANSWER: A (1, 2, and 3 are correct.)

SUMMARY:

This is a classic boards question that tests knowledge of an interesting but rare condition that can affect anesthetic care. The porphyrias are a group of enzymatic disorders in the production of heme from δ-aminolaevulinic acid (δ-ALA). The heme formed by these enzymatic reactions is used in the synthesis of hemoglobin and cytochrome P450s. Importantly, anything inducing the formation of hemoglobin or cytochrome P450s will induce δ-ALA synthetase, causing the buildup of harmful porphyrin precursors.[1] Acute intermittent porphyria is a specific type of porphyria in which the enzyme porphobilinogen deaminase is defective, leading to the buildup of porphobilinogen when δ-ALA synthetase is induced. Similar to other porphyrins, porphobilinogen is neurotoxic and can cause autonomic dysfunction, electrolyte abnormalities, neuropsychiatric disturbances, cranial nerve palsies, and muscle weakness severe enough to progress to respiratory failure. Attacks are precipitated by drugs or physiologic factors such as menstruation, fasting, dehydration, infection, and stress that can induce heme synthesis. It is important to avoid drugs such as barbiturates and etomidate that can trigger attacks during anesthesia. The stress of surgery and anesthesia can precipitate an attack in the absence of triggering agents.

EXPLANATION:

(1) **Correct.** The following drugs have been used safely in patients with porphyria or are unlikely to provoke an attack: inhaled anesthetics, propofol, ketamine, neuromuscular blockers, anticholinergics, acetylcholinesterase inhibitors, local anesthetics, benzodiazepines, H_2 blockers, α- and β-agonists, epinephrine, and diltiazem.
(2) **Correct.** See above.
(3) **Correct.** See above.

(4) *Incorrect.* Possible triggering agents include all barbiturates (thiopental, thiamylal, and methohexital), etomidate, ketorolac, phenacetin, pentazocine, and nifedipine. Etomidate is the only choice listed that can precipitate an attack, and choice 4 is incorrect.

REASONING:

This is a difficult question to answer because the well-known triggering agents, barbiturates, are not listed as one of the answer choices. Nonetheless, knowledge that anything inducing cytochrome P450s can incite acute intermittent porphyria allows choices 2 and 3 to be chosen as correct answers because neither isoflurane nor pancuronium induces cytochrome P450s. Thus answers B, C, and D can be eliminated. This allows a 50 percent chance at obtaining the correct answer if you are not sure about etomidate, which can induce liver enzymes and precipitate an attack. A is the best answer.

REFERENCES:

1. Barash PG, Cullen BF, Stoelting RK. Clinical Anesthesia, 4th ed. Philadelphia, Lippincott Williams & Wilkins, 2001, p. 541.
2. Stoelting RK, Dierdorf SF. Anesthesia and Co-existing Disease, 4th ed. New York, Churchill Livingston, 2002, pp. 455–460.
3. Morgan GE, Mikhail MS, Murray MJ. Clinical Anesthesiology, 3d ed. New York, McGraw-Hill, 2002, p. 159.

BOOK A:

QUESTION 63

Answer E

Physiology

QUESTION (K-type):

Recurrent laryngeal nerve paralysis is a recognized complication of which of the following procedures?

(1) Ligation of a patent ductus arteriosus.
(2) Stellate ganglion block.
(3) Mediastinoscopy.
(4) Use of a topical ice slush during heart surgery.

CORRECT ANSWER: E (All are correct.)

SUMMARY:

The recurrent laryngeal nerve is a branch of the vagus nerve. It innervates all the muscles of the larynx except the cricothyroid muscle, which is innervated by the superior laryngeal branch of the vagus nerve. Unilateral injury to the recurrent laryngeal nerve may result in paralysis of the ipsilateral vocal cord and can present as hoarseness. Acute bilateral injury to the nerve may result in stridor or respiratory distress because the unopposed adduction of the vocal cord by the cricothyroid muscle keeps the vocal cords in a paramedian position. Chronic bilateral injury may result in aphonia because the vocal cord eventually is positioned more medially.[1] The vagus nerve or any of its branches may be injured during many different types of cardiothoracic surgery or nonthoracic surgery owing to endotracheal intubation, positioning, central line placement, or surgical dissection.[1,2]

EXPLANATION:

(1) *Correct.* Recurrent laryngeal nerve paralysis is a reported complication of ligation of patent ductus arteriosus (PDA), along with inadvertent ligation of left pulmonary artery or descending aorta and bleeding from PDA disruption.[1]
(2) *Correct.* Recurrent laryngeal nerve paralysis is a reported complication of stellate ganglion block, along with hematoma, pneumothorax, brachial plexus blockade, in-

travascular or subarachnoid injection, osteitis, or mediastinitis following esophageal puncture.

(3) **Correct.** Recurrent laryngeal nerve paralysis is a reported complication of mediastinoscopy, along with cerebral ischemia from compression innominate artery, pneumothorax, air embolism, and phrenic nerve injury.

(4) **Correct.** Recurrent laryngeal nerve paralysis is a reported complication of use of topical ice slush during heart surgery, along with phrenic nerve injury.[2]

REASONING:

Key concepts to answering this question include understanding the anatomy of the recurrent laryngeal nerve and the brachial plexus, as well as the factors that contribute to nerve injuries. Each choice listed is a procedure in which the surgeon operates in the thorax and is in proximity to the course of the recurrent larygneal nerve. Paralysis is a recognized complication of each of the procedures

REFERENCES:

1. Miller RD, Miller ED, Reves JG, et al. Anesthesia, 5th ed. New York, Churchill Livingstone, 2000, pp. 1839, 2183.
2. Sharma AD, Parmley CL, Sreeram G, Grocott H. Peripheral nerve injuries during cardiac surgery: Risk factors, diagnosis, prognosis, and prevention. Anesth Analg 91:1358–1368, 2000.
3. Morgan GE, Mikhail MS, Murray MJ. Clinical Anesthesiology, 3d ed. New York, McGraw-Hill, 2002, pp. 59–63, 333, 545–546.

BOOK A:

Answer A

Physiology

QUESTION 64

QUESTION (K-type):

Clinical situations associated with an increase in parasympathetic activity include

(1) Manipulation of the carotid sinus.
(2) Intestinal insufflation during colonoscopy.
(3) Traction on the superior oblique muscle during strabismus surgery.
(4) Caudal anesthesia for excision of a pilonidal cyst.

CORRECT ANSWER: A (1, 2, and 3 are correct.)

SUMMARY:

Manipulation of the carotid sinus often will increase parasympathetic tone and in fact is known as a vagal maneuver. *Intestinal insufflation during colonoscopy also can provoke increases in parasympathetic tone and so-called vasovagal reactions. Strabismus surgery also may provoke bradycardia as a result in increased parasympathetic tone owing to traction on the ocular musculature. This has been termed the* oculocardiac reflex. *Caudal anesthesia is not typically associated with increases in parasympathetic tone.*

EXPLANATION:

(1) **Correct.** Manipulation of the carotid sinus is often done deliberately during paroxysmal supraventricular tachycardia and may end atrioventricular (AV) junctional tachyarrhythmias by increasing parasympathetic tone to the AV node.

(2) **Correct.** Approximately 17 percent of patients undergoing colonoscopy experience some type of vasovagal reaction during colonoscopy, often associated with insufflation of the colon.

(3) **Correct.** The oculocardiac reflex is mediated by afferent impulses traveling via V_1 and efferent parasympathetic impulses mediated by the vagus. It may be seen in asso-

ciation with retrobulbar block, pressure on the eyeball, or traction of the extraocular muscles. It is most common in pediatric patients undergoing strabismus surgery. The severity of the oculocardiac reflex is variable and ranges from bradycardia to sinus arrest or ventricular fibrillation. Management of the oculocardiac reflex involves cessation of the surgical stimulation, intravenous atropine, and possible infiltration with local anesthetic. Adequate depth of anesthesia also should be confirmed.

(4) **Incorrect.** Typical complications of caudal anesthesia do not include vasovagal reactions.

REASONING:

This question tests knowledge of mediators of parasympathetic activity. Unlike the sympathetic nervous system, preganglionic parasympathetic fibers terminate near the end organ they innervate. There are fewer postganglionic synapses (1:1 to 3:1) compared with the sympathetic nervous system (20:1). This accounts for the more localized actions of parasympathetic effects.[1] The key to this question is differentiating choice 4 from the other three likely causes of increased parasympathetic activity. A is the best answer.

REFERENCES:

1. Barash PG, Cullen BF, Stoelting RK. Clinical Anesthesia, 4th ed. Philadelphia, Lippincott Williams & Wilkins, 2001, p. 265.
2. Herman LL, Kurtz RC, McKee KJ, et al. Risk factors associated with vasovagal reactions during colonoscopy. Gastrointest Endosc 39:388–391, 1993.
3. Morgan GE, Mikhail MS, Murray MJ. Clinical Anesthesiology, 3d ed. New York, McGraw-Hill, 2002, p. 657.

BOOK A: **QUESTION 65**

Answer A

Physiology

QUESTION (K-type):

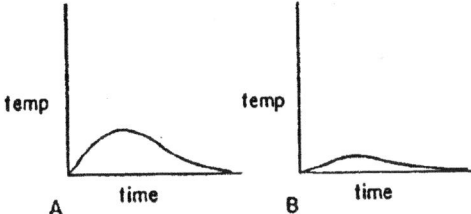

Curve *A* shown above is an accurate thermodilution curve from a patient with a cardiac output of 4 L/min. Curve *B* was obtained at the same time from the same patient. Curve *B* is consistent with

(1) An opening at the syringe-catheter junction that allows some injectate to leak out of the system.
(2) Use of room-temperature injectate when the computer is programmed for iced injectate.
(3) Injection of cold indicator solution through a long extension tube rather than directly into the correct catheter lumen.
(4) Use of 10 mL cold indicator solution when the cardiac output computer is programmed for 5 mL injectate.

CORRECT ANSWER: A (1, 2, and 3 are correct.)

SUMMARY:

Measurement of cardiac output can be determined by the thermodilution technique. This technique must be performed correctly for accurate results. Measurement of cardiac output is based on injection of solution at a proximal site and measuring its change in temperature at a distal site. This involves a system free of leaks, knowledge of correct injection sites, and the correct volume and temperature of the injected solution. If any of these are compromised, the results will be inaccurate.

EXPLANATION:

(1) **Correct.** A leak in the system at the syringe-catheter junction would cause less of the solution to reach the temperature probe and result in a lower temperature spike. This would result in a lower measured cardiac output.

(2) **Correct.** When room-temperature solution is used instead of iced solution, the measured temperature spike will be smaller, and the measured cardiac output will be falsely low.

(3) **Correct.** Use of a long extension tube for injection would result in a falsely low temperature spike owing to increased thermal loss from the extra length.

(4) **Incorrect.** Added volume of injectate would result in a greater temperature spike. This would display a falsely high cardiac output.

REASONING:

To answer this question correctly, one must have a good understanding of the mechanism by which thermodilution cardiac output is measured. Choices 1 through 3 correctly predict curve *B*. All these options cause less predicted (volume or temperature) injectate to reach the final probe. All result in a smaller (area under the curve) calculated cardiac output. Choice 4 is incorrect because a greater volume of cold solution would cause an elevated temperature spike and a falsely high cardiac output.

REFERENCE:

1. Barash PG, Cullen BF, Stoelting RK. Clinical Anesthesia, 4th ed. Philadelphia, Lippincott Williams & Wilkins, 2001, p. 678.
2. Morgan GE, Mikhail MS, Murray MJ. Clinical Anesthesiology, 3d ed. New York, McGraw-Hill, 2002, pp. 106–107.

BOOK A:

Answer C

Cardiovascular

QUESTION 66

QUESTION (K-type):

While evaluating oliguria following operative repair of an aortic aneurysm, large "V" waves are noted in a pulmonary artery occlusion pressure trace. This finding is consistent with which of the following disorders?

(1) Tricuspid regurgitation.
(2) Mitral regurgitation.
(3) Aortic regurgitation.
(4) Coronary artery disease.

CORRECT ANSWER: C (2 and 4 are correct.)

SUMMARY:

Large "V" waves are seen in any condition that can produce acute mitral regurgitation. This can be seen with rupture of chordea tendinae or papillary muscle dysfunction sec-

ondary to ischemia. The height of the "V" wave correlates with the regurgitant volume and pulmonary blood flow and is indicative of the severity. It is inversely related to compliance of the atrium and pulmonary vasculature. The "V" wave may not be very prominent in chronic mitral regurgitation (MR).

EXPLANATION:

(1) *Incorrect.* Tricuspid regurgitation does not produce large "V" waves. Most often it may be challenging to pass the pulmonary artery (PA) catheter.
(2) *Correct.* Acute MR of any etiology, including ischemia, endocarditis, and trauma, is associated with large "V" waves.
(3) *Incorrect.* Aortic regurgitation does not produce large "V" waves.
(4) *Correct.* Coronary artery disease can produce MR from various mechanisms. It can produce papillary muscle dysfunction from ischemia causing restriction of leaflet motion, chordal rupture, and papillary muscle rupture from infarction.[1]

REASONING:

This question tests knowledge of pulmonary artery catheter interpretation and causes of "V" waves. It is important to understand the mechanism of normal and abnormal waveforms during invasive monitoring. The important points to remember include the association of "V" waves on pulmonary artery catheter tracing with mitral regurgitation, as well as the causes of acute MR. The best answer is C.

REFERENCE:

Barash PG, Cullen BF, Stoelting RK. Clinical Anesthesia, 4th ed. Philadelphia, Lippincott Williams & Wilkins, 2001, pp. 886, 900–903.
Morgan GE, Mikhail MS, Murray MJ. Clinical Anesthesiology, 3d ed. New York, McGraw-Hill, 2002, pp. 412–415.

BOOK A: **QUESTION 67**

Answer B

Equipment/Physics

QUESTION (K-type):

The output of an agent-specific vaporizer is higher than the dial setting under which of the following conditions?

(1) The vaporizer is filled with an agent of higher vapor pressure.
(2) Ambient temperature increases from 20°C to 24°C.
(3) The vaporizer is used at an elevation of 5000 ft.
(4) The inspiratory valve is incompetent.

CORRECT ANSWER: B (1 and 3 are correct.)

SUMMARY:

The agent-specific vaporizer or variable-bypass vaporizer is designed to deliver a constant concentration of volatile anesthetic regardless of ambient temperature or flow through the vaporizer. Each vaporizer is calibrated for each specific agent and atmospheric pressure. Based on the concentration set on the dial, a certain percentage of total gas flow is directed over the anesthetic, whereas the balance exits the chamber unchanged, yielding the concentration set on the agent-specific vaporizer. The amount of vapor output for each anesthetic is determined by the following equation:

$$\text{Vapor output} = \frac{\text{carrier gas} \times \text{vapor pressure}}{(\text{barometric pressure} - \text{vapor pressure})}$$

EXPLANATION:

(1) **Correct.** Using the preceding equation above, assume that a sevoflurane vaporizer is used for both sevoflurane (vapor pressure = 160 mm Hg) and isoflurane (vapor pressure = 240 mm Hg). The same amount of carrier gas will be used for each because the vaporizer is set for sevoflurane. For simplicity, we will use 100 mL of carrier gas. Using the preceding equation this would yield

$$\text{For sevoflurane: Vapor output} = \frac{100 \text{ mL} \times 160 \text{ mm Hg}}{(760 \text{ mm Hg} - 240 \text{ mm Hg})} = 27 \text{ mL}$$

$$\text{For isoflurane: Vapor output} = \frac{100 \text{ mL} \times 240 \text{ mm Hg}}{(760 \text{ mm Hg} - 240 \text{ mm Hg})} = 46 \text{ mL}$$

Clearly, the vaporizer filled with an agent of higher vapor pressure has a higher output.

(2) **Incorrect.** Agent-specific vaporizers are not affected by changes in ambient temperature. The vaporizers contain a metallic strip composed of two metals that expand or contract based on ambient temperature, controlling the amount of gas flow into the vaporizer and keeping the flow constant.

(3) **Correct.** At an elevation of 5000 ft, the barometric pressure decreases to roughly 700 mm Hg. Using the preceding equation and the same example as in answer choice 1, the sevoflurane vaporizer with 100 mL of carrier gas, the following numbers are obtained:

$$\text{Vapor output} = \frac{100 \text{ mL} \times 160 \text{ mm Hg}}{(700 \text{ mm Hg} - 160 \text{ mm Hg})} = 30 \text{ mL}$$

which is greater than the 27 mL of output at sea level.

(4) **Incorrect.** An incompetent inspiratory valve would not change the output of a variable-bypass vaporizer because typically there is a valve located after the vaporizers and prior to the common gas outlet to prevent backflow of gases into the anesthesia machine.

REASONING:

This question tests knowledge of anesthetic vaporizers and calculation of vapor output. Choice 2 is clearly incorrect because ambient temperature does not affect vaporizer output. This allows answers A, C, and E to be eliminated. Knowledge of the equation for vapor output allows some simple calculations to obtain the correct answer because choices 1 and 3 are correct. Choice 4 is incorrect because an incompetent inspiratory valve does not change vaporizer output. This leaves only B as the best answer.

REFERENCE:

Miller RD, Miller ED, Reves JG, et al. Anesthesia, 5th ed. New York, Churchill Livingstone, 2000, pp. 183–191.
Morgan GE, Mikhail MS, Murray MJ. Clinical Anesthesiology, 3d ed. New York, McGraw-Hill, 2002, pp. 47–50.

BOOK A:

No Answer

Clinical Anesthesia

QUESTION 68 (OPTIONAL)

QUESTION (K-type):

The advantages of colloid over crystalloid for massive volume replacement include

(1) Lower incidence of pulmonary edema.
(2) Greater urine output.
(3) Less disruption of hemostasis.
(4) Greater potency in restoring circulatory homeostasis.

CORRECT ANSWER: No answer (1 and 4 are correct.)

SUMMARY:

An ongoing controversy exists over whether crystalloid or colloid solutions should be used in fluid replacement therapy. Crystalloids such as normal saline or lactated Ringer's are cheaper, more ubiquitous, and lack the risk of exposure to infectious agents, coagulopathy, or transfusion reactions. However, three to four times the volume as compared with colloid solutions must be given to obtain the equivalent intravascular replacement.[1] Also, normal saline given in large amounts can cause a dilutional hyperchloremic metabolic acidosis. Colloid solutions such as blood-derived albumin or synthetic hetastarch maintain plasma oncotic pressure better and have an intravascular half-life of 3 to 6 hours compared with the 20- to 30-minute half-life of crystalloids. Whether crystalloid or colloid is used, the practitioner also must be cognizant of the appropriate indications for blood product transfusion.

EXPLANATION:

(1) *Correct.* There is a greater risk of developing pulmonary edema with massive crystalloid infusions because the dilution of plasma proteins results in reduction of plasma oncotic pressure and subsequent movement of fluid from the intravascular into the interstitial compartment.[1]

(2) *Incorrect.* When given in sufficient amounts, crystalloids are just as effective in restoring intravascular volume, which is the main determinant in preserving urine output. Infusions of dextran have been associated with renal failure.

(3) *Incorrect.* Infusion of dextran has been associated with prolonged bleeding time. In fact, dextran is often used for its antiplatelet effects and to decrease blood viscosity in microvascular surgery. Hetastarch also has been associated with abnormal coagulation studies when more than 25 mL/kg has been given.

(4) *Correct.* Three to four times the volume of crystalloids as compared with colloids usually are required to replace the equivalent intravascular volume. Thus colloids are more "potent" in restoring circulatory homeostasis. The statement does not claim that colloids are better, just that less volume is required to achieve the same intravascular replacement.

REASONING:

This is a very controversial topic in clinical anesthesiology. Key concepts for answering this question include understanding the different types of crystalloid and colloid solutions and their clinical applications. Choice 4 is clearly correct based on the criteria of potency. Choice 3 is clearly incorrect because certain colloids have been associated with coagulopathies. Choice 2 is also incorrect because dextran has been associated with renal failure, and with adequate fluid resuscitation with either solutions, renal function should be preserved. Finally, in K-type questions, choices 1 and 3 are tied together. For this question, the evidence that choice 1 is correct is at least as convincing as the evidence that choice 3 is incorrect. This leaves the question unanswerable in its current form.

REFERENCE:

1. Miller RD, Miller ED, Reves JG, et al. Anesthesia, 5th ed. New York, Churchill Livingstone, 2000, pp. 1601–1604.
2. Morgan GE, Mikhail MS, Murray MJ. Clinical Anesthesiology, 3d ed. New York, McGraw-Hill, 2002, pp. 628–630.

Answer E

Pain

QUESTION (K-type):

A 24-year-old man has constant burning pain 3 months after sustaining a crush injury to the arm. The injured muscles and joints are healed. Findings consistent with a diagnosis of causalgia include

(1) Beads of perspiration on the skin.
(2) Skin discoloration.
(3) Hypersensitivity to touch.
(4) Warm extremity.

CORRECT ANSWER: E (All are correct.)

SUMMARY:

Causalgia is now known as complex regional pain syndrome type II *(CRPS type II). Reflex sympathetic dystrophy is now known as* complex regional pain syndrome type I *(CRPS type I). Both are characterized by chronic pain disproportionate to an initial inciting event, with symptoms not confined to the distribution of a single nerve and associated with signs of sympathetic dysfunction such as edema, color changes, sweating changes, or skin and hair changes that cannot be explained by another disease process. Both diseases may be accompanied by allodynia (pain to a nonnoxious stimuli), hyperalgesia (exaggerated pain response to a noxious stimuli), and hyperpathia (progressively more intense and longer pain caused by repetitive stimulation). CRPS type II differs from CRPS type I in that CRPS type II, or causalgia, should be diagnosed only in the presence of a known injury to a distinct nerve.*

EXPLANATION:

(1) **Correct.** Sudomotor dysfunction is consistent with causalgia.
(2) **Correct.** Skin discoloration is consistent with the vasomotor dysfunction of causalgia.
(3) **Correct.** Allodynia is seen often in causalgia.
(4) **Correct.** In causalgia, the affected extremity may be warm or cold as a function of vasomotor dysfunction. This is not confined to an acute or chronic phase.

REASONING:

This question tests knowledge of the findings associated with CRPS (types I and II). Signs of sympathetic dysfunction can be thought of as vasomotor, sudomotor, and pilomotor signs referring to aberrant blood vessel tone, sweat activity, and cutaneous hair activity (goosebumps), respectively. Beads of perspiration on the skin clearly can be a sign of sudomotor dysfunction, especially when seen only in the distribution of the pain. Skin discoloration and a warm extremity both may be caused by changes in cutaneous blood vessel diameter as a result of sympathetic dysfunction. Hypersensitivity to the touch (allodynia) is also frequently, though not necessarily, seen in CRPS type II (causalgia). Given the history provided in the question, a diagnosis of CRPS type I (reflex sympathetic dystrophy) is more appropriate than CRPS type II (causalgia) because a single nerve injury is not identified.

REFERENCE:

Benzon R, Borsook M, Strichartz. Essentials of Pain Medicine and Regional Anesthesia. New York, Churchill Livingstone, 1999, pp. 245–246.

Morgan GE, Mikhail MS, Murray MJ. Clinical Anesthesiology, 3d ed. New York, McGraw-Hill, 2002, p. 308.

Answer B

Pharmacology

QUESTION (K-type):

A 45-year-old patient who takes tranylcypromine (Parnate), a monoamine oxidase (MAO) inhibitor, is scheduled for elective surgery under general anesthesia. True statements include

(1) Meperidine can produce hyperthermia.
(2) Surgery must be delayed for 2 weeks after discontinuation of MAO inhibitor therapy.
(3) An exaggerated response to ephedrine should be expected.
(4) A decrease in pressor response to phenylephrine should be expected.

CORRECT ANSWER: B (1 and 3 are correct.)

SUMMARY:

MAO inhibitors are used for the treatment of depression and panic disorder. There are two types of MAOs, A and B, that oxidatively deaminate naturally occurring monoamines such as dopamine, serotonin, norepinephrine, and epinephrine. The MAO inhibitors phenelzine (Nardil) and tranylcypromine block MAO irreversibly, causing an increase in monoamines.[1] Certain drugs used during anesthesia can interact adversely with MAO inhibitors, such as opiates, especially meperidine, and ephedrine.[2] Adverse reactions can manifest as hypertensive crisis, hyperpyrexia, agitation, seizures, and coma.

EXPLANATION:

(1) ***Correct.*** Meperidine and other opiates can precipitate either an excitatory response characterized by agitation, headache, skeletal muscle rigidity, and hyperthermia or a depressive response characterized by hypotension, depressed ventilation, and coma. Meperedine causes the excitatory response by blocking neuronal uptake of serotonin. MAO inhibitors slow the breakdown of meperedine, causing the depressive response.

(2) ***Incorrect.*** Previously, in an attempt to prevent possibly life-threatening cardiovascular and neurologic instability, elective surgery was delayed for 2 weeks after discontinuation of MAO inhibitors to allow sufficient time for MAO regeneration. This places the patient at risk of his or her primary psychiatric disturbance. Anesthesia has been administered safely to patients taking MAO inhibitors by avoiding drugs that trigger adverse reactions. Current clinical opinion supports continuing MAOI therapy up to the time of surgery.[2]

(3) ***Correct.*** Ephedrine acts indirectly at α and β receptors by causing the release of catecholamines. Since MAO inhibitors decrease the breakdown of catecholamines, concomitant administration of ephedrine will cause an exaggerated response.

(4) ***Incorrect.*** An exaggerated response to phenylephrine would be expected, and lower doses should be used.

REASONING:

This question tests knowledge of drug interactions associated with MAO inhibitor therapy. Choice 3 obviously is correct because ephedrine causes an exaggerated response. This allows answers C and D to be eliminated. Choice 4 is incorrect because any sympathomimetic agents should be used in small doses owing to the potential for an exaggerated response. This leaves only answers A and B as possibilities. B is correct because surgery need not be delayed for patients taking MAO inhibitors.

REFERENCES:

1. Barash PG, Cullen BF, Stoelting RK. Clinical Anesthesia, 4th ed. Philadephia, Lippincott Williams & Wilkins, 2001, p. 308.
2. Ibid., p. 1315.
3. Stoelting RK. Pharmacology and Physiology in Anesthetic Practice, 3d ed. Philadelphia, Lippincott Raven Publishers, 1999, pp. 364–367.
4. Morgan GE, Mikhail MS, Murray MJ. Clinical Anesthesiology, 3d ed. New York, McGraw-Hill, 2002, pp. 591–593.

BOOK A:

Answer C

Clinical Anesthesia

QUESTION 71

QUESTION (K-type):

A 52-year-old man with a chronic cough associated with a long history of smoking is scheduled for elective cholecystectomy. Cessation of smoking for 48 hours will result in

(1) Decreased bronchial secretions.
(2) Shift of the oxyhemoglobin dissociation curve to the right.
(3) Decreased airway irritability.
(4) Decreased carboxyhemoglobin level.

CORRECT ANSWER: C (2 and 4 are correct.)

SUMMARY:

Cigarette smoking causes many potentially reversible adverse effects on respiratory function and oxygen delivery such as decreased mucociliary clearance, increased mucous production, and increased carboxyhemoglobin levels. Smoking cessation can lead to improvements in these effects but can take between 4 and 8 weeks for maximal benefit and improved outcomes in patients undergoing surgery. In fact, smoking cessation 2 days prior to surgery causes increased bronchial secretions, airway irritability, and patient anxiety. However, the benefits of such acute smoking cessation include decreased carboxyhemoglobin levels promoting increased oxygen-carrying capacity and improved oxygen delivery and decreased nicotine-induced tachycardia.

EXPLANATION:

(1) **Incorrect.** Bronchial secretions and airway irritability (bronchospasticity) increase in the first few days after smoking cessation, leading to potential respiratory problems during anesthesia.
(2) **Correct.** Decreased carboxyhemoglobin levels improve both oxygen-carrying capacity and oxygen delivery to tissues because hemoglobin has a 200-fold greater affinity for carbon monoxide than oxygen, and carbon monoxide interferes with oxygen release from hemoglobin. Therefore, decreasing levels of carbon monoxide shift the oxyhemoglobin curve to the right.
(3) **Incorrect.** See above.
(4) **Correct.** Carboxyhemoglobin levels decrease within 12 to 48 hours after smoking cessation.

REASONING:

This question tests knowledge of the physiologic effects of acute smoking cessation. Choice 4 is obviously correct because carboxyhemoglobin levels decrease rapidly with smoking cessation. This allows answers A and B to be eliminated. Choices 1 and 3 are both incorrect because airway irritability and bronchial secretions both increase 2 days after smoking cessation. Answer B can be eliminated. The only question is whether or not choice 2 is correct. Choice 2 is correct because carboxyhemoglobin worsens oxygen delivery, shifting the oxyhemoglobin dissociation curve to the left. C is the best answer.

REFERENCE:

Miller RD, Miller ED, Reves JG, et al. Anesthesia, 5th ed. New York, Churchill Livingstone, 2000, p. 1673.

Morgan GE, Mikhail MS, Murray MJ. Clinical Anesthesiology, 3d ed. New York, McGraw-Hill, 2002, pp. 501–502, 516–517.

BOOK A:

Answer B

Physiology

QUESTION 72

QUESTION (K-type):

A 55-year-old woman has a urine output of 15 mL during the first 2 hours following a radical hysterectomy. Findings consistent with a prerenal cause include

(1) Urine osmolality of 590 mOsm/L.
(2) Plasma creatinine concentration of 1.1 mg/dL.
(3) Urine specific gravity of 1.025.
(4) Urine sodium concentration of 40 mEq/L.

CORRECT ANSWER: B (1 and 3 are correct.)

SUMMARY:

Azotemia can be defined as either prerenal, renal, or postrenal. The most common cause of prerenal azotemia is decreased renal perfusion. A fall in arterial pressure, an increase in venous pressure, or an increase in renal vascular tone can lead to decreased renal perfusion. Laboratory tests can be useful in differentiating prerenal from other forms of azotemia. Specific gravity and osmolality are high, and the amount of sodium being excreted by the kidney is low, reflecting the kidney's attempt to maintain intravascular volume.

EXPLANATION:

(1) **Correct.** The osmolality in prerenal azotemia is greater than 500 mmol/kg. This is in contrast to renal azotemia, where the osmolality is less than 350 mmol/kg.
(2) **Incorrect.** The plasma creatinine concentration may be elevated from baseline in prerenal azotemia, but a single number does not help to differentiate prerenal from other forms of azotemia. A trend, not an isolated number, is important for monitoring renal function. In addition, creatinine can be elevated in all forms of azotemia.
(3) **Correct.** The urine specific gravity is increased greater than 1.018 in prerenal azotemia. It is less than 0.012 in renal azotemia.
(4) **Incorrect.** The urine sodium concentration in prerenal azotemia is less than 10 mEq/L as the kidney attempts to hold onto sodium to maintain intravascular volume.

REASONING:

This question tests knowledge of oliguria and the laboratory values associated with various etiologies. It is clear that in a prerenal state the kidney will attempt to maintain intravascular volume through sodium retention and concentrating urinary output. However, the specific numbers for each test need to be memorized. B is the best answer.

REFERENCE:

Barash PG, Cullen BF, Stoelting RK. *Clinical Anesthesia,* 4th ed. Philadelphia, Lippincott Williams & Wilkins, 2001, pp. 1008–1010, 1393.

Morgan GE, Mikhail MS, Murray MJ. Clinical Anesthesiology, 3d ed. New York, McGraw-Hill, 2002, pp. 976–977, Table 50-8, Urinary Indices in Azotemia.

BOOK A:

Answer E

Pediatrics

QUESTION 73

QUESTION (Choose single best answer):

An 8-kg, 1-year-old child has a measured blood loss of 50 mL during the first 2 hours of a rectal pull-through operation. Preoperative hematocrit was 31%. Balanced saline solution 150 mL has been administered for replacement. Urine output has been 2 mL for the last hour, heart rate is 160 bpm, and blood pressure is 40/15 mm Hg. The most appropriate fluid therapy is

(A) 25% albumin.
(B) Balanced salt solution.
(C) Balanced salt solution and mannitol.
(D) 5% dextrose in 0.45% saline solution.
(E) Packed red blood cells.

CORRECT ANSWER: E

SUMMARY:

In estimating maximal allowable blood loss (MABL) before needing to transfuse red blood cells (RBCs), multiple factors must be taken into consideration, including the patient's age, weight, cardiovascular status, metabolic needs, and potential for ongoing blood loss. The following formula may be used to estimate MABL

$$MABL = \frac{EBV \times (starting\ Hct - minimal\ acceptable\ Hct)}{starting\ Hct}$$

where Hct = hematocrit, and EBV = estimated blood volume.[1] EBV varies with age, ranging from 95 mL/kg for a premature infant to 65 mL/kg for an adult woman. For infants, it is approximately 80 mL/kg. Blood loss may be replaced with crystalloid or colloid solution initially, but neither can replace the oxygen-carrying ability of red blood cells. Most healthy children tolerate hematocrit levels in the 20 to 25 percent range.[1,2] However, premature infants and patients with cyanotic heart disease or severe pulmonary disease may require higher baseline hematocrits. Because of the risk of transmission of infectious diseases, administration of blood products clearly must be indicated.

EXPLANATION:

(A) ***Incorrect.*** Twenty-five percent albumin is a hypertonic solution that is used to treat hypoalbuminemia. Five percent albumin is an isotonic colloid solution that may be used as replacement fluid.[3]

(B) ***Incorrect.*** Balanced salt solution such as lactated Ringer's is appropriate initial fluid replacement for hypovolemia. Because of equilibration into the extravascular space, crystalloid should be administered three parts for every one of blood lost. However, if evidence of shock (hypotension, tachycardia, oliguria) persists, consideration must be given to transfusing red blood cells.

(C) ***Incorrect.*** Mannitol is a six-carbon sugar used to treat raised intracranial pressure and as an osmotic diuretic. In a patient who is oliguric, it will increase urinary output but may worsen hypovolemia.

(D) ***Incorrect.*** Dextrose-containing solutions may be used as maintenance fluids in neonates and children but should not be used as replacement fluids because they are hypotonic and may result in hyperglycemia.[4]

(E) **Correct.** The patient is already showing signs of inadequate oxygen delivery despite appropriate crystalloid replacement. Therefore, packed red blood cell transfusion is indicated.

REASONING:

This question is challenging because it tests clinical judgment rather than scientific fact. Answers A, C and D can be ruled out because they are not appropriate choices for isotonic fluid resuscitation. The question that remains is whether the clinical situation warrants the risk of blood transfusion. Based on calculation of MABL and fluid replaced, the answer would be no. But based on clinical signs of hypotension, tachycardia, oliguria, and the potential for ongoing blood loss, the answer should be E.

REFERENCES:

1. Miller RD, Miller ED, Reves JG, et al. Anesthesia, 3d ed. New York, Churchill Livingstone, 2000, p. 2104.
2. Cote CJ. A Practice of Anesthesia for Infants and Children, 3d ed. Philadelphia, Saunders, 2001, pp. 236–237.
3. Stoelting RK, Dierdorf SF. Anesthesia and Co-existing Diseases, 3d ed. New York, Churchill Livingstone, 1993, p. 420.
4. Miller RD, Miller ED, Reves JG, et al. Anesthesia, 3d ed. New York, Churchill Livingstone. 2000, pp. 1606–1607.
5. Morgan GE, Mikhail MS, Murray MJ. Clinical Anesthesiology, 3d ed. New York, McGraw-Hill, 2002, pp. 628–633, 673–674.

BOOK A:

Answer C

Pharmacology

QUESTION 74

QUESTION (Choose single best answer):

An increased initial dose and a decreased maintenance dose of pancuronium are required in patients with

(A) Advanced age.
(B) Burns.
(C) Cirrhosis.
(D) Chronic renal failure.
(E) Fever.

CORRECT ANSWER: C

SUMMARY:

Pancuronium is a long-acting nondepolarizing neuromuscular blocking agent that is (up to 80 percent) eliminated primarily unchanged by the kidneys. The liver metabolizes 10 to 40 percent of pancuronium into several metabolites. One has about 50 percent of the activity of pancuronium at the neuromuscular junction, and the other has only minimal activity. Renal and liver functions primarily govern the clearance and appropriate initial and maintenance dosages of pancuronium. Cirrhotic patients with decreased liver function require greater initial doses of pancuronium because of their greater volume of distribution but decreased maintenance doses because clearance is slightly decreased. In contrast, patients with chronic renal failure should receive smaller initial and maintenance doses because clearance is severely affected.

EXPLANATION:

(A) **Incorrect.** Advanced age does not alter the receptor affinity for pancuronium, so the initial dose is unchanged; however, the maintenance dose is decreased because renal function worsens with aging.

(B) *Incorrect.* Burn patients are resistant to nondepolarizing agents and require increased doses. This is so because burn patients have altered protein binding and an increased number of extrajunctional acetycholine receptors that bind nondepolarizing neuromuscular blocking drugs.

(C) *Correct.* Cirrhotic patients have an increased volume of distribution for neuromuscular blocking drugs, increasing the initial dose required. Cirrhotics also have decreased maintenance requirement for pancuronium because of impaired hepatic clearance.

(D) *Incorrect.* Patients with chronic renal failure require decreased initial and maintenance doses of pancuronium because the kidneys are primarily responsible for its excretion.

(E) *Incorrect.* Fever does not decrease the maintenance requirements of pancuronium.

REASONING:

This question requires knowledge of the elimination pathways of pancuronium. It is important to understand that pancuronium is eliminated primarily through the kidney, with a small amount of hepatic elimination. Knowledge of the pharmacokinetic and pharmacodynamic differences associated with aging and different physiologic states is also important. The best answer is C.

REFERENCE:

Stoelting RK. Pharmacology and Physiology in Anesthetic Practice, 3d ed. Philadelphia, Lippincott Raven Publishers, 1999, pp. 202–204.
Morgan GE, Mikhail MS, Murray MJ. Clinical Anesthesiology, 3d ed. New York, McGraw-Hill, 2002, pp. 194–195, 687–688, 802.

BOOK A:

Answer C

Clinical Anesthesia

QUESTION 75

QUESTION (Choose single best answer):

Which of the following statements concerning banked blood is true?

(A) Red blood cells preserved with CPDA-1 have a shelf life of approximately 21 days.

(B) Packed red blood cells deliver oxygen normally immediately after administration.

(C) Packed red blood cells contain most of the leukocytes present in the donated unit.

(D) Citrate is used as a source of energy for whole blood.

(E) Stored whole blood contains all coagulation factors except II and VIII.

CORRECT ANSWER: C

SUMMARY:

Storage of blood is achieved by adding CPDA-1, which contains citrate for chelation of calcium to prevent clotting, phosphate as a buffer, dextrose as a fuel source, and adenine as a substrate for the synthesis of ATP. CPDA-1 allows red blood cells (RBCs) to be stored for 35 days. Without adenine, RBCs can be stored for only 21 days. The longer blood is stored, the lower are the levels of 2,3-DPG, shifting the oxyhemoglobin dissociation curve to the left, which impairs oxygen delivery. Packed red blood cells (PRBCs) are derived from whole blood from which the plasma has been removed. PRBCs contain leukocytes unless they have been specifically leukoreduced.

EXPLANATION:

(A) *Incorrect.* RBCs stored with CPDA-1 can be stored for 35 days, not 21.

(B) *Incorrect.* RBCs deliver oxygen abnormally because 2,3-DPG levels are depleted in stored blood, shifting the oxyhemoglobin dissociation curve to the left.[1]

(C) **Correct.** PRBCs, unless leukodepleted, contain all the leukocytes found in a donated unit.[1]

(D) **Incorrect.** Citrate is used as an anticoagulant, and dextrose is used as an energy source.[1]

(E) **Incorrect.** Stored whole blood initially contains all coagulation factors, but factor V and VIII activity decline rapidly with storage.

REASONING:

This question tests knowledge of blood banking and transfusion practices. Answer B, D, and E are obviously incorrect because stored RBCs do not deliver oxygen normally, citrate is an anticoagulant, and whole blood contains all clotting factors, albeit some with decreased activity. Answer A is incorrect because stored blood with CPD is good for 21 days, but stored blood with CPDA-1 is good for 35 days. C is the best choice because RBCs contain leukocytes unless specifically leukodepleted.

REFERENCES:

1. Barash PG, Cullen BF, Stoelting RK. Clinical Anesthesia, 4th ed. Philadelphia, Lippincott Williams & Wilkins, 2001, pp. 204–209.
2. Miller RD, Miller ED, Reves JG, et al. Anesthesia, 5th ed. New York, Churchill Livingstone, 2000, pp. 1618–1621.
3. Morgan GE, Mikhail MS, Murray MJ. Clinical Anesthesiology, 3d ed. New York, McGraw-Hill, 2002, pp. 634–635.

BOOK A:

Answer C

Physiology

QUESTION 76

QUESTION (Choose single best answer):

A 73-year-old woman with a preoperative serum creatinine concentration of 2.1 mg/dL develops oliguria during enflurane anesthesia. Urine sodium concentration is 10 mEq/L, and urine osmolality is 450 mOsm/L. The most likely cause of these findings is

(A) Acute renal failure.
(B) Chronic renal insufficiency.
(C) Decreased renal perfusion.
(D) Fluoride nephrotoxicity.
(E) Intraoperative administration of furosemide.

CORRECT ANSWER: C

SUMMARY:

Inhalational agents decrease renal blood flow, which can lead to decreased urinary output. The accumulation of fluoride is more pronounced in patients with renal failure, but this does not necessarily translate into increased renal impairment. Decreased urine production with laboratory values indicating a prerenal cause (low urine sodium and concentrated urine) is an appropriate physiologic response to low renal perfusion.

EXPLANATION:

(A) **Incorrect.** The low urine sodium level combined with increased osmolality points to a kidney able to scavenge sodium and concentrate urine, not a failing kidney.

(B) **Incorrect.** Chronic renal insufficiency predisposes to acute renal failure but should not in itself lead to oliguria.

(C) **Correct.** Inhalational anesthetics decrease renal blood flow, glomerular filtration rate, and urinary output.

(D) *Incorrect.* Fluoride toxicity manifests as polyuric renal failure.

(E) *Incorrect.* Furosemide increases sodium excretion and urinary output.

REASONING:

This question is challenging because the patient has preexisting renal impairment, is given an inhalational agent that is associated with fluoride nephrotoxicity, and develops signs of renal impairment during anesthesia. There are multiple factors at work.[1] Fortunately, we can eliminate answers D and E easily. Acute renal failure may be caused by prolonged hypoperfusion of the kidneys, but we do not have evidence of this yet. The *most likely cause* of oliguria, to which all patients are susceptible, is decreased renal perfusion.

REFERENCE:

1. Barash PG, Cullen BF, Stoelting RK. Clinical Anesthesia, 4th ed. Philadelphia, Lippincott Williams & Wilkins, 2001, p. 1010, Fig. 36-5.

2. Morgan GE, Mikhail MS, Murray MJ. Clinical Anesthesiology, 3d ed. New York, McGraw-Hill, 2002, pp. 138, 142, 976–979.

BOOK A:

QUESTION 77

Answer C

OB/Regional

QUESTION (Choose single best answer):

During active labor, 10 mL bupivacaine 0.5% with epinephrine 1:200,000 is administered epidurally. Fifteen minutes later, maternal blood pressure is 70/50 mm Hg, and heart rate is 70 bpm; fetal heart rate is 90 bpm for 45 seconds, with loss of beat-to-beat variability. The most likely explanation for the fetal vital signs is

(A) Fetal bupivacaine cardiotoxicity.

(B) Maternal bupivacaine cardiotoxicity.

(C) Maternal hypotension.

(D) Uterine artery vasoconstriction.

(E) Umbilical cord compression.

CORRECT ANSWER: C

SUMMARY:

Complications associated with epidural anesthesia with local anesthetics include hypotension and bradycardia from sympathectomy, unintended dural puncture, catheter migration into the intrathecal or intravascular space, epidural abscess or hematoma, and failed block. In obstetric practice, hypotension associated with epidural anesthesia can decrease placental perfusion and oxygen delivery to the fetus. Fetal heart rate monitoring is the best means of assessing fetal well-being. Changes in fetal oxygen delivery would be manifested by heart rate decelerations, loss of beat-to-beat variability, and changes in the fetal baseline heart rate.[1]

EXPLANATION:

(1) *Incorrect.* The question states that the bupivicaine was injected epidurally. Owing to the high protein binding of bupivicaine, maternal bupivicaine toxicity (from an intravenous injection) would manifest as cardiac arrest before fetal effects are seen.

(2) *Incorrect.* Maternal bupivicaine toxicity would result from intravenous injection, and the question states that the medication was administered epidurally. The absence of tachycardia in the presence of an epinephrine-containing injection is further evidence that the injection was not intravascular.

(3) *Correct.* A known side effect of epidural analgesia is hypotension. The onset of the hypotension is 15 minutes, which is consistent with the onset of epidural

bupivicaine. Low maternal blood pressure can cause decreased oxygen delivery to the fetus, leading to bradycardia and loss of beat-to-beat variability.

(4) **Incorrect.** Although uterine artery vasoconstriction can occur with the administration of intravascular epinephrine, this is an epidural injection.

(5) **Incorrect.** While fetal bradycardias can result from umbilical cord compression, the temporal nature of the change in fetal status suggests that it is related to the hypotension. Furthermore, umbilical cord compression usually is associated with variable decelerations and likely would not have such a long duration (45 seconds) until after a long period of fetal compromise.[1]

REASONING:

The key to answering this question is the temporal nature of the hypotension and fetal bradycardia. Think as if you had just placed this epidural catheter. Rule out an intravascular injection. The onset of hypotension is 15 minutes, and there is no increase in blood pressure or heart rate with the epinephrine-containing solution. Most likely this is not intravascular, and the solution is epidural. This eliminates answers A, B, and D. The fact that the bradycardia coincides with the hypotension makes C the best answer.

REFERENCE:

1. Hughes SC, Levinson G, Rosen MA. Shnider and Levinson's Anesthesia for Obstetrics, 4th ed. Philadelphia, Lippincott Williams & Wilkins, 2002, p. 367.
2. Morgan GE, Mikhail MS, Murray MJ. Clinical Anesthesiology, 3d ed. New York, McGraw-Hill, 2002, pp. 274–280, 840–842, Fig. 43-3 (p. 841), Periodic Changes in Fetal Heart Rate Related to Uterine Contractions.

BOOK A:

Answer D

Pharmacology

QUESTION 78

QUESTION (Choose single best answer):

Compared with diazepam, midazolam

(A) Is more lipid-soluble.
(B) Has a longer elimination half-life.
(C) Has a larger volume of distribution.
(D) Has a greater clearance.
(E) Undergoes slower hepatic metabolism.

CORRECT ANSWER: D

SUMMARY:

Both midazolam and diazepam are benzodiazepines that act by binding to gamma-aminobutyric acid (GABA) receptors, facilitating the action of GABA. These drugs cause anxiolysis, sedation, and anterograde amnesia. Although both midazolam and diazepam are used in anesthetic practice, midazolam is administered much more commonly. Midazolam has an imidazole ring in its structure that is open at acidic pH, allowing it to be water-soluble, but closed at physiologic pH, making it more lipid-soluble. This allows midazolam to be water-soluble for painless injection yet still rapidly cross the blood–brain barrier to achieve clinical effect. Diazepam is more lipid-soluble, requiring a propylene glycol soublizer that causes venoirritation on injection. Both drugs are metabolized by the liver. Midazolam is metabolized much more quickly than diazepam, accounting for its faster clearance and shorter elimination half-life.

EXPLANATION:

(A) **Incorrect.** Diazepam is more lipid-soluble than midazolam.
(B) **Incorrect.** Diazepam has a longer elimination half-life.

(C) *Incorrect.* Diazepam and midazolam have similar volumes of distribution.
(D) *Correct.* Midazolam has a greater clearance than diazepam.
(E) *Incorrect.* Diazepam undergoes slower hepatic metabolism.

REASONING:

This commonly asked question tests knowledge of the similarities and differences between midazolam and diazepam. Answers B and E can be eliminated because diazepam has a longer elimination half-life and undergoes slower hepatic metabolism. Answer D is the opposite of these and is correct because midazolam is cleared more rapidly than diazepam. Answer A is incorrect because midazolam is less lipid-soluble and more soluble in aqueous solutions. Answer C is incorrect because the two drugs have similar volumes of distribution. The best answer is D.

REFERENCE:

Stoelting RK. Pharmacology and Physiology in Anesthetic Practice, 3d ed. Philadelphia, Lippincott Raven Publishers, 1999, pp. 126–136.
Morgan GE, Mikhail MS, Murray MJ. Clinical Anesthesiology, 3d ed. New York, McGraw-Hill, 2002, pp. 160–164.

BOOK A: **QUESTION 79**

Answer E

OB/Regional

QUESTION (Choose single best answer):

A 30-year-old woman has difficulty talking 15 minutes after initiation of interscalene block for closed reduction of a dislocated shoulder. The most likely cause is

(A) Cervical sympathetic block.
(B) Delayed systemic toxic reaction.
(C) Phrenic nerve paralysis.
(D) Pneumothorax.
(E) Recurrent laryngeal nerve block.

CORRECT ANSWER: E

SUMMARY:

Interscalene blocks are used for shoulder, arm, and forearm procedures and block the nerves of the brachial plexus. The brachial trunks are located between the anterior and middle scalene muscles at the level of the cricoid cartilage. Complications related to placement of this block include (1) inadvertent blockade of the recurrent laryngeal nerve (hoarseness), phrenic nerve (dyspnea), or stellate ganglion (Horner's syndrome), (2) intraarterial injection (seizure), (3) epidural or spinal injection (neuraxial block or total spinal), and more rarely, (4) pneumothorax.

EXPLANATION:

(A) *Incorrect.* This is also known as a *stellate ganglion block.* It causes increased temperature of the ipsilateral arm, nasal congestion, and Horner's syndrome: ipsilateral ptosis, miosis, and facial anhidrosis.
(B) *Incorrect.* Local anesthetic toxicity usually presents as central nervous system (CNS) complaints: tinnitus, blurred vision, circumoral numbness, and dizziness.
(C) *Incorrect.* Phrenic nerve paralysis is usually asymptomatic and probably very common in interscalene nerve blocks. Patients with preexisting pulmonary disease are more likely to complain of dyspnea following phrenic nerve blockade.
(D) *Incorrect.* Pneumothorax is a rare complication of interscalene block.

(E) **Correct.** Almost all laryngeal muscles are innervated by the recurrent laryngeal nerve. Unilateral nerve blockade leads to paralysis of the ipsilateral vocal cord, causing hoarseness.

REASONING:

While all choices are possible complications of the interscalene block, some are less probable, namely, pneumothorax (based on frequency) and toxicity (based on presentation). Knowing the complications involved with blockade of the remaining nerves leads to phrenic versus recurrent laryngeal nerve paralysis. The difficulty talking is most likely vocal cord dysfunction and not dyspnea. E is the single best answer.

REFERENCE:

Barash PG, Cullen BF, Stoelting RK. Clinical Anesthesia, 4th ed. Philadelphia, Lippincott Williams & Wilkins, 2001, pp. 724–725.
Morgan GE, Mikhail MS, Murray MJ. Clinical Anesthesiology, 3d ed. New York, McGraw-Hill, 2002, pp. 288–289.

BOOK A:

Answer C

Physiology

QUESTION 80

QUESTION (Choose single best answer):

An acutely ill 65-year-old-man with sepsis has severe hypophosphatemia. Which of the following is most likely to result from this electrolyte disorder?

(A) Bronchospasm.
(B) Diarrhea.
(C) Muscle weakness.
(D) Seizures.
(E) Ventricluar ectopy.

CORRECT ANSWER: C

SUMMARY:

Hypophosphatemia can cause several sequelae; the most common include muscle weakness, myopathy, and respiratory failure. In addition, a low phosphorus level (<1.0 mg/dL) also can cause cardiomyopathy with impaired oxygen delivery, decreased levels of 2,3-DPG, hemolysis, impaired leukocyte and platelet function, encephalopathy, rhabdomyolysis, hepatic dysfunction, and metabolic acidosis.[1]

EXPLANATION:

(A) **Incorrect.** Patients with hypocalcemia (not hypophosphatemia) tend to develop laryngospasm or laryngeal stridor. Bronchospasm is not usually associated with hypophosphatemia.
(B) **Incorrect.** Diarrhea frequently results from the abuse of phosphorus-containing laxatives, causing the patient to become hyperphosphatemic.
(C) **Correct.** Patients with low phosphorus levels suffer from weakness and subsequent respiratory failure and skeletal muscle myopathies.
(D) **Incorrect.** Hypophosphatemia first leads to muscle weakness. Other electrolyte imbalances, such as hyponatremia, are associated more commonly with seizures.
(E) **Incorrect.** Phosphorus does not produce ventricular ectopy principally, as do imbalances in other electrolytes such as calcium and potassium.

This question tests knowledge of the pathophysiology of hypophosphatemia. Of the choices given, phosphorus is most clearly related to muscle weakness. Frequently, patients on prolonged total parenteral nutrition (TPN) are difficult to wean from mechanical ventilation because of inadequate phosphorus supplementation and, subsequently, develop weakness of respiratory muscles. Recent carbohydrate or insulin administration shifts phosphorus intracellularly. Other circumstances that may cause low phosphorus levels include diabetic ketoacidosis, aluminum- or magnesium-containing antacids, severe burns, alcohol withdrawal, and prolonged respiratory alkalosis. With respiratory alkalosis, there is an intracellular shift of phosphorus to counteract the decrease in bicarbonate. C is the best answer.

REFERENCE:

1. Barash PG, Cullen BF, Stoelting RK. Clinical Anesthesia, 4th ed. Philadelphia, Lippincott Williams & Wilkins, 2001, pp. 193, 724–725.
2. Morgan GE, Mikhail MS, Murray MJ. Clinical Anesthesiology, 3d ed. New York, McGraw-Hill, 2002, pp. 528–540.

BOOK A: **QUESTION 81**

Answer E

Clinical Anesthesia

QUESTION (Choose single best answer):

During a right lower lobe resection, SpO_2 decreases from 99 to 70 percent after institution of one-lung ventilation. FIO_2 is 1.0. The most appropriate management is to

(A) Administer an inhaled bronchodilator.
(B) Apply continuous positive airway pressure (CPAP) to the right lung.
(C) Apply positive end-expiratory pressure (PEEP) to the left lung.
(D) Increase tidal volume.
(E) Reinflate the right lung.

CORRECT ANSWER: E

SUMMARY:

An acute drop in oxygen saturation after institution of one-lung ventilation requires a rigorous, systematic management plan. First, reinflate the lung and keep the patient on 100% FIO_2. Check the position of the double-lumen tube with a fiberoptic scope, and listen for breath sounds on clamping each side of the tube. Hypoxemia during one-lung ventilation can be a result of inadequate FIO_2, alveolar hypoventilation, or a large alveolar-to-arterial oxygen tension gradient. In addition to ruling out malposition of the tube, check for mechanical problems (i.e., obstruction or bronchospasm) and ensure hemodynamic stability (i.e., no arrythmias or hypotension).

EXPLANATION:

(A) *Incorrect.* An inhaled bronchodilator may help somewhat with a sudden onset of wheezing and worsening asthma. However, with such an acute drop in SpO_2 to 70 percent, the next-best maneuver is to reinflate the right lung and rule out other causes of hypoxemia.

(B) *Incorrect.* With such an acute drop in saturation on starting one-lung ventilation, ensure that the tube is positioned correctly, and rule out mechanical problems before instituting this CPAP. Applying CPAP to the nondependent, or collapsed, lung is the most efficacious maneuver to improve arterial oxygenation during one-lung ventilation once other causes have been ruled out. Unfortunately, CPAP is most efficacious with partial reexpansion of the nondependent lung, and this can interfere with surgical exposure.

(C) **Incorrect.** A low level of PEEP to the ventilated, dependent lung can help to improve arterial oxygenation. However, this also can increase pulmonary resistance and shunt more blood to the collapsed, nondependent lung. With such an acute drop in saturation, reinflating the lung should be done first.

(D) **Incorrect.** With one-lung ventilation, try to keep tidal volumes the same as prior to lung isolation. Monitor peak pressures carefully because they should rise 3 to 5 cm H_2O with the initiation of one-lung ventilation. If peak inspiratory pressures are within normal limits (i.e., below 35 to 40 cm H_2O), small adjustments in tidal volumes can be made, but this will not correct such a rapid desaturation to 70 percent.

(E) **Correct.** If a sudden drop in SpO_2 occurs on initiating one-lung ventilation, first reexpand the nondependent lung and rule out tube malposition and mechanical problems (i.e., obstruction, bronchospasm, hemodynamic instability). After maximizing oxygen delivery with both lungs inflated, attempt one-lung ventilation again, possibly using CPAP or PEEP if necessary.

REASONING:

This question requires detailed knowledge of the management of hypoxia during one-lung ventilation. Ultimately, if a patient cannot tolerate one-lung ventilation despite these maneuvers and surgeons are unwilling to reinflate the lung, the ipsilateral pulmonary artery can be ligated to shunt all blood to the ventilated lung. E is the best answer.

REFERENCE:

Miller R, Stoeling R. Basics of Anesthesia, 3d ed. New York, Churchill Livingstone, 1994, pp. 284–285.

Morgan GE, Mikhail MS, Murray MJ. Clinical Anesthesiology, 3d ed. New York, McGraw-Hill, 2002, pp. 464–465.

BOOK A:

Answer Unknown

Physiology

QUESTION 82 (OPTIONAL)

QUESTION (Choose single best answer):

Carbon dioxide retention first occurs when the ratio of forced expiratory volume in 1 second to vital capacity (FEV_1/VC) decreases below

(A) 15 percent.
(B) 35 percent.
(C) 50 percent.
(D) 65 percent.
(E) 75 percent.

CORRECT ANSWER: The answer to this question is unknown.

SUMMARY:

Pulmonary function testing provides valuable information on airflow disease states such as chronic obstructive pulmonary disease (COPD). FEV_1 is a measure of the volume of gas expired during the first second of forced expiration from total lung capacity (TLC). It is measured by asking the patient to take a maximal inspiratory breath followed by a maximal forced expiration. The volume of gas expired in the first second is measured. Vital capacity (VC) is the volume change in the lung between maximal inspiration (TLC) and maximal expiration (RV).[1] It can be measured by several methods. If the subject takes a maximal inspiratory breath (TLC) and then exhales forcefully to maximum expiration (RV), forced expiratory vital capacity (FEVC or FVC) is measured. If the subject begins at end-tidal volume (FRC), expires maximally (RV), and then inspires to full TLC, inspi-

ratory vital capacity (IVC) is measured. If the subject begins at end-tidal inspiration, makes a full expiration, and then exhales maximally, expiratory vital capacity (EVC) or "slow vital capacity" is measured. In healthy patients, all three measurements should produce approximately similar values. In patients with COPD, IVC > EVC > FVC. We assume that FVC has been measured in this question. A normal FEV_1/FVC ratio is usually greater than or equal to 75 percent.[2]

EXPLANATION:

(A) **Unknown.** The degree of airflow obstruction measured by the FEV_1/FVC ratio that is associated with the first onset of clinically significant CO_2 retention is unknown.

(B) **Unknown.** See below.

(C) **Unknown.** See below.

(D) **Unknown.** See below.

(E) **Unknown.** The reader might assume that any degree of obstruction will lead to some "theoretical" amount of hypoventilation and CO_2 retention (even if is not clinically significant). Since this is a normal ratio, the reader might assume that CO_2 retention might "first occur" when the ratio decreases below this value. However, there is no scientific evidence to support this assumption.

REASONING:

This question is extremely challenging because it is not clear if the examiners are referring to the first onset of *any amount* of CO_2 retention or if they are referring to *clinically significant* retention. There are no data in the literature to support either hypothesis.

In general, carbon dioxide retention is caused by impairment of pulmonary gas exchange. There are four major processes that can impair pulmonary gas exchange: hypoventilation, diffusion limitation, shunt, and ventilation-perfusion inequality.[3] Hypoventilation has many etiologies, including obstructive lung disease. The severity of obstruction can be measured by pulmonary function testing, with a normal FEV_1/FVC ratio that is greater than or equal to 75 percent. This question asks us to determine what FEV_1/VC ratio (i.e., degree of obstruction/hypoventilation) corresponds to the first onset of carbon dioxide retention. We presume that the only cause of CO_2 retention in this patient stems from airway obstruction/hypoventilation owing to COPD. The severity of the associated obstruction can be quantified by the FEV_1/VC ratio.

However, no clinical studies have correlated FEV_1/VC with Pa_{CO_2}. Indeed, Montes de Oca and colleagues studied a cohort of 33 patients with COPD and stratified them into eucapneic ($Pa_{CO_2} < 44$ mm Hg) and hypercapneic ($Pa_{CO_2} > 45$ mm Hg) patients.[4] They found that the FEV_1 and FVC measurements were signficantly lower for the hypercapnic group compared with the eucapneic group (FEV_1 was 0.9 versus 0.6; FVC was 2.6 versus 1.7). However, their FEV_1/FVC ratios were virtually identical (0.346 versus 0.353). This evidence suggests that the FEV_1/FVC ratio is a poor predictor of Pa_{CO_2} in patients with COPD. Interestingly, the authors found that ventilatory drive in response to CO_2 was significantly lower in the hypercapneic cohort.[4] This is an important feature of the disease that is independent of level of obstruction (although the two components clearly can combine to make hypercapnea more likely).

The reader should not be discouraged by the difficulty of this question. Critical care faculty in the department of anesthesia and expert pulmonologists from the faculty of medicine at Stanford agree that the answer to this question is unknown.

REFERENCES:

1. Barash PG, Cullen BF, Stoelting RK. Clinical Anesthesia, 4th ed. Philadelphia, Lippincott Williams & Wilkins, 2001, p. 805.
2. Ibid.
3. Murray JF, Nadel JA. Textbook of Respiratory Medicine, 3d ed. Philadelphia, Saunders, 2000, p. 71.
4. Montes de Oca M, Celli BR. Mouth occlusion pressure, CO_2 response and hypercapnia in severe chronic obstructive pulmonary disease. Eur Respir J 12:666–671, 1998.

5. Morgan GE, Mikhail MS, Murray MJ. Clinical Anesthesiology, 3d ed. New York, McGraw-Hill, 2002, p. 516.

BOOK A:

Answer D

Pharmacology

QUESTION 83 (OPTIONAL)

QUESTION (Choose single best answer):

During recovery from halothane anesthesia, an alveolar concentration of 0.1% will have the greatest effect on

(A) Myocardial contractility.
(B) Ventilatory response to hypercarbia.
(C) Atrioventricular conduction.
(D) Ventilatory response to hypoxia.
(E) Neuromuscular transmission.

CORRECT ANSWER: D

SUMMARY:

Halothane is an inhalational anesthetic that is now used rarely in clinical anesthesia. At anesthetic levels (1 MAC and higher), halothane can cause dose-dependent myocardial depression, junctional rhythms, skeletal muscle relaxation, and a reduction in hypercarbic and hypoxic ventilatory drive. During recovery from halothane anesthesia, the hypoxic ventilatory drive remains depressed even at concentrations as low as 0.1 MAC. Patients in the postanesthesia care unit may be at risk for hypoventilation despite the presence of arterial hypoxemia.

EXPLANATION:

(A) *Incorrect.* Halothane causes a decrease in blood pressure secondary to direct myocardial depression. This effect is dose-dependent, with a 50 percent decrease in blood pressure at 2 MAC.
(B) *Incorrect.* Halothane can reduce hypercarbic respiratory drive and increase the apneic threshold, but this effect is dose-dependent, and subanesthetic concentrations do not alter the normal ventilatory response to CO_2.[1]
(C) *Incorrect.* Patients anesthetized with halothane may develop a junctional rhythm as a result of slow sinoatrial node conduction. Junctional rhythm can occur with all inhalational anesthetics.[1]
(D) *Correct.* Even at 0.1 MAC, which occurs during recovery from anesthesia, halothane severely blunts hypoxic respiratory drive. At greater than 1 MAC, halothane eliminates the ventilatory response to hypoxia.[1]
(E) *Incorrect.* Halothane potentiates the effects of nondepolarizing muscle relaxants at anesthetic levels.

REASONING:

Of the many effects that halothane has on the cardiovascular and respiratory systems, nearly all of them occur at anesthetic levels and recover rapidly following emergence. Depression of the hypoxic ventilatory drive is the most sensitive to the effects of volatile anesthetic agents and persists into the recovery period.[1] The best answer is D.

REFERENCE:

1. Stoelting RK, Miller RD. Basics of Anesthesia, 4th ed. New York, Churchill Livingstone, 2000, pp. 51, 55–56.
2. Morgan GE, Mikhail MS, Murray MJ. Clinical Anesthesiology, 3d ed. New York, McGraw-Hill, 2002, pp. 138–140, Table 7-6 (p. 138), Clinical Pharmacology of Inhalational Anesthetics.

Answer B

Cardiovascular

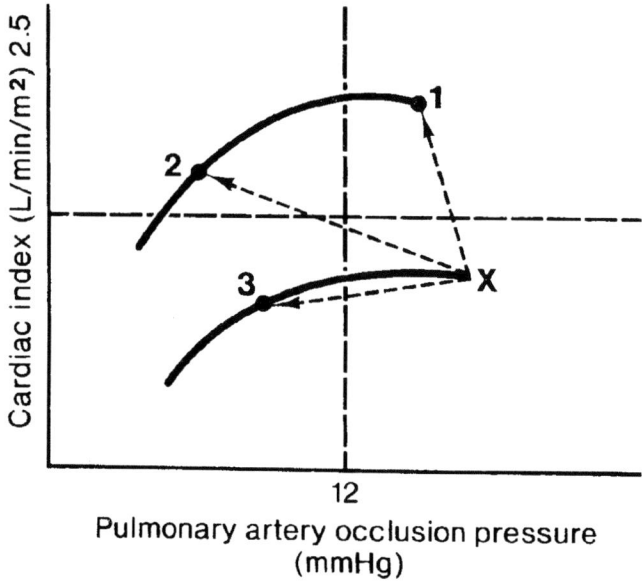

In the diagram above, point X represents a patient with severe left ventricular dysfunction. The points labeled 1, 2, and 3 each represent the results of a different therapeutic intervention. Which of the following represents the most likely intervention at each point?

	Point 1	**Point 2**	**Point 3**
(A)	Dopamine	Furosemide	Nitroprusside
(B)	Dopamine	Nitroprusside	Furosemide
(C)	Furosemide	Dopamine	Nitroprusside
(D)	Nitroprusside	Dopamine	Furosemide
(E)	Nitroprusside	Furosemide	Dopamine

CORRECT ANSWER: B

SUMMARY:

The graph represents a patient with severe left ventricular (LV) dysfunction with a PAOP of approximately 18 mm Hg and a cardiac index of less than 2 L/min/m². Dopamine is an adrenergic agent with dose-dependent β and α activity that increases cardiac output and cardiac index and slightly decreases PAOP. Furosemide is a loop diuretic that produces diuresis and reduces preload. This results in decreased PAOP. Sodium nitroprusside causes both arteriolar and venodilation. This decreases both preload and afterload. The decrease in afterload improves LV stroke volume, cardiac output, renal perfusion, and diuresis. The net effect is a decrease in PAOP and an increase in cardiac output (CO).

EXPLANATION:

(A) *Incorrect.*

(B) *Correct.* Point 1 on the graph illustrates an increase in cardiac index from point X and a small reduction in PAOP. This effect can be seen after treatment with an inotropic agent such as dopamine. Point 2 on the graph shows greater reduction in PAOP and improvement in cardiac index seen with sodium nitroprusside. Point 3 on graph shows a large reduction in PAOP and even a very small decrease in cardiac index. This is produced by furosemide, which reduces preload by diuresis.

(C) *Incorrect.*

(D) *Incorrect.*

(E) *Incorrect.*

REASONING:

This complex question tests knowledge of the pathophysiology of LV dysfunction and the associated hemodynamic responses to pharmacologic therapy. It is important to understand the pathophysiology of congestive heart failure with its attendant maladaptive changes, such as increased activity in the sympathetic and renin-angiotensin systems leading to excess water and sodium accumulation and increased afterload on a failing heart. The pharmacologic therapy in heart failure is directed toward correcting these changes. The best answer is B.

REFERENCE:

Stoelting R. Anesthesia and Co-existing Diseases, 3d ed. New York, Churchill Livingstone, 1993, pp. 91–95.

BOOK A:

Answer A

Pharmacology

QUESTION 85

QUESTION (Choose single best answer):

With long-term administration, which of the following drugs produces the most prolonged sedative effect of diazepam?

(A) Cimetidine.

(B) Famotidine.

(C) Metoclopramide.

(D) Ranitidine.

(E) Warfarin.

CORRECT ANSWER: A

SUMMARY:

Diazepam is metabolized via the cytochrome P450 enzyme system in the liver and has a slow hepatic extraction and a large volume of distribution. This results in a long elimination half-life. Cimetidine also binds to cytochrome P450 and reduces hepatic blood flow, thereby producing a more prolonged sedative effect with diazepam.

EXPLANATION:

(A) **Correct.** Cimetidine is an H_2-receptor antagonist that binds to the cytochrome P450 system, thereby reducing the metabolism of diazepam. Approximately 30 percent is slowly inactivated by the liver's microsomal oxygenase system, whereas the other 70 percent is excreted unchanged in the urine.

(B) **Incorrect.** Famotidine is also an H_2-receptor antagonist; however, it does not inhibit the cytochrome P450 system in the liver. It is more similar to ranitidine in its pharmacologic action. However, it is 3 to 20 times more potent than ranitidine.

(C) **Incorrect.** Metaclopromide binds dopaminergic receptors both peripherally and centrally and increases LES tone and gastric motility and decreases gastric fluid volume. Owing to its antagonism at the dopaminergic receptors, metaclopramide may cause some sedation and extrapyramidal side effects. It does not interact with the P450 system.

(E) **Incorrect.** Warfarin uses the cytochrome P450 system for metabolism, and with concurrent administration of diazepam, warfarin acts as an enzyme inducer to the speed the catabolism of diazepam rather than prolonging its effects.

REASONING:

The key to this question is understanding that the elimination mechanism of diazepam occurs via the cytochrome P450 enzyme system. Cimetidine binds this enzyme, slowing elimination and prolonging the clinical effect. The best answer is A.

REFERENCE:

Mycek M, Harvey A, Champe P. Pharmacology, 2d ed. Philadelphia, Lippincott Raven Publishers, 1999 pp. 238–239.

Morgan GE, Mikhail MS, Murray MJ. Clinical Anesthesiology, 3d ed. New York, McGraw-Hill, 2002, pp. 137, 203.

BOOK A:

Answer B

Pediatrics

QUESTION 86

QUESTION (Choose single best answer):

During uncomplicated mask induction with halothane and 50% nitrous oxide in oxygen in a 6-month-old infant with a large ventricular septal defect and valvular pulmonic stenosis, SpO_2 decreases from 85 (room air) to 60 percent, heart rate is 100 bpm, and blood pressure is 62/40 mm Hg. The most appropriate management is to

(A) Administer atropine.
(B) Administer phenylephrine.
(C) Administer propranolol.
(D) Increase anesthetic depth.
(E) Intubate the trachea.

CORRECT ANSWER: B

SUMMARY:

Ventricular septal defects (VSDs) are the most common congenital heart lesions and comprise up to 25 to 35 percent of all defects. The balance between pulmonary vascular resistance (PVR) and systemic vascular resistance (SVR) determines the direction of shunting and therefore whether the blood is oxygenated in the lungs prior to circulation to the rest of the body. Blood always flows down the path of least resistance. Beyond the first few days to weeks of life, the resistance in the pulmonary bed drops so that shunting in most VSDs occurs left to right. Left uncorrected, a large VSD with chronic left-to-right shunting will result in vascular changes in the pulmonary circulation that raise PVR. Eventually, PVR increases relative to SVR, and the shunt is reversed right to left, resulting in what is termed Eisenmenger's syndrome.

EXPLANATION:

(A) **Incorrect.** There is no need to administer an anticholinergic agent. The patient is not bradycardic, and there is no reason to make him tachycardic. One could argue that bronchospasm is the cause of the desaturation, but the initial room air saturations were already 85 percent, and there is another more likely explanation.

(B) **Correct.** Phenylephrine is the drug of choice to raise the systemic vascular resistance. This selective α_1-adrenergic agonist will increase systemic vascular resistance relative to pulmonary vascular resistance, decrease the amount of blood shunted through the VSD, and route some blood to the lungs to be oxygenated. Alternatively, one could put the patient's knees to chest or apply pressure to the femoral arteries.

(C) *Incorrect.* Propranolol, a β-adrenergic antagonist, has been used in the past to relieve dynamic infundibular spasm in hypercyanotic spells but is unlikely to be effective in relieving a fixed valvular pulmonic stenosis.

(D) *Incorrect.* Increasing anesthetic depth may be effective in treating dynamic infundibular spasm but will not affect a fixed pulmonic stenosis. Also, in this case it also might lower systemic vascular resistance, which could worsen shunting.

(E) *Incorrect.* Intubating the trachea alone without increasing the F_{IO_2} will not help, especially if little blood is reaching the pulmonary circulation to be oxygenated. Increasing the F_{IO_2} to 100 percent will maximize oxygen in the lungs to be absorbed once pulmonary circulation has been reestablished.

REASONING:

This patient has fixed pulmonic stenosis, so any decrease in cardiac output or SVR will change the shunt across the VSD profoundly, as manifested by the observed decrease in Sao_2 and blood pressure. The clinical situation described is similar to that of a patient with tetrology of Fallot—a congenital heart defect consisting of ventricular septal defect, right ventricular outflow tract obstruction (pulmonic stenosis), right ventricular hypertrophy, and overriding aorta. The first two lesions are primarily responsible for the hypercyanotic (or "tet") spells that may occur in these patients. During a hypercyanotic spell, deoxygenated blood from the right side of the heart is preferentially shunted through the VSD out the aorta owing to obstruction along the right ventricular outflow tract. In other words, PVR is greater than SVR. Immediate interventions are directed at raising SVR relative to PVR. B is the only answer that will raise SVR. Administration of oxygen also would be helpful, but this is not a choice. The other choices have no direct effect or an undesirable effect on SVR.

REFERENCE:

Barash PG, Cullen BF, Stoelting RK. Clinical Anesthesia, 4th ed. Philadelphia, Lippincott Williams & Wilkins, 2001, pp. 1360–1361.
Morgan GE, Mikhail MS, Murray MJ. Clinical Anesthesiology, 3d ed. New York, McGraw-Hill, 2002, pp. 216, 423–426.

BOOK A:

QUESTION 87

Answer A

OB/Regional

QUESTION (Choose single best answer):

Which of the following statements concerning variable decelerations of fetal heart rate is true?

(A) It indicates compression of the umbilical cord.
(B) It indicates compression of the fetal head.
(C) It indicates prematurity.
(D) It is obliterated by atropine.
(E) It occurs normally following epidural anesthesia.

CORRECT ANSWER: A

SUMMARY:

Monitoring of the fetal heart rate is currently the best indicator of fetal oxygenation and tolerance of labor. Heart rate decelerations are evaluated with respect to uterine contractions. Early decelerations occur at the onset of the contraction, nadir at the peak of the contrac-

tion, and return to baseline at the end. They are due to a vagal response to fetal head compression and can be blocked by atropine.[1] *Late decelerations are thought to be due to utero-placental insufficiency and begin after the onset of the contraction, nadir after the peak, and return to baseline after the contraction has terminated. Late decelerations are associated with uteroplacental insufficiency. Variable contractions are variable in onset, duration, and relationship to contractions. Typically, this pattern is vagally mediated and due to umbilical cord compression, although repeated hypoxia due to cord compression can result in bradycardia owing to intrinsic myocardial depression. While early decelerations are not associated with fetal hypoxia, variable and late patterns can be associated with fetal hypoxia and acidosis, especially when associated with tachycardia and loss of beat-to-beat variability.*[2]

EXPLANATION:

(A) **Correct.** Variable decelerations are thought to be a vagal response to the increased afterload associated with umbilical cord compression.
(B) **Incorrect.** Early decelerations are associated with fetal head compression.
(C) **Incorrect.** Variable decelerations are more common in preterm fetuses but are also seen frequently in term pregnancies.[1]
(D) **Incorrect.** The efferent component of variable decelerations is vagally mediated and can be blocked by atropine.[1] However, the variable decelerations also can occur due to intrinsic myocardial depression from prolonged hypoxia, and this response will not be blocked by atropine.[1]
(E) **Incorrect.** Decelerations are not normal after epidural anesthesia. If fetal heart rate changes occur after institution of epidural anesthesia, causes include maternal hypotension or uterine hypertonus.[2]

REASONING:

Correctly answering this question requires knowledge of commonly occurring fetal heart rate patterns. Answer E can be eliminated because decelerations do not normally occur after epidural anesthesia. Answers B and D are associated with early decelerations. Answer C can be eliminated because variable decelerations are also seen in term fetuses. A is the single best answer.

REFERENCES:

1. Freeman RK, Garite TJ, Nageotte MP. Fetal Heart Rate Monitoring, 2d ed. Baltimore, Williams & Wilkins, 1991, pp. 13–17, 151–155.
2. Hughes SC, Levinson G, Rosen MA. Shnider and Levinson's Anesthesia for Obstetrics, 4th ed. Philadelphia, Lippincott Williams & Wilkins, 2002, pp. 130, 628–632.
3. Morgan GE, Mikhail MS, Murray MJ. Clinical Anesthesiology, 3d ed. New York, McGraw-Hill, 2002, pp. 840–842, Fig. 43-3 (p. 841), Periodic Changes in Fetal Heart Rate Related to Uterine Contractions.

BOOK A:

Answer E

Clinical Anesthesia

QUESTION 88 (OPTIONAL)

QUESTION (Choose single best answer):

During enflurane anesthesia for colectomy in a 75-year-old man with sepsis, urine output decreases to 10 mL/h. Heart rate is 120 bpm, blood pressure is 100/50 mm Hg, central venous pressure is 10 mm Hg, and pulmonary artery occlusion pressure is 15 mm Hg. The most appropriate management at this time is to

(A) Measure cardiac output.
(B) Increase fluid administration.
(C) Infuse dopamine.
(D) Administer propanolol.
(E) Switch from enflurane to isoflurane.

CORRECT ANSWER: E

SUMMARY:

Sepsis and the associated intraoperative hypotension are common occurrences. A patient with sepsis may demonstrate hypotension for several different reasons, including decreased SVR, intravascular volume depletion from third spacing, or direct myocardial depression from toxins associated with the septic state. Treatment would involve maintaining adequate filling pressures with volume replacement, maintaining SVR with medications, and avoiding myocardial depressants such as halothane and enflurane.

EXPLANATION:

(A) *Incorrect.* Although obtaining a cardiac output would provide some useful information, it is not the most important nor most appropriate next step in treating this patient's hypotension.

(B) *Incorrect.* Fluid administration is vitally important in maintaining an adequate preload in septic patients, but in this case the CVP is 10 mm Hg, indicating that the preload should be adequate. A different treatment choice would be warranted.

(C) *Incorrect.* Dopamine would be a valid choice if other treatable options have been rule out. The patient is already tachycardic, and the addition of dopamine will only worsen the tachycardia.

(D) *Incorrect.* The patient's tachycardia is a direct result of the septic state and is needed to maintain perfusion. Administering a β-blocker at this point may precipitate cardiovascular collapse.

(E) *Correct.* Enflurane both depresses myocardial contractility and decreases systemic vascular resistance. This combination is detrimental to a patient with sepsis. Changing from enflurane to isoflurane theoretically would be useful because isoflurane causes minimal cardiac depression and maintains cardiac output.[1]

REASONING:

This is a challenging question that tests knowledge of hemodynamic management during sepsis and the pharmacologic effects of inhalational anesthetics. One could argue that the appropriate response would be to give additional fluid even with an adequate CVP because septic patients have increased fluid requirements. In addition, one could argue that despite the tachycardia, dopamine should be started to improve overall cardiac performance. The isoflurane versus enflurane question is a more theoretical consideration than a practical one.

REFERENCE:

1. Miller RD, Miller ED, Reves JG, et al. Anesthesia, 5th ed. New York, Churchill Livingstone, 2000, p. 1482.
2. Morgan GE, Mikhail MS, Murray MJ. Clinical Anesthesiology, 3d ed. New York, McGraw-Hill, 2002, pp. 142–143.

BOOK A:

Answer B

Pharmacology

QUESTION 89

QUESTION (Choose single best answer):

The effect of neomycin at the neuromuscular junction is

(A) Decreased by depolarizing relaxants.
(B) Partially reversed by calcium.
(C) Potentiated by anticholinesterases.
(D) Prevented by pretreatment with magnesium.
(E) Primarily prejunctional.

CORRECT ANSWER: B

SUMMARY:

Antibiotics, especially aminoglycosides such as neomycin, potentiate neuromuscular blockade. Neomycin impairs neuromuscular transmission and produces clinically significant weakness. The mechanism responsible is a decrease in both the release of acetylcholine from prejunctional nerve endings and the sensitivity of the postsynaptic site. Studies also have shown that neomycin preferentially interacts with the open state of the acetylcholine receptor ion channel complex. Cholinesterase inhibitors (i.e., neostigmine), the infusion of calcium, and aminopyridines can partially reverse the weakness.

EXPLANATION:

(A) ***Incorrect.*** Neomycin potentiates the effect of depolarizing agents, and its action at the neuromuscular junction is not decreased by the administration of paralytics.

(B) ***Correct.*** Calcium can partially reverse the effect of neomycin at the neuromuscular junction. Intravenous calcium gluconate or calcium chloride supplementation should be administered, especially since neomycin decreases the intestinal absorption of calcium in patients.

(C) ***Incorrect.*** Anticholinesterases can partially reverse the effect of neomycin at the neuromuscular junction rather than potentiating any muscle weakness.

(D) ***Incorrect.*** Magnesium will not prevent the effect of neomycin at the neuromuscular junction. Hypermagnesemia actually decreases the release of acetylcholine and can potentiate neuromuscular blockade.

(E) ***Incorrect.*** Studies have proven that neomycin acts to decrease acetylcholine release at prejunctional sites. It also stabilizes the effects of some functional components on postsynaptic membranes, resulting in decreased neuromuscular transmission.

REASONING:

This is a somewhat difficult question that requires good knowledge of the effects of neomycin at the neuromuscular junction. Most readers recognize that neomycin can impair neuromuscular transmission. However, to answer this question correctly, it is important to understand its mechanism of action. Only then can the correct answer, B, be identified.

REFERENCES:

Fiekers JF. Sites and mechanisms of antibiotic-induced neuromuscular blockade: Pharmacological analysis using quantal content, voltage clamped end-plate currents, and single channel analysis. Acta Physiol Pharmacol 49:242–250, 1999.

Karatas Y. Possible postsynaptic action of aminoglycosides in frog rectus abdominis. Acta Med Okayama 54:49–56, 2000.

Mycek M, Harvey R, Champe P. Pharmacology, 2d ed. Philadelphia, Lippincott Raven, 1997, p. 317.

Singh YN. Antibiotic-induced paralysis of mouse phrenic nerve hemidiaphragm preparation and reversibility by calcium and by neostigmine. Anesthesiology 48:418–424, 1978.

Morgan GE, Mikhail MS, Murray MJ. Clinical Anesthesiology, 3d ed. New York, McGraw-Hill, 2002, p. 155.

QUESTION (Choose single best answer):

A patient is bleeding excessively after routine transurethral resection of the prostate (TURP). Reexploration discloses diffuse oozing. The most appropriate management is administration of

(A) Platelets.
(B) Fresh frozen plasma.
(C) Desmopressin.
(D) ε-Aminocaproic acid.
(E) Cryoprecipitate.

CORRECT ANSWER: Several answers are possibly correct.

SUMMARY:

Abnormal bleeding is rare after TURP.[1] Less than 1 percent of patients develop abnormal bleeding after TURP. Disseminated intravascular coagulation (DIC) has been reported and is thought to be secondary to release of thromboplastins from the prostate cancer tissue. Others believe that primary fibrinolysis can occur from prostatic tumors that excrete plasminogen activator, which converts plasminogen to plasmin.[2] Treatment of DIC involves supportive care and repletion of coagulation factors and platelets. If primary fibrinolysis is suspected, administration of ε-aminocaproic acid and cryoprecipitate may be beneficial.

EXPLANATION:

(A) ***Possibly correct.*** If DIC is suspected and the patient is thrombocytopenic, transfusion of platelets would be beneficial. We do not have enough information to determine the etiology of the bleeding.

(B) ***Possibly correct.*** DIC after TURP can lead to depletion of coagulation factors and platelets. It would be important to determine the coagulation profile for this patient. The release of thromboplastin from cancerous prostate tissue will trigger a hypercoagulable state initially. After coagulation factors have been exhausted, a coagulopathic state ensues. Abnormal (prolonged) coagulation tests and low fibrinogen and platelet levels would increase clinical suspicion of DIC. We do not have enough information to determine the etiology of the bleeding.

(C) ***Incorrect.*** The use of desmopressin would only be indicated if the patient had dysfunctional platelets. This patient's oozing is most likely due to DIC or primary fibrinolysis, not platelet dysfunction.

(D) ***Possibly correct.*** The use of ε-aminocaproic acid would be indicated if the patient were undergoing primary fibrinolysis from a cancerous prostate.[3] Clinical suspicion would be heightened if laboratory studies showed low fibrinogen levels in the presence of normal coagulation tests and platelet counts. We do not have enough information to determine the etiology of the bleeding.

(E) ***Possibly correct.*** The use of cryoprecipitate would be indicated if the patient's fibrinogen level was low. If primary fibrinolysis is suspected, cyoprecipitate may be beneficial.

REASONING:

This question is very difficult because there is little information to help narrow down the etiology of the bleeding. There are several different causes of abnormal bleeding after TURP, and more laboratory data would be helpful to determine the cause. Answers A, B, D, and E seem plausible and are well-known causes of bleeding diatheses after TURP. We cannot determine the correct answer without additional information.

REFERENCES:

1. Barash PG, Cullen BF, Stoelting RK. Clinical Anesthesia, 4th ed. Philadelphia, Lippincott Williams & Wilkins, 2001, pp. 1020–1021.

2. Miller RD, Miller ED, Reves JG, et al. Anesthesia, 5th ed. New York, Churchill Livingstone, 2000, p. 1948.

3. Hatch PD. Surgical and anaesthetic considerations in transurethral resection of the prostate. Anaesth Intensive Care 15:203, 1987.

4. Morgan GE, Mikhail MS, Murray MJ. Clinical Anesthesiology, 3d ed. New York, McGraw-Hill, 2002, p. 696.

BOOK A:

Answer B

Physiology

QUESTION 91

QUESTION (Choose single best answer):

Which of the following statements concerning functional residual capacity is true?

(A) It decreases linearly during a 3-hour anesthetic.
(B) It decreases in pregnancy primarily because of a decrease in the expiratory reserve volume.
(C) It increases in patients with a history of heavy smoking.
(D) It increases with pulmonary contusions.
(E) It is smaller (mL/kg) in children than in adults.

CORRECT ANSWER: B

SUMMARY:

Functional residual capacity (FRC) is the volume remaining in the lung at the end of normal exhalation. Factors that decrease FRC include the supine or prone position, obesity, restrictive lung disease, and pregnancy. In pregnancy, FRC is reduced primarily as a result of decreased expiratory reserve volume. Neonates and infants have lower FRC owing to a limited number of alveoli, but development of the respiratory system is nearly complete by early childhood, when FRC resembles adult values.

EXPLANATION:

(A) *Incorrect.* Induction of anesthesia reduces FRC by 15 to 20 percent. This reduction in FRC is not related to duration or depth of anesthesia and continues for several hours after emergence from anesthesia.
(B) *Correct.* By term, FRC in the pregnant patient is reduced by 20 percent primarily owing to a reduction in expiratory reserve volume. Decreased FRC puts the pregnant patient at risk for rapid desaturation due to diminished apneic times.
(C) *Incorrect.* Patients with chronic obstructive pulmonary disease (COPD) have increased residual volume and FRC. Patients with a history of heavy smoking will not necessarily have increased FRC unless they have COPD.
(D) *Incorrect.* Chest trauma with rib fractures and underlying pulmonary contusion tends to reduce lung volumes secondary to splinting. Pulmonary contusion can lead to progressive respiratory failure.
(E) *Incorrect.* Although infants tend to have reduced FRC as a result of immature alveoli, the respiratory system approaches complete development by childhood. A 5-year-old patient will have an FRC of 35 mL/kg, which is almost equal to the average adult.[1]

REASONING:

This is a challenging question because multiple answers seem possible. Only answer D is clearly incorrect. Answer A is incorrect because the reduction in FRC with general anesthesia occurs on induction and is not related to the duration of the anesthetic. Answer C is incorrect because not all smokers develop COPD. Answer E is incorrect because children and adults have nearly the same FRC in milliliters per kilogram, although infants tend to have a lower FRC. B is the correct answer. Pregnant patients take larger tidal volumes but have a lower expiratory reserve volume.

REFERENCE:

1. Stoelting RK, Miller RD. Basics of Anesthesia, 4th ed. New York, Churchill Livingstone, 2000, p. 365, Table 27-2.
2. Morgan GE, Mikhail MS, Murray MJ. Clinical Anesthesiology, 3d ed. New York, McGraw-Hill, 2002, pp. 483–484, 489–490, 516, 799, 806, 850.

BOOK A:

Answer A

Pharmacology

QUESTION 92

QUESTION (Choose single best answer):

After 2 hours of anesthesia with halothane 1.2% and oxygen, nitrous oxide 75% is added to the inspired gas mixture. This addition would

(A) Increase the alveolar halothane and oxygen concentrations above inspired.
(B) Increase the alveolar halothane concentration only.
(C) Cause no change in alveolar gas concentrations compared with inspired.
(D) Decrease alveolar oxygen concentration compared with inspired.
(E) Decrease alveolar oxygen and halothane concentrations below inspired.

CORRECT ANSWER: A

SUMMARY:

The rapid uptake of nitrous oxide augments the uptake of a concurrently administered potent anesthetic gas. This phenomenon is referred to as the second-gas effect.[1] For example, if 75% (75 parts/100) nitrous is administered with 1.2% (1.2 parts/100) halothane and the remainder oxygen 23.8% (23.8 parts/100) and two-thirds of the nitrous is taken up (50 parts), then the remaining 1.2 parts of halothane and 23.8 parts of oxygen are at a higher concentration. The gas mixture now becomes 1.2 parts halothane per 50 total parts or 2.4% halothane and 23.8 parts oxygen per 50 total parts or 47.6% oxygen. Therefore, when nitrous oxide is administered initially and taken up rapidly, it increases the alveolar partial pressure of the other agents.

EXPLANATION:

(A) **Correct.** The second-gas effect causes an increase in alveolar concentration of both oxygen and halothane when it is added because of its rapid uptake.
(B) **Incorrect.** The alveolar partial pressures of both oxygen and halothane are increased because of the second-gas effect.
(C) **Incorrect.** See above.
(D) **Incorrect.** See above.
(E) **Incorrect.** See above.

REASONING:

Understanding the second-gas effect is the key to answering this question correctly. As nitrous oxide at a high concentration of 75% is added to the system, a large portion of the gas will be taken up, concentrating the remaining gases in the lungs in comparison with the inspired gases. Answer A describes the effect and is correct.

REFERENCE:

Barash PG, Cullen BF, Stoelting RK. Clinical Anesthesia, 4th ed. Philadelphia, Lippincott Williams & Wilkins, 2001, p. 384.
Morgan GE, Mikhail MS, Murray MJ. Clinical Anesthesiology, 3d ed. New York, McGraw-Hill, 2002, pp. 131–132.

Answer D

Basic Science

QUESTION (Choose single best answer):

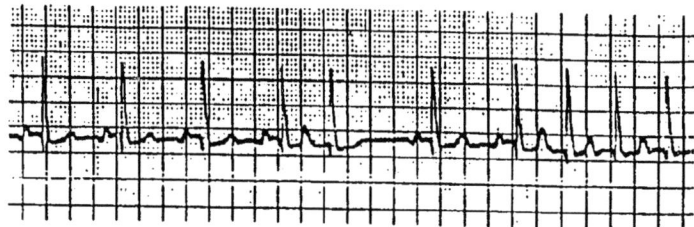

The ECG tracing above shows

(A) Aberrant intraventricular conduction.
(B) Acceleration of phase 4 depolarization of the sinus node.
(C) A compensatory pause.
(D) Initiation of reentrant supraventricular tachycardia (SVT).
(E) Paroxysmal atrial fibrillation.

CORRECT ANSWER: D

SUMMARY:

The ECG shows a normal pattern in first half with normal PR interval and QRS complex and a rate of approximately 75 beats per minute. The midsection shows a single junctional beat with a normal QRS complex without a P wave. The end segment shows a normal-looking QRS complex at the rate of 150 beats per minute without discernible P waves. SVT usually occurs at a rate of 130 to 220 beats per minute and often is initiated by a premature supraventricular beat (atrial or junctional).

EXPLANATION:

(A) *Incorrect.* Aberrant intraventricular conduction has a widened, abnormal-looking QRS complex.
(B) *Incorrect.* Unlike cardiac ventricular muscle cells, pacemaker cells of the heart (SA and AV nodes) undergo a slow, spontaneous depolarization during phase 4 owing to pacemaker currents.[1] The tracing shows a reentrant supraventricular tachycardia. The mechanism of the tachycardia is reentry, not increased rate of spontaneous depolarization of the SA node.
(C) *Incorrect.* A compensatory pause follows a premature ventricular beat.
(D) *Correct.* The ECG shows a narrow-complex tachycardia with a rate of 150 beats per minute.
(E) *Incorrect.* Atrial fibrillation occurs with an irregular heart rate without P waves.

REASONING:

There are several different causes of reentrant supraventricular tachycardias. Etiologies include Wolff-Parkinson-White (WPW) syndrome, AV reentrant tachycardia, AV nodal reentrant tachycardia, and SA node and atrial reentrant tachycardias. Reentry is usually triggered by a premature cardiac impulse. The salient features of this ECG are the triggering junctional beat followed by regular narrow-complex tachycardia at a rate of 150 beats per minute. D is the best answer.

REFERENCES:

1. Barash PG, Cullen BF, Stoelting RK. Clinical Anesthesia, 4th ed. Philadelphia, Lippincott Williams & Wilkins, 2001, p. 863.
2. Stoelting RK, Dierdorf SF. Anesthesia and Co-existing Diseases, 3d ed. New York, Churchill Livingstone, 1993, pp. 69–70.
3. Morgan GE, Mikhail MS, Murray MJ. Clinical Anesthesiology, 3d ed. New York, McGraw-Hill, 2002, p. 383.

BOOK A:

Answer C

Physiology

QUESTION 94

QUESTION (Choose single best answer):

One hour after an open cholecystectomy, a 42-year-old patient is hemodynamically stable and breathing spontaneously (rate 10 breaths per minute and regular) at an FIO_2 of 0.4. Fentanyl, isoflurane, nitrous oxide, and pancuronium were used during the procedure. Analysis of arterial blood gases is most likely to show

	pH	P_{CO_2} (mm Hg)	P_{O_2} (mm Hg)
(A)	7.18	40	100
(B)	7.18	60	140
(C)	7.28	50	85
(D)	7.40	26	220
(E)	7.40	40	40

CORRECT ANSWER: C

SUMMARY:

General anesthesia and abdominal surgery have a number of adverse effects on pulmonary mechanics. These include increased shunting, decreased vital capacity, decreased functional residual capacity, and increased dead space. These changes are accentuated by upper abdominal surgery and may persist for days. Respiratory function is optimized in the operating room by increasing the delivered FIO_2 and minute ventilation during controlled positive-pressure ventilation. In the immediate postoperative period, impaired respiratory mechanics will be reflected by a mild respiratory acidosis and larger than normal arterial-alveolar oxygen gradient.

EXPLANATION:

(A) *Incorrect.* In a hemodynamically stable patient 1 hour following an open upper abdominal procedure, one would expect a mild respiratory acidosis owing to the ventilatory depression of the opiates and lingering volatile anesthetics. This patient has a normal P_{CO_2}, reflecting a metabolic acidosis.

(B) *Incorrect.* Although this patient has a respiratory acidosis, we also would expect to see a diminished PaO_2 as a result of shunting caused by altered ventilatory mechanics and subsequent atelectasis.

(C) *Correct.* This gas correctly reflects the expected respiratory acidosis and decreased PaO_2. A pH of 7.28, P_{CO_2} of 50 mm Hg, and P_{O_2} of 85 mm Hg are consistent with the expected mild acute mixed respiratory and metabolic acidosis, as well as decreased lung volumes and shunting.

(D) *Incorrect.* A pH of 7.18 would be unusual in a spontaneous breathing patient who is hemodynamically stable following an open cholycystecomy. This degree of acidemia would tend to cause some hemodynamic instability.

(E) *Incorrect.* See above. General anesthesia consistently produces a decrease in functional residual capacity of 15 to 20 percent. This, in turn, results in increased intrapulmonary shunting as blood continues to perfuse unventilated regions. This may be augmented by the impairment in hypoxic pulmonary vasoconstriction that accompanies general anesthesia. Decreased lung volumes, including vital capacity and functional residual capacity, remain depressed for 10 to 14 days following upper abdominal surgery with general anesthesia.

REASONING:

This question tests knowledge of the expected changes in respiratory function following general acidemia for an open abdominal procedure. Answers A and B are wrong owing to the severity of the acidemia, which is life-threatening and not consistent with a hemodynamically stable patient breathing regularly at 10 breaths per minute. Answers D and E are also incorrect because they do not reflect the expected respiratory acidosis. One would expect a mild respiratory acidosis as a result of the lingering anesthetic and opioids. The P_{CO_2} of 50 mm Hg would be expected to decrease the pH to approximately 7.32. The lower pH of 7.28 would suggest a mild metabolic acidosis as well. The P_{O_2} of 85 mm Hg is consistent with the splinting, atelectasis, and intrapulmonary shunting expected following upper abdominal surgery resulting in an increase in the A–a gradient. C is the best answer.

REFERENCE:

Stoelting RK, Dierdorf SF. Anesthesia and Co-existing Disease, 3d ed. New York, Churchill Livingstone, 1993, p. 142.
Morgan GE, Mikhail MS, Murray MJ. Clinical Anesthesiology, 3d ed. New York, McGraw-Hill, 2002, pp. 421–425, 559–574.

BOOK A:

Answer B

Pharmacology

QUESTION 95

QUESTION (Choose single best answer):

A 6-year-old child with asthma begins wheezing during anesthesia with halothane and nitrous oxide in oxygen. A loading dose of aminophylline is administered, followed by continuous infusion. Premature ventricular contractions appear on the ECG. The most appropriate management is to

(A) Administer fentanyl.
(B) Discontinue aminophylline.
(C) Increase exhalation time.
(D) Increase the inspired concentration of halothane.
(E) Switch the inhalational agent to isoflurane.

CORRECT ANSWER: B

SUMMARY:

Aminophylline is an older intravenous drug used in the treatment of asthma. It is a methylxanthine that increases the level of cAMP, resulting in bronchodilation.[1] Its major side effects, ventricular dysrhythmias and seizures, warrant close monitoring of blood level. Acute administration of aminophylline decreases the threshold of epinephrine to induce arrhythmias. Halothane also sensitizes the myocardium to arrythmias from epinephrine.

EXPLANATION:

(A) *Incorrect.* Fentanyl will not affect the interaction between halothane and aminophylline. It may be appropriate to increase the depth of anesthesia if light level is suspected. However, the temporal relationship of aminophylline and premature ventricular contraction (PVC) is the suspect here.

(B) **Correct.** The onset of ventricular arrhythmias with administration of amino-phylline should be scrutinized, especially given its narrow therapeutic window. In addition, studies suggest that aminophylline does not improve outcomes and can cause adverse effects in children with acute asthma.[2] There are several other more effective treatments for bronchospasm, including sympathomimetic agents (aerosolized β_2-selective drugs such as albuterol) and parasympatholytics such as ipratropium. It would be best to terminate aminophylline therapy and initiate other safer and more efficacious treatments.

(C) **Incorrect.** Exhalation time has no effect on the PVCs. It is a reasonable maneuver in asthma with airway obstruction.

(D) **Incorrect.** This maneuver will further exacerbate the arrhythmogenic effect of halothane.

(E) **Incorrect.** Isoflurane does not sensitize the myocardium to catecholamines. Although switching from halothane to isoflurane theoretically might minimize arrhythmias, it does not address the primary concern—aminophylline toxicity. In reality, we probably also would discontinue halothane; however, the *most appropriate management* is to first address the potential aminophylline toxicity by terminating the infusion.

REASONING:

The key elements to this question are the toxicity profile of aminophylline and the drug interaction between halothane and aminophylline. Aminophylline has a narrow therapeutic range and variable clearance, mandating close attention to drug interactions that can compound its toxicity. This question is made somewhat challenging by two seemingly plausible answers (B and E). However, the key is to recognize that the examination is asking for the "most appropriate management." In this case, addressing the potential aminophylline toxicity is the primary concern. The best answer is B.

REFERENCES:

1. Barash PG, Cullen BF, Stoelting RK. Clinical Anesthesia, 4th ed. Philadelphia, Lippincott Williams & Wilkins, 2001, p. 817.

2. Strauss RE, Wertheim DL, Bonagura VR, Valacer DJ. Aminophylline therapy does not improve outcome and increases adverse effects in children hospitalized with acute asthmatic exacerbations. Pediatrics 93:205–210, 1994.

3. Stoelting RK, Dierdorf SF. Anesthesia and Co-existing Diseases, 3d ed. New York, Churchill Livingstone, 1993, p. 153.

BOOK A:

QUESTION 96

Answer B

Equipment/Physics

QUESTION (Choose single best answer):

Oxygen 100 mL/min is bubbled through a vaporizer containing an anesthetic with a vapor pressure of 150 mm Hg, and this mixture is added to a fresh gas flow of 5 L/min. The delivered anesthetic concentration is

(A) 0.25%.
(B) 0.5%.
(C) 1%.
(D) 2.5%.
(E) 5%.

CORRECT ANSWER: B

SUMMARY:

The amount of vapor leaving a copper kettle type of vaporizer depends on the vapor pressure of the anesthetic agent, the flow rate of the carrier gas (i.e., oxygen), and the barometric pressure at which the vaporizer is used. Thus we can compute the delivered vapor output by the equation:

$$Vapor\ output = \frac{carrier\ gas\ flowrate \times vapor\ pressure\ of\ gas}{barometric\ pressure - vapor\ pressure\ of\ gas}$$

$$= \frac{100(cc/mL) \times 150(mm\ Hg)}{760(mm\ Hg) - 150(mm\ Hg)} = 24.6\ cc/min$$

This calculation equals 24.6 cc/min of anesthetic. This is the amount of anesthetic gas picked up by the oxygen carrier gas. To determine the final anesthetic concentration, add 24.6 cc/min to 100 cc/min of carrier gas flow and to 5000 cc/min of fresh gas flow (5124.6 cc/min total). Finally, divide actual anesthetic gas flow by the total as follows:

$$\frac{24.6\ cc/min}{5124.6\ cc/min} = 0.5\%$$

EXPLANATION:

(A) **Incorrect.** See above.

(B) **Correct.** To compute the answer, four variables must be defined: (a) the barometric pressure, (b) the vapor pressure of the anesthetic gas, (c) the carrier flow rate, and (d) the fresh gas flow. Often the carrier gas rate is 100 cc/min of oxygen, and the barometric pressure is set at sea level (760 mm Hg). With these values, one can determine the final anesthetic concentration of any anesthetic gas using the following equation:

$$Vapor\ output = \frac{carrier\ gas\ flow \times vapor\ pressure\ of\ gas}{barometric\ pressure - vapor\ pressure\ of\ gas}$$

$$Final\ anesthetic\ concentration = \frac{vapor\ output}{carrier\ gas\ flow + vapor\ output + fresh\ gas\ flow}$$

(C) **Incorrect.** See above.

(D) **Incorrect.** See above.

(E) **Incorrect.** See above.

REASONING:

The copper kettle was developed by Lucien Morris in 1948 as the first temperature-compensated, accurate vaporizer of anesthetic agents.[1] Although it is taught routinely in many residency programs and review texts, the copper kettle is a fairly esoteric and obsolete topic that probably will not be tested on current board examinations. It is, however, important for the reader to review other factors that can influence vaporizer output, such as changes in temperature, intermittent backpressure (i.e., pumping effect), and changes in carrier gas composition.[2] It is also important to note that unlike other modern variable bypass vaporizers, the Tec-6 vaporizer that is used for desflurane is electrically heated and pressurized and requires compensation when used at altitudes above sea level.[2] Congratulations if you got the answer correct!

REFERENCES:

1. Morris LE. A new vaporizer for liquid anesthetic agents. Anesthesiology 13:587, 1952.
2. Barash PG, Cullen BF, Stoelting RK. Clinical Anesthesia, 4th ed. Philadelphia, Lippincott Williams & Wilkins, 2001, pp. 13, 575–578.
3. Morgan GE, Mikhail MS, Murray MJ. Clinical Anesthesiology, 3d ed. New York, McGraw-Hill, 2002, pp. 40–41.

Answer D

Physiology

QUESTION (Choose single best answer):

A 50-year-old man who takes aspirin and nifedipine is scheduled for thoracotomy with one-lung ventilation. Which of the following is associated with the greatest risk for intraoperative hypoxemia?

(A) Preoperative withdrawal of nifedipine therapy.
(B) Intraoperative mild respiratory acidosis.
(C) Intraoperative administration of isoflurane.
(D) Intraoperative administration of nitroglycerin.
(E) Intraoperative thoracic epidural morphine.

CORRECT ANSWER: D

SUMMARY:

Shunting (perfusion in the absence of ventilation) and hypoxemia during one-lung ventilation are minimized through hypoxic pulmonary vasoconstriction (HPV). Factors that impair HPV will increase the risk of hypoxemia. HPV directs blood away from poorly oxygenated lung regions to areas of the lung that are better ventilated. This results in better matching of blood flow to ventilated lung regions (better $\dot{V}/\dot{Q}$ matching). This is especially important during one-lung ventilation. Oxygen-poor blood from the nonventilated lung will mix with oxygenated blood traveling from the ventilated lung and reduce systemic Pa_{O_2}. This process is minimized by HPV, which preferentially reduces blood flow to the nonventilated lung. Factors known to inhibit HPV and increase the risk of hypoxemia during one-lung ventilation include (1) hypocapnia from hyperventilation, (2) extremes of mixed venous P_{O_2}, (3) extremes of pulmonary artery pressure, (4) systemic vasodilators such as calcium channel blockers, nitroglycerin, and sodium nitroprusside, (5) infection, and (6) at high doses some inhaled anesthetics, particularly halothane.[1] Nonetheless, studies in humans have either failed to demonstrate or have demonstrated only very slight changes in Pa_{O_2} during one-lung ventilation with up to 1 MAC of isoflurane. There is no clear association between epidural opiates and hypoxic pulmonary vasoconstriction.

EXPLANATION:

(A) *Incorrect.* Calcium channel blockers impair HPV, and their withdrawal preoperatively will reduce the risk of intraoperative hypoxemia.
(B) *Incorrect.* Hypocapnia (respiratory alkalosis), not respiratory acidosis, can impair HPV, increasing the risk of intraoperative hypoxemia.
(C) *Incorrect.* Isoflurane at clinically useful doses does not significantly impair HPV.
(D) *Correct.* Nonspecific vasodilators such as nitroglycerin can impair HPV significantly and increase the risk of intraoperative hypoxia.
(E) *Incorrect.* Thoracic epidural morphine would not be expected to have an effect on intraoperative hypoxemia.

REASONING:

This question tests knowledge of pharmacologic effects on hypoxic pulmonary vasoconstriction during one-lung ventilation. It is important to understand the factors that directly impair HPV, such as vasodilator agents, infection, hypocarbia, and metabolic alkalosis.[1] Factors that increase pulmonary artery pressures also can indirectly antagonize the effects of HPV, such as mitral stenosis, volume overload, thromboembolism, and vasoconstrictor drugs.[1] Finally, there are certain drugs that actually can enhance HPV. Almitrine, prostaglandin inhibitors, and even lidocaine have been found to have some potentiating properties. However, their use is largely experimental, and their value during one-lung ventilation has not been established.[1]

REFERENCE:

1. Barash PG, Cullen BF, Stoelting RK. Clinical Anesthesia, 4th ed. Philadelphia, Lippincott Williams & Wilkins, 2001, pp. 831–833.
2. Morgan GE, Mikhail MS, Murray MJ. Clinical Anesthesiology, 3d ed. New York, McGraw-Hill, 2002, pp. 455–456.

BOOK A:

Answer C

Physiology

QUESTION 98

QUESTION (Choose single best answer):

A 35-year-old woman with severe myasthenia gravis is scheduled for thymectomy. Which of the following preoperative pulmonary function tests is most likely to be normal?

(A) Forced expiratory volume in 1 second (FEV_1).
(B) Forced vital capacity (FVC).
(C) FEV_1/FVC.
(D) Maximum voluntary ventilation.
(E) Peak inspiratory force.

CORRECT ANSWER: C

SUMMARY:

Myasthenia gravis is an autoimmune skeletal muscle disease that causes weakness and fatigability by destruction of postsynaptic acetylcholine receptors at the neuromuscular junction. In approximately 80 percent of patients, the thymus gland is the origin of the antibodies to the acetylcholine receptors. Pulmonary function tests (PFTs) measure muscle strength and endurance and will be below normal in a patient with myasthenia gravis.

EXPLANATION:

(A) *Incorrect.* A patient weak with myasthenia will have an impaired ability to forcefully exhale.
(B) *Incorrect.* Again, the severe myasthenic will not have a normal forced capacity.
(C) *Correct.* If both FEV_1 and FVC are lowered, the ratio may be normal.
(D) *Incorrect.* MVV measures muscle endurance and is likely to be abnormal.
(E) *Incorrect.* PIF requires good muscle strength. This number has predictive value for postoperative respiratory complications and impending respiratory failure in the myasthenic patient.

REASONING:

This question tests knowledge of pulmonary function testing in the setting of myasthenia gravis. The answer to this question relies in part on your mathematical prowess. It does not take much knowledge of myasthenia and PFTs. Weak patients have below normal PFTs for effort-dependent assessments such as FEV_1, FVC, MVV, and PIF. However, answer C is a ratio that eliminates units (liters) and seemingly corrects for impaired patient effort. With both FEV_1 and FVC decreased in the myasthenic patient, the ratio may be normal.

REFERENCE:

Miller RD, Miller ED, Reves JG, et al. Anesthesia, 5th ed. New York, Churchill Livingstone, 2000, p. 887.
Morgan GE, Mikhail MS, Murray MJ. Clinical Anesthesiology, 3d ed. New York, McGraw-Hill, 2002, pp. 753–754.

Answer E

Physiology

QUESTION (Choose single best answer):

A 66-year-old man with aortic regurgitation is brought to the operating room for aortic valve replacement after having received morphine and scopolamine premedication. The P_{O_2} is 40 mm Hg in a sample of pulmonary artery blood drawn 10 minutes after the patient started breathing pure oxygen. This finding is compatible with

(A) Wedging of the catheter tip.
(B) Left-to-right intracardiac shunting.
(C) Increased intrapulmonary shunting.
(D) Excessively depressed ventilation.
(E) Normal cardiac output.

CORRECT ANSWER: E

SUMMARY:

Mixed venous saturation represents the global oxygen supply and demand balance and is useful in assessing overall blood supply and tissue demand. In the absence of increased oxygen demand, hypoxia, and anemia, a drop in mixed venous saturation is indicative of decreased blood flow in relation to tissue requirements. This results in increased extraction and a drop in mixed venous oxygen saturation. This relationship allows mixed venous saturation to be used as a surrogate measure of adequate cardiac output. Normal mixed venous saturation is 75 percent with a partial pressure of 40 mm Hg.[1]

EXPLANATION:

(A) *Incorrect.* Wedging of the catheter tip is diagnosed by PA catheter tracing.
(B) *Incorrect.* Left-to-right shunt would exhibit a higher P_{O_2} and saturation.
(C) *Incorrect.* Intrapulmonary shunt would contribute toward hypoxia and thus further decrease mixed venous saturation and partial pressure.
(D) *Incorrect.* Excessively depressed ventilation would affect CO_2 elimination. Unless extreme, it would not affect oxygenation or S_{VO_2}.
(E) *Correct.* The P_{O_2} of 40 mm Hg is normal and indicates a saturation near 75 percent. This is consistent with an adequate cardiac output.

REASONING:

The relationship between $S\bar{v}_{O_2}$, $\dot{V}_{O_2}$, and $\dot{D}_{O_2}$ is described by the equation

$$S\bar{v}_{O_2} = S_{aO_2} - \frac{\dot{V}_{O_2}}{Hb \times 13.8 \times CO}$$

where S_{aO_2} is the arterial O_2 saturation, Hb is the hemoglobin concentration, $\dot{V}_{O_2}$ is the rate of oxygen consumption, 13.8 represents the volume of O_2 carried by 1 g Hb/L, and CO is the cardiac output.[1] In clinical practice, $S\bar{v}_{O_2}$ can be measured continuously using reflectance spectrophotometry of blood at the tip of a pulmonary artery catheter.[1] It is important to understand that $S\bar{v}_{O_2}$ represents global tissue oxygen extraction in the body, with a normal value of 75 percent indicating 25 percent tissue extraction. Various end organs, however, have different extraction ratios that can vary from 55 to 70 percent for myocardium to 7 to 10 percent for the kidney and skin.[1] It is important for the reader to be familiar with the relationship of cardiac output and mixed venous oxygen saturation and the factors that influence mixed venous saturation. The best answer is E.

REFERENCE:

1. Barash PG, Cullen BF, Stoelting RK. Clinical Anesthesia, 4th ed. Philadelphia, Lippincott Williams & Wilkins, 2001, pp. 201–202, 678. (Note that the equation is printed incorrectly in this text.)
Morgan GE, Mikhail MS, Murray MJ. Clinical Anesthesiology, 3d ed. New York, McGraw-Hill, 2002, pp. 499–502.

BOOK A:

Answer A

Pharmacology

QUESTION 100

QUESTION (Choose single best answer):

Which of the following statements concerning metoclopramide is true?

(A) It is antagonized by concomitant administration of atropine.
(B) It decreases gastrointestinal motility.
(C) It decreases gastric secretion.
(D) It lacks antiemetic properties.
(E) It stimulates dopamine receptors.

CORRECT ANSWER: A

SUMMARY:

Metoclopramide, a commonly used antiemetic and prokinetic agent functions (1) centrally as a dopamine antagonist (antiemetic mechanism) and (2) peripherally by facilitating muscarinic acetylcholine transmission (resulting in its gastrointestinal effects: increased lower esophageal sphincter tone, increased gastric emptying, and decreased gastric fluid volume). Note that metoclopramide does not effect gastric pH or the secretion of gastric acid. Also, because its peripheral mechanism is cholinomimetic in nature, its gastrointestinal effects can be inhibited by antimuscarinic agents such as atropine and glycopyrrolate.

EXPLANATION:

(A) **Correct.** Metoclopramide exerts its gastrointestinal effects by facilitating acetylcholine transmission at muscarinic receptors. These actions can be inhibited by antimuscarinic agents such as atropine and glycopyrrolate.
(B) **Incorrect.** Metoclopramide increases upper gastrointestinal motility, resulting in increased gastric emptying.
(C) **Incorrect.** Metoclopramide does not effect gastric secretion. However, it does lower gastric volume by facilitating gastric emptying. Metoclopramide does not alter the pH of the stomach.
(D) **Incorrect.** Metoclopramide is used commonly for its antiemetic properties, which are mediated via antagonism of dopamine receptors.
(E) **Incorrect.** Metoclopramide antagonizes dopamine receptors.

REASONING:

This question tests knowledge of the mechanism of metoclopramide, which acts both peripherally (cholinomimetic) and centrally (antidopaminergic). It is important to understand the effects of metoclopramide on the upper gastrointestinal tract. Metoclopramide increases upper gastrointestinal motility and gastroesophageal sphincter tone but does not affect gastric acid secretion or pH.[1] The best answer is A.

REFERENCES:

1. Barash PG, Cullen BF, Stoelting RK. Clinical Anesthesia, 4th ed. Philadelphia, Lippincott Williams & Wilkins, 2001, p. 559.
2. Morgan GE, Mikhail MS, Murray MJ. Clinical Anesthesiology, 3d ed. New York, McGraw-Hill, 2002, pp. 245–246.

Answer C

Physiology

QUESTION (Choose single best answer):

During halothane anesthesia with spontaneous ventilation, the most reliable sign of malignant hyperthermia is

(A) Hypertension.
(B) Increased temperature.
(C) Increased minute ventilation.
(D) Muscle rigidity.
(E) Tachycardia.

CORRECT ANSWER: C

SUMMARY:

Malignant hyperthermia (MH) is a rare and potentially fatal complication of general anesthesia. It is a hypermetabolic state that results from abnormal calcium release from the sarcoplasmic reticulum in myocytes. The clinical signs of MH are the result of the associated hypermetabolism, increased sympathetic activity, muscle damage, and hyperthermia. Treatment includes stopping the triggering agent, supportive care, and administration of intravenous dantrolene.

EXPLANATION:

(A) *Incorrect.* Although sympathetic activation is a sign of MH, it is not the most sensitive sign. Other signs of increased sympathetic activity associated with MH include tachycardia and arrhythmias.

(B) *Incorrect.* An elevated temperature is a late sign of MH. The temperature rise can be as much as $1°C$ every 5 minutes.

(C) *Correct.* The most reliable sign for MH is an increasing end-tidal CO_2 reflecting the increased CO_2 production from the hypermetabolic state. In a patient who is breathing spontaneously, the increased CO_2 will result in increased minute ventilation.

(D) *Incorrect.* Muscle rigidity is a sign of MH but does not have to be present for the diagnosis of MH.

(E) *Incorrect.* Once again, sympathetic activation is a sign of MH, but tachycardia is not specific or sensitive for the diagnosis of MH.

REASONING:

This question tests knowledge of the clinical signs of malignant hyperthermia. Although all the choices may occur during MH, we are asked to select the *most sensitive* indicator of the disease. Increased Pa_{CO_2} with the resulting increased minute ventilation is the best answer. It is also important for the reader to review appropriate management of suspected MH. Treatment includes (1) cessation of all triggering agents (inhalational anesthetics and succinylcholine), (2) hyperventilation, (3) administration of intravenous dantrolene, (4) active cooling with external ice packs and/or gastric, wound, or rectal lavage, (5) treatment of metabolic acidosis with bicarbonate, and (6) monitoring and treatment of electrolyte abnormalities such as hyperkalemia.[1] Prophylactic administration of dantrolene in MH-susceptible patients prior to administration of a nontriggering anesthetic is not necessary.[1]

REFERENCE:

1. Barash PG, Cullen BF, Stoelting RK. Clinical Anesthesia, 4th ed. Philadelphia, Lippincott Williams & Wilkins, 2001, pp. 529–530.
2. Morgan GE, Mikhail MS, Murray MJ. Clinical Anesthesiology, 3d ed. New York, McGraw-Hill, 2002, pp. 869–870.

QUESTION 102

QUESTION (Choose single best answer):

Which of the following is the most appropriate action after an anesthetic vaporizer is tipped?

(A) Return to the manufacturer for recalibration.
(B) Flush the vaporizer with oxygen at 5 L/min for 24 hours.
(C) Store the vaporizer for 24 hours at room temperature.
(D) Set the vaporizer at low concentration and flush with oxygen at 10 L/min for 30 minutes.
(E) Verify the vaporizer output with mass spectrography.

CORRECT ANSWER: D

SUMMARY:

Tipping of a vaporizer sometimes can occur when the vaporizer is moved incorrectly or changed from an anesthetic machine. Tipping a vaporizer can cause the anesthetic agent to flood the bypass area of the vaporizer that is usually only crossed by the carrier gas.[1] This could lead to a dangerously high concentration of vapor output because the carrier gas picks up more of the agent as it crosses the bypass chamber. The appropriate action after the tipping of a vaporizer is to set it at a low concentration and flush the vaporizer with the carrier gas or oxygen at high flows (10 L/min) for 20 to 30 minutes.[1]

EXPLANATION:

(A) *Incorrect.* Returning the vaporizer to the manufacturer is not necessary. The problem is solved easily by flushing out any excess vapor from the bypass chamber and running the vaporizer at low concentrations to be assured that equilibrium is reestablished. After such a maneuver, we can be fairly certain that the dialed concentration is the same as the amount of anesthetic vapor being delivered to the patient.

(B) *Incorrect.* Flushing the vaporizer with oxygen for 24 hours is not necessary because it will not take that long to rid the bypass chamber of any excess volatile agent. In addition, keeping a vaporizer on for this amount of time with medium to high flows will rid the vaporizer of all inhalational agent.

(C) *Incorrect.* Storing the vaporizer for 24 hours at room temperature does nothing to rid the vaporizer of potential agents in the bypass chamber. Thus, restarting the vaporizer after this time may put the patient in jeopardy of receiving more vapor output than dialed on the vaporizer.

(D) *Correct.* By setting the vaporizer on a low concentration and flushing it with oxygen at 10 L/min for 30 minutes, any excess agent is flushed through the vaporizer, and the bypass chamber reestablishes an equilibrium with the dialed concentration on the vaporizer. Only then can one be reassured that the patient is receiving the appropriate concentration of vapor output.

(E) *Incorrect.* Mass spectrography will identify an increased amount of vapor output going to the patient compared with that dialed into the vaporizer. However, this number will vary minute to minute until the bypass chamber is cleared of any excess anesthetic agent. Also, it is inconvenient to follow mass spectrography continuously until equilibrium is reestablished.

REASONING:

Vaporizers have two chambers through which gases pass prior to entering the inspiratory limb of the anesthetic circuit to deliver gas to the patient. The carrier gas, which is frequently oxygen, goes through the liquid anesthetic agent to pick up vapor. A portion of the carrier gas flow is not exposed to anesthetic agent and passes through a bypass chamber. The amount of vapor output is controlled by varying the ratio of gas that flows through the bypass chamber. When a vaporizer is tipped, there is potential for the agent to cross over into the bypass chamber and for the oxygen carrier gas to pick up more anesthetic than is dialed into the vaporizer. The first action that must be taken when this occurs is to flush the vaporizer while dialed on low concentrations to clear that bypass chamber, minimizing the waste of anesthetic agent. After approximately half an hour at high carrier flow rate, the vaporizer once again can be used safely without fear of delivering a dangerously high amount of vapor to the patient. The best answer is choice D.

REFERENCE:

1. Barash PG, Cullen BF, Stoelting RK. Clinical Anesthesia, 4th ed. Philadelphia, Lippincott Williams & Wilkins, 2001, p. 576.
2. Morgan GE, Mikhail MS, Murray MJ. Clinical Anesthesiology, 3d ed. New York, McGraw-Hill, 2002, p. 42.

BOOK A:

Answer A

Physiology

QUESTION 103

QUESTION (Choose single best answer):

Following pneumonectomy, a paralyzed patient being ventilated mechanically has the following arterial blood gas values: Pa_{O_2} 71 mm Hg, Pa_{CO_2} 55 mm Hg, pH 7.29, and $S\bar{v}_{O_2}$ 45 percent. The most likely explanation for this $S\bar{v}_{O_2}$ is

(A) Decreased red cell mass.
(B) high cardiac output.
(C) Hypothermia.
(D) Peripheral left-to-right arteriovenous shunt.
(E) Ventilation-perfusion mismatch.

CORRECT ANSWER: A

SUMMARY:

Mixed venous oxygen saturation ($S\bar{v}_{O_2}$) is the percent saturation of venous blood prior to entering the lungs. A normal $S\bar{v}_{O_2}$ typically is around 75 percent. Many factors can cause an alteration in the $S\bar{v}_{O_2}$, as demonstrated by the following equation derived from the Fick relationship:

$$S\bar{v}_{O_2} = Sa_{O_2} - [\dot{V}_{O_2}/(Hb \times 13.8 \times CO)]$$

where Sa_{O_2} is the arterial O_2 saturation, Hb is the hemoglobin concentration, $\dot{V}_{O_2}$ is the rate of oxygen consumption, 13.8 represents the volume of O_2 carried by 1 g Hb/L, and CO is the cardiac output.[1] Based on this equation, it is easy to see how each variable can affect $S\bar{v}_{O_2}$.

EXPLANATION:

(A) *Correct.* A decreased red cell mass, according to the preceding equation, will lead to a decreased $S\bar{v}_{O_2}$. Since there is less hemoglobin to carry oxygen, more oxygen will be extracted from the hemoglobin by tissues, causing a decreased $S\bar{v}_{O_2}$.
(B) *Incorrect.* A high cardiac output would deliver more oxygen to tissue, leading to less extraction and a greater $S\bar{v}_{O_2}$.
(C) *Incorrect.* Hypothermia would decrease oxygen consumption, leading to less oxygen extraction and a greater $S\bar{v}_{O_2}$.

(D) *Incorrect.* A left-to-right arteriovenous shunt would prevent the shunted blood from coming into contact with tissue, decreasing oxygen extraction for the shunted blood and leading to a greater $S\bar{v}O_2$ and likely increased cardiac output.

(E) *Incorrect.* A $\dot{V}/\dot{Q}$ mismatch would cause hypoxemia and decrease SaO_2, causing a decrease in $S\bar{v}O_2$. However, a PaO_2 of 71 mm Hg is not sufficiently hypoxemic to explain the observed $S\bar{v}O_2$ of 45 percent.

REASONING:

This question tests knowledge of the factors that influence $S\bar{v}O_2$. Knowing that a decreased $S\bar{v}O_2$ can occur with either a decreased supply of oxygen or increased demand allows answers, B, C, and D to be eliminated because they either increase supply or decrease demand. Choice E is tempting, but it is hard to explain a very low $S\bar{v}O_2$ with a PaO_2 of 71 mm Hg, which corresponds to a SaO_2 above 90 percent saturation. The only answer remaining is decreased red cell mass, which can be explained easily by bleeding during the procedure.

REFERENCE:

1. Barash PG, Cullen BF, Stoelting RK. Clinical Anesthesia, 4th ed. Philadelphia, Lippincott Williams & Wilkins, 2001, p. 678. (Note that equation is printed incorrectly in the text).
2. Morgan GE, Mikhail MS, Murray MJ. Clinical Anesthesiology, 3d ed. New York, McGraw-Hill, 2002, p. 503.

BOOK A:

Answer C

Pharmacology

QUESTION 104

QUESTION (Choose single best answer):

Which of the following is a sign of cyclosporine toxicity?

(A) Abnormal hepatic enzyme activity.
(B) Decreased hemoglobin concentration.
(C) Increased serum creatinine concentration.
(D) Nodular density on radiograph of the chest.
(E) ST-T wave changes on ECG.

CORRECT ANSWER: C

SUMMARY:

Cyclosporine is an immunosupressant associated with multiple toxicities that include seizures, hypertension, elevated liver enzymes, gingival hyperplasia, and renal toxicity resulting in elevated blood urea nitrogen (BUN) and creatinine concentrations. Nephrotoxicity can occur with either acute or chronic use and is due to renal fibrosis and tubular atrophy. Cyclosporine works by (1) inhibiting interleukin 1 (IL-1) production, (2) inhibiting IL-2 secretion, and (3) blocking activation of CD4 helper cells.

EXPLANATION:

(A) *Incorrect.* Cyclosporine can result in elevated liver enzymes, not abnormal liver enzyme function.

(B) *Incorrect.* Unlike other immunosupressant drugs, cyclosporine does not suppress bone marrow cellular production.

(C) *Correct.* Cyclosporine can elevate serum creatinine by causing interstitial renal fibrosis and tubular atrophy. Cyclosporine nephrotoxicity renders the kidney sensitive to acute insults such as radiographic dye and hypotension-induced nephropathy.

(D) *Incorrect.* This is not a toxicity of cyclosporine.

(E) *Incorrect.* This is not a toxicity of cyclosporine.

REASONING:

This question tests knowledge of cyclosporine toxicity. It is important for the reader to be familiar with the side effects of other antirejection medications as well.[1] Tacrolimus has a similar side-effect and toxicity profile. Glucocorticoids can produce adrenal suppression, glucose intolerance, cushingoid appearance, and exacerbation of peptic ulcer disease. Azathioprine can produce anemia, thrombocytopenia, and hepatitis and can increase the requirement for nondepolarizing muscle relaxants.

REFERENCE:

1. Barash PG, Cullen BF, Stoelting RK. Clinical Anesthesia, 4th ed. Philadelphia, Lippincott Williams & Wilkins, 2001, Table 52-16, p. 1367.

BOOK A: QUESTION 105

Answer D

Pain

QUESTION (Choose single best answer):

Myofascial pain is an example of

(A) A central pain state.
(B) Neuropathic pain.
(C) Psychogenic pain.
(D) Somatic pain.
(E) Visceral pain.

CORRECT ANSWER: D

SUMMARY:

Myofascial pain originates from muscle. It is therefore a type of somatic pain that refers to all types of pain originating from the structures of the body wall (e.g., muscle, tendon, ligament, and bone) rather than a type of visceral pain originating from internal organs (e.g., the pain of pancreatitis). It is distinct from the pain caused by direct injury to the central nervous system (central pain states) and the peripheral nervous system (neuropathic pain). Psychogenic pain refers to pain caused by psychological conflict rather than pathology in the structure felt to be in pain.

EXPLANATION:

(A) *Incorrect.* Central pain states and neuropathic pain are the result of pain caused by injury to nervous system tissue.

(B) *Incorrect.* See above.

(C) *Incorrect.* The term *psychogenic pain* specifically excludes pain caused by pathology in the muscles and only refers to pain stemming entirely from psychological factors.

(D) *Correct.* Myofascial pain is a subset of somatic pain that also includes pain from bones (fractures), joints (arthritis), tendons (tendonitis), and other structures of the body wall.

(E) *Incorrect.* Visceral pain comes from structures such as internal organs.

REASONING:

Myofascial pain is pain originating from a muscle group. It is often associated with trigger points. These trigger points are tender to palpation and when stimulated refer pain along stereotypical distributions that are nondermatomal in nature. Trigger point injection with local anesthetic or without (dry-needling) in conjunction with physical therapy may provide relief. The cause of myofascial pain and trigger points is not clear but is not associated with overt central or peripheral nervous system injury, as in central pain states or neuropathic pain. Psychogenic pain is also different and refers to pain based purely on psychological factors such as a need to suffer because of extreme guilt or other psychological conflict. Visceral pain refers to pain arising from the internal organs. Myofascial pain is a type of somatic pain that refers to pain originating from structures in the body wall (as opposed to internal viscera) or skeletal structures such as muscle, bone, tendon, and joint.

REFERENCE:

Barash PG, Cullen BF, Stoelting RK. Clinical Anesthesia, 4th ed. Philadelphia, Lippincott Williams & Wilkins, 2001, p. 1445.

Morgan GE, Mikhail MS, Murray MJ. Clinical Anesthesiology, 3d ed. New York, McGraw-Hill, 2002, pp. 309–310.

BOOK A:

Answer B

Pediatrics

QUESTION 106

QUESTION (Choose single best answer):

In children with preoperative upper respiratory tract infection (URI), which of the following is associated with the greatest risk for postoperative airway obstruction?

(A) Age less than 1 year.
(B) Endotracheal intubation.
(C) Head and neck injury.
(D) Inadequate airway humidification.
(E) Surgery for more than 2 hours.

CORRECT ANSWER: B

SUMMARY:

Children commonly present for elective surgery with symptoms of an active URI or with a recent history of one. There are many conflicting studies that disagree regarding whether children are at increased risk from general anesthesia during or after a URI.[1] Taken as a whole, most studies agree that there is a higher incidence of minor respiratory events (e.g., hypoxemia, bronchospasm, and laryngospasm) but that these events are not more severe than if they were to occur in a patient who did not have a URI.[1] Since children can develop 5 to 10 URIs a year,[2] this places the clinician in a difficult situation regarding postponing surgery because studies have documented that changes in pulmonary reactivity and spirometry can last as long as 7 weeks after a URI.[1] Most clinicians will not anesthetize a child who is acutely "ill" (i.e., with fever, rhinorrhea, and respiratory difficulty) and will postpone surgery for 2 weeks after resolution of symptoms.

EXPLANATION:

(A) *Incorrect.* Children younger than 1 year of age actually have less risk of postoperative airway obstruction. The greatest incidence of croup is in children between the ages of 1 and 4 years. Beyond age 4, the incidence decreases.[3]
(B) *Correct.* Endotracheal intubation has been associated consistently with an increased risk of bronchospasm, laryngospasm, and desaturation events. Most of these events are not severe and are treated easily.[1,3]
(C) *Incorrect.* Neck surgery is associated with increased risk of postoperative airway obstruction, but not head surgery.[3]
(D) *Incorrect.* Humidified air is used to treat croup, but its lack of use is not associated with increased risk of airway obstruction.[3]

(E) *Incorrect.* Duration of surgery in and of itself is not associated with postoperative airway obstruction. Increased duration of endotracheal intubation, however, is directly correlated with an increased incidence of airway obstruction.[3]

REASONING:

This is a challenging question because all the answers appear to be reasonable. The literature itself is inconclusive and often conflicting. The one factor that was most consistently associated with increased postoperative airway obstruction in previous studies was endotracheal intubation. The final decision whether to anesthetize a child should take into consideration factors that include other medical problems, severity of symptoms, urgency of surgery, availability of postoperative care, and the family wishes.

REFERENCES:

1. Cote CJ. A Practice of Anesthesia for Infants and Children, 3d ed. Philadelphia, Saunders, 2001, pp. 43–44.
2. Cohen MM, Cameron CB. Should you cancel the operation when a child has an upper respiratory tract infection? Anesth Analg 72:282–288, 1991.
3. Koka BV, Jeon IS, Andre JM, et al. Postintubation croup in children. Anesth Analg 56:501–505, 1977.
4. Morgan GE, Mikhail MS, Murray MJ. Clinical Anesthesiology, 3d ed. New York, McGraw-Hill, 2002, pp. 856–857.

BOOK A:

QUESTION 107

Answer B

Equipment/Physics

QUESTION (Choose single best answer):

In an anesthetized patient being ventilated mechanically, end-expired carbon dioxide is 58 mm Hg, and peak inspiratory airway pressure is 15 cm H_2O. Ventilator settings indicate a delivered tidal volume of 800 mL, but the expiratory flowmeter shows a tidal volume of 360 mL. Which of the following is the most likely cause of this discrepancy?

(A) Fresh gas flow of 0.5 L/min.
(B) Incompetence of the pressure-relief valve.
(C) Low ventilatory rate.
(D) Presence of a hole in the ventilator bellows.
(E) Prolongation of the inspiratory phase.

CORRECT ANSWER: B

SUMMARY:

Ventilators contain their own pressure-relief valve because the circle system's pressure-relief valve is functionally removed from the circuit. During inspiration, the valve remains closed, allowing positive-pressure ventilation to occur. During expiration, the valve opens when sufficient expiratory pressure is generated. If the valve is stuck and does not open, the patient can be exposed to high airway pressures. If the valve is incompetent, airway pressures may be too low to ventilate the patient.

EXPLANATION:

(A) *Incorrect.* If there were insufficient fresh gas flow, the ventilator settings would indicate a delivered tidal volume roughly equal to the expired tidal volume. High fresh gas flows would increase the exhaled tidal volume.

(B) *Correct.* An incompetent ventilator pressure-relief valve allows some of the tidal volume to leak out the valve as opposed to being delivered to the patient, as is the case in this question.

(C) **Incorrect.** A low ventilatory rate does not explain the difference between set and expired tidal volumes.

(D) **Incorrect.** Presence of a hole in the ventilator bellows would cause a decrease in both the indicated delivered tidal volume and the measured expiratory tidal volume.

(E) **Incorrect.** Prolonging the inspiratory phase would lead to an increase in expired tidal volume relative to the ventilator settings as more of the fresh gas flows in.

REASONING:

The key to answering this question is recognizing that the ventilator settings indicate an adequate tidal volume but that the expired tidal volume is significantly less. In addition, the peak airway pressure is relatively low for a tidal volume of 800 mL. Factors that can influence discordance between set and exhaled tidal volumes include flowmeter settings, inspiratory time, breathing circuit compliance, and leakage in the system.[1] Only choice B explains this. Choices A, C, and D could lead to inadequate ventilation, but the ventilator settings would show low tidal volumes equivalent to expired volumes. Choice E is incorrect because an increase in the inspiratory time would increase the expired tidal volume relative to the ventilator settings.

REFERENCE:

1. Barash PG, Cullen BF, Stoelting RK. Clinical Anesthesia, 4th ed. Philadelphia, Lippincott Williams & Wilkins, 2001, p. 584.
2. Morgan GE, Mikhail MS, Murray MJ. Clinical Anesthesiology, 3d ed. New York, McGraw-Hill, 2002, p. 53.

BOOK A:

Answer D

Pharmacology

QUESTION 108 (OPTIONAL)

QUESTION (Choose single best answer):

Which of the following statements concerning pipecuronium is true?

(A) It has a faster onset than pancuronium.
(B) It increases systemic vascular resistance.
(C) It induces tachycardia.
(D) It is eliminated by the kidney.
(E) It induces histamine release.

CORRECT ANSWER: D

SUMMARY:

Pipecuronium is a long-acting steroid-based nondepolarizing muscle relaxant that is similar to pancuronium. Like pancuronium, it is eliminated primarily unchanged by the kidney. The two drugs also share a similar onset and duration of action. However, unlike pancuronium, pipecuronium does not release histamine and does not have any significant cardiovascular side effects (e.g., tachycardia or altered systemic vascular resistance).

EXPLANATION:

(A) **Incorrect.** The onset of pipecuronium is similar to that of pancuronium.
(B) **Incorrect.** Pipecuronium is devoid of significant cardiovascular side effects.
(C) **Incorrect.** See above.
(D) **Correct.** Pipecuronium is excreted primarily unchanged by the kidney (70 percent) and has a small amount of biliary secretion (20 percent).
(E) **Incorrect.** Unlike pancuronium, pipecuronium does not cause histamine release.

REASONING:

This question tests knowledge of pipecuronium, an old and now uncommonly used non-depolarizing muscle relaxant. It is best answered by process of elimination. In general, pipecuronium and pancuronium have similar onset, duration, and metabolism but differ in their side-effect profiles. Like many board examination questions, the key is being able to compare one drug with another and knowing the specific differences between them. It is unlikely that future board examinations will test knowledge of this outdated nondepolarizing muscle relaxant. Choice D is the best answer.

REFERENCE:

Barash PG, Cullen BF, Stoelting RK. Clinical Anesthesia, 4th ed. Philadelphia, Lippincott Williams & Wilkins, 2001, p. 422.

Morgan GE, Mikhail MS, Murray MJ. Clinical Anesthesiology, 3d ed. New York, McGraw-Hill, 2002, pp. 194–196.

BOOK A:

QUESTION 109

Answer B

Cardiovascular

QUESTION (Choose single best answer):

Left ventricular end-diastolic volume is most likely to be underestimated by pulmonary artery occlusion pressure in patients with

(A) Acute myocardial ischemia.
(B) Aortic insufficiency.
(C) Mitral stenosis.
(D) Primary pulmonary hypertension.
(E) Tricuspid stenosis.

CORRECT ANSWER: B

SUMMARY:

Left ventricular end-diastolic volumes rarely are measured directly in clinical practice. Instead, pulmonary artery catheters are used to measure a pulmonary artery occlusion pressure (PAOP) that provides an estimate of left ventricular end-diastolic pressure (LVEDP). Clinicians use LVEDP as a surrogate measure of left ventricular end-diastolic volume (LVEDV). This interpretation is based on certain assumptions. For example, we assume that a given unit increase in pressure corresponds to a proportional increase in volume or that end-diastolic left atrial pressures equal end-diastolic left ventricular pressures.[1] In reality, these assumptions are not always valid. Indeed, there are multiple factors that influence the PAOP-LVEDV relationship and can cause over- or underestimation of LVEDV. Factors that lead to an underestimation of LVEDV by PAOP stem from decreased left ventricular compliance, aortic or pulmonic valve regurgitation, right bundle-branch block, and decreased pulmonary vascular bed (e.g., after pneumonectomy).[1] Many clinical scenarios can alter the relationship between LV preload (LVEDV) and PAOP, and it is important to review these carefully.[1]

EXPLANATION:

(A) **Incorrect.** Acute myocardial ischemia is associated with mitral regurgitation that can cause "V" waves on pulmonary artery occlusion tracing. Systolic "V" waves raise mean PAOP and can lead to an overestimation of PAOP.[1]

(B) **Correct.** Aortic insufficiency is a classic example of PAOP underestimating LVEDV. Because of the incompetent aortic valve, diastolic ventricular filling begins before the mitral valve opens. More important, diastolic ventricular filling continues *after* atrial contraction and closure of the mitral valve. Because the mitral valve closes before diastolic filling is complete (and LVEDP is maximal), PAOP underestimates the true LVEDP/LVEDV.[1]

(C) *Incorrect.* Mitral stenosis leads to an overestimate of LVEDP because the PAOP is greater than the LVEDP.

(D) *Incorrect.* Pulmonary hypertension increases pulmonary vascular resistance and pulmonary artery diasolic pressures. However, the PAOP should provide an accurate estimate of LVEDP.[1]

(E) *Incorrect.* Tricuspid stenosis does not alter the relationship between PAOP and LVEDP.

REASONING:

It is important to remember that PAOP is an indirect surrogate measure of LVEDV. There are many factors that can challenge the validity of the assumptions used for the interpretation of PAOP as an estimate of LVEDV. The reader should review these carefully.[1] Choice B is the best answer.

REFERENCE:

1. Mark JB. Atlas of Cardiovascular Monitoring, New York, Churchill-Livingstone, 1998, pp. 60–79, 248–259.

2. Morgan GE, Mikhail MS, Murray MJ. Clinical Anesthesiology, 3d ed. New York, McGraw-Hill, 2002, p. 106.

BOOK A:

Answer A

Pharmacology

QUESTION 110

QUESTION (Choose single best answer):

Which of the following statements concerning the cardiovascular effects of intravenous bupivacaine is true?

(A) Bretylium is effective in treating bupivacaine-induced ventricular arrhythmias.
(B) Cardiovascular toxicity is decreased during pregnancy.
(C) Cardiovascular toxicity occurs at lower blood levels than central nervous system toxicity.
(D) Systemic vascular resistance is unchanged.
(E) The rate of impulse conduction through the heart is increased.

CORRECT ANSWER: A

SUMMARY:

Bupivacaine is distinguished among local anesthetics for its cardiotoxicity. It has a high binding affinity for myocardial sodium and potassium channels, inhibits calcium channels and release of calcium from the sarcoplasmic reticulum, inhibits intracellular cAMP production, and may act centrally in the central nervous system to elicit dysrhythmias that are resistant to resuscitation.[1] Bupivicaine toxicity also causes vasodilation and decreased myocardial contractility and can lead to cardiovascular collapse. Purturients are more prone to local anesthetic toxicity. Bretyllium and isoprenaline should be considered in the treatment of ventricular arrhythmia and heart block, respectively. Patients with bupivicaine toxicity benefit from early hyperventilation because hypocarbia raises the seizure threshold.

EXPLANATION:

(A) *Correct.* Bretyllium is the drug of choice in the treatment of ventricular tachyarrhythmia in bupivacaine toxicity.
(B) *Incorrect.* Local anesthetic sensitivity is increased during pregnancy, including toxic reactions.

(C) **Incorrect.** Symptoms of central nervous system toxicity are first to appear in the awake patient.

(D) **Incorrect.** Arteriolar dilation occurs with intravenous bupivacaine, resulting in decreased systemic vascular resistance (SVR).

(E) **Incorrect.** The rate of impulse conduction is depressed owing to blocking of myocyte sodium channels.

REASONING:

This question tests knowledge of the diagnosis and treatment of bupivacaine toxicity. Lidocaine is not a preferred drug for the management of bupivacaine-induced ventricular tachyarrhythmias. Treatment of bupivacaine-induced dysrhythmias may require aggressive treatment with large amounts of bretyllium, epinephrine, and magnesium and multiple attempts at electrical cardioversion.[1] A is the best answer.

REFERENCE:

1. Barash PG, Cullen BF, Stoelting RK. Clinical Anesthesia, 4th ed. Philadelphia, Lippincott Williams & Wilkins, 2001, pp. 460–462.
2. Morgan GE, Mikhail MS, Murray MJ. Clinical Anesthesiology, 3d ed. New York, McGraw-Hill, 2002, pp. 238–241.

BOOK A:

Answer E

Equipment/Physics

QUESTION 111

QUESTION (Choose single best answer):

Which of the following is indicated by an alarm condition in the line-isolation monitor?

(A) An electric shock to the patient.
(B) A power surge in the main hospital power supply.
(C) Disconnection of the patient from an electrocautery grounding pad.
(D) Overload of the operating room circuits.
(E) The presence of a current leak between an operating room electrical device and ground.

CORRECT ANSWER: E

SUMMARY:

Most operating rooms have special power supplies that isolate electric current from the ground using an isolation transformer. Isolated power supplies decrease the risk of electric shock by eliminating the ground as a return route to complete an electrical circuit (a common cause of inadvertent household electrocutions). Despite this transformer, faults can occur in all electrical equipment (leakage current). A line-isolation monitor measures the potential for electricity to flow from an isolated electric circuit to the ground. If electrical flow to the ground (leakage current) is greater than 2 to 5 mA, the alarm will sound. The alarm does not indicate that the patient is being shocked, only that the potential exists if a second fault in the circuit develops.

EXPLANATION:

(A) **Incorrect.** The line-isolation monitor serves as a warning and alarms when a single fault in an isolated electric circuit develops. The alarm does not mean that current is flowing through the patient or that a shock is occurring. It simply means that a faulty piece of electrical equipment has caused the isolated operating room (OR) electrical system to be essentially "converted" to a grounded power system such as those found in most residential services.[1] The patient is at risk of a shock if a second fault in the system occurs. Once the line-isolation monitor alarm is activated, try to postpone the procedure if it is not yet started or unplug each electrical device in the OR (starting with whichever one was plugged in last). The goal is to remove the defective device from the circuitry.

(B) **Incorrect.** A line-isolation monitor measures leakage current in the OR. A power surge in the main hospital power supply would not be expected to affect the leakage current in the OR.

(C) **Incorrect.** An electrocautery grounding pad must be placed on a patient to provide a large surface area for this current to return to the Bovie and prevent burns to the patient. The line-isolation monitor has nothing to do with such a grounding pad.

(D) **Incorrect.** Line-isolation monitors do not alarm based on the amount of current within OR circuits or the amount of equipment used in one OR. They alarm only if leakage current exceeds 2 to 5 mA.

(E) **Correct.** The line-isolation monitor will alarm if a fault in the electrical circuitry develops that results in a leakage current greater than 2 to 5 mA. Its main purpose is to advise the OR personnel that there is a potential for electric shock to occur if a second fault in the system develops. Surgery should be stopped and electrical devices systematically unplugged to discover the source of the leakage current.

REASONING:

Each operating room has a main isolation transformer to isolate its electricity from the hospital's main power supply. It has a primary circuit that is grounded and a secondary circuit that is not. Unfortunately, every electrical device has a small amount of leakage current to ground and thus has the potential to turn an ungrounded circuit into a grounded one. Line-isolation monitors (LIMs) alarm when the secondary circuit of a main isolation transformer becomes grounded. This acts as a forewarning before one or more faults occur to complete a circuit and cause potential electrical hazard to OR personnel and the patient. Usually, 2 to 5 mA of leakage current will activate the alarm. A line-isolation monitor does not prevent electrical shock. Only a vigilant anesthesiologist with a thorough understanding of the LIM can protect the patient and the OR staff from electrical injury. The single best answer is E.

REFERENCE:

1. Barash PG, Cullen BF, Stoelting RK. Clinical Anesthesia, 4th ed. Philadelphia, Lippincott Williams & Wilkins, 2001, pp. 152–154.

2. Morgan GE, Mikhail MS, Murray MJ. Clinical Anesthesiology, 3d ed. New York, McGraw-Hill, 2002, pp. 17–19.

BOOK A:

Answer E

Pharmacology

QUESTION 112

QUESTION (Choose single best answer):

Which of the following statements concerning ketorolac is true?

(A) It binds to opioid receptors.
(B) It causes dose-related thrombocytopenia.
(C) It decreases heart rate during isoflurane anesthesia.
(D) It is eliminated unchanged in urine.
(E) It reversibly inhibits cyclooxygenase.

CORRECT ANSWER: E

SUMMARY:

Ketorolac is a nonsteroidal anti-inflammatory drug (NSAID) that works by reversibly inhibiting cyclooxygenase activity and inhibiting prostaglandin production. It is metabo-

lized by hepatic enzymes and eliminated by the kidney (both unchanged and in the form of metabolites). Ketorolac is a known inhibitor of platelet function (not number) and can result in prolonged bleeding time.

EXPLANATION:

(A) *Incorrect.* Ketorolac binds to cyclooxygenase and blocks prostaglandin synthesis. It does not exert its analgesic effect by binding to opioid receptors.

(B) *Incorrect.* Ketorolac inhibits platelet function, not platelet number. Therefore, it does not result in thrombocytopenia.

(C) *Incorrect.* This is not a known effect of ketorolac. Ketorolac does not affect minimum alveolar concentration (MAC).

(D) *Incorrect.* Ketorolac is metabolized in the liver and then eliminated by the kidney. Although some ketorolac is eliminated renally as whole drug, most is metabolized by the liver.

(E) *Correct.* Ketorolac reversibly inhibits the cyclooxygenase enzyme, like most NSAIDs.

REASONING:

Ketorolac is a safe and effective analgesic that avoids respiratory depression, sedation, and constipation associated with opioid analgesics. Ketorolac reversibly inhibits the cyclooxygenase enzyme, blocking prostaglandin synthesis. Because of its inhibitory effects on platelet function, some surgeons prefer to avoid the use of ketorolac for postoperative pain control. Potential adverse effects of NSAID use include exacerbation of bronchospasm in patients with a history of nasal polyps, asthma, and rhinitis.[1] Although D is partly true, E is the single best answer.

REFERENCES:

1. Barash PG, Cullen BF, Stoelting RK. Clinical Anesthesia, 4th ed. Philadelphia, Lippincott Williams & Wilkins, 2001, p. 1412.

2. Gilman AG, Jardman JG, Limbird LE. Goodman & Gilman's The Pharmacological Basis of Therapeutics, 10th ed. New York, McGraw-Hill, 2001, pp. 691–692.

3. Morgan GE, Mikhail MS, Murray MJ. Clinical Anesthesiology, 3d ed. New York, McGraw-Hill, 2002, p. 248.

BOOK A:

Answer D

Equipment/Physics

QUESTION 113

QUESTION (Choose single best answer):

Postoperatively, a patient is being ventilated mechanically by a constant-flow, pressure-cycled ventilator with the following initial settings: inspiratory–expiratory (I:E) ratio of 1:2, peak inspiratory pressure (PIP) of 25 cm H_2O, and rate of 10 breaths per minute. One hour later, the I:E ratio is 1:4. Which of the following would ensure that the minute ventilation is the same as that set initially?

(A) Inflate the endotracheal tube cuff to prevent leakage.
(B) Double the respiratory rate.
(C) Decrease the expiratory pause until the I:E ratio is 1.0.
(D) Increase the PIP until the I:E ratio is 1:2.
(E) Increase the PIP to 50 cm H_2O.

CORRECT ANSWER: D

SUMMARY:

Pressure-cycled ventilators, also referred to as pressure-controlled ventilators, are a ventilatory mode in which ventilation is controlled completely by the ventilator, and a set airway pressure is delivered to the patient. With this mode of ventilation, the tidal volume varies with airway resistance and lung compliance. If airway resistance increases and/or lung compliance decreases, the set peak airway pressure is reached earlier, and a smaller tidal volume is delivered.[1] In addition, the time in inspiration relative to expiration decreases.

EXPLANATION:

(A) *Incorrect.* A leak in the cuff does not explain the problem. Leakage of air from the endotracheal tube cuff would make it more difficult for the ventilator to reach the set inspiratory pressure, increasing the time in inspiration, not decreasing it.

(B) *Incorrect.* Doubling the respiratory rate would increase the time in inspiration, but dead-space ventilation increases more than alveolar ventilation with smaller tidal volumes and higher respiratory rates.

(C) *Incorrect.* Decreasing the expiratory pause to obtain an I:E ratio of 1.0 likely will increase the minute ventilation because more time is spent in inspiration.

(D) *Correct.* Increasing the PIP until the I:E ratio is 1:2 will allow for the same tidal volumes to be delivered as before because it is a constant-flow ventilator. Since it is a constant flow ventilator, the same time in inspiration will yield the same total amount of flow and tidal volume.

(E) *Incorrect.* Increasing the PIP to 50 cm H_2O will increase the tidal volume delivered and minute ventilation, but it likely will not be the same as set initially because we are not sure how much the compliance and/or airway resistance of the lungs has changed.

REASONING:

The key to answering this question is knowing how a pressure-cycled ventilator functions. Choice A can be eliminated easily because a cuff leak would increase the inspiratory time, not decrease it. Choices B, C, and E do increase the minute ventilation, but not to the same minute ventilation as the initial settings. Only choice D ensures the same minute ventilation as the previous setting. The best answer is D.

REFERENCE:

1. Barash PG, Cullen BF, Stoelting RK. Clinical Anesthesia, 4th ed. Philadelphia, Lippincott Williams & Wilkins, 2001, p. 1471.
2. Morgan GE, Mikhail MS, Murray MJ. Clinical Anesthesiology, 3d ed. New York, McGraw-Hill, 2002, pp. 961–964.

BOOK A:

Answer B

Physiology

QUESTION 114

QUESTION (Choose single best answer):

Left ventricular subendocardial perfusion pressure is best estimated by the difference between

(A) Mean arterial and central venous pressures.
(B) Diastolic arterial and pulmonary artery occlusion pressures.
(C) Mean arterial and pulmonary artery occlusion pressures.
(D) Systolic arterial and pulmonary artery occlusion pressures.
(E) Diastolic arterial and central venous pressures.

CORRECT ANSWER: B

SUMMARY:

Myocardial perfusion is intermittent and occurs primarily during diastole for the left ventricle. Left ventricular pressures during systole are high enough to occlude coronary ves-

sels, preventing any flow during systole. Since right ventricular systolic pressures are lower, the right ventricle is perfused during both systole and diastole. The majority of right ventricular perfusion occurs during systole.[1] Left ventricular subendocardial perfusion pressure is determined by the difference between aortic diastolic pressure and left ventricular end-diastolic pressure (or pulmonary artery occlusion pressure [PAOP] as an estimate of LVEDP).

EXPLANATION:

(A) *Incorrect.* See above.
(B) *Correct.* Coronary flow occurs during diastole; thus the difference between diastolic and left ventricular end-diastolic pressure determines coronary perfusion pressure.
(C) *Incorrect.* See above.
(D) *Incorrect.* See above.
(E) *Incorrect.* Subendocardial perfusion pressure is determined by the difference between aortic diastolic pressure and left ventricular end-diastolic pressure or PAOP.

REASONING:

This question tests knowledge of the determinants of left ventricular coronary perfusion pressure. Left ventricular coronary perfusion occurs primarily during diastole, when the aortic valve closes and diastolic aortic pressures drive blood through the coronary ostia to perfuse myocardium. Coronary perfusion pressure for the left ventricle is defined as aortic diastolic pressure minus LVEDP (or PAOP as an estimate of LVEDP).[1] The best answer is B.

REFERENCE:

1. Barash PG, Cullen BF, Stoelting RK. Clinical Anesthesia, 4th ed. Philadelphia, Lippincott Williams & Wilkins, 2001, Fig. 32-1, pp. 883–884.
2. Morgan GE, Mikhail MS, Murray MJ. Clinical Anesthesiology, 3d ed. New York, McGraw-Hill, 2002, p. 376.

BOOK A:　　　　　　　　**QUESTION 115**

Answer C

Clinical Anesthesia

QUESTION (Choose single best answer):

A 29-year-old man who has been nasotracheally intubated for 2 weeks following a motor vehicle accident has a fever (39°C) and a constant headache. Leukocyte count is 18,000/mm³. The most likely cause is

(A) Fractured nasal septum.
(B) Retropharyngeal abscess.
(C) Maxillary sinusitis.
(D) Meningitis.
(E) Rhinovirus infection.

CORRECT ANSWER: C

SUMMARY:

Patients in an intensive care unit require mechanical ventilation for many reasons, most commonly for respiratory failure. Endotracheal intubation may be accomplished via the oral or nasal route. Nasal intubation often is considered more comfortable for the patient and more secure from accidental extubation. There are, however, complications associated with nasotracheal intubation, including nasal necrosis,[1] bacteremia, epistaxis, sinusitis, otitis media, submucosal dissection of the nasopharynx that can develop into retropharyngeal abcesses,[2] *and accidental insertion of the endotracheal tube into the cranial vault through a basilar skull fracture.*[2] *The decision on the route of intubation should be based on the clinical situation, experience of the practitioner, and expected duration of ventilation. Tracheostomy may be considered for periods of prolonged ventilation (>2 to 3 weeks) in adults.*

EXPLANATION:

(A) *Incorrect.* There is inadequate evidence for a fractured nasal septum. One would not expect a fever and increased leukocyte count with just a fractured nasal septum.

(B) *Incorrect.* Retropharyngeal abcess is a reported complication with nasal intubations.[2] However, it would cause a sore throat rather than a constant headache.

(C) *Correct.* Sinusitis is a reported common complication of nasal intubation.[1,2] The signs and symptoms are consistent with this diagnosis.

(D) *Incorrect.* While all the symptoms listed are consistent with an ongoing infection, meningitis is not a reported common complication of nasotracheal intubation.

(E) *Incorrect.* The most common organisms associated with nasal intubations are bacteria that colonize the nasopharynx, e.g., *Streptococcus viridans.*[2] Rhinovirus infection, while a common cause of upper respiratory infections, is not associated with nasal intubations.

REASONING:

This question tests knowledge of the complications of nasotracheal intubation and symptoms of infection. A fractured nasal septum, choice A, might occur after a motor vehicle accident but by itself would not explain the signs and symptoms of infection. Meningitis, choice D, is not a common complication of motor vehicle accidents or nasotracheal intubation. Rhinovirus infection, choice E, also can cause fever, headache, and increased leukocyte count but is not necessarily associated with motor vehicle accidents or nasotracheal intubation. This leaves, choices B and C. Both are reported complications of nasotracheal intubation and can cause fever and increased white blood cell count. A constant headache is more consistent with maxillary sinusitis than retropharyngeal abcess. Thus C is the more likely correct answer.

REFERENCES:

1. Miller RD, Miller ED, Reves JG, et al. Anesthesia, 5th ed. New York, Churchill Livingstone, 2000, pp. 1445–1446.
2. Benumof JL, Saidman LJ. Anesthesia and Perioperative Complications, 2d ed. St Louis, Mosby, 1999, pp. 5–6.
3. Morgan GE, Mikhail MS, Murray MJ. Clinical Anesthesiology, 3d ed. New York, McGraw-Hill, 2002, pp. 965–966.

BOOK A:

QUESTION 116

Answer D

OB/Regional

QUESTION (Choose single best answer):

Surgery is canceled 10 minutes after initiation of intravenous regional anesthesia with 50 mL lidocaine 0.5%. To terminate anesthesia safely, what is the most appropriate timing for deflating the tourniquet?

(A) Immediately if benzodiazepines have been administered.
(B) Immediately after intravenous administration of ephedrine 10 mg.
(C) Immediately, followed by repeated reinflation and deflation.
(D) In no less than 20 minutes after initial injection.
(E) In no less than 45 minutes after initial injection.

CORRECT ANSWER: D

SUMMARY:

Intravenous regional anesthesia (Bier block) is an excellent anesthetic for short surgeries involving the forearm and hand. The block involves placing an intravenous catheter in the distal extremity, followed by exsanguination and inflation of a tourniquet placed on the upper arm. Once cessation of arterial inflow into the extremity has been established, 40 mL 0.5% lidocaine is injected through the distal intravenous catheter. The anesthesia is intense and develops within 10 minutes. The patient eventually starts to experience tourniquet pain, which is the limiting factor for the duration of the block. Once the surgery is complete, the tourniquet is deflated, and the residual lidocaine is taken up into the systemic circulation. The principal risk of this type of anesthetic is local anesthetic toxicity from premature release of the tourniquet. The generally agreed on minimal time that the tourniquet needs to remain inflated is 20 minutes regardless of the duration of surgery.[1]

EXPLANATION:

(A) ***Incorrect.*** Signs of local anesthetic toxicity include circumoral numbness, tongue paresthesia, dizziness, tinnitus, blurred vision, central nervous system (CNS) excitation, CNS depression, and tonic-clonic seizures. Prior benzodiazipine administration does not decrease the risk of developing these complications significantly. It has only been 10 minutes, and no maneuver is safe at this point.

(B) ***Incorrect.*** The dangers of local anesthetic toxicity are not eliminated by administration of intravenous ephedrine. It has only been 10 minutes, and no maneuver is safe at this point.

(C) ***Incorrect.*** It has only been 10 minutes, and no maneuver is safe at this point.

(D) ***Correct.*** The minimal time that should transpire is at least 20 minutes prior to tourniquet release to minimize a large bolus of drug into the systemic circulation.

(E) ***Incorrect.*** Within the 20- to 40-minute period, one can slowly deflate the tourniquet or deflate the tourniquet and rapidly reinflate it followed by a second deflation to decrease the initial bolus of local anesthetic. After 40 minutes, the tourniquet simply can be released with little risk of toxicity.

REASONING:

This question tests knowledge of local anesthetic toxicity and Bier block regional anesthesia. It is a classic example that illustrates the need to read choices carefully. On first pass, you might think that choice C could be correct, but it states *immediately*. Even though repeated deflation and reinflation is a correct strategy for early tourniquet release, it is still only safe after at least 20 minutes.

REFERENCE:

1. Barash PG, Cullen BF, Stoelting RK. Clinical Anesthesia, 4th ed. Philadelphia, Lippincott Williams & Wilkins, 2001, p. 728.
2. Morgan GE, Mikhail MS, Murray MJ. Clinical Anesthesiology, 3d ed. New York, McGraw-Hill, 2002, pp. 297–298.

BOOK A:

QUESTION 117

Answer D

Pediatrics

QUESTION (Choose single best answer):

A 2500-g, 12-hour-old infant is tracheally intubated and mechanically ventilated at a rate of 20 breaths per minute with an FiO_2 of 0.4 and peak inspiratory pressure of 25 cm H_2O. At birth, amniotic fluid was meconium-stained, and Apgar scores were 2 and 7. The most recent arterial blood gas levels are PaO_2 50 mm Hg, $PaCO_2$ 55 mm Hg, and pH 7.20. The most appropriate management is to

(A) Administer sodium bicarbonate.
(B) Begin intravenous infusion of prostaglandin E_1.
(C) Increase FiO_2.
(D) Increase ventilation.
(E) Perform bronchial lavage.

CORRECT ANSWER: D

SUMMARY:

Meconium is present in up to 26 percent of all deliveries and is correlated with gestational age (i.e., postdate neonates are at greater risk). Aspiration of meconium particles produces mechanical obstruction, chemical pneumonitis, and symptoms of obstructive lung disease, e.g., hyperinflation and increased dead space.[1] The meconium aspiration syndrome is often complicated by hypoxia, pulmonary hypertension, inactivated surfactant, and air leak, (e.g., pneumothorax). Prevention begins at delivery with immediate suctioning of the oropharynx and continues with endotracheal intubation and suctioning of meconium from the lungs. With severe meconium aspiration pneumonia, surfactant therapy, inhaled nitric oxide, high-frequency ventilation, and even extracorporeal membrane oxygenation may be necessary.

EXPLANATION:

(A) *Incorrect.* Sodium bicarbonate may be used to treat metabolic acidosis but actually may worsen respiratory acidosis when the bicarbonate is converted to carbon dioxide and water. It also increases risk of intracranial hemorrhage.

(B) *Incorrect.* Prostaglandin E_1 is used to maintain patency of the ductus arteriosus in ductal-dependent congenital cardiac lesions. It also may be used to decrease pulmonary vascular resistance in pulmonary hypertension. There is not enough evidence that either of these situations exists in this patient.

(C) *Incorrect.* The fetus tolerates intrauterine Pao_2 levels in the high 20s owing to fetal hemoglobin, polycythemia, and a rightward shift of the hemoglobin-oxygen dissociation curve in response to increased amounts of 2,3-DPG. Increasing Fio_2 in a neonate may not be desirable because hyperoxia may increase the risk of retinopathy of prematurity, especially in infants younger than 32 weeks' gestation.[1]

(D) *Correct.* A pH of 7.20 and a $Paco_2$ of 55 mm Hg indicate a respiratory acidosis. Treatment involves increasing the minute ventilation, which can be accomplished by increasing either respiratory rate or tidal volume.

(E) *Incorrect.* Treatment of meconium aspiration includes chest physiotherapy and warmed humidified oxygen. Bronchial lavage is contraindicated because it may worsen lung function.[1]

REASONING:

This is a difficult question that tests the reader's ability to analyze multiple clinical data and prioritize treatment. One can rule out choice B immediately because there is inadequate information supporting the presence of congenital cardiac disease. Choice A also can be ruled out because the blood gas indicates a primarily respiratory acidosis. If the reader does not know that bronchial lavage may exacerbate lung function in meconium aspiration pneumonia, one should recognize that a rate of 20 breaths per minute and a $Paco_2$ of 55 mm Hg demonstrate inadequate ventilation and that improving ventilation also may improve oxygenation. Thus D is the best answer.

REFERENCE:

1. Taeusch HW, Ballard RA. Avery's Diseases of the Newborn, 7th ed. Philadelphia, Saunders, 1998, pp. 619–622, 720–721, 1384.
2. Morgan GE, Mikhail MS, Murray MJ. Clinical Anesthesiology, 3d ed. New York, McGraw-Hill, 2002, pp. 652, 846, 864.

Answer C

Clinical Anesthesia

QUESTION (Choose single best answer):

A 60-year-old woman who is taking propranolol for hypertension and is allergic to penicillin is anesthetized with thiopental and halothane for resection of an abdominal aortic aneurysm. Shortly after intubation, she is given vancomycin 500 mg intravenously, after which her blood pressure decreases from 140/80 to 70/50 mm Hg, and her heart rate remains steady at 64 beats per minute. The most likely explanation for the decrease in blood pressure is

(A) Cross-sensitivity of penicillin and vancomycin.
(B) Interaction of vancomycin and propranolol.
(C) Vancomycin-induced anaphylactoid reaction.
(D) Interaction of halothane and propranolol.
(E) Interaction of halothane and vancomycin.

CORRECT ANSWER: C

SUMMARY:

Administration of vancomycin is commonly associated with "red man syndrome." This anaphylactoid-type reaction consists of flushing, pruritus, and hypotension. Alternatively, patients may develop isolated hypotension without the other symptoms. The rate of administration is a key factor in the development of these symptoms. Vancomycin should never be given by bolus administration. In a patient on chronic beta-blocker therapy, tachycardia may not develop as a compensating response to hypotension.

EXPLANATION:

(A) *Incorrect.* Vancomycin is a glycopeptide antibiotic and is not cross-sensitive with the beta-lactam antibiotics such as penicillin and cephalosporins.
(B) *Incorrect.* Chronic beta-blockade prevents an increase in heart rate but does not interact with vancomycin to produce hypotension.
(C) *Correct.* This hypotension most likely is mediated by histamine release secondary to rapid administration of vancomycin.
(D) *Incorrect.* The myocardial depressant effects of halothane may be exacerbated by beta-blockade. However, halothane has a slow uptake and would not cause such severe hypotension immediately after induction.
(E) *Incorrect.* The concentration of halothane immediately after induction would likely be negligible and would not interact with the vancomycin to cause hypotension.

REASONING:

The temporal relationship of the administration of vancomycin and the development of hypotension is incriminating. While the use of propranolol and halothane may cause hypotension, the rapid decrease in blood pressure points to a drug reaction. Patients can develop anaphylaxis to vancomycin, but it is more common to develop "red man syndrome" or simply hypotension from administration. C is the best answer.

REFERENCE:

Barash PG, Cullen BF, Stoelting RK. Clinical Anesthesia, 4th ed. Philadelphia, Lippincott Williams & Wilkins, 2001, Table 49-5, p. 1302.
Levy JH, Kettlekamp N, Goertz P. Histamine release by vancomycin: A mechanism for hypotension in man. Anesthesiology 67:122, 1987.
Morgan GE, Mikhail MS, Murray MJ. Clinical Anesthesiology, 3d ed. New York, McGraw-Hill, 2002, p. 907.

Answer E

Clinical Anesthesia

QUESTION (Choose single best answer):

During a reoperative total hip arthroplasty requiring transfusion of 8 units of packed red blood cells, blood begins to ooze from the operative field and intravenous catheter sites. The urine is pink. The most likely cause is

(A) Citrate intoxication.
(B) Factor V and VIII deficiencies.
(C) Rhabdomyolysis.
(D) Thrombocytopenia.
(E) Transfusion reaction.

CORRECT ANSWER: E

SUMMARY:

Pink urine in the setting of a blood transfusion is indicative of an acute hemolytic transfusion reaction owing to destruction of the donor red blood cells by the patient's antibodies.[1] It is usually due to ABO blood incompatibility and occurs in 1 in 6000 transfusions. Awake patients present with fever, chills, nausea, and chest pain, whereas anesthetized patients present with fever, tachycardia, hypotension, hemoglobinuria, and diffuse oozing in the surgical field. Once such signs are detected, the transfusion should be stopped immediately. The transfused unit should be rechecked to verify the correct patient identification and ABO compatibility. Samples should be sent to identify hemoglobin in the plasma, and full clotting studies should be done owing to the potential of disseminated intravascular coagulation (DIC). Diuresis should be attempted to try to prevent acute renal failure.

EXPLANATION:

(A) *Incorrect.* There is a potential for citrate intoxication with a large amount of transfused blood owing to the citrate preservative that binds calcium. Usually, anesthetized patients would not exhibit signs of hypocalcemia unless the transfusion rate exceeded 1 unit every 5 minutes. Clinical signs of hypocalcemia include cardiac arrythmias with a prolonged QT interval, hypotension, and a decreased cardiac output.

(B) *Incorrect.* Clinically significant dilution of procoagulant factors, such as factors V and VIII, is unusual in otherwise healthy people and only becomes an important consideration with massive transfusions of over 10 to 12 units. These two particular factors are not as stable as all others in stored red blood and have the highest likelihood of being diluted with massive transfusions.

(C) *Incorrect.* Rhabdomyolysis signals acute muscle breakdown owing to such things as succinylcholine being given to patients with Duchenne muscular dystrophy. Such muscle deterioration would not cause generalized oozing or hematuria, as with this patient. Instead, it can cause acute renal failure with hyperphosphatemia and subsequent hypocalcemia.

(D) *Incorrect.* Thrombocytopenia is the most common cause of bleeding following massive transfusions that usually exceed one to two times a patient's blood volume. Platelets are extremely sensitive to cold temperatures and become nonviable if stored at low temperatures. The answer is incorrect because only 8 units were transfused in this patient. A dilutional thrombocytopenia would result in bleeding and oozing from the surgical site and probably not cause hematuria.

(E) *Correct.* An acute hemolytic blood transfusion reaction is the most likely cause of the hematuria and oozing in this patient. It is probably due to ABO incompatibility, and the transfusion must be stopped immediately. The physician should attempt to prevent acute renal failure and support the patient through possible DIC and potential cardiovascular collapse.

REASONING:

This question tests knowledge of the diagnosis of acute hemolytic transfusion reactions. A constellation of symptoms that includes pink urine, oozing, fever, tachycardia, and hypotension after transfusion of blood product should raise clinical suspicion of an acute hemolytic transfusion reaction. E is the single best answer.

REFERENCE:

1. Barash PG, Cullen BF, Stoelting RK. Clinical Anesthesia, 4th ed. Philadelphia, Lippincott Williams & Wilkins, 2001, pp. 207–208.
2. Morgan GE, Mikhail MS, Murray MJ. Clinical Anesthesiology, 3d ed. New York, McGraw-Hill, 2002, pp. 551–554, 622–623.

BOOK A:

Answer C

OB/Regional

QUESTION 120

QUESTION (Choose single best answer):

Eight hours after abdominal surgery, a 51-year-old patient becomes increasingly somnolent. Epidural morphine 5 mg was administered immediately following the procedure. Postoperatively, respiratory rate has not decreased below 12 breaths per minute, and SpO_2 has remained greater than 92 percent. Arterial blood gas (ABG) analysis shows a PaO_2 of 80 mm Hg, a $PaCO_2$ of 82 mm Hg, and a pH of 7.1. Which of the following is the most appropriate conclusion?

(A) Analysis of the blood sample was delayed.
(B) The blood sample was venous rather than arterial.
(C) The patient is receiving supplemental oxygen.
(D) The pulse oximeter readings are falsely high.
(E) No treatment is required at this time.

CORRECT ANSWER: C

SUMMARY:

The patient is hypercarbic with a respiratory acidosis caused by opioid-induced respiratory depression. The patient's CO_2 response curve has shifted to the right. The SpO_2 is a measure of oxygenation not ventilation. It appears to be in the low-normal range despite hypoventilation, suggesting that the patient is receiving supplemental oxygen. An SpO_2 of 92 percent is consistent with a PaO_2 of 80 mm Hg. Despite titration of epidural morphine to a respiratory rate above 12, this patient is experiencing acidosis and CO_2 narcosis with CNS depression and must be treated.

EXPLANATION:

(A) *Incorrect.* The ABGs suggest respiratory acidosis secondary to hypoventilation consistent with the patient's current clinical state. There is nothing in the question to suggest a delayed analysis of the blood sample.

(B) *Incorrect.* Normal mixed venous oxygen tension (PvO_2) and carbon dioxide tension ($PvCO_2$) are 40 and 46 mm Hg, respectively. The SpO_2 would be 100 percent with a PvO_2 value of 80 mm Hg.

(C) *Correct.* Despite hypoventilation secondary to a reduced hypercarbic and hypoxic respiratory drive, this patient is being oxygenated adequately. The patient must be receiving supplemental oxygen.

(D) *Incorrect.* There is nothing to suggest that the SpO_2 reading is inaccurate because it correlates with the PaO_2 of 80 mm Hg. There is no suggestion of other conditions (e.g., carbon monoxide poisoning) that may falsely elevate oximeter readings.

(E) *Incorrect.* This patient is acidotic and experiencing CNS depression from CO_2 narcosis. Acidosis causes a rightward shift in the hemoglobin-oxygen binding curve, as well as cardiac, smooth muscle and CNS depression. The patient should be treated with an opioid antagonist or mechanically ventilated to correct the respiratory acidosis.

REASONING:

The key to answering this question is recognizing that the patient is experiencing CO_2 narcosis and respiratory acidosis secondary to opioid administration. Since the SpO_2 and PaO_2 correlate, there is nothing in the question to suggest that the analysis was delayed, that a venous sample was erroneously analyzed, or that the pulse oximeter was reading falsely high. The severe respiratory acidosis with CO_2 narcosis must be treated. C is the single best answer.

REFERENCE:

Barash PG, Cullen BF, Stoelting RK. Clinical Anesthesia, 4th ed. Philadelphia, Lippincott Williams & Wilkins, 2001, pp. 1385–1386.

Morgan GE, Mikhail MS, Murray MJ. Clinical Anesthesiology, 3d ed. New York, McGraw-Hill, 2002, pp. 167, 168ff, 344, 499–500, 652, 658–659.

BOOK A:

Answer B

Clinical Anesthesia

QUESTION 121

QUESTION (Choose single best answer):

A 76-year-old patient is restless and hallucinating in the preoperative holding area. He received morphine 5 mg and scopolamine 0.4 mg intramuscularly as premedication and is now breathing oxygen 2 L/min through nasal prongs. The SpO_2 is 98 percent. Which of the following is the most appropriate next step?

(A) Administration of naloxone.
(B) Administration of physostigmine.
(C) Induction of general anesthesia.
(D) Determination of serum electrolyte concentrations.
(E) Computed tomographic (CT) scan of the head.

CORRECT ANSWER: B

SUMMARY:

This question describes central anticholinergic syndrome, *caused in this case by scopolamine. Atropine also can produce the syndrome when administered in high doses.[1] CNS symptoms range from sedation or stupor to restlessness, disorientation, and hallucinations. Elderly patients and those in pain may have an increased likelihood to develop the syndrome.[1] Physostigmine, by virtue of it being a tertiary amine (unlike glycopyrrolate, a quaternary amine, neostigmine, and edrophonium) readily crosses the blood–brain barrier and reverses these symptoms.*

EXPLANATION:

(A) *Incorrect.* Restlessness can be a symptom of hypoxia caused by respiratory depression from morphine. However, the patient is not hypoxic (SpO_2 is 98 percent). In addition, morphine rarely causes hallucinations.

(B) **Correct.** The patient most likely has central anticholinergic syndrome from scopolamine. Adminstration of physiostigmine is the most appropriate therapy.

(C) **Incorrect.** Induction of general anesthesia is not indicated.

(D) **Incorrect.** It may be reasonable to check serum electrolyte concentrations to rule out abnormalities such as hyponatremia. However, the most likely cause of this patient's symptoms is scopolamine, and the most appropriate next step is treatment with physiostigmine.

(E) **Incorrect.** A CT scan of the head would help to rule out anatomic reasons for acute mental status changes, such as acute stroke or intracranial bleeding. However, these are unlikely causes of the patient's symptoms. If the symptoms did not resolve with physostigmine, electrolytes were normal, and the patient were oxygenating well, further investigation with CT scan might be warranted.

REASONING:

This question tests knowledge of the diagnosis and treatment of central anticholinergic syndrome. Choice A is a "distracter" answer to suggest that the morphine is to blame. Choices D and E are other causes of mental status changes that do not fit the clinical picture. This leaves choice B and C to consider for management. B is the best answer.

REFERENCE:

1. Barash PG, Cullen BF, Stoelting RK. Clinical Anesthesia, 4th ed. Philadelphia, Lippincott Williams & Wilkins, 2001, p. 561.

2. Morgan GE, Mikhail MS, Murray MJ. Clinical Anesthesiology, 3d ed. New York, McGraw-Hill, 2002, pp. 173–175.

BOOK A:

QUESTION 122

Answer E

Physiology

QUESTION (Choose single best answer):

For any given FIO_2 and $PaCO_2$, the PaO_2 is lower in a healthy paralyzed patient anesthetized with isoflurane than in the same patient unanesthetized and breathing spontaneously. The primary cause of this difference is

(A) Controlled ventilation.

(B) Increased airway resistance.

(C) Inhibition of hypoxic pulmonary vasoconstriction.

(D) Intraoperative hypothermia.

(E) Preferential ventilation of nondependent lung.

CORRECT ANSWER: E

SUMMARY:

When compared with a nonanesthetized patient, the PaO_2 will be lower in anesthetized patients for several reasons. General anesthesia causes a 20 percent reduction in functional residual capacity, a 10 percent increase in venous admixture, $\dot{V}/\dot{Q}$ mismatch, and inhibition of hypoxic pulmonary vasoconstriction.

EXPLANATION:

(A) **Incorrect.** Controlled ventilation tends to recruit alveoli, which helps to prevent hypoxia.

(B) **Incorrect.** Airway resistance would not contribute significantly to hypoxia unless the resistance was significant enough to cause a dramatic decrease in airflow.

(C) **Incorrect.** All anesthetics cause an inhibition of hypoxic pulmonary vasoconstriction. This, however, is only usually clinically significant at high concentrations.

(D) **Incorrect.** Intraoperative hypothermia will decrease oxygen consumption but will not cause a hypoxia.

(E) **Correct.** Under normal negative-pressure spontaneous ventilation, the dependent areas of the lung get both an increased perfusion and increased ventilation secondary to the effects of gravity and a more negative intrapleural pressure. Under positive-pressure ventilation, the less dependent areas of the lung will get more ventilation, and the dependent areas will get more perfusion, resulting in an increased $\dot{V}/\dot{Q}$ mismatch and a resulting lower Pao_2.

REASONING:

This question tests knowledge of the changes in pulmonary physiology associated with controlled ventilation and anesthesia with an inhalational anesthetic agent. On first pass, it would seem that the correct answer would be inhibition of hypoxic pulmonary vasoconstriction. The examiners would like you to understand a more subtle difference between positive- and negative-pressure ventilation. In reality, there are many reasons why the Pao_2 is lower in an anesthetized patient. Here, the board asks for the single best answer, which for this question is E.

REFERENCE:

Barash PG, Cullen BF, Stoelting RK. Clinical Anesthesia, 4th ed. Philadelphia, Lippincott Williams & Wilkins, 2001, Chap. 29, pp. 791–812.

Morgan GE, Mikhail MS, Murray MJ. Clinical Anesthesiology, 3d ed. New York, McGraw-Hill, 2002, pp. 491, 493, 495.

BOOK A:

Answer D

Basic Science

QUESTION 123

QUESTION (Choose single best answer):

Normal pseudocholinesterase

(A) Is highly concentrated at the motor end plate.
(B) Hydrolyzes succinylcholine by Hofmann elimination.
(C) Is produced primarily at nerve terminals.
(D) Is antagonized by acetylcholinesterase inhibitors.
(E) Resists dibucaine inhibition more than its atypical variant.

CORRECT ANSWER: D

SUMMARY:

Both pseudocholinesterase and acetylcholinesterase are enzymes that catalyze the ester hydrolysis of acetylcholine and succinylcholine. Pseudocholinesterase is a soluble enzyme that circulates in the blood (made primarily in the liver), whereas acetylcholinesterase is a membrane-bound enzyme present at the motor end plate. Both these enzymes are inhibited by acetylcholinesterase (or just cholinesterase) inhibitors because these drugs are nonspecific in mechanism. Dibucaine is an amide local anesthetic that can inhibit normal pseudocholinesterase activity by 80 percent. It also inhibits variant pseudocholinesterase, but to a lesser degree. Dibucaine inhibition can be used to identify patients with low pseudocholinesterase activity and those with enzyme variants.[1] Clinically significant prolongation of succinylcholine neuromuscular blockade only occurs after pseudocholinesterase activity decreases more than 75 percent from normal levels.[1]

EXPLANATION:

(A) **Incorrect.** Pseudocholinesterase is a soluble enzyme found in the plasma, not at the motor end plate.

(B) *Incorrect.* Pseudocholinesterase degrades succinylcholine by ester hydrolysis, producing succinic acid and choline. Hoffmann elimination is not involved in succinylcholine metabolism.

(C) *Incorrect.* Pseudocholinesterase is produced in the liver and then circulates in the plasma. Acetylcholinesterase, however, is produced and functions at the motor end plate.

(D) *Correct.* Cholinesterase inhibitors are nonspecific agents that block both acetylcholinesterase and pseudocholinesterase.

(E) *Incorrect.* Normal pseudocholinesterase in more sensitive to dibucaine inhibition than its abnormal variant.

REASONING:

This question tests knowledge of cholinesterase enzymes. It is important to understand that pseudocholinesterase and acetylcholinesterase are separate enzymes that catalyze similar reactions and that both are inhibited by cholinesterase inhibitors. The reader also should understand that acetylcholinesterase resides at the motor end plate and that pseudocholinesterase is present in the plasma and produced by the liver. The best answer is D.

REFERENCE:

1. Miller RD, Miller ED, Reves JG, et al. Anesthesia, 5th ed. New York, Churchill Livingstone, 2000, p. 546.
2. Morgan GE, Mikhail MS, Murray MJ. Clinical Anesthesiology, 3d ed. New York, McGraw-Hill, 2002, pp. 183, 712.

BOOK A: **QUESTION 124**

Answer E

Pediatrics

QUESTION (Choose single best answer):

Thirty-six hours after primary repair of a meningomyelocele, a term newborn has frequent periods of apnea lasting 25 seconds and associated with oxygen desaturation to 80 percent. The most likely explanation is

(A) Hyperglycemia.
(B) Loss of cerebrospinal fluid.
(C) Obstructive hydrocephalus.
(D) Residual anesthetic effect.
(E) Normal postoperative events.

CORRECT ANSWER: E

SUMMARY:

Neural tube defects occur from failed closure of the neural tube in utero and include spina bifida, myelomeningocele, encephalocele, and tethered cord. Myelomeningocele is a defect of the vertebral column of neural tissue partially covered by epithelial tissue and occurs in the lumbosacral region 75 percent of the time. Ninety-five percent of patients with myelomeningocele also have Arnold-Chiari malformation type II, which is abnormal development of the cerebellum and brain stem into the foramen magnum and even the lower cervical vertebrae. Associated problems include obstructive hydrocephalus, vocal cord paralysis, swallowing problems, and central respiratory dysfunction (e.g., apnea, stridor, and aspiration).[1] Treatment involves surgical resection of the myelomeningocele, ventriculoperitoneal shunting, and decompression of the cerebellum and brain stem.

EXPLANATION:

(A) *Incorrect.* Hyperglycemia is not associated with meningomyelocele or apnea.
(B) *Incorrect.* There is no evidence of loss of cerebrospinal fluid (CSF). And moderate loss of CSF should not cause apnea or desaturation.

(C) *Incorrect.* Obstructive hydrocephalus occurs in 85 percent of patients with myelomeningocele and is treated surgically with ventriculoperitoneal shunting, usually at the time of repair. Central respiratory dysfunction occurs in approximately 6 percent of such patients and is due to abnormal development of the brain stem, not hydrocephalus.[1]

(D) *Incorrect.* Residual anesthetic effects should not last 36 hours.

(E) *Correct.* Neonates (especially ex-preterm infants) are at increased risk of postoperative apnea until they are 50 to 60 weeks postconceptual age. Furthermore, infants who have had repair of meningomyelocele are at risk of central respiratory dysfunction despite cervical decompression for Arnold-Chiari malformation or ventriculoperitoneal shunting for hydrocephalus.[2]

REASONING:

The key concepts tested here are that patients are at risk of central respiratory problems even after repair of myelomeningocele and even with a working ventriculoperitoneal shunt in place. Choices A and B do not explain the apnea. Choice C, while it may cause apnea, is usually treated at the time of surgery. Choice D is unlikely 36 hours postoperatively. Finally, while not normal for a healthy patient, central respiratory dysfunction can continue even after surgical repair and therefore is "normal" in patients with meningomyelocele.

REFERENCES:

1. Peterson MC, Wolraich M, Sherbondy A, Wagener J. Abnormalities in control of ventilation in newborn infants with myelomeningocele. J Pediatr 126:1011–1015, 1995.

2. Oren J, Kelly DH, Todres ID, Shannon DC. Respiratory complications in patients with myelodysplasia and Arnold-Chiari malformation. Am J Dis Child 140:221–224, 1986.

3. Cote CJ. A Practice of Anesthesia for Infants and Children, 3d ed. Philadelphia, Saunders, 2001, pp. 45–48, 513–514, 516–517.

4. Morgan GE, Mikhail MS, Murray MJ. Clinical Anesthesiology, 3d ed. New York, McGraw-Hill, 2002, p. 864.

BOOK A:

Answer A

Pediatrics

QUESTION 125

QUESTION (Choose single best answer):

Inhalation induction of anesthesia is more rapid in a 6-month-old infant than in an adult because infants have

(A) A greater ratio of alveolar ventilation to functional residual capacity.
(B) A greater ratio of blood volume to body weight.
(C) A greater solubility of anesthetic in blood.
(D) A lower anesthetic requirement.
(E) A lower distribution of cardiac output to vessel-rich organs.

CORRECT ANSWER: A

SUMMARY:

Various factors contribute to a more rapid uptake of inhalational anesthetic agents and therefore the rate of inhalational induction in children. First, there is greater alveolar minute ventilation along with a lower functional residual capacity compared with adults. In addition, children have a higher cardiac index that correlates with increased alveolar blood flow compared with adults. Neonates and infants also have lower blood/gas partition coefficients, which translate into lower solubility and more rapid uptake.[1] Finally, a greater proportion of the cardiac output is delivered to vessel-rich organs, which extract a greater amount of anesthetic more quickly. Even though minimum alveolar concentration (MAC) is greater in infants and children, care must be taken with induction because the margin of safety between adequate anesthesia and cardiopulmonary depression is decreased.

EXPLANATION:

(A) *Correct.* Infants have greater alveolar ventilation and smaller functional residual capacity compared with adults. This results in more rapid uptake of anesthetic agents.[1]

(B) *Incorrect.* Infants do have a greater ratio of blood volume to body weight, but this does not affect rate of induction. However, cardiac output, the rate at which the blood is pumped throughout the body, does affect rate of induction.

(C) *Incorrect.* Greater solubility in blood would *slow* induction. The blood/gas coefficients, and thus solubility, for isoflurane and halothane actually are *lower* in children than in adults.

(D) *Incorrect.* MAC (preterm infant < term infant < 3- to 6-month-old infant) >> older child > adult > elderly.[1]

(E) *Incorrect.* Children have a *higher* distribution of cardiac output to vessel-rich organs.

REASONING:

This question tests understanding of the determinants of the rate of induction with inhaled anesthetic agents and the physiologic differences between children and adults. Choice B is misleading because it is a true statement. However, blood-volume-to-body-weight ratio does not affect rate of induction. Choice C can be eliminated because it is false and because greater solubility actually slows induction. The reader should be able to recognize that children have greater anesthetic requirements and a greater distribution to vessel-rich organs and rule out choices D and E. This leaves A, which is true, and explains why induction is more rapid in children.

REFERENCES:

1. Miller RD, Miller ED, Reves JG, et al. Anesthesia, 5th ed. New York, Churchill Livingstone, 2000, Fig. 59-6, p. 2093.

2. Cote CJ. A Practice of Anesthesia for Infants and Children, 3d ed. Philadelphia, Saunders, 2001, pp. 133–134.

3. Morgan GE, Mikhail MS, Murray MJ. Clinical Anesthesiology, 3d ed. New York, McGraw-Hill, 2002, pp. 852–854.

BOOK A:

Answer B

Pediatrics

QUESTION 126

QUESTION (Choose single best answer):

Which of the following findings is most hazardous in premature infants?

(A) Hematocrit of 55 percent.
(B) Rectal temperature of 35°C.
(C) Umbilical arterial blood P_{O_2} of 50 mm Hg.
(D) Umbilical arterial blood P_{CO_2} of 45 mm Hg.
(E) Umbilical arterial systolic pressure of 60 mm Hg.

CORRECT ANSWER: B

SUMMARY:

Children born before 37 weeks' gestation are termed premature infants *and include low-birth-weight (<2500 g), very low-birth-weight (<1500 g), and the extremely low-birth-weight (<1000 g) infants. All may have immature physiologic systems, including immature pulmonary (e.g., surfactant deficiency, apnea), renal, gastrointestinal (e.g., feeding* *intolerance, inadequate absorption), hematopoetic (e.g., anemia), and immune function (e.g., increased susceptibility to infection); immature cerebral vasculature (e.g., increased risk of hemorrhage); patent ductus arteriosus (e.g., left-to-right shunt); and impaired thermoregulation. These high-risk newborns require meticulous supportive care just so that they can use all their energy to grow.*

EXPLANATION:

(A) *Incorrect.* A hematocrit of 55 percent is acceptable for a premature infant. Hyperviscosity is not a concern until the hematocrit exceeds 65 to 70 percent.[1]

(B) *Correct.* A temperature of 35°C is considered hypothermic and should be corrected because it increases oxygen consumption, forces the infant to use calories for heat production instead of growth, and increases the risk of hypoglycemia, bradycardia, apnea, and metabolic acidosis. Taking rectal temperatures in premature infants is relatively contraindicated because there is a risk of rectal perforation.[2]

(C) *Incorrect.* Drawn with the patient on room air, an umbilical artery blood Po_2 of 50 mm Hg is acceptable as long as there is no acidosis. In fact, the Pao_2 should be kept as low as possible but at least less than 150 mm Hg to avoid the risk of retinopathy of prematurity.[3]

(D) *Incorrect.* An umbilical artery blood Pco_2 of 45 mm Hg is acceptable.

(E) *Incorrect.* Umbilical artery systolic blood pressure of 60 mm Hg may be slightly high for an extremely low-birth-weight infant but is normal and not concerning in most preterm and term infants.[1]

REASONING:

This question test knowledge of neonatal physiology and the range of normal values for premature infants. Choices A and D are well within normal ranges, so they can be eliminated. Choice C is acceptable. While a Pao_2 of 50 mm Hg is not ideal, we have no evidence that it is inadequate for this patient. In fact, for patients with mixing congenital cardiac lesions, this may be normal. Finally, a systolic blood pressure of 60 mm Hg is neither high nor low enough to be concerning, so choice E can be eliminated. This leaves B, which is concerning because premature infants have decreased ability for thermoregulation.

REFERENCES:

1. Cote CJ. A Practice of Anesthesia for Infants and Children, 3d ed. Philadelphia, Saunders, 2001, pp. 16 (Table 2-10), 19–20, 142–143.

2. Hay WW, Groothuis JR, Hayward AR, Levin MJ: Current Pediatric Diagnosis and Treatment, 12th ed. Norwalk, CT, Appleton & Lange, 1995, pp. 24–26.

3. Miller RD, Miller ED, Reves JG, et al. Anesthesia, 5th ed. New York, Churchill Livingstone, 2000, p. 2092.

4. Morgan GE, Mikhail MS, Murray MJ. Clinical Anesthesiology, 3d ed. New York, McGraw-Hill, 2002, pp. 851, 864.

BOOK A:

QUESTION 127

Answer E

Clinical Anesthesia

QUESTION (Choose single best answer):

A 40-year-old patient has pain following injection of 8 mL thiopental 2.5% through a right radial artery catheter. His hand remains pink. Which of the following is the most appropriate next step?

(A) Injection of lidocaine through the catheter.
(B) Injection of nitroglycerin though the catheter.
(C) Injection of papaverine through the catheter.
(D) Right stellate ganglion block.
(E) No intervention.

CORRECT ANSWER: E

SUMMARY:

Inadvertant intraarterial injection of thiopental causes vasospasm owing to the local re-lease of norepinephrine. Local tissue injury can occur. Furthermore, there is potential for ischemia, gangrene, and loss of tissue or a limb. There are no well-controlled studies that clearly demonstrate the effectiveness of any given therapy.[1] Any drug that promotes blood flow, such as the vasodilators papaverine and lidocaine, or any procedure to improve blood flow, such as a brachial plexus or stellate ganglion block, could be helpful. In ad-dition, intravenous heparin potentially can prevent any thrombosis. Because the hand is still pink, the most appropriate next step is to watch the hand carefully and hold off on any interventions. If the hand subsequently becomes cyanotic and pain persists, different therapies can be attempted, such as elevation of the hand to improve flow, local anes-thetic infiltration, extremity sympatholysis, or other medical therapies.

EXPLANATION:

(A) *Incorrect.* Although lidocaine may help to vasodilate an artery exposed to thiopental and prevent reflex vasospasm, there are also risks to its administration, such as arterial laceration or tissue damage contributing to thrombosis. In addition, there also have been isolated case reports of lidocaine-induced vasospasm.[2] Thus it is best to wait and watch the hand very closely.

(B) *Incorrect.* Nitroglycerin generally is a venodilator more so than an arterial dilator. In addition, injecting nitroglycerin intraarterially can cause profound systemic hy-potension and is not the best choice to improve blood flow to the affected limb.

(C) *Incorrect.* Although papaverine could promote blood flow to the limb after acci-dental intraarterial thiopental administration, again, there is a risk to its intraarterial administration, and it is best not to intervene yet because the hand is still pink.

(D) *Incorrect.* An ipsilateral stellate ganglion block can produce a sympathectomy in the affected arm, causing vasodilation for a prolonged period of time and improving blood flow to the right arm. However, since the hand is still pink, it is not worth the risk of a pneumothorax, nerve paralysis, local anesthetic toxicity, or spinal injection.

(E) *Correct.* The hand is still pink and presumably well perfused. It is best not to in-tervene and to watch the extremity closely. Only if the hand appears ischemic or continues to be quite painful should something be done. Vasospasm of the artery can develop with subsequent gangrene and loss of tissue.

REASONING:

Thiopental is a water-soluble barbiturate prepared in an alkaline solution with a pH of 10.5. Because of its alkaline state, thiopental has the potential of forming crystals and can cause subsequent occlusion in the smaller arteries and arterioles to which it is acciden-tally administered through an arterial catheter. Extravasation into subcutaneous tissue can cause necrosis, and inadvertent intraarterial injection can cause vasospasm, pain, ischemia, gangrene, and the potential loss of tissue or a limb. Although lidocaine and papaverine can be helpful in causing vasodilation in the affected limb, an ipsilateral stellate ganglion block probably is the most efficacious in promoting increased blood flow to the arm with a sympathectomy. However, in this situation, the hand is still pink with good perfusion. It is not yet worth incurring the risks of such therapies.

REFERENCES:

1. Ghouri A, Mading W, Prabaker K. Accidental intraarterial drug injections via intravascular catheters placed on the dorsum of the hand. Anesth Analg 95:487–491, 2002.

2. Azma T, Okida M. Does lidocaine provoke clinically significant vasospasm? Acta Anaesthesiol Scand 47(9):1174, 2003.

3. Stoelting RK, Miller RD. Basics of Anesthesia, 3d ed. New York, Churchill Livingstone, 1994, p. 62.

4. Morgan GE, Mikhail MS, Murray MJ. Clinical Anesthesiology, 3d ed. New York, McGraw-Hill, 2002, p. 72.

Answer D

Equipment/Physics

QUESTION (Choose single best answer):

During nitrous oxide anesthesia, which of the following expands most rapidly?

(A) Air bubble in the blood.
(B) Air in the intestine.
(C) Endotracheal tube cuff.
(D) Pneumothorax.
(E) Sulfahexafluoride bubble in the vitreal cavity.

CORRECT ANSWER: D

SUMMARY:

Nitrous oxide is 35 times more soluble than nitrogen in blood. Thus it will diffuse into air-containing cavities more rapidly than nitrogen is absorbed by the bloodstream. The magnitude of volume increase is influenced by the alveolar partial pressure of nitrous oxide, blood flow to the air-filled cavity, and the duration of the nitrous oxide anesthetic. Nitrous oxide exposed to those places which are noncompliant, such as a gas space created in the eye by a sulfur hexafluoride injection, will cause a rapid increase in pressure rather than volume. Conversely, volume rather than the pressure will expand rapidly within more compliant places, such as a pneumothorax, bowel, air embolus, and the endotracheal cuff. The volume of gas in the bowel expands slowly, and rarely can such expansion cause a clinically significant difference in an hour. Likewise, the cuff of an endotracheal tube will increase its volume rather slowly because the nitrous oxide must penetrate different materials.

EXPLANATION:

(A) ***Incorrect.*** An air bubble in blood will increase its volume rather quickly with a nitrous oxide anesthetic. However, the bubble must remain intact within the circulation for the nitrous oxide to diffuse into this compliant space from the blood. There is no secondary mechanism for nitrous oxide uptake into the bubble as there is with a pneumothorax. With the latter, there is direct diffusion of nitrous oxide from the alveoli rather than just vascular delivery of this gas into a closed space.

(B) ***Incorrect.*** The increase in bowel gas is slow compared with the increase in the size of a pneumothorax. Normally, there is only approximately 100 mL of air in the bowel. Thus, after several hours, the nitrous oxide in the blood may be delivered to the bowel to double its gaseous contents. This may not even be appreciated by the surgeon.

(C) ***Incorrect.*** An endotracheal tube cuff is filled with 5 to 7 mL of air. Only after several hours of a nitrous oxide anesthetic will some of the nitrous oxide diffuse into the cuff and potentially increase the pressure exerted on tracheal mucosa. The nitrous oxide must penetrate the cuff first and slowly increase the volume within this compliant, closed space.

(D) ***Correct.*** A pneumothorax will expand the rather quickly because the insoluble nitrous oxide gas will leave the blood rapidly and enter the air-filled cavity 35 times faster than nitrogen would exit the pneumothorax. The more rapid change with a pneumothorax probably results from the movement of nitrous oxide across the visceral pleura rather than just from the transport of the nitrous oxide into this space from blood alone.

(E) ***Incorrect.*** Sulfahexafluoride is an inert gas that is less soluble in blood than nitrogen and much less soluble than nitrous oxide. Thus its longer duration of action compared with an air bubble can be advantageous to the ophthalmologist. If a patient is breathing a nitrous oxide anesthetic, the nitrous oxide will entrain the bubble quickly and increase its size before the sulfahexafluoride has a chance to diffuse into the blood. A 70% nitrous oxide technique will almost double the pressure in a closed eye within 30 minutes. Because it is a rather noncompliant space, its pressure rather than its volume increases quickly.

REASONING:

Nitrous oxide will cause an increase in pressure in noncompliant spaces, such as those created by sulfahexafluoride injections and, on the contrary, will cause an increase in volume in compliant spaces, such as the bowel, a pneumothorax, an air embolus, and an endotracheal tube cuff. Of these, a pneumothorax expands the most rapidly probably owing to diffusion of nitrous oxide through the visceral pleura besides the delivery and diffusion of the nitrous oxide in the circulation. Nitrous oxide is quite insoluble in blood. However, it is 35 times more soluble than nitrogen in blood. Hence, anywhere there is air (the majority of which is nitrogen), it will attempt to fill the space more quickly than the nitrogen can escape. Both the bowel and endotracheal cuff fill with nitrous oxide rather slowly. An air bubble has the potential to expand rapidly with nitrous oxide if the nitrous oxide is able to diffuse into the bubble before it is dissipated within the circulation. D is the best answer.

REFERENCES:

Eger E. Nitrous Oxide. New York, Elsevier Science, 1985, pp. 95–99.

Kaur S, Cortiella J, Vacanti C. Diffusion of nitrous oxide into the pleural cavity. Br J Anaesthesiol 87:894–896, 2001.

Stoelting RK, Miller RD. Basics of Anesthesia, 3d ed. New York, Churchill Livingstone Publishers, 1994, p. 21.

Morgan GE, Mikhail MS, Murray MJ. Clinical Anesthesiology, 3d ed. New York, McGraw-Hill, 2002, pp. 117, 658.

BOOK A:

QUESTION 129

Answer C

Equipment/Physics

QUESTION (Choose single best answer):

While checking an anesthesia machine, opening the oxygen flow-control valve yields no oxygen flow, although the wall-mounted oxygen pipeline supply gauge reads 50 psig. Opening the backup oxygen cylinder results in normal oxygen flow. The most likely cause is

(A) Failure of the oxygen pipeline supply.
(B) Failure of the second-stage oxygen pressure regulator.
(C) A malfunctioning check valve in the oxygen pipeline supply inlet.
(D) A malfunctioning fail-safe valve.
(E) A malfunctioning oxygen flow-control valve.

CORRECT ANSWER: C

SUMMARY:

The oxygen flow-valve assembly receives gas input from the pipeline directly or from a second-stage pressure regulator. The only valve that lies close to the beginning of the oxygen supply from the pipeline is the check valve from the pipeline supply inlet. A faulty valve could prevent oxygen from reaching the flowmeters. If the cylinder is opened, oxygen could bypass this faulty valve and enter the flowmeter. Because the gauge reads 50 psig, there is no failure with the pipeline. In addition, the oxygen flow-control valve is working appropriately because opening the backup oxygen cylinder results in normal oxygen flow. The second-stage oxygen pressure regulator and the fail-safe valve lie downstream of the oxygen supply from both the pipeline and cylinder and would not prevent oxygen from flowing entirely if they are faulty.

EXPLANATION:

(A) *Incorrect.* The oxygen pipeline supply has not failed because the supply gauge still reads 50 psig, which is normal.

(B) *Incorrect.* Ohmeda machines usually have a second-stage oxygen regulator located downstream from the oxygen sources (pipeline and cylinders). The regulator limits the pressure from the high-pressure oxygen source to 12 to 19 psig.[1] Pressures upstream from the regulator must be greater than 12 psig to deliver flow through the oxygen flow-valve assembly. Because it lies downstream from both oxygen sources, a defect here could not explain why the backup oxygen cylinder restored normal oxygen flow.

(C) *Correct.* The check valve in the oxygen pipeline supply inlet prevents transfilling of gas cylinders or flow of gas from cylinders into the central supply and lies directly after the start of the pipeline supply into the anesthesia machine. A faulty valve may prevent oxygen from the pipeline supply from reaching the flowmeters.

(D) *Incorrect.* The fail-safe valve lies downstream from the oxygen supply from both the pipeline and cylinder. This valve automatically closes all other gas lines if oxygen pressure falls below 25 psig or 50 percent of normal to help prevent the possibility of delivering a hypoxic gas mixture.

(E) *Incorrect.* The oxygen flow-control valve on the flowmeter is not malfunctioning because there is oxygen flow once the source is changed from the pipeline supply to the cylinder.

REASONING:

This questions tests knowledge of the anesthesia machine, valves, and differences in the high- and low-pressure systems. It is important to review the anesthesia machine schematic to ensure a thorough understanding of the system.[1] There are several valves within the anesthesia machine, each positioned in a different place within the "circuit" of the machine. The check valve in the pipeline supply inlet prevents backfilling from the cylinders into the pipeline supply and is the only valve directly downstream from the pipeline supply. Thus its malfunction could prevent any oxygen from being delivered from this one source, which is functioning appropriately with a pressure of 50 psig. Both the fail-safe valve and the second-stage pressure regulator lie further downstream from both the pipeline supply and the oxygen cylinder. A malfunction in either of these valves probably would prevent oxygen flow entirely. In this particular situation, oxygen flow was restored to the opened oxygen flow-control valve assembly once the cylinder was opened. C is the best answer.

REFERENCE:

1. Barash PG, Cullen BF, Stoelting RK. Clinical Anesthesia, 4th ed. Philadelphia, Lippincott Williams & Wilkins, 2001, Fig. 22-3, p. 569.

2. Morgan GE, Mikhail MS, Murray MJ. Clinical Anesthesiology, 3d ed. New York, McGraw-Hill, 2002, pp. 35–36.

BOOK A: **QUESTION 130**

Answer A

Physiology

QUESTION (Choose single best answer):

Which of the following statements concerning pulmonary function in patients with pulmonary fibrosis is true?

(A) Diffusion capacity is decreased.
(B) Pulmonary artery diastolic-to-occlusion pressure gradients are normal.
(C) Ventilation-perfusion relationships are normal.
(D) Static pulmonary compliance is unchanged.
(E) Mechanical ventilation with a slow rate and a large tidal volume is optimal.

CORRECT ANSWER: A

SUMMARY:

Pulmonary fibrosis is a disease state that has significant anesthetic implications. There are many different causes, but the end result is the same—progressive scarring of the lungs with eventual respiratory failure. The scarring causes chronic hypoxia and pulmonary hypertension that eventually results in death unless the patient receives a lung transplant.

EXPLANATION:

(A) **Correct.** The ongoing fibrosis in the lung causes a decrease in diffusing capacity of the alveoli.

(B) **Incorrect.** Patients with pulmonary fibrosis have pulmonary hypertension, but left-sided pressures in the heart are normal. Pulmonary artery diastolic pressures will be significantly higher than pulmonary artery occlusive pressure.

(C) **Incorrect.** The ventilation-perfusion ratio is will be abnormal owing to increased $\dot{V}/\dot{Q}$ mismatch from lung damage.

(D) **Incorrect.** Static and dynamic lung compliance will be decreased from the continued scarring of the lung.

(E) **Incorrect.** Large tidal volumes increase the risk of barotrauma that could result in a lethal pneumothorax. The patient should be ventilated with smaller tidal volumes at a rate that does not cause air trapping.

REASONING:

This question tests knowledge of the pathophysiology of pulmonary fibrosis. Patients with pulmonary fibrosis develop restrictive lung physiology, leading to decreased FRC and FVC with a relatively normal FEV_1.[1] The decrease in diffusion capacity observed with restrictive lung disease such as pulmonary fibrosis can be due to thickening of the alveolar membrane (gas/blood barrier) in addition to loss of lung volume associated with the restrictive disease state.[1] The single best answer is A.

REFERENCE:

1. Barash PG, Cullen BF, Stoelting RK. Clinical Anesthesia, 4th ed. Philadelphia, Lippincott Williams & Wilkins, 2001, pp. 806, 815 (Fig. 30-2).
2. Morgan GE, Mikhail MS, Murray MJ. Clinical Anesthesiology, 3d ed. New York, McGraw-Hill, 2002, pp. 519–520.

BOOK A:

QUESTION 131

Answer E

Physiology

QUESTION (Choose single best answer):

Mismatching of ventilation to perfusion in the lung is greatest in which of the following situations?

(A) Awake patient, spontaneous ventilation, lateral decubitus position.
(B) Anesthetized patient, controlled ventilation, supine position.
(C) Anesthetized patient, controlled ventilation, lateral decubitus position.
(D) Anesthetized patient, controlled ventilation, sitting position.
(E) Anesthetized patient, spontaneous ventilation, prone position.

CORRECT ANSWER: E

SUMMARY:

Dependent areas of the lung receive more blood flow than nondependent areas owing to gravity regardless of body position or anesthesia. In contrast, ventilation is affected by body position and anesthesia. In the awake, spontaneously ventilating patient, nondependent alveoli are near maximally expanded, and less compliant but dependent alveoli are more compliant. Awake, spontaneously ventilating patients tend to have better matching of ventilation and perfusion even in the lateral position. Anesthesia reduces functional residual capacity (FRC), improving compliance of nondependent alveoli and worsening compliance of dependent alveoli. The supine and prone positions further decrease FRC and reduce compliance of dependent lung areas.

EXPLANATION:

(A) *Incorrect.* The lateral decubitus position in an awake, spontaneously breathing patient preserves ventilation-perfusion matching. The dependent lung receives greater perfusion owing to gravity and greater ventilation owing to compliance.[1]

(B) *Incorrect.* Induction of anesthesia decreases FRC by 15 to 20 percent, and the supine position further reduces pulmonary compliance by allowing abdominal viscera to push up against the diaphragm.

(C) *Incorrect.* Anesthesia decreases FRC, worsening dependent lung compliance but improving compliance of the upper lung. Controlled ventilation under anesthesia favors the upper lung owing to increased compliance. Therefore, significant ventilation-perfusion mismatching occurs in this position.

(D) *Incorrect.* FRC is minimally reduced in the sitting position under anesthesia compared with other positions.

(E) *Correct.* FRC is decreased in the prone position as a result of abdominal pressure impeding diaphragmatic movement. Inhalational anesthetics induce a rapid, shallow breathing pattern that further exacerbates atelectasis and intrapulmonary shunting.[1]

REASONING:

Ventilation-perfusion mismatching increases under anesthesia and in positions other than the upright position. This makes choice A least likely. Choices B, C, and D all involve controlled ventilation. Choice E presents a patient under anesthesia breathing spontaneously. The resulting atelectasis combined with the negative effects of anesthesia and prone position on FRC will produce the greatest ventilation-perfusion mismatching. The single best answer is E.

REFERENCE:

1. Barash PG, Cullen BF, Stoelting RK. Clinical Anesthesia, 4th ed. Philadelphia, Lippincott Williams & Wilkins, 2001, Chap. 29, pp. 641–659, 821–824.
2. Morgan GE, Mikhail MS, Murray MJ. Clinical Anesthesiology, 3d ed. New York, McGraw-Hill, 2002, pp. 484–495, 526–527.

BOOK A:

Answer C

Cardiovascular

QUESTION 132

QUESTION (Choose single best answer):

The hemodynamic profile below is from a 62-year-old man in the ICU after coronary artery bypass grafting.

	Entering ICU	+30 Minutes
Heart rate (beats/min)	90	120
Blood pressure (mm Hg)	125/75	80/30
PADP (mm Hg)	12	25
PAOP (mm Hg)	10	25
CVP (mm Hg)	6	8

Which of the following is the most likely cause of the changes occurring after 30 minutes?

(A) Anaphylactic reaction.
(B) Left ventricular ischemia.
(C) Pericardial tamponade.
(D) Pulmonary embolism.
(E) Septic shock.

CORRECT ANSWER: C

SUMMARY:

Cardiac tamponade after heart surgery is a common perioperative complication that requires surgical reexploration. Tamponade can occur even if the pericardium is left open after surgery. Loculated bleeding and clot formation can cause obstruction to diastolic filling of the right or left sides of the heart independently. The differential diagnosis includes right or left ventricular dysfunction. Classic signs of tamponade are hypotension, tachycardia, shock, and equalization of pressures in the heart such that CVP = PAD = PCWP = 25 mm Hg (although not all signs are always seen). Echocardiography (TTE or TEE) can be helpful in establishing the diagnosis.

EXPLANATION:

(A) *Incorrect.* Anaphylactic reaction would cause distributive shock with low CVP, PAD, and PCWP. Associated symptoms such as rash and bronchospasm may be seen.
(B) *Incorrect.* Electrocardiographic (ECG) changes of ischemia may be noted. It is unusual for left ventricular dysfunction to cause pressure equalization of PAD and PCWP. Echocardiography will help to differentiate these findings.
(C) *Correct.* Tamponade is consistent with these hemodynamic findings.
(D) *Incorrect.* Pulmonary embolus will give rise to elevated right-sided pressures, right ventricular failure, bronchospasm, and hypoxia. It will not cause equalization of pressures across the heart chambers.
(E) *Incorrect.* Septic shock will have a clinical picture significant for a source of infection, fever, elevated white blood cell count, and distributive shock. Unless there was an ongoing active infection, it would be unusual to see septic shock immediately after surgery.

REASONING:

It is important to have a thorough differential diagnosis for postoperative hypotension after cardiac surgery. Some causes include hypovolemia, biventricular failure, bleeding, tamponade, or pneumothorax. Clinical signs and symptoms can create a confusing picture. Tamponade is the most likely cause of the observed findings in this patient with acute hypotension in ICU after a short period of stability who has pressure equalization without increased chest tube drainage.

REFERENCE:

Hensley F, Martin DE, Gravlee FP. Practical Approach to Cardiac Anesthesia, 3d ed. Philadelphia, Lippincott Williams & Wilkins, 2002, p. 265.
Morgan GE, Mikhail MS, Murray MJ. Clinical Anesthesiology, 3d ed. New York, McGraw-Hill, 2002, p. 459.

BOOK A: **QUESTION 133**

Answer D

Equipment/Physics

QUESTION (Choose single best answer):

The odor of isoflurane is noted during isoflurane anesthesia with an endotracheal tube and mechanical ventilation. Mean airway pressure is unchanged. A scavenging system with an open interface and an active disposal system is being used. The most likely cause of the isoflurane odor is

(A) A leak in the inspiratory limb of the anesthesia circuit.
(B) Application of an excessive negative pressure to the scavenging interface.
(C) Malfunction of the pop-off valve of the anesthesia machine.
(D) Obstruction of the gas disposal tubing leading from the scavenging interface.
(E) Obstruction of the transfer tubing to the scavenging interface.

CORRECT ANSWER: D

SUMMARY:

The scavenging system collects waste gases from the anesthetic machine gas collecting assembly and transfers them to a scavenging interface that serves as a collection reservoir. In most operating rooms, the scavenging interface is connected to an active disposal system that uses constant negative vacuum pressure to eliminate waste gas from the operating room. An open interface describes a scavenging system reservoir that lacks valves and provides a direct connection to the atmosphere.[1] A leak in the inspiratory limb would cause a drop in mean airway pressures and thus could not be the source of the operating room pollution. Application of excessive negative pressure to the scavenging system would cause entrainment of atmospheric air through the open interface of the reservoir, helping to protecting the patient from untoward negative pressure in the circuit. This would not cause the atmospheric pollution of waste gases described. Malfunction of the APL valve would not cause a leak into the atmosphere, and obstruction of the transfer tubing to the scavenging interface could cause an increase in mean airway pressure. Thus an obstruction of the gas disposal tubing leading from the scavenging interface most likely would cause the venting of gases into the operating room. The interface is open to the atmosphere without any valves to prevent escape of waste gas from the reservoir.

EXPLANATION:

(A) *Incorrect.* A leak in the inspiratory limb would cause a drop in mean airway pressures. Pressure alarms would be activated, and appropriate tidal volumes would not be achieved.

(B) *Incorrect.* By applying excessive negative pressure to the scavenging system, atmospheric air would be entrained through the open interface of the scavenging reservoir. Truly excessive pressure may produce negative pressure in the breathing circuit or ventilator. Gaseous wastes would not be vented into the operating room in this circumstance.

(C) *Incorrect.* Malfunction of the pop-off valve would result in excessive buildup of pressure in the breathing circuit rather than venting of gaseous waste into the environment.

(D) *Correct.* An obstruction in the gas disposal tubing leading from the scavenging interface into the hospital's vacuum system would cause waste gases to escape into the operating room. There are no valves with an open interface, so waste gas will escape from the reservoir into the atmosphere.

(E) *Incorrect.* Obstruction in the transfer tubing going to the scavenging interface can cause a buildup of pressure and gases into the patient's circuit with a potential for barotrauma.

REASONING:

The questions tests knowledge of the anesthesia machine and scavenging system. There are various reasons for operating room pollution. The most common cause is kinking or obstruction of the tubing leading from the scavenging interface. An obstruction at this point also would cause the venting of gases into the operating room through an open interface because there are no valves to protect against this hazard. A leak in the inspiratory limb would lead to a decrease in mean airway pressures and obstruction of the transfer tubing, or malfunction of the pop-off valve could lead to barotrauma in the patient. The best answer is D.

REFERENCE:

1. Barash PG, Cullen BF, Stoelting RK. Clinical Anesthesia, 4th ed. Philadelphia, Lippincott Williams & Wilkins, 2001, Figs. 22-27 and 22-28, p. 587.
2. Morgan GE, Mikhail MS, Murray MJ. Clinical Anesthesiology, 3d ed. New York, McGraw-Hill, 2002, p. 45.

Answer E

Pharmacology

QUESTION (Choose single best answer):

Which of the following statements concerning the volume of distribution of a drug is true?

(A) It is equal to the sum of the volumes of the tissue spaces into which it diffuses.
(B) It is equal to the volume to which it is distributed outside the plasma volume.
(C) It is unaltered by the amount bound to red blood cells and plasma proteins.
(D) It depends on elimination from plasma.
(E) It relates the total amount of the drug in the body to the plasma concentration.

CORRECT ANSWER: E

SUMMARY:

Volume of distribution *is defined as the volume of plasma that would be necessary to account for a drug's observed plasma concentration. It can be calculated by dividing the dose of the drug in the body by its plasma concentration,*[1] *where*

$$V_d = \frac{\text{total amount of drug present}}{\text{plasma concentration}}$$

Causes for a small volume of distribution include anything that increases plasma concentration, such as high protein binding or ionization. Conversely, anything that decreases plasma concentration will increase the volume of distribution, such as high solubility or binding of the drug in tissues other than plasma (e.g., fentanyl in adipose tissue). The volume of distribution does not depend on elimination from the plasma.

EXPLANATION:

(A) *Incorrect.* The volume of distribution only reflects the volume of plasma necessary to account for the observed plasma concentration of the drug and has nothing to do with volumes of other tissues into which the drug diffuses.
(B) *Incorrect.* The volume of plasma into which the drug is distributed is key to calculating the volume of distribution, and the volume outside the plasma is irrelevant to the calculation.
(C) *Incorrect.* The binding of drug to plasma proteins increases its distribution within the plasma and therefore decreases its volume of distribution.
(D) *Incorrect.* A drug's elimination from the plasma does not affect its volume of distribution.
(E) *Correct.* The volume of distribution of a drug can be calculated by the total amount of drug administered and the proportion that resides in the plasma.

REASONING:

Volume of distribution is a quantitative measure of drug distribution in the body. If a drug is distributed extensively, it will have a lower plasma concentration for a given dose. However, if a drug is limited to a small compartment (e.g., highly plasma-bound drugs), it will have a small volume of distribution. There are many factors that affect drug distribution in the body, including ionization, protein binding, and lipophilicity. The best answer is E.

REFERENCE:

1. Barash PG, Cullen BF, Stoelting RK. Clinical Anesthesia, 4th ed. Philadelphia, Lippincott Williams & Wilkins, 2001, p. 250.
2. Morgan GE, Mikhail MS, Murray MJ. Clinical Anesthesiology, 3d ed. New York, McGraw-Hill, 2002, p. 129.

Answer E

Pharmacology

QUESTION (Choose single best answer):

Which of the following statements concerning propofol is true?

(A) Active metabolites can produce residual postoperative sedation.
(B) It causes less cardiovascular depression than an equivalent induction dose of thiopental.
(C) It causes less respiratory depression than an equivalent induction dose of thiopental.
(D) It has analgesic properties.
(E) The vehicle emulsion is associated with hypersensitivity reactions.

CORRECT ANSWER: E

SUMMARY:

Propofol (2,6-diisopropylphenol) is one of the most commonly used modern intravenous induction agents. It is formulated in a soybean oil–egg lecithin–glycerol emulsion (Diprivan) that is capable of causing hypersensitivity reactions.[1] Propofol can cause cardiovascular and respiratory depression, and these effects are more pronounced than with thiopental administration. Propofol is thought to work by facilitation of neurotransmission by gamma-aminobutyric acid (GABA). Propofol does not have any analgesic properties (but can synergize with fentanyl and alfentanil). Propofol is metabolized by the liver, and its subsequent inactive metabolites are eliminated by the kidneys.

EXPLANATION:

(A) *Incorrect.* Propofol is metabolized in the liver by conjugation with glucuronide and sulfate into inactive water-soluble compounds that are eliminated by the kidneys.
(B) *Incorrect.* Propofol causes more cardiovascular depression than an equivalent dose of thiopental.
(C) *Incorrect.* Propofol causes more respiratory depression than an equivalent dose of thiopental.
(D) *Incorrect.* Propofol has no analgesic properties.
(E) *Correct.* Propofol is packaged as an emulsion containing 10 percent soybean oil, 2.25 percent glycerol, and 1.2 percent egg yolk phospholipid. Allergic hypersensitivity reactions can occur to these additives.[1]

REASONING:

This question tests knowledge of the pharmacologic properties of propofol. It is important for the reader to review the multisystemic effects of propofol and how they differ compared with other anesthetic agents. Propofol does not have analgesic properties, and its metabolites are not active. Propofol is profoundly insoluble in aqueous solution and requires the use of solubilizing agents. Early clinical formulations of propofol (e.g., propofol EL) contained a cremophor-EL solubilizer that produced a high incidence of allergic reactions and was withdrawn subsequently from clinical testing.[2] Diprivan uses an egg lecithin emulsion to solubilize propofol. Allergic reactions to these components can occur but are rare and reported at 1 in 45,000 anesthetics for propofol-related immune reactions.[3]

REFERENCES:

1. Bassett CW, Talusan-Canlas E, Holtzin L, et al. An adverse reaction to propofol in a patient with egg hypersensitivity (abstract 476). J Allergy Clin Immunol 93(1):242, 1994.

2. Barash PG, Cullen BF, Stoelting RK. Clinical Anesthesia, 4th ed. Philadelphia, Lippincott Williams & Wilkins, 2001, pp. 332–333.

3. Laxenaire MC, Maten-Bermejo E, Moneret-Vautrin DA, Gueant JL. Life-threatening anaphylactoid reactions to propofol (Diprivan). Anesthesiology 77:275–280, 1992.

4. Miller RD, Miller ED, Reves JG, et al. Anesthesia, 5th ed. New York, Churchill Livingstone, 2000, pp. 250, 256.

5. Morgan GE, Mikhail MS, Murray MJ. Clinical Anesthesiology, 3d ed. New York, McGraw-Hill, 2002, pp. 173–174.

BOOK A: | **QUESTION 136**

Answer C

Cardiovascular

QUESTION (Choose single best answer):

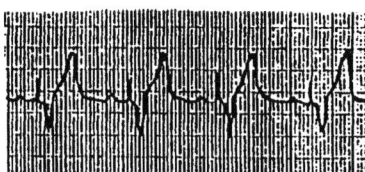

The ECG strip shown above is recorded as a patient with a permanent transvenous DDD pacemaker enters the operating room. These changes indicate that the pacemaker is

(A) Sensing the T waves.
(B) Sensing the retrograde P waves.
(C) Triggering off the intrinsic atrial activity.
(D) Malfunctioning in the atrial pacing mechanism.
(E) Prematurely stimulating the ventricle.

CORRECT ANSWER: C

SUMMARY:

Pacemakers are identified by a five-letter coding system. The first letter stands for the chambers being paced, and the second letter indicates the chambers sensed for inherent electrical activity. The third letter indicates the pacemaker response to the sensed P and R waves. The fourth letter denotes the programmability of pacemaker, and the last letter denotes the antitachyarrhythmia therapy. The DDD pacemaker in this patient is dual-chamber paced and dual-chamber sensed and has a dual response to sensing (i.e., triggered and inhibited).[1] On ECG, normal intrinsic P waves are visible followed by a pacer spike for QRS stimulation. The pacemaker is triggering off the intrinsic atrial activity.

EXPLANATION:

(A) *Incorrect.* Pacemakers sense atrial and ventricular depolarizing activity as P and R waves, not repolarizing T waves.
(B) *Incorrect.* Retrograde P waves would have different morphology from a sinus node P wave.
(C) *Correct.* A normal P wave is followed by a pacer spike and QRS complex.
(D) *Incorrect.* With atrial pacer malfunction, one may not see P waves or a pacer spike for P waves, and atrial-ventricular synchrony would be lost.
(E) *Incorrect.* The PR interval is normal in this patient and is not consistent with premature simulation of the ventricle.

REASONING:

This is a challenging question because it requires interpretation of the ECG to assess pacemaker performance. The reader should review the pacermaker letter coding system to fully understand the function expected of any pacer. Besides clinical history, the ECG is good way to evaluate the pacer activity.

REFERENCE:

1. Barash PG, Cullen BF, Stoelting RK. Clinical Anesthesia, 4th ed. Philadelphia, Lippincott Williams & Wilkins, 2001, p. 1515.
2. Morgan GE, Mikhail MS, Murray MJ. Clinical Anesthesiology, 3d ed. New York, McGraw-Hill, 2002, pp. 431–432.

BOOK A:

Answer A

Pediatrics

QUESTION 137

QUESTION (Choose single best answer):

Acute epiglottitis usually

(A) Requires a lateral radiograph of the neck for diagnosis.
(B) Occurs in children 2 to 4 years of age.
(C) Is treated effectively with racemic epinephrine.
(D) Has a viral etiology.
(E) Requires immediate awake intubation by direct laryngoscopy in the emergency department.

CORRECT ANSWER: A

SUMMARY:

Acute epiglottitis usually is caused by a bacterial infection with Hemophilus influenzae. *It was seen classically in 2- to 6-year-old children but has now become a disease of adults since the introduction of the Hib vaccine in the 1980s.[1] Acute epiglottitis progresses from a sore throat to dysphagia and complete airway obstruction with progressive supraglottic inflammation. A presumptive diagnosis often is made simply based on clinical history and presentation. A thickened and swollen epiglottis ("thumb sign") is the classic lateral radiographic finding. At no time should direct laryngoscopy be attempted in an unanesthetized patient because agitation may precipitate collapse of an already compromised airway.*

EXPLANATION:

(A) ***Correct.*** While fever, drooling, and a "hot potato" voice are characteristic of acute epiglottitis (especially in children), a lateral radiograph of a thickened epiglottis (the classic finding in 73 to 86 percent of cases) is diagnostic.[1]
(B) ***Incorrect.*** Acute epiglottitis was formerly a disease of children but now occurs mainly in adults at a rate of 2 to 3 per 100,000 per year. The incidence in children is 0.3 to 0.6 per 100,000 per year.[1]
(C) ***Incorrect.*** Racemic epinephrine is of limited usefulness in acute epiglottitis.[2]
(D) ***Incorrect.*** The most common etiologic agent is *H. influenza*, although various *Streptococcus* and *Staphylococcus* species also have been implicated.[1]
(E) ***Incorrect.*** Only up to 20 percent of cases of acute epiglottitis have required an artificial airway.[1] Impending or actual airway obstruction is treated with careful inhalation induction of general anesthesia prior to rigid bronchoscopy or endotracheal intubation.[2]

REASONING:

This question test knowledge of diagnosis and management of the airway in the setting of acute epiglottits. Although presumptive diagnosis often is made based on history and presentation alone, radiographic evidence of a "thumb sign" on lateral radiograph is diagnostic. Important management issues in pediatric acute epiglottitis include avoiding provoking anxiety in the child because this can precipitate sudden airway compromise. A caregiver should be present at all times to calm the child, and blood draws and placement of intravenous lines should be avoided. Airway issues should be addressed in the operating room, not the emergency room. Emergency airway equipment, including a wide assortment of endotracheal tubes and a tracheostomy kit, and a surgeon (ideally scrubbed with scalpel in hand) should be in the room prior to attempting intubation. Answers B, C, and D are factually incorrect. Answer E is contraindicated in acute epiglottitis. A is the best answer.

REFERENCES:

1. Bansal A, Miskoff J, Lis RJ. Otolaryngological critical care. Crit Care Clin 19:55–72, 2003.
2. Miller RD, Miller ED, Reves JG, et al. Anesthesia, 5th ed. New York, Churchill Livingstone, 2000, p. 2189.
3. Morgan GE, Mikhail MS, Murray MJ. Clinical Anesthesiology, 3d ed. New York, McGraw-Hill, 2002, p. 867.

BOOK A:

Answer E

OB/Regional

QUESTION 138 (OPTIONAL)

QUESTION (Choose single best answer):

Characteristics of postdural puncture headache include

(A) Incidence unrelated to the timing of ambulation.
(B) Increased severity with addition of vasoconstrictors to the anesthetic.
(C) Less frequent occurrence if the needle bevel is perpendicular to the direction of dural fibers.
(D) More frequent occurrence in men.
(E) Prevention by prophylactic epidural blood patch.

CORRECT ANSWER: E

SUMMARY:

Post–dural puncture headache (PDPH) can occur after spinal anesthesia, inadvertent dural puncture while placing an epidural, subarachnoid migration of an epidural catheter, diagnostic lumbar puncture, and myelograms. Characterized as throbbing, the pain typically is frontal, occipital, and retroorbital and extends to the neck. Postural changes are key to the diagnosis of PDPH, with the headache worsened when assuming the upright position and relieved with lying supine. The incidence of PDPH is highest in young women, especially during pregnancy. Technical factors such as needle direction parallel to dural fibers, decreased needle size, and use of pencil point (Whitacre) rather than cutting (Qunicke) needles decrease the incidence of PDPH. Treatment ranges from conservative management with hydration and caffeine to epidural blood patch.

EXPLANATION:

(A) **Incorrect.** There is no relationship between the timing of ambulation and incidence of PDPH.
(B) **Incorrect.** There is no evidence that the intensity of the headache is increased in patients who have had vasoconstrictors added to the spinal anesthetic.
(C) **Incorrect.** Dural fibers are longitudinal. The incidence of headache is increased if the needle bevel is perpendicular to the direction of the dural fibers. This is likely due to increased leakage of CSF with more traumatic injury to the dura.
(D) **Incorrect.** The incidence of PDPH is higher in women.
(E) **Correct.** Epidural blood patch is an effective treatment for PDPH in 90 percent of patients. Studies examining the efficacy of prophylactic blood patch show promis-

ing results, especially for patients who may have difficulty returning to the hospital for an additional procedure.[1]

REASONING:

This is a difficult question because controversy exists about the efficacy of prophylactic blood patch. Choices A, C, and D can be eliminated because they are not characteristic of PDPH. Differentiating between choices B and E is difficult because prophylactic blood patch has not been proven to be definitively effective. However, at the time the question was written (1993), the study by Colonna-Romano and colleagues showed promise that this might become a standard treatment. Choice B has not been studied in isolation, but studies examining the efficacy of different local anesthetic combination do not show an increase in intensity in patients who receive epinephrine or other vasoconstrictors in the anesthetic. E is the best answer.

REFERENCE:

1. Colonna-Romano P, Shapiro B. Unintentional dural puncture and prophylactic epidural blood patch in obstetrics. Anesth Analg 69:522–523, 1989.
2. Morgan GE, Mikhail MS, Murray MJ. Clinical Anesthesiology, 3d ed. New York, McGraw-Hill, 2002, pp. 275–276.

BOOK A:

Answer B

Physiology

QUESTION 139

QUESTION (Choose single best answer):

Which of the following statements concerning the superior laryngeal nerve is true?

(A) It provides sensory innervation to the subglottic surface of the vocal cord.
(B) It provides sensory innervation to the inferior surface of the epiglottis.
(C) It is a branch of the glossopharyngeal nerve.
(D) It is blocked by injection of anesthetic near the lateral portion of the cricothyroid membrane.
(E) It is the most commonly injured nerve during thyroid surgery.

CORRECT ANSWER: B

SUMMARY:

The superior laryngeal nerve is a branch of the vagus nerve (X) and has two terminal branches: the internal and external. The internal branch is sensory and innervates the supra-glottic area, including the vocal folds, base of the tongue, and epiglottis. The external branch is motor and innervates the cricothyroid muscle. This nerve is blocked by injection of local anesthetic at the thyrohyoid junction. The recurrent laryngeal nerve is also a branch of the vagus nerve (X). It has sensory innervation below the level of the vocal cords and controls motor function for all muscles of the larynx except the cricothyroid muscle. The recurrent laryngeal nerve is the most commonly injured nerve during thyroid surgery.

EXPLANATION:

(A) *Incorrect.* The superior laryngeal nerve provides sensory innervation to the supra-glottic surface of the vocal cords.
(B) *Correct.* The internal branch of the superior laryngeal nerve provides sensory innervation to the epiglottis.
(C) *Incorrect.* The superior laryngeal nerve is a branch of the vagus nerve.
(D) *Incorrect.* It is blocked by injection of local anesthetic at the lateral aspect of the thyrohyoid membrane.

(E) **Incorrect.** The recurrent laryngeal nerve is the most commonly injured nerve during thyroid surgery.

REASONING:

This question tests knowledge of the differences in sensory and motor innervation between the superior and recurrent laryngeal nerves. This knowledge would eliminate choice A and make B correct. Also knowing that both these nerves are branches of the vagus would eliminate choice C. Knowledge of the anatomy of the larynx and its associated structures enables elimination of choice D. Choice E is incorrect because the recurrent laryngeal nerve is the most commonly injured. The best answer is B.

REFERENCE:

Barash PG, Cullen BF, Stoelting RK. Clinical Anesthesia, 4th ed. Philadelphia, Lippincott Williams & Wilkins, 2001, pp. 722–723.
Morgan GE, Mikhail MS, Murray MJ. Clinical Anesthesiology, 3d ed. New York, McGraw-Hill, 2002, p. 83.

BOOK A:

Answer D

Pharmacology

QUESTION 140

QUESTION (Choose single best answer):

Which of the following is a complication of glycine used for irrigation during transurethral resection of the prostate (TURP)?

(A) Epileptiform activity on EEG.
(B) Peripheral neuropathy.
(C) Tachycardia.
(D) Transient blindness.
(E) Transient deafness.

CORRECT ANSWER: D

SUMMARY:

The use of 1.5% glycine during a TURP procedure is common. Glycine is used as an irrigant to distend the bladder and facilitate removal of blood and dissected prostatic tissue. Glycine is inexpensive, nonelectrolytic, and slightly hypo-osmolar. Absorption of large amounts of glycine can result in visual disturbances and transient blindness. This is thought to occur because of glycine's inhibitory neurotransmitter properties. (See also Question 35, Book B.)

EXPLANATION:

(A) **Incorrect.** Glycine is an inhibitory neurotransmitter.
(B) **Incorrect.** Glycine irrigation during TURP has not been associated with an increased incidence of perpheral neuropathy.
(C) **Incorrect.** This is not a common side effect of glycine irrigation.
(D) **Correct.** Glycine toxicity is a known cause of visual disturbances and transient blindness.
(E) **Incorrect.** Hyperglycinemia can result in visual disturbances but not deafness.

REASONING:

This question tests knowledge of the toxicity of glycine used as an irrigant for TURP. In addition to transient blindness, glycine also is associated with ammonia toxicity. Ammonia is a major by-product of glycine metabolism. Elevated ammonia levels can result in nausea and vomiting, followed by encephalopathy. Absorption of irrigant depends on the duration of resection and the pressure of the irrigation. D is the best answer.

REFERENCE:

Faust RJ. Anesthesiology Review, 3d ed. New York, Churchill Livingstone, 2002, pp. 529–530.
Morgan GE, Mikhail MS, Murray MJ. Clinical Anesthesiology, 3d ed. New York, McGraw-Hill, 2002, pp. 695–696.

BOOK A:

Answer C

Equipment/Physics

QUESTION 141

QUESTION (Choose single best answer)

In the event of a leak in the air flowmeter, which flowmeter arrangement produces the lowest risk for delivering hypoxic gas mixtures?

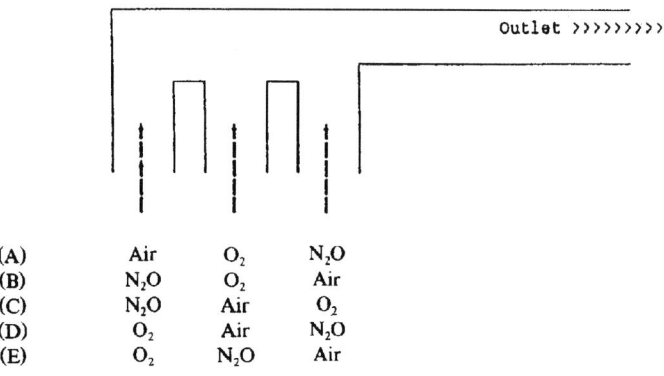

(A)	Air	O_2	N_2O
(B)	N_2O	O_2	Air
(C)	N_2O	Air	O_2
(D)	O_2	Air	N_2O
(E)	O_2	N_2O	Air

CORRECT ANSWER: C

SUMMARY:

There are many safety features built into the anesthesia machine. Flowmeters are arranged to maximize safety by differences in control knob feel, color, and position for each gas. The oxygen knob is large and fluted, whereas the N_2O knob is small and non-fluted. The oxygen control knob is green in color, whereas the N_2O knob is blue. Finally, the oxygen control knob usually is located closest to the common gas outlet, whereas the N_2O knob is located upstream from the oxygen knob. This arrangement ensures that oxygen flow is delivered close to the gas outlet.

EXPLANATION:

(A) *Incorrect.* This arrangement is more likely to deliver a hypoxic mixture because oxygen is located upstream from the gas outlet.
(B) *Incorrect.* This arrangement is more likely to deliver a hypoxic mixture because oxygen is located upstream from the gas outlet.
(C) *Correct.* This arrangement produces the lowest risk for a hypoxic mixture because oxygen is located closest to the gas outlet.
(D) *Incorrect.* This arrangement is more likely to deliver a hypoxic mixture because oxygen is upstream from the gas outlet.
(E) *Incorrect.* This arrangement is more likely to deliver a hypoxic mixture because oxygen is upstream from the gas outlet.

REASONING:

The key to answering this question correctly is identifying choice C as the only correct option because it places the oxygen flowmeter the furthest downstream and closest to the gas outlet. If a flowmeter leak occurs, delivery of a hypoxic gas mixture is less likely if the oxygen flowmeter is located furthest downstream.[1,2] The other choices are incorrect because they place the oxygen flowmeter upstream from either air or nitrous oxide and further from the outlet. Situations such as choice D are dangerous. If the air flowmeter develops a large leak, most of the oxygen flow upstream will leak out the air flowmeter. The patient will receive a hypoxic gas mixture of predominately nitrous oxide because the nitrous oxide flowmeter is placed downstream from the leak and is closest to the gas outlet. C is the best answer.

REFERENCES:

1. Barash PG, Cullen BF, Stoelting RK. Clinical Anesthesia, 4th ed. Philadelphia, Lippincott Williams & Wilkins, 2001, Fig. 29-2, p. 572.
2. Eger EI, Hylton RR, Irwin RH. Anesthetic flowmeter sequence: A cause for hypoxia. Anesthesiology 24:396, 1963.
3. Morgan GE, Mikhail MS, Murray MJ. Clinical Anesthesiology, 3d ed. New York, McGraw-Hill, 2002, pp. 43–44.

BOOK A:　　　　**QUESTION 142**

Answer D

Neuroanesthesia

QUESTION (Choose single best answer):

A 100-kg, 42-year-old woman received enflurane and oxygen for clipping of an intracranial aneurysm lasting 8 hours. In the first 2 postoperative hours, urine output is 2 L. Serum sodium concentration is 152 mEq/L. Urine osmolarity and central venous pressure are low. Which of the following is best used to establish the diagnosis?

(A) Pulmonary artery occlusion pressure.
(B) Serum fluoride concentration.
(C) Serum osmolarity.
(D) Response to antidiuretic hormone.
(E) Response to fluid restriction.

CORRECT ANSWER: D

SUMMARY:

Dilute polyuria, polydipsia, and hypernatremia following a neurosurgical procedure in the absence of hyperglycemia should suggest the diagnosis of central diabetes insipidus.[1] The diagnosis is confirmed by an increase in urine osmolarity after the administration of antidiuretic hormone (ADH). A positive response to ADH also will differentiate central from nephrogenic diabetes insipidus. Fluoride toxicity may impair renal concentrating ability and can produce a syndrome of polyuric renal failure most often associated with methoxyflurane. However, renal dysfunction owing to high fluoride concentrations is unlikely with enflurane even after almost 10 MAC-hours.

EXPLANATION:

(A) *Incorrect.* While pulmonary artery occlusion pressure (PAOP) may be a better indicator of left ventricular filling pressure than central venous pressure (CVP), PAOP does not aid in establishing a diagnosis.

(B) *Incorrect.* Fluoride concentrations associated with renal dysfunction are reported to be 40 to 50 μmol/L.[1] Although high plasma fluoride concentrations may result from enflurane anesthesia, especially in obese patients, this has little clinical significance. Fluoride toxicity should be a diagnosis of exclusion.

(C) *Incorrect.* Serum osmolarity may be higher than urine osmolarity in both diabetes insipidus and fluoride toxicity. Therefore, measuring serum osmolarity will not help establish a diagnosis.

(D) **Correct.** A positive response to antidiuretic hormone results in an increase in urine osmolarity and confirms the diagnosis of central diabetes insipidus.

(E) **Incorrect.** Fluid restriction can be helpful in the treatment of the syndrome of inappropriate ADH secretion.[1] It is not useful in the diagnosis of this patient's disease process.

REASONING:

The scenario of high urinary output and dehydration following enflurane anesthesia for cerebral aneurysm clipping sets up the differential diagnosis: diabetes insipidus versus fluoride toxicity. Since central diabetes insipidus is most likely following neurosurgery, the administration of ADH should either rule it in or out. Renal dysfunction owing to fluoride toxicity is a diagnosis of exclusion. D is the single best answer.

REFERENCE:

1. Barash PG, Cullen BF, Stoelting RK. Clinical Anesthesia, 4th ed. Philadelphia, Lippincott Williams & Wilkins, 2001, pp. 1137–1138, 1376.
2. Morgan GE, Mikhail MS, Murray MJ. Clinical Anesthesiology, 3d ed. New York, McGraw-Hill, 2002, pp. 142, 577, 605, 672.

BOOK A:

Answer C

Neuroanesthesia

QUESTION 143

QUESTION (Choose single best answer):

The drug that causes does-dependent electroencephalographic (EEG) evidence of both central nervous system excitation and depression is

(A) Lidocaine.
(B) Halothane.
(C) Thiopental.
(D) Nitrous oxide.
(E) Midazolam.

CORRECT ANSWER: C

SUMMARY:

EEG monitoring is a valuable tool used during neurosurgical procedures and controlled hypotension and for assessing depth of anesthesia. Anesthetic agents have variable effects on the EEG ranging from activation, depression, and other unique patterns. Barbiturates (including thiopental), etomidate, and propofol are the only intravenous agents capable of producing burst suppression and electrical silence at high doses. Among inhalational agents, halothane produces a biphasic (activation at low doses followed by depression at high doses) pattern, and isoflurane produces an isoelectric EEG at high doses. Both desflurane and enflurane produce burst suppression at high doses, and nitrous oxide produces an increase in both frequency and amplitude at escalating doses.

EXPLANATION:

(A) **Incorrect.** Lidocaine does not produce an excitation/depression pattern.
(B) **Incorrect.** Halothane produces a biphasic pattern on the EEG, with initial fast activation followed by dose-dependent slowing.
(C) **Correct.** Thiopental produces both excitation and depression in a dose-dependent manner, with periods of burst suppression at higher doses, followed by eventual electrical silence at even higher doses.
(D) **Incorrect.** Nitrous oxide produces an increase in both amplitude and frequency.
(E) **Incorrect.** Midazolam produces a biphasic pattern on the EEG, with initial fast activation followed by dose-dependent slowing.

REASONING:

This question tests knowledge of the effects of common anesthetic agents on EEG. It is important to understand that the question asks for the drug that causes both activation and depression in a dose-dependent manner (as opposed to a drug that causes activation followed by depression in a dose-dependent manner). Both halothane and midazolam fit this last description, so they can be eliminated. Nitrous oxide produces nothing but increasing frequency and amplitude (high-amplitude activation), so it can be eliminated. Lidocaine does not cause the kinds of EEG changes this question seeks. We are left with thiopental, which does cause dose-dependent activation and depression with characteristic burst suppression patterns. C is the best answer.

REFERENCES:

Faust RJ. Anesthesiology Review, 3d ed. New York, Churchill Livingstone, 2002, pp. 60–63.

Miller RD, Miller ED, Reves JG, et al. Anesthesia, 5th ed. New York, Churchill Livingstone, 2000, p. 1329.

Morgan GE, Mikhail MS, Murray MJ. Clinical Anesthesiology, 3d ed. New York, McGraw-Hill, 2002, pp. 563–564.

BOOK A:

Answer A

Physiology

QUESTION 144

QUESTION (Choose single best answer):

Which of the following findings differentiates the pickwickian syndrome from morbid obesity?

(A) Carbon dioxide retention.
(B) Upper airway obstruction.
(C) Decreased forced expiratory volume.
(D) Increased shunt fraction.
(E) Increased functional residual capacity.

CORRECT ANSWER: A

SUMMARY:

Obesity is a growing epidemic in the United States.[1] Approximately 27 percent of the U.S. population is obese (body mass index $\geq$ 30). Obesity is associated with many diseases and has special physiologic consequences and anesthetic implications. Changes in respiratory physiology associated with obesity include increased oxygen demand, increased CO_2 production, decreased chest wall compliance, decreased FRC, $\dot{V}/\dot{Q}$ mismatch, and hypoxemia. A special subset of morbidly obese patients has a hypoventilation state characterized by CO_2 retention and hypercarbia. First described by Charles Dickens as a condition afflicting the character "Fat Boy" in his serial "The Pickwick Papers" published between 1836 and 1837, pickwickian syndrome is characterized by hypoventilation from obstructive sleep apnea leading to chronic hypoxemia and hypercarbia.[2] Other associated findings can include polycythemia, hypersomnolence, pulmonary hypertension, and eventual biventricular failure.[3]

EXPLANATION:

(A) *Correct.* Pickwickian syndrome is uniquely characterized by carbon dioxide retention.
(B) *Incorrect.* Upper airway obstruction can be present with both morbid obesity and pickwickian syndrome.
(C) *Incorrect.* Both can cause decreased forced expiratory volume.
(D) *Incorrect.* Both can cause an increased shunt fraction.
(E) *Incorrect.* Decreased FRC is a characteristic of both morbid obesity and pickwickian syndrome.

REASONING:

This question tests knowledge of the pathophysiology of morbid obesity and pickwickian syndrome. Morbidly obese patients with pickwickian syndrome develop chronic hypoxemia and hypercarbia owing to alveolar hypoventilation (unlike the classic morbidly obese patient with normocarbia and alveolar hyperventilation). This knowledge leads to choice A as the correct answer. Choices B through D are common to both disorders and can be eliminated. Finally, decreased, not increased, FRC is a feature of both disorders. The best answer is A.

REFERENCES:

1. Yanovski SZ, Yanovski JA. Obesity. N Engl J Med 346(8):591–602, 2002.
2. Dickens C. The Pickwick Papers. New York, Penguin Books, 2000; originally published in serial form between 1836 and 1837.
3. Barash PG, Cullen BF, Stoelting RK. Clinical Anesthesia, 4th ed. Philadelphia, Lippincott Williams & Wilkins, 2001, p. 1035.
4. Miller RD, Miller ED, Reves JG, et al. Anesthesia, 5th ed. New York, Churchill Livingstone, 2000, p. 914.
5. Morgan GE, Mikhail MS, Murray MJ. Clinical Anesthesiology, 3d ed. New York, McGraw-Hill, 2002, p. 748.

BOOK A:

Answer B

OB/Regional

QUESTION 145

QUESTION (Choose single best answer):

Which of the following is the most likely sequela of interscalene brachial plexus block?

(A) Cervical epidural block.
(B) Hemidiaphragmatic paralysis.
(C) Pneumothorax.
(D) Seizure.
(E) Vocal cord paralysis.

CORRECT ANSWER: B

SUMMARY:

The interscalene brachial plexus block is performed most commonly for surgical procedures involving the shoulder, upper arm, and forearm. Urmey demonstrated with ultrasonography that ipsilateral hemidiaphragmatic paresis occurred in 100 percent of interscalene blocks.[1] Therefore, interscalene block should be used with caution in patients with significant respiratory impairment. Other common sequelae from this block include stellate ganglion block resulting in Horner's syndrome and hoarseness from ipsilateral recurrent laryngeal nerve blockade. Intravenous, intraarterial, epidural, spinal, and subdural injection of local anesthetic and pneumothorax are rare complications of the interscalene block.

EXPLANATION:

(A) *Incorrect.* Inadvertent epidural injection of local anesthetic is possible but not the most likely sequela following interscalene block.[2]

(B) *Correct.* Hemidiaphragmatic paralysis from blockade of the phrenic nerve is the most likely sequela following interscalene block.[1]

(C) *Incorrect.* Pneumothorax is a rare complication that may occur from advancing the needle too far and lateral to the interscalene groove.

(D) *Incorrect.* Intraarterial injection into the vertebral artery is a rare complication of placement of an interscalene block. However, as little as 1 mL of local anesthetic injected in the vertebral artery can result in the rapid onset of seizures.

(E) **Incorrect.** Vocal cord paralysis from blockade of the recurrent laryngeal nerve is a common sequela of interscalene brachial plexus block but is not the *most* common complication.

REASONING:

Since all the choices are potential sequelae of the interscalene block, the key to answering this question correctly is knowing which one is the *most common*. The proximity of the phrenic nerve results in its blockade 100 percent of the time, making hemidiaphragmatic paresis an expected sequela of interscalene block rather than a "complication."[1]

REFERENCES:

1. Urmey WF, Talts KH, Sharrock NE. One hundred percent incidence of hemidiaphragmatic paresis associated with interscalene brachial plexus anesthesia as diagnosed by ultrasonography. Anesth Analg 72(4):498–503, 1991.
2. Stoelting RK, Miller RD. Basics of Anesthesia, 4th ed. New York, Churchill Livingstone, 2000, pp. 187–188.
3. Morgan GE, Mikhail MS, Murray MJ. Clinical Anesthesiology, 3d ed. New York, McGraw-Hill, 2002, pp. 288–289, Fig. 17-4 (p. 289), Interscalene Approach to Brachial Plexus Block.

BOOK A: **QUESTION 146**

Answer B

Physiology

QUESTION (Choose single best answer):

Which of the following is the most reliable indicator of adequate reversal of neuromuscular block?

(A) Inspiratory force equal to –30 cm H_2O.
(B) Sustained head lift for 5 seconds.
(C) Train-of-four ratio of 0.7.
(D) Twitch height at 100 percent of control.
(E) Vital capacity of 15 mL/kg.

CORRECT ANSWER: B

SUMMARY:

Assessment of adequate recovery from neuromuscular blockade is important for patients emerging from anesthesia. Inadequate reversal and subsequent weakness can result in postoperative morbidity and mortality from hypoxia, hypercarbia, and aspiration. The motivation for this question appears to stem from a seminal paper by Pavlin and colleagues, who exposed a cohort of healthy unanesthetized volunteers to partial neuromuscular blockade with D-tubocurarine. They used this group to examine the correlation between a range of maximum inspiratory pressures (MIPs) that gradually diminished with increasing paralysis and various clinical outcome measures such as vital capacity (VC), hand grip strength, PETCO_2, and functional assessment of the muscles of airway protection.[1] They found that while a MIP of –25 cm H_2O may be adequate to prevent hypoventilation, the MIP$_{50}$ for return of protective airway muscles was –42 cm H_2O. Pavlin and colleagues concluded by agreeing with the findings originally reported by Miller— the ability to sustain a head lift for 5 seconds is the most sensitive indicator of residual muscle paresis.[2] In addition, they concluded that it is also associated with adequate strength to both protect the airway and ensure adequate ventilation.

EXPLANATION:

(A) **Incorrect.** While an MIP of –30 cm H_2O may be sufficient to ensure adequate ventilation, it does not ensure return of adequate muscle function necessary to protect the airway from aspiration.

(B) **Correct.** Miller originally reported the 5-second head lift as the most sensitive indicator of residual neuromuscular blockade.[2] Pavlin and colleagues found that the MIP_{50} for a 5-second head lift is –53 cm H_2O. This is much more negative inspiratory pressure than the MIP_{50} of –43 cm H_2O associated with return of muscles of airway protection and the MIP of –25 cm H_2O associated with adequate ventilation.

(C) **Incorrect.** The train-of-four ratio of 0.7 has been associated with decreased grip strength, decreased pharyngeal muscle tone, and inability to sit up without assistance.

(D) **Incorrect.** The twitch height can be at 100 percent of baseline but could demonstrate significant fade that would indicate residual paralysis.

(E) **Incorrect.** Normal vital capacity is approximately 60 mg/kg and is reduced with ventilatory muscle weakness.[3] This vital capacity is approximately 25 percent of normal and does not indicate adequate reversal of neuromuscular blockade. Pavlin and colleagues found that an MIP of –38 cm H_2O corresponds to a vital capacity that is 77 percent of control.[1] This observation implies that a patient can have a vital capacity almost 80 percent of normal and still have inadequate muscle strength to protect the airway.

REASONING:

This question tests knowledge of clinical indicators of adequate reversal of neuromuscular blockade. The answer stems from the seminal work of Pavlin and colleagues, who performed a quantitative study correlating MIP with various clinical measures of muscle function. It is important to remember that a 5-second head lift is the most sensitive indicator of residual neuromuscular blockade and that return of muscle function sufficient to ensure adequate ventilation *and* to protect the airway from aspiration can be best assessed by this maneuver.

REFERENCES:

1. Pavlin EG, Holle RH, Schoene RB. Recovery of airway protection compared with ventilation in humans after paralysis with curare. Anesthesiology 70:381–385, 1989.
2. Miller RD. Antagonism of neuromuscular blockade. Anesthesiology 44:318–329, 1976.
3. Miller RD. How should residual neuromuscular blockade be detected? Anesthesiology 70:379–380, 1989.
4. Miller RD, Miller ED, Reves JG, et al. Anesthesia, 5th ed. New York, Churchill Livingstone, 2000, pp. 1361–1362, Table 36-1.
5. Morgan GE, Mikhail MS, Murray MJ. Clinical Anesthesiology, 3d ed. New York, McGraw-Hill, 2002, p. 182.

BOOK A:

QUESTION 147

Answer D

Physiology

QUESTION (Choose single best answer):

A 25-year-old man requires exploratory laparotomy following a motor vehicle accident. He is acutely intoxicated with alcohol. Which of the following is the most likely result of the alcohol ingestion?

(A) Hyperdynamic circulation.
(B) Hyperglycemia.
(C) Hyperthermia.
(D) Increased respiratory depression from opioids.
(E) Increased sensitivity to neuromuscular blocking drugs.

CORRECT ANSWER: D

SUMMARY:

The anesthetic implications of alcohol depend on the acuity of its use. Chronic use of alcohol often has end-organ effects such as hyperdynamic circulation, hypoglycemia, in-

creased MAC requirements, increased depressant effects of opioids, and a resistance to neuromuscular blockade. Acute intoxication lowers MAC and can synergize with other depressant drugs such as opioids.

EXPLANATION:

(A) *Incorrect.* Chronic not acute alcohol usage results in a hyperdynamic circulation and elevated cardiac output.

(B) *Incorrect.* Hypoglycemia is a consequence of chronic alcohol use.

(C) *Incorrect.* Hyperthermia is not a known consequence of either chronic or acute alcohol ingestion. If anything, hypothermia is a more likely consequence of alcohol intoxication (e.g., due to unplanned physical exposure to environmental elements).

(D) *Correct.* Acute alcohol intoxication can synergize with opioids, resulting in increased respiratory depression.

(E) *Incorrect.* Chronic alcohol use results in resistance to neuromuscular blockers.

REASONING:

This question tests knowledge of the physiologic differences between acute and chronic alcohol ingestion. Choices B, C, and E can be eliminated because they are not associated with alcohol ingestion. Choice A is a consequence of chronic use, so it also can be eliminated. Choice D remains and is by default the correct answer. Interestingly, acute alcohol intoxication causes respiratory depression by synergizing with opioids, whereas chronic use can cause respiratory depression by impairing the elimination of opioids.

REFERENCE:

Faust RJ. Anesthesiology Review, 3d ed. New York, Churchill Livingstone, 2002, pp. 523–524.
Morgan GE, Mikhail MS, Murray MJ. Clinical Anesthesiology, 3d ed. New York, McGraw-Hill, 2002, p. 594.

BOOK A:

Answer A

Pharmacology

QUESTION 148

QUESTION (Choose single best answer):

The decreased duration of action of an intravenous dose of fentanyl compared with an intravenous dose of morphine is best explained by

(A) Greater lipid solubility.
(B) Increased hepatic metabolism.
(C) Less protein binding.
(D) Shorter elimination half-life.
(E) Smaller volume of distribution.

CORRECT ANSWER: A

SUMMARY:

Both fentanyl and morphine are used commonly for perioperative analgesia. Compared with morphine, fentanyl has a characteristically shorter duration of action. Fentanyl has a much greater lipid solubility. This accounts for both its rapid onset and offset. Fentanyl can easily cross cell membranes and is taken up rapidly by highly perfused tissues such as the brain, heart, and lung.[1] Elimination from these tissues is also rapid because fentanyl distributes to other tissues such as muscle and fat.[1] Compared with morphine, fentanyl has more protein binding and a larger volume of distribution. Both morphine and fentanyl have similar hepatic metabolism.

EXPLANATION:

(A) **Correct.** Fentanyl does have a greater lipid solubility than morphine. This explains its rapid onset and decreased duration of action. Redistribution of fentanyl to muscle and fat compartments occurs rapidly and is responsible for its short duration of action.

(B) **Incorrect.** Both fentanyl and morphine have an equal degree of hepatic metabolism.

(C) **Incorrect.** Fentanyl has more protein binding compared with morphine

(D) **Incorrect.** Fentanyl actually has a somewhat longer elimination half-life than morphine (2 to 7 hours versus 1 to 4 hours). However, fentanyl has faster initial redistribution to muscle and fat compartments compared with morphine. This explains its shorter duration of action.

(E) **Incorrect.** Fentanyl has a larger volume of distribution than morphine.

REASONING:

This question tests knowledge of the pharmacokinetic differences between fentanyl and morphine. Realizing that both fentanyl and morphine have equal hepatic metabolism eliminates choice B. Compared with morphine, fentanyl has more protein binding, a longer elimination half-life, and a larger volume of distribution. This eliminates choices C through E as potential answers. It is important to understand that fentanyl's short duration of action is due to its rapid distribution phase compared with morphine. A is the best answer.

REFERENCE:

1. Barash PG, Cullen BF, Stoelting RK. Clinical Anesthesia, 4th ed. Philadelphia, Lippincott Williams & Wilkins, 2001, pp. 251, 358.
2. Morgan GE, Mikhail MS, Murray MJ. Clinical Anesthesiology, 3d ed. New York, McGraw-Hill, 2002, p. 165.

BOOK A:

Answer D

Pediatrics

QUESTION 149 (OPTIONAL)

QUESTION (Choose single best answer):

Which of the following complications of caudal anesthesia with 0.25% bupivacaine is more likely in children than in adults?

(A) Intravascular injection.
(B) Neurotoxicity.
(C) Profound motor block.
(D) Systemic toxicity.
(E) Total spinal block.

CORRECT ANSWER: D

SUMMARY:

Caudal anesthesia is a common and valuable regional technique in infants and children. While the potential for inadvertent intrathecal or intravenous injection is always present, the overall rate of complications of pediatric caudal anesthesia is low.[1] Intravascular injection does not occur at a higher rate in children compared with adults, but lower protein binding leading to a greater free fraction of bupivacaine in children younger than 6 months of age puts these patients at increased risk for systemic toxicity.[2]

EXPLANATION:

(A) **Incorrect.** The risk of intravascular injection should not be increased in pediatric patients. A negative aspiration for blood should precede injection of local anesthetic.[2]

244

(B) *Incorrect.* Local anesthetics readily cross the blood-brain barrier.[2] Therefore, the risk of CNS toxicity should be the same in adults and children.

(C) *Incorrect.* In a study of 750 caudal anesthetics, the incidence of motor block in children following caudal anesthesia with 0.25% bupivacaine was 54 percent.[1] There have been no studies demonstrating a greater rate of motor block in children compared with adults using the same concentration and milligram per kilogram dose of local anesthetic. The incidence of motor block is lower using concentrations of less than 0.25%.

(D) *Correct.* After intercostal blocks, caudal blocks result in the highest peak plasma levels of local anesthetic.[2] Owing to lower plasma binding, children younger than 6 months of age develop a greater free fraction of drug and more potential for systemic toxicity compared with adults at the same milligram per kilogram dose.[2]

(E) *Incorrect.* Although the distance to the intrathecal space is more superficial in children,[2] children have not been shown to have a greater risk of total spinal block. Injection of local anesthetic should take place only after a negative aspiration for cerebrospinal fluid (CSF). Some clinicians advocate the administration of a test dose, whereas others simply dose the caudal incrementally.

REASONING:

This is a very challenging question. Few studies have been done to compare the same regional technique in adults and children. Since the overall rate of complications of caudal anesthesia is low, it is difficult to show a significant difference in complication rates. While the dura is more superficial, the sacral hiatus is also easier to identify in children. The only difference between children and adults with respect to a given dose of bupivacaine is a greater free fraction of drug that puts children at higher risk of systemic toxicity.[2]

REFERENCES:

1. Dalens B, Hasnaoui A. Caudal anesthesia in pediatric surgery. Anesth Analg 68(2):83–89, 1989.
2. Cote CJ, Ryan JF, Todres ID, Goudsouzian NG, eds. A Practice of Anesthesia for Infants and Children, 2d ed., Philadelphia, Saunders, 1993, pp. 430–433, 464–466.
3. Morgan GE, Mikhail MS, Murray MJ. Clinical Anesthesiology, 3d ed. New York, McGraw-Hill, 2002, p. 863.

BOOK A:

QUESTION 150

Answer B

OB/Regional

QUESTION (Choose single best answer):

After an axillary brachial plexus block, the patient feels pain when the surgeon clips the skin over the thenar eminence. The most likely cause is inadequate anesthesia in the distribution of the

(A) Intercostobrachial nerve.
(B) Median nerve.
(C) Musculocutaneous nerve.
(D) Radial nerve.
(E) Ulnar nerve.

CORRECT ANSWER: B

SUMMARY:

A complete understanding of brachial plexus anatomy and patterns of innervation is important for the application of this block in clinical practice. A potential complication of an axillary block is failure to block the median nerve. The median nerve is derived from the lateral and medial cords of the brachial plexus. It runs medial to the brachial artery and the insertion of the biceps tendon at the level of the elbow. The median nerve provides sensory innervation to most of the palmer surface of the hand, including the thenar eminence.

EXPLANATION:

(A) *Incorrect.* The intercostobrachial nerve provides sensory innervation to the medial aspect of the arm, not the hand.

(B) *Correct.* The median nerve supplies the thenar eminence of the hand and is a common cause of a failed axillary block.

(C) *Incorrect.* The musculocutaneous nerve supplies the lateral half of the forearm.

(D) *Incorrect.* The radial nerve supplies the lateral aspect of the lower arm, a middle strip on the posterior forearm, and most of the posterior aspect of the hand.

(E) *Incorrect.* The ulnar nerve supplies about half the palmer surface but not the thenar eminence.

REASONING:

This question tests knowledge of the sensory innervation of the brachial plexus. A complete knowledge of upper extremity innervation is required to eliminate wrong answers. The reader should review this information carefully because it is commonly tested.[1] Choices A and C can be eliminated because they supply the arm/forearm and not the hand. Choice E can be eliminated because, although it does have palmer innervation, it does not supply the thenar eminence. Choice D can be eliminated because, although it does supply some of the thenar eminence, it does not supply the bulk of it. The median nerve supplies this distribution, and B is the best answer.

REFERENCE:

1. Barash PG, Cullen BF, Stoelting RK. Clinical Anesthesia, 4th ed. Philadelphia, Lippincott Williams & Wilkins, 2001, pp. 723–729.

2. Morgan GE, Mikhail MS, Murray MJ. Clinical Anesthesiology, 3d ed. New York, McGraw-Hill, 2002, pp. 295–296.

BOOK A: **QUESTION 151**

Answer E

Equipment/Physics

QUESTION (Choose single best answer)

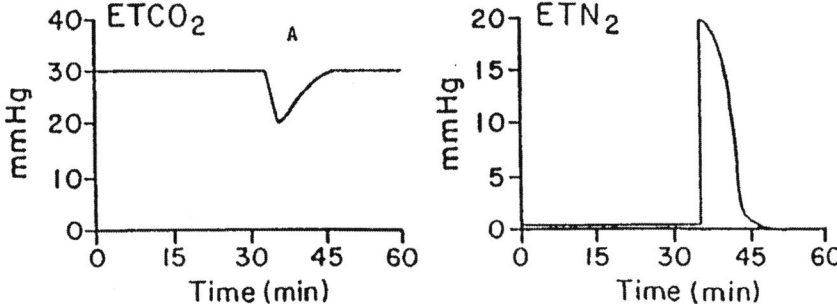

The trend plot above shows end-tidal gases measured during a radical neck dissection. The event occurring at *A* is most likely

(A) Acute hypotension.

(B) Endobronchial intubation.

(C) Kinking of the endotracheal tube.

(D) Rupture of the endotracheal tube cuff.

(E) Venous air embolism.

CORRECT ANSWER: E

SUMMARY:

Analysis of expired gases in an anesthetized patient can provide valuable clinical information. In addition to confirming endotracheal intubation, it also provides information on expired anesthetic concentration and the amount of expired oxygen and carbon dioxide. A sudden increase in expired nitrogen is highly specific for detecting the presence of air embolism, although it is somewhat less sensitive than a decrease in expired carbon dioxide for the detection of subclinical air embolism.[1] Measurement of expired nitrogen also enables the volume of the air embolism to be calculated.[2]

EXPLANATION:

(A) *Incorrect.* Acute hypotension can cause a sudden drop in $ETco_2$ owing to increased dead space ventilation from decreased perfusion of the lung. However, it would not be associated with an increase in expired nitrogen.

(B) *Incorrect.* Endobronchial intubation would not cause a change in $ETco_2$, especially an acute drop. It also would not be associated with an increase in expired nitrogen.

(C) *Incorrect.* Kinking of the endotracheal tube might cause a decreased $ETco_2$, but it would not be associated with an increase in expired nitrogen.

(D) *Incorrect.* Rupture of the endotracheal tube cuff can result in a drop in $ETco_2$ from the large leak that would develop. This leak also could produce an increase in end-tidal nitrogen, but it would not be transient. A cuff rupture would cause a continued leak with the associated lower CO_2 and high nitrogen from the entrainment of air around the leak.

(E) *Correct.* A sudden drop in $ETco_2$ with an associated rise in end-tidal nitrogen is highly suspicious for a venous air embolism.

REASONING:

This question tests knowledge of the interpretation of expired gas analysis for the detection of air embolism. There are many causes of decreased end-tidal carbon dioxide that the reader should review carefully.[2] However, a sudden rise in end-tidal nitrogen is highly specific for air embolism and is the key to establishing the diagnosis in this patient. The best answer is E.

REFERENCES:

1. Matjasko J, Petrozza P, Mackenzie CF. Sensitivity of end-tidal nitrogen in venous air embolism detection in dogs. Anesthesiology 63(4):418–423, 1985.

2. Barash PG, Cullen BF, Stoelting RK. Clinical Anesthesia, 4th ed. Philadelphia, Lippincott Williams & Wilkins, 2001, pp. 669 (Table 25-1), 766–767.

3. Morgan GE, Mikhail MS, Murray MJ. Clinical Anesthesiology, 3d ed. New York, McGraw-Hill, 2002, p. 575.

BOOK A:

Answer C

Clinical Anesthesia

QUESTION 152

QUESTION (Choose single best answer):

A 36-year-old woman develops acute airway obstruction 24 hours after total thyroidectomy. The most likely cause is

(A) Bilateral recurrent laryngeal nerve injury.
(B) Unilateral recurrent laryngeal nerve injury.
(C) Hypocalcemia.
(D) Subglottic edema.
(E) Tracheomalacia.

CORRECT ANSWER: C

SUMMARY:

Anesthesiologists should be vigilant for signs of airway compromise after thyroid surgery. Airway obstruction after thyroidectomy can occur in the immediate postoperative period, 24 hours after surgery, or even several days postoperatively. Complications such as recurrent laryngeal nerve damage and hematoma often can lead to immediate compromise of the airway. Hypocalcemia owing to inadvertent removal of parathyroid tissue can lead to airway compromise and usually presents 24 to 96 hours after surgery.[1] Other problems, such as tracheomalacia, can lead to airway issues several days to months postoperatively.

EXPLANATION:

(A) *Incorrect.* Bilateral injury of the recurrent laryngeal nerve can result in stridor and airway problems but usually occurs immediately after extubation or before the first postoperative day.

(B) *Incorrect.* Unilateral injury of the recurrent laryngeal nerve often results in hoarseness or unilateral vocal cord dysfunction but not airway compromise.

(C) *Correct.* Hypocalcemia owing to inadvertent removal of the parathyroid gland can lead to stridor that can progress to laryngospasm and acute airway obstruction.

(D) *Incorrect.* Subglottic edema also can result in airway obstruction. However, the timing and acuity of the airway obstruction in this patient suggest that it is more likely due to hypocalcemia.

(E) *Incorrect.* Tracheomalacia can lead to airway obstruction but usually beyond the 24- to 48-hour period.

REASONING:

The clinical presentation of acute airway obstruction 24 hours after thyroid surgery helps to narrow down the options. Choices A and B can be readily eliminated because they are more likely to manifest immediately after surgery. Choices D and E can be eliminated because they are more likely to occur after 24 hours. This leaves choice C, a classic complication that is the most likely cause of airway obstruction 24 hours after surgery.

REFERENCE:

1. Barash PG, Cullen BF, Stoelting RK. Clinical Anesthesia, 4th ed. Philadelphia, Lippincott Williams & Wilkins, 2001, p. 1122.
2. Morgan GE, Mikhail MS, Murray MJ. Clinical Anesthesiology, 3d ed. New York, McGraw-Hill, 2002, p. 742.

BOOK A:

Answer D

Cardiovascular

QUESTION 153

QUESTION (Choose single best answer):

Arterial pressure in the radial artery is 155/70 mm Hg measured by a correctly calibrated catheter-transducer system. At the same time, aortic pressure is 140/75 mm Hg using a high-fidelity catheter tip transducer. The most likely cause of this discrepancy is

(A) A large amount of air in the dome of the radial artery transducer.
(B) Coarctation of the aorta.
(C) Peripheral vascular constriction produced by sympathetic stimulation.
(D) Physiologic amplification of the waveform from the aorta to the radial artery.
(E) Too high a frequency response in the catheter-transducer system.

CORRECT ANSWER: D

SUMMARY:

Arterial pressure waveforms change as they move from the aortic root to the peripheral vasculature.[1] The waveform is a combination of an incident wave (forward pressure of blood traveling from the heart) and a reflected wave (pressure reflected back to the heart from the peripheral vasculature). The reflected waves produce a greater additive effect in the peripheral arterial circulation presumably because they are closer to the reflecting site. This phenomenon of pulse wave amplification (PWA) explains why the arterial pressure waveform has increased amplitude and systolic pressure and reduced MAP and lower diastolic pressures in the distal peripheral circulation.[1]

EXPLANATION:

(A) *Incorrect.* The presence of a large air bubble in the transducer dome reduces the natural frequency of the transducing system and can lead to overdamping, which underestimates systolic blood pressure.[1]

(B) *Incorrect.* Coarctation of the aorta is a congenital defect that narrows a segment of aorta, impeding forward blood flow distal to the lesion. Preductal (infantile) lesions occur proximal to the opening of the ductus arteriosis and can lead to marked hypoperfusion and cyanosis of the lower body. Postductal lesions have variable symptoms depending on the location and severity of the narrowing. A diagnostic finding associated with coarctation of the aorta is discordance of blood pressures measured from the upper extremities compared with measurements obtained from the lower extremities.

(C) *Incorrect.* It is not clear from the question that this patient has a reason for sympathetic stimulation. Regardless, the effect of sympathetic stimulation (i.e., strenuous exercise) on PWA has been studied. Roswell and colleagues examined changes in radial artery and aortic arch pressure waveforms at rest and during upright exercise requiring up to 100 percent maximal oxygen uptake in a cohort of young healthy men.[2] They found that mean arterial pressures were essentially the same when measured at both sites, ranging from 87 to 104 mm Hg from mild to maximal exercise. However, systolic pressures were higher and diastolic pressures were lower at the radial artery site. In addition, while pulse pressures at the central aortic arch site increased 1.95-fold with maximal exercise, the measured radial pulse pressure increased 2.60-fold. The authors postulate that the *increased* PWA observed at the peripheral site is due to local vasoconstriction. They corroborate their theory with the finding that reactive hyperemia and peripheral vasodilatation from increased heat load during exercise significantly decrease peripheral amplification. Thus, while local vasoconstriction may be responsible for *increased* peripheral PWA observed with sympathetic stimulation, we have no reason to suspect that PWA in this patient should be increased above baseline. It is certainly not the *most likely* cause of the observed discrepancy.

(D) *Correct.* Physiologic PWA causes the observed changes in systolic and diastolic blood pressure.

(E) *Incorrect.* An excessive high-frequency response leads to underdamping that could cause falsely elevated systolic blood pressures in the radial artery catheter-transducer system. This would not explain the lower diastolic radial artery pressure.

REASONING:

This is a challenging question that tests knowledge of pulse wave amplification and its effects on arterial pressure waveforms in the peripheral circulation. The question is made more difficult because choices C and D are plausibly correct. Each choice describes aspects of PWA. However, we have no reason to suspect that PWA is increased above baseline in this patient, and the simplest and most likely cause of the observed discrepancy is simply PWA. The best answer is D.

REFERENCES:

1. Barash PG, Cullen BF, Stoelting RK. Clinical Anesthesia, 4th ed. Philadelphia, Lippincott Williams & Wilkins, 2001, pp. 673, 825, 875 (Fig. 31-20).

2. Roswell LB, Brengelmann GL, Blackmon JR, et al. Disparaties between aortic and peripheral pulse pressures induced by upright exercise and vasomotor changes in man. Circulation 38:954–964, 1968.
3. Morgan GE, Mikhail MS, Murray MJ. Clinical Anesthesiology, 3d ed. New York, McGraw-Hill, 2002, p. 375.

QUESTION 154

Answer A

Neuroanesthesia

QUESTION (Choose single best answer):

During insertion of a Harrington rod with deliberate hypotension for correction of spinal scoliosis, accurate interpretation of somatosensory evoked potentials requires

(A) Core temperature greater than 35°C.
(B) Hematocrit of at least 25 percent.
(C) Mean arterial pressure greater than 70 mm Hg.
(D) P_{O_2} of at least 80 mm Hg.
(E) Reversal of neuromuscular block.

CORRECT ANSWER: A

SUMMARY:

Accurate interpretation of somatosensory evoked potentials (SSEPs) requires a stable anesthetic technique with a limited amount of inhalational agent, stable hemodynamics and oxygenation, and normothermia. Hypothermia can increase latency and decrease amplitude. A core temperature of greater than 35°C is required. As long as the hematocrit is reasonable and stable and the mean arterial pressure and saturation do not fluctuate dramatically, SSEPs are reliable indicator of neurologic sensory function. Neuromuscular blockade will not affect SSEPs because motor potentials from the ventral spinal cord are not being monitored.

EXPLANATION:

(A) **Correct.** Below 35°C, the amplitude is reduced and latency of SSEPs is increased. In addition, marked hyperthermia also can alter SSEPs.
(B) **Incorrect.** A hematocrit of 25 percent would not interfere with SSEPs interpretation as long as this blood level has been relatively stable throughout the operation. If the patient has suffered an acute loss of blood from a hematocrit of 45 to 25 percent within minutes, this change could alter SSEPs.
(C) **Incorrect.** Hemodynamic stability is key to accurate interpretation of SSEPs. If a MAP of 70 mm Hg remains stable throughout the surgery, SSEP monitoring is reliable. Frequently, deliberate hypotension is requested by the surgeon, and a MAP of 70 mm Hg is common in this type of surgery. However, if the patient had a MAP of 110 mm Hg throughout the surgery and it suddenly drops to 70 mm Hg, there may be a change in the SSEPs.
(D) **Incorrect.** A P_{O_2} of 80 mm Hg corresponds to a saturation greater than 90 percent. Although hypoxia will alter SSEPs, this oxygen tension and a corresponding saturation greater than 90 percent should not significantly affect SSEP monitoring.
(E) **Incorrect.** Neuromuscular blockade will not interfere with SSEPs. Most of the blood supply to the motor tracts derives from the anterior spinal artery. The spinal tracts monitored by SSEP are supplied by posterior spinal arteries. SSEPs do not monitor changes in motor tracts, and neuromuscular blockade is not contraindicated.

REASONING:

SSEPs are produced by application of small electric currents that stimulate a peripheral nerve. The evoked potential reflects the integrity of neurologic pathways from the periphery to the spinal cord and then to the somatocortex. Multiple factors, including anesthetic agents and temperature, can affect the accurate interpretation of SSEPs. Nitrous oxide does not affect latency, etomidate increases both latency and amplitude, and ketamine only increases amplitude. In addition, large changes in hemodynamics, oxygenation, and hematocrit levels must be avoided to ensure reliable monitoring. Extreme hypotension (MAP below 50 to 60 mm Hg), severe anemia, and oxygen saturations below 90 percent will interfere with SSEPs. It is important to ensure adequate oxygenation, ventilation, and perfusion in the setting of acute SSEP changes. Surgeons should be informed immediately of any changes so that effects of surgical manipulation can be assessed.

REFERENCE:

Stoelting RK, Miller R. Basics of Anesthesia, 3d ed. New York, Churchill Livingstone, 1994, p. 213.

Morgan GE, Mikhail MS, Murray MJ. Clinical Anesthesiology, 3d ed. New York, McGraw-Hill, 2002, pp. 100, 313, 403, 502, 680.

BOOK A:

QUESTION 155

Answer E

Clinical Anesthesia

QUESTION (Choose single best answer):

During insufflation of the peritoneal cavity with carbon dioxide at the start of laparoscopy, heart rate increase to 140 beats per minute, blood pressure decreases to 70/40 mm Hg, and a loud murmur is heard through the esophageal stethoscope. The most appropriate immediate step is to

(A) Administer a vasoconstrictor.
(B) Infuse crystalloid solution rapidly.
(C) Discontinue the inhaled anesthetic.
(D) Insert a central venous catheter.
(E) Deflate the abdomen.

CORRECT ANSWER: E

SUMMARY:

Laparoscopy is common surgical procedure. The technique relies on the creation of a pneumoperitoneum using CO_2 gas that is insufflated percutaneously into the peritoneal cavity. This is usually achieved by blindly passing a Veress needle through the abdominal wall into the peritoneal cavity, followed by insufflation of CO_2 gas through the needle. Inadvertent intravascular needle placement can lead to massive venous gas embolism and subsequent hemodynamic collapse. Other adverse effects associated with laparoscopy include cardiopulmonary effects of the pneumoperitoneum, systemic carbon dioxide absorption, and extraperitoneal gas insufflation.[1]

EXPLANATION:

(A) *Incorrect.* A patient experiencing a venous gas embolism (VGE) may undergo circulatory depression and collapse. It is appropriate to support the pressure with a vasoconstrictor, but this is not the first step in the management of VGE. The source of the VGE first must be identified and terminated promptly.

(B) *Incorrect.* Infusing crystalloid solution will increase central filling pressures but will not help prevent to further entrainment of pressurized CO_2 gas.

(C) *Incorrect.* This could help to prevent further cardiovascular depression and hypotension, but it is not the first treatment.

(D) *Incorrect.* Once again, this is a valid treatment option to attempt to remove the gas from the right side of the heart, but this is not the first step in the treatment.

(E) *Correct.* This should be the first step. The gas is entering the venous system through the pressure created by insufflation of CO_2 gas. Deflation of the abdomen will prevent further gas entrainment into the venous system.

REASONING:

This question tests knowledge of management of venous gas embolism in the setting of laparoscopic surgery. This question ask for the *most appropriate immediate step.* Several of the answers are helpful in the treatment of VGE. However, the first step should be to deflate the abdomen to prevent further gas entrainment. E is the best answer.

REFERENCE:

1. Barash PG, Cullen BF, Stoelting RK. Clinical Anesthesia, 4th ed. Philadelphia, Lippincott Williams & Wilkins, 2001, Table 38-5, p. 1057.
2. Morgan GE, Mikhail MS, Murray MJ. Clinical Anesthesiology, 3d ed. New York, McGraw-Hill, 2002, pp. 523–524.

BOOK A:

Answer E

Pain

QUESTION 156

QUESTION (Choose single best answer):

A 35-year-old man has acute onset of low back pain, lower extremity weakness, and bladder dysfunction. He had a lumbar laminectomy 2 years ago. A myelogram shows disk herniation at L4–5. The most appropriate management is

(A) Bed rest.
(B) Administration of a nonsteroidical anti-inflammatory agent.
(C) Epidural administration of a corticosteroid.
(D) Epidural administration of a local anesthetic.
(E) Surgical decompression.

CORRECT ANSWER: E

SUMMARY:

A patient with acute low back pain and signs of neurologic compromise (both new lower extremity weakness and bladder dysfunction) requires emergent surgical decompression. Failure to decompress expeditiously may lead to permanent neurologic injury. Short-term bed rest is appropriate for low back sprain marked by low back pain. NSAID use may relieve some pain associated with low back sprain but is not the primary intervention in a patient with neurologic compromise. Epidural corticosteroid appears to be effective in reducing the time to resolution of lumbar radiculopathy (pain radiating from the back below the knee). Epidural local anesthetic has an unclear role in back pain and in this case might only mask further neurologic deterioration.

EXPLANATION:

(A) *Incorrect.* Bed rest, NSAIDs, and epidural corticosteroids are reasonable approaches to acute low back pain without severe or rapidly progressive neurologic signs but are inadequate in the face of acute onset of low back pain, lower extremity weakness, and bladder dysfunction.
(B) *Incorrect.* See above.
(C) *Incorrect.* See above.
(D) *Incorrect.* Epidural local anesthetics are contraindicated in this case because they do not address the emergent nature of the injury and could mask further neurologic compromise.
(E) *Correct.* Spinal cord compression from disk herniation with acute neurologic changes requires immediate surgical decompression to prevent further neurologic compromise.

REASONING:

Indications for emergent surgical decompression of a herniated lumbar disk are severe or rapidly progressive radicular neurologic deficit or the cauda equina syndrome (i.e., bladder, bowel, and sexual dysfunction). In properly selected patients, lumbar diskectomy has an 80 to 90 percent success rate. In the absence of these symptoms, conservative treatment can be pursued. Conservative treatment includes bed rest (2 to 3 days) and NSAIDs. The sooner patients resume normal activity, the more likely they are to recover fully. They should be encouraged to pursue aerobic exercise and avoid heavy lifting. Most patients will experience resolution of symptoms within 4 to 6 weeks if there is no distinct underlying pathology. While most patients (90 percent) will experience relief with these measures, the use of epidural steroids reduces the amount of time until resolution of symptoms.

REFERENCE:

Gordon D. Diagnosis and management of lumbar disk disease. Mayo Clin Proc 71(3):283–287, 1996.

Morgan GE, Mikhail MS, Murray MJ. Clinical Anesthesiology, 3d ed. New York, McGraw-Hill, 2002, pp. 311–313.

BOOK A:

Answer B

OB/Regional

QUESTION 157

QUESTION (Choose single best answer):

A patient with chronic obstructive pulmonary disease (COPD) is undergoing spinal anesthesia to a T6 sensory level. The most pronounced effect on pulmonary function will be a decrease in

(A) Minute ventilation.
(B) Peak expiratory flow.
(C) Physiologic dead space.
(D) Tidal volume.
(E) Vital capacity.

CORRECT ANSWER: B

SUMMARY:

The respiratory effects of neuraxial blockade are relatively minimal. Tidal volume, minute ventilation, dead space, arterial blood gas tensions, and shunt fraction are minimally affected.[1] Sensory levels affecting abdominal and intercostal musculature can have an effect on respiratory function by decreasing active exhalation and therefore decreasing expiratory reserve volume (ERV). Patients with impaired respiratory function owing to obstructive or restrictive pulmonary disease may depend on active exhalation and have compromised oxygenation with neuraxial anesthesia extending to a high thoracic sensory level.

EXPLANATION:

(A) *Incorrect.* Minute ventilation is not changed with spinal anesthesia to a T6 sensory level.
(B) *Correct.* Peak expiratory flow is accomplished by active exhalation, which requires mainly abdominal muscle function. Blockade of these muscles owing to a T6 sensory level will cause paralysis of the abdominal musculature and significantly impair active exhalation.
(C) *Incorrect.* Anatomic dead space is the gas in nonrespiratory airways, and alveolar dead space is the gas in alveoli that are not perfused. The sum of the two is the physiologic dead space, and it is not changed with neuraxial anesthesia to thoracic sensory levels.

(D) *Incorrect.* Tidal volume is the volume of air in each normal breath. It is unchanged with thoracic neuraxial anesthesia.

(E) *Incorrect.* Vital capacity is the maximum volume of gas that can be exhaled following maximal inspiration. While this maneuver depends on intercostal and abdominal muscular function, vital capacity changes less than 10 percent with neuraxial blockade.[2]

REASONING:

This question tests changes in respiratory function associated with neuraxial anesthesia. Choices A, C, and D could be eliminated early because these parameters do not change with neuraxial anesthesia. Choices B and E both decrease with high sensory levels, but this question asks what would have the *most pronounced effect.* Vital capacity will be decreased in this situation. However, the effect is minimal compared with the decrease in peak expiratory flow, a maneuver that requires abdominal muscular strength. The best answer is B.

REFERENCES:

1. Barash PG, Cullen BF, Stoelting RK. Clinical Anesthesia, 4th ed. Philadelphia, Lippincott Williams & Wilkins, 2001, p. 663.
2. Miller RD, Miller ED, Reves JG, et al. Anesthesia, 5th ed. New York, Churchill Livingstone, 2000, p. 1497.
3. Morgan GE, Mikhail MS, Murray MJ. Clinical Anesthesiology, 3d ed. New York, McGraw-Hill, 2002, pp. 260–261, 484–489, Fig. 22-5 (p. 484), Spirogram Showing Static Lung Volumes.

BOOK A: **QUESTION 158**

Answer D

Cardiovascular

QUESTION (Choose single best answer):

A 70-year-old patient is shivering and has chest pain in the PACU following a cholecystectomy. Heart rate is 120 beats per minute, and blood pressure is 220/120 mm Hg. SpO_2 is 97 percent at an FIO_2 of 0.4. An ECG shows ST-T wave changes which are not affected by intravenous administration of nitroglycerin. Which of the following is the most appropriate next step?

(A) Administration of esmolol.
(B) Administration of hydralazine.
(C) Administration of nitroprusside.
(D) Application of a warming blanket.
(E) Increasing FIO_2.

CORRECT ANSWER: D

SUMMARY:

Postoperative shivering causes an enormous rise in oxygen consumption (up to 800 percent), CO_2 production, and myocardial oxygen demand. These physiologic responses are not well tolerated in patients with limited cardiopulmonary reserve.[1] The patient in this clinical scenario is likely developing myocardial ischemia owing to increased demand placed on the compromised heart. Treatment should be directed at correcting the inciting event, in this case shivering.

EXPLANATION:

(A) *Incorrect.* Esmolol would decrease myocardial oxygen demand by lowering the heart rate but would not treat the underlying cause of the event.

(B) *Incorrect.* Hydralazine would decrease myocardial oxygen demand by lowering the blood pressure but again would not treat the underlying cause of the ischemia.

(C) *Incorrect.* See above.

(D) *Correct.* Application of a warming blanket would treat the hypothermia causing the shivering that is thought to be the root cause of the increased myocardial oxygen demand responsible for the ischemia.

(E) *Incorrect.* Increasing the F_{IO_2} would improve oxygenation but would not treat the underlying cause of the ischemia.

REASONING:

This question tests knowledge of the physiologic response to hypothermia and the consequence of such a response in patients with a compromised cardiopulmonary system. It is important to direct efforts initially at correcting hypothermia with forced-air warming and small doses of meperidine. Intubation with paralysis and mechanical ventilation while actively rewarming should be considered if the hypothermia and myocardial oxygen supply-demand imbalance is profound or hemodynamic instability insues. D is the best answer.

REFERENCE:

1. Barash PG, Cullen BF, Stoelting RK. Clinical Anesthesia, 4th ed. Philadelphia, Lippincott Williams & Wilkins, 2001, p. 1397.
2. Morgan GE, Mikhail MS, Murray MJ. Clinical Anesthesiology, 3d ed. New York, McGraw-Hill, 2002, pp. 940–941.

BOOK A:

QUESTION 159

Answer E

Clinical Anesthesia

QUESTION (Choose single best answer):

A 24-year-old man who sustained multiple rib fractures in a motor vehicle accident has air leaks through bilateral chest tubes. Which of the following is most likely following initiation of high-frequency jet ventilation?

(A) Airway pressure will be measured most reliably at the proximal (external) end of the endotracheal tube.

(B) Atelectatic areas of the lungs will reexpand.

(C) Changes in end-tidal carbon dioxide tension measured at the tip of the endotracheal tube will match changes in Pa_{CO_2}.

(D) Hypercarbia will develop.

(E) The air leaks will be proportional to peak airway pressure.

CORRECT ANSWER: E

SUMMARY:

This patient has bilateral pneumothoraces that can present significant ventilation challenges owing to poor lung compliance resulting from the injury and the need to keep airway pressures low. High-frequency jet ventilation (HFJV) uses a small catheter to send a jet of gas from a high-pressure source into the airway. The small gas jet entrains additional gas via the Venturi effect to provide ventilation. The lower airway pressures and smaller tidal volumes produced by HFJV would be beneficial in this patient and help to reduce the amount of air leakage from the pneumothoraces.

EXPLANATION:

(A) *Incorrect.* The small high-pressure jet at the proximal end of the endotracheal tube generates a subatmospheric pressure gradient via the Venturi principle that entrains additional gas to achieve ventilation. Airway pressures at the proximal (external) end would not accurately reflect tracheal airway pressures at the tip of the endotracheal tube.[1,2]

(B) *Incorrect.* HFJV provides high-frequency (100 to 400 breaths per minute) low-tidal-volume breaths to achieve lower peak airway pressures. These small tidal volumes would not likely significantly reexpand areas of atelectatic lung. Gas transport in HFJV may depend more on molecular diffusion, high-velocity flow, and coaxial gas flow in the airways.[3]

(C) *Incorrect.* Gottschalk and colleagues demonstrated that a significant gradient between arterial and end-tidal CO_2 tension exists during supraglottic jet ventilation (13.4 ± 6.8 mm Hg) compared with conventional ventilation through an endotracheal tube (5.7 ± 5.2 mm Hg).[4]

(D) *Incorrect.* HFJV can be an effective method of ventilation in this situation, and hypercarbia would not be likely with adequate ventilation.

(E) *Correct.* The air leaks from the chest tube represent air moving through the bronchial airways out the pneumothorax and into the chest tube. Higher peak airway pressures would generate larger air leaks. This is why HFJV is beneficial for this patient.

REASONING:

This is a challenging question that test knowledge of the management of high-frequency jet ventilation in a patient who cannot tolerate high peak airway pressures. Many of the finer points of this question involve detailed knowledge of the principles of HFJV, and thus HFJV should be reviewed carefully. However, most readers would be able to reason that air leakage from the pneumothoraces would be proportional to peak airway pressures, even without detailed knowledge of HFJV. E is the single best answer.

REFERENCES:

1. Baer G. Complications and technical aspects of jet ventilation for endolaryngeal procedures. Acta Anaesthesiol Scand 44(10):1273, 2000.
2. Patel C, Diba A. Measuring tracheal airway pressures during transtracheal jet ventilation: An observational study. Anaesthesia 59(3):248–251, 2004.
3. Barash PG, Cullen BF, Stoelting RK. Clinical Anesthesia, 4th ed. Philadelphia, Lippincott Williams & Wilkins, 2001, p. 839.
4. Gottschalk A, Mirza N, Weinstein GS, Edwards MW. Capnography during jet ventilation for laryngoscopy. Anesth Analg 85(1):155–159, 1997.

BOOK A:

Answers B and D

Clinical Anesthesia

QUESTION 160

QUESTION (Choose single best answer):

Which of the following statements concerning the risk of acquiring hepatitis from a blood transfusion is true?

(A) Most patients with posttransfusion hepatitis become clinically jaundiced.
(B) Most cases of posttransfusion hepatitis are caused by the hepatitis B virus.
(C) The risk for hepatitis is less than the risk for acquired immune deficiency syndrome (AIDS).
(D) The risk for posttransfusion hepatitis is less than 1 percent per unit transfused.
(E) The incidence of posttransfusion hepatitis has remained unchanged over the past decade.

CORRECT ANSWERS: B and D

SUMMARY:

Within the last 10 years, the incidence of posttransfusion hepatitis has decreased from 7 to 10 percent to less than 1 percent per unit of blood transfused. Most posttransfusion hepatitis is now due to the hepatitis B virus because of improved virus nucleic acid testing for hepatitis C. Although rare, patients who do present with posttransfusion hepatitis usually are not jaundiced. The transmission of human immunodeficiency virus (HIV) following blood transfusions has an estimated incidence of 1 in 1,215,000 transfusions.

EXPLANATION:

(A) **Incorrect.** Most patients with posttransfusion hepatitis do not become clinically jaundiced. About 75 percent of patients are anicteric, 50 percent develop chronic liver disease, and of the latter, 10 to 20 percent develop cirrhosis.

(B) **Correct.** Most cases of posttransfusion hepatitis are caused by the hepatitis B virus. Most recent statistics from the American Red Cross in 2003 reveal that the incidence of transfusion-transmitted hepatitis C is 1 in 1,935,000 transfusions and the incidence of hepatitis B is 1 in 205,000 transfusions. Although the numbers have decreased dramatically, hepatitis B now accounts for most cases of posttransfusion hepatitis owing to new and improved virus nucleic acid testing for hepatitis C.

(C) **Incorrect.** The risk for HIV (1 in 1,215,000 transfusions) is much less than the risk for hepatitis B following a blood transfusion according to the 2003 statistics from the American Red Cross.

(D) **Correct.** The risk for posttransfusion hepatitis is significantly less than 1 percent per unit transfused.

(E) **Incorrect.** The incidence of posttransfusion hepatitis has decreased dramatically over the past decade owing to improved blood screening methods involving virus nucleic acid testing.

REASONING:

Over the last decade, testing the blood supply has decreased the potential risk of transfusion-transmitted infections dramatically. With virus nucleic acid testing, hepatitis C transmission has decreased to 1 in 1,935,000 transfusions according to the American Red Cross in 2003, making its transmission even more rare than hepatitis B (1 in 205,000 transfusions). HIV testing also has improved drastically, with a transfusion-related incidence of infection that is 1 in 1,215,000. Overall, the risk of posttransfusion hepatitis is much less than 1 percent, and most of those who do get infected do not become jaundiced. One needs to remember that this examination was written in 1993. Current statistics make *both* B and D correct.

REFERENCE:

Pomper GJ, Wu Y, Snyder EL. Risks of transfusion-transmitted infections: 2003. Curr Opin Hematol 10:412–418, 2003.

Morgan GE, Mikhail MS, Murray MJ. Clinical Anesthesiology, 3d ed. New York, McGraw-Hill, 2002, p. 553.

BOOK A:

QUESTION 161

Answer D

Pharmacology

QUESTION (Choose single best answer):

Which of the following is more likely to occur with use of trimethaphan to induce hypotension than with use of nitroprusside?

(A) A predictable decrease in mean arterial pressure.
(B) Increased mixed venous P_{O_2}.
(C) Increased serum lactate concentration.
(D) Mydriasis.
(E) Reflex tachycardia.

CORRECT ANSWER: D

SUMMARY:

Trimethaphan and nitroprusside are intravenous agents used to induce hypotension. Trimethaphan works by producing a selective nondepolarizing blockade of acetylcholine receptors in autonomic ganglia without causing neuromuscular blockade. This blockade causes decreased sympathetic nervous system output, relaxing vascular smooth muscle to produce peripheral vasodilatation. Major side effects of trimethaphan are fixed dilated pupils and rapid tachyphylaxis.[1] Nitroprusside relaxes both arteriolar and venous smooth muscle through the production of nitric oxide.

EXPLANATION:

(A) *Incorrect.* Both nitroprusside and trimethaphan produce a reliable and predictable decrease in blood pressure.

(B) *Incorrect.* Unlike nitroprusside, trimethaphan does not inhibit hypoxic pulmonary vasoconstriction and will not affect mixed venous P_{O_2}.

(C) *Incorrect.* Trimethaphan is eliminated through hydrolysis by the pseudo-cholinesterase enzyme.[1] Unlike nitroprusside, its metabolism does not result in cyanide production and is not associated with increased serum lactate levels. (*See also Question 5, Book B.*)

(D) *Correct.* Trimethaphan blocks parasympathetic ganglia and can cause mydriasis.

(E) *Incorrect.* Trimethaphan is associated with an increased heart rate, but it is caused by parasympathetic ganglionic blockade rather than reflex tachycardia.

REASONING:

This question tests knowledge of the pharmacologic differences between trimethaphan and nitroprusside. Unlike nitroprusside, trimethaphan is not used commonly in the operating room. Mydriasis is a well-known side effect that makes trimethaphan a poor choice for intraoperative blood pressure control, especially for neurosurgical procedures where eye signs have significant clinical value. D is the best answer.

REFERENCE:

1. Barash PG, Cullen BF, Stoelting RK. Clinical Anesthesia, 4th ed. Philadelphia, Lippincott Williams & Wilkins, 2001, p. 284.

2. Morgan GE, Mikhail MS, Murray MJ. Clinical Anesthesiology, 3d ed. New York, McGraw-Hill, 2002, pp. 225, 229.

BOOK A:

Answer E

Basic Science

QUESTION 162

QUESTION (Choose single best answer):

Local anesthetics block nerve conduction by

(A) Closing calcium channels.
(B) Decreasing intracellular calcium concentration.
(C) Decreasing potassium conductance.
(D) Causing extrusion of intracellular potassium.
(E) Inhibiting cellular influx of sodium.

CORRECT ANSWER: E

SUMMARY:

Local anesthetics slow the rate of depolarization of nerve membranes by binding to specific receptors inside of sodium channels in their inactivated state. This prevents the sodium channel from opening and also prevents subsequent membrane depolarization and propagation of the action potential. Local anesthetics do not block nerve conduction by closing calcium channels, decreasing intracellular calcium, decreasing potassium conductance, or causing the extrusion of intracellular potassium. The resting membrane potential of the nerve is also unaffected.

EXPLANATION:

(A) *Incorrect.* Calcium channel blockers, but not local anesthetics, close intracellular calcium channels by blocking them (nifedipine) or binding them in their depolarized inactivated state (verapamil).

(B) *Incorrect.* Local anesthetics do not decrease intracellular calcium concentrations.

(C) *Incorrect.* The nerve cell membrane is much more permeable to potassium than to sodium, accounting for a negative resting membrane potential of –70 mV. With decreased intracellular sodium, there will be a decrease in potassium conductance outside the cell and a slowing of the rate of depolarization. However, a slow outflow of potassium is not the mechanism of action of local anesthetics.

(D) *Incorrect.* Local anesthetics do not cause an extrusion of intracellular potassium.

(E) *Correct.* Local anesthetics inhibit sodium channel activation. Without influx of sodium, the membrane potential does not sufficiently depolarize to reach threshold, and there is no propagation of the action potential.

REASONING:

This question tests knowledge of the molecular mechanism for local anesthetic blockade of neuronal conduction. It is important for the reader to review this mechanism carefully because it is tested frequently on board examinations.[1] The mechanism of action for clinically used tertiary amine local anesthetics is based on the modulated receptor theory. Lipophilic neutral base forms of the local anesthetic cross the lipid bilayer membrane. Once intracellular, the neutral base can be protonated to a charged form that interacts directly with sodium channels at the negatively charged membrane surface to inhibit channel function. In addition, the neutral base also can cause sodium channel closure through expansion of the membrane.[1] E is the best answer.

REFERENCE:

1. Barash PG, Cullen BF, Stoelting RK. Clinical Anesthesia, 4th ed. Philadelphia, Lippincott Williams & Wilkins, 2001, pp. 450–453, Fig. 17-4.
2. Morgan GE, Mikhail MS, Murray MJ. Clinical Anesthesiology, 3d ed. New York, McGraw-Hill, 2002, pp. 234, 363–364.

BOOK A: **QUESTION 163**

Answer B

Pharmacology

QUESTION (Choose single best answer):

Which of the following drugs decreases lower esophageal sphincter tone?

(A) Edrophonium
(B) Glycopyrrolate
(C) Metoclopramide
(D) Prochlorperazine
(E) Succinylcholine

CORRECT ANSWER: B

SUMMARY:

The lower esophageal sphincter (LES) is a 2- to 3-cm segment of the gastrointestinal (GI) tract located above and below the diaphragm that is under increased pressure. The likelihood for reflux is related to the barrier pressure or the difference between the LES pres-

sure and gastric pressure. The LES is innervated by vagal and sympathethic nerves. Certain drugs with anticholinergic effects, including atropine, glycopyrrolate, and tricyclic antidepressants, have been shown to relax the LES. Decreased LES tone is associated with pregnancy, obesity, hiatal hernia, and gastroesophageal reflux disease (GERD). A number of medications that increase acetylcholine activity, including succinylcholine, prochlorperazine, metoclopramide, edrophonium, and neostigmine, also will increase LES tone.[1]

EXPLANATION:

(A) *Incorrect.* Edrophonium is an acetylcholinesterase inhibitor. It stimulates gastrointestinal Ach receptors, leading to increased LES tone.

(B) *Correct.* Glycopyrrolate is an anticholinergic agent. It has been shown to lower LES tone.

(C) *Incorrect.* Metoclopramide acts centrally as a dopamine antagonist and peripherally as a cholinomimetic, increasing Ach transmission in receptors on intestinal smooth muscle as well as increasing LES tone.

(D) *Incorrect.* Prochlorperazine (Compazine) is a phenothiazine that antagonizes dopaminergic receptors in the chemoreceptor trigger zone in the medulla. Like metoclopramide, it also increases LES tone peripherally.[1]

(E) *Incorrect.* Succinylcholine is a depolarizing muscle relaxant that mimics Ach receptors and causes abdominal wall fasciculations that increase intragastric pressure and LES tone.

REASONING:

This question tests knowledge of the effects of drugs on lower esophageal sphincter tone. Even if the reader did not know the correct answer, a guess can be made on the basis that one of the drugs listed (glycopyrrolate) antagonizes acetylcholine activity, whereas all the others have a cholinomimetic effect. B is the best answer.

REFERENCE:

1. Barash PG, Cullen BF, Stoelting RK. Clinical Anesthesia, 4th ed. Philadelphia, Lippincott Williams & Wilkins, 2001, pp. 560, 1042, 1042t.
2. Morgan GE, Mikhail MS, Murray MJ. Clinical Anesthesiology, 3d ed. New York, McGraw-Hill, 2002, pp. 186–187, 202–205, 209, 245.

BOOK A:

Answer A

Basic Science

QUESTION 164

QUESTION (Choose single best answer):

In patients homozygous for atypical pseudocholinesterase, which of the following best explains the prolonged action of succinylcholine?

(A) An increased proportion of the dose reaches the neuromuscular junction.
(B) Diffusion away from the neuromuscular junction is slowed.
(C) Hepatic clearance of succinylcholine is decreased.
(D) Prejunctional activity is unopposed.
(E) Succinylmonocholine induces neuromuscular block.

CORRECT ANSWER: A

SUMMARY:

Most of the succinylcholine administered to a patient is metabolized by pseudocholinesterase in the bloodstream to succinylmonocholine, a metabolite with minimal neuromuscular blocking properties. Only 5 percent of the injected drug ever reaches the neuromuscular junction. Neuromuscular blockade ends when succinylcholine diffuses into the extracellular space. Prolonged blockade occurs in individuals who are homozygous for atypical pseudocholinesterase, which has 1/100 the affinity of the normal enzyme for succinylcholine. As a consequence, more succinylcholine reaches the neuromuscular junction. In these individuals, urinary excretion and protein binding contribute to the clearance of the drug.[1]

EXPLANATION:

(A) **Correct.** In patients who are homozygous for atypical pseudocholinesterase, less succinylcholine is metabolized in the plasma, and a larger percentage of the drug reaches the neuromuscular junction, resulting in prolonged block.

(B) **Incorrect.** It is the higher drug concentration at the neuromuscular junction and not a slower diffusion away that accounts for the prolonged effects of succinylcholine in patients who are homozygous for atypical pseudocholinesterase.

(C) **Incorrect.** While pseudocholinesterase is produced by the liver, succinylcholine does not undergo hepatic metabolism.

(D) **Incorrect.** Prejunctional activity is opposed by the inhibition of motor end plate repolarization by succinylcholine.

(E) **Incorrect.** Succinylmonocholine, the metabolite of succinylcholine produced by pseudocholinesterase, is a very weak neuromuscular blocker with 1/20 to 1/80 the potency of succinylcholine. It is quickly hydrolyzed to succinic acid in the plasma. Patients homozygous for atypical pseudocholinesterase would have reduced levels of succinylmonocholine in the plasma.[2]

REASONING:

This question tests knowledge of the mechanism of succinylcholine and its effects in patients with atypical pseudocholinesterase enzyme. It is important for the reader to review the mechanism of action and pharmacology of succinylcholine.[1] Answers B, C, D, and E are clearly incorrect. Prolonged block is due mainly to the increased proportion of the dose of drug reaching the neuromuscular junction. A is the best answer.

REFERENCES:

1. Barash PG, Cullen BF, Stoelting RK. Clinical Anesthesia, 4th ed. Philadelphia, Lippincott Williams & Wilkins, 2001, pp. 421–424, 538–540.
2. Stoelting RK: Pharmacology and Physiology in Anesthetic Practice, 2d ed. Philadelphia, Lippincott, 1991, p. 178.
3. Morgan GE, Mikhail MS, Murray MJ. Clinical Anesthesiology, 3d ed. New York, McGraw-Hill, 2002, pp. 181–187.

BOOK A:

QUESTION 165

Answer E

OB/Regional

QUESTION (Choose single best answer):

Recognized side effects of magnesium sulfate used for the treatment of preeclampsia that would be of anesthetic concern include each of the following *except*

(A) Maternal pulmonary edema.
(B) Neonatal hypotonia.
(C) Increased maternal sensitivity to succinylcholine.
(D) Increased maternal sensitivity to vecuronium.
(E) Maternal hypokalemia.

CORRECT ANSWER: E

SUMMARY:

Magnesium sulfate is used commonly for eclamptic seizure prophylaxis in preeclamptic patients.[1] *The therapeutic range for intravenous magnesium administered to preeclamptic parturients is from 4.8 to 9.6 mg/dL. Side effects of magnesium therapy include (1) loss of patellar reflex (8 to 12 mg/dL), (2) somnolence (10 to 12 mg/dL), (3) slurred speech (10 to 12 mg/dL), (4) muscular paralysis (15 to 17 mg/dL), (5) respiratory difficulty (15 to 17 mg/dL), and (6) cardiac arrest (30 to 35 mg/dL).*[1] *These patients are also at an increased risk of pulmonary edema, increased sensitivity to neuromuscular blocking agents, and fetal depression with fetal hypotonia. Parturients who receive magnesium infusions should have deep tendon reflexes and vital signs assessed hourly. Calcium gluconate should be readily available to treat magnesium intoxication.*[1]

EXPLANATION:

(A) **Incorrect.** The combination of preeclampsia and magnesium increases the risk for maternal pulmonary edema.

(B) **Incorrect.** Magnesium crosses the placenta, increasing the risk of fetal hypotonia.

(C) **Incorrect.** There is an increased sensitivity to both depolarizing and nondepolarizing neuromuscular agents in patients receiving magnesium.

(D) **Incorrect.** There is an increased sensitivity to both depolarizing and nondepolarizing neuromuscular agents in patients receiving magnesium.

(E) **Correct.** Hypokalemia typically is not associated with magnesium tocolysis. Other beta-adrenergic tocolytic agents such as terbutaline and ritodrine are more commonly associated with hyperglycemia and the subsequent hypokalemia (owing to increased intracellular K^+ uptake). These effects result from $beta_1$- and $beta_2$-adrenergic effects on lipolysis, glycogenolysis, and gluconeogenesis.

REASONING:

This question tests knowledge of magnesium for seizure prophylaxis in preeclamptic women. It is important to review the therapeutic and toxic range of magnesium levels in parturients. In addition to its tocolytic properties, magnesium is effective in the prevention and treatment of eclamptic seizures and has been shown to be superior to phenytoin.[2] E is the best answer.

REFERENCES:

1. Gabbe SG. Obstetrics: Normal and Problem Pregnancies, 4th ed. New York, Churchill Livingstone, 2002, pp. 966, 969–970.
2. Lucas MJ, Leveno KJ, Cunningham FG. A comparison of magnesium sulfate with phenytoin for the prevention of eclampsia. N Engl J Med 333:201, 1995.
3. Morgan GE, Mikhail MS, Murray MJ. Clinical Anesthesiology, 3d ed. New York, McGraw-Hill, 2002, p. 813.

BOOK A:

QUESTION 166

Answer B

Neuroanesthesia

QUESTION (Choose single best answer):

A comatose 40-year-old man is to undergo evacuation of an acute subdural hematoma. His left pupil is dilated, and blood is present behind the left tympanic membrane. Each of the following is an acceptable intervention *except*

(A) Application of 5 cm H_2O positive end-expiratory pressure (PEEP).

(B) Blind nasotracheal intubation.

(C) Use of isoflurane.

(D) Use of nitrous oxide.

(E) Use of succinylcholine.

CORRECT ANSWER: B

SUMMARY:

Patients with neurologic injury often have competing indications and contraindications for the use of medications and anesthetic techniques. Management of increased intracranial pressure (ICP) must be considered when assessing clinical techniques for managing and securing the airway. Cerebral perfusion pressure (CPP) must be maintained. CPP = mean arterial pressure (MAP) – ICP (or CVP, whichever is greater). Interventions that reduce ICP increase CPP. These maneuvers include hyperventilation, elevating the head of the bed, administration of mannitol and lasix, and placement of interventricular drains. The dilated pupil of this patient suggests an elevated ICP, whereas hemotympanum is associated with a basilar skull fracture.

EXPLANATION:

(A) *Incorrect.* PEEP increases central venous pressure, which potentially can decrease CPP, but it is not contraindicated.

(B) *Correct.* Blind nasotracheal intubation (BNTI) in this patient may result in inadvertent placement of an endotracheal tube into the cranial vault. One case report in the anesthesia literature has described inadvertent intracranial placement during BNTI in a patient with fracture of the nasal fossa and a complex skull fracture.[1] There have been numerous reports of inadvertent placement of nasogastric tubes into the cranial vault after basilar skull fractures.[2–4] Therefore, BNTI is relatively contraindicated in the setting of severe facial trauma or basilar skull fracture.[5,6]

(C) *Incorrect.* Isoflurane is perfectly acceptable for patients with increased ICP.

(D) *Incorrect.* The effects of nitrous oxide on ICP are mild.

(E) *Incorrect.* Succinylcholine can cause a transient increase in ICP. In a trauma situation this risk is outweighed by the importance of quickly and safely securing the airway.

REASONING:

This question tests knowledge of the anesthetic management of a patient with signs of increased ICP and possible skull fracture. The choices for this question vary from perfectly acceptable (isoflurane), to acceptable (nitrous), to less than ideal but acceptable (succinylcholine), to not necessarily harmful (PEEP), to an unacceptable intervention (BNTI). One must use clinical judgment when weighing several alternatives in anesthetic management. B is the best answer.

REFERENCES:

1. Horellou MF, Mathe D, Feiss P. A hazard of nasotracheal intubation. Anaesthesia 33:73–74, 1978.

2. Bouzarth WF. Intracranial nasogastric tube intubation. J Trauma 18:818–819, 1978.

3. Fremstad JD, Martin SH. Lethal complication from insertion of nasogastric tube after severe basilar skull fracture. J Trauma 18:820–822, 1978.

4. Gregory A, Turner P, Reynolds A. A complication of nasogastric intubation: Intracranial penetration. J Trauma 18:823–824, 1978.

5. Morris IR. Airway management. In Rosen P, Barkin RM, Braen GR, et al., eds. Emergency Medicine Concepts and Clinical Practice, 3d ed. St Louis, Mosby, 1992, pp. 79–105.

6. Pointer JE. Nasotracheal intibation. In Dailey RH, Simon B, Young CP, Stewart RD, eds. The Airway Emergency Management. St Louis, Mosby, 1992, pp. 101–110.

7. Morgan GE, Mikhail MS, Murray MJ. Clinical Anesthesiology, 3d ed. New York, McGraw-Hill, 2002, pp. 557–564, 575–577.

Answer C

Clinical Anesthesia

QUESTION (Choose single best answer):

A jaundiced patient requires general anesthesia for portocaval shunt. He has a long history of alcohol abuse and is cirrhotic with ascites. Special considerations relevant to induction of anesthesia for this patient include each of the following *except*

(A) Denitrogenation by mask may be more rapid than expected.
(B) The risk of aspiration is increased.
(C) The dose of thiopental necessary for induction will be predictably reduced.
(D) The duration of succinylcholine action may be prolonged.
(E) Alfentanil would be an appropriate supplement.

CORRECT ANSWER: C

SUMMARY:

Cirrhosis is a multisystem disease. There are many unique considerations relevant to the induction of anesthesia for patients with chronic alcoholism, cirrhosis, and ascites. There is an increased risk of aspiration and a slower clearance of drugs that are metabolized hepatically (e.g.. alfentanil) or that are degraded by pseudocholinesterase, an enzyme manufactured in the liver (e.g., succinylcholine). These patients often have a primary respiratory alkalosis from hyperventilation and hypoxemia secondary to intrapulmonary shunting, a decreased function residual capacity (FRC), and a restrictive ventilatory defect resulting from large amounts of ascites. Additionally, there is often an unpredictable CNS response to anesthetic agents such as thiopental, and the dose cannot be reduced predictably.

EXPLANATION:

(A) *Incorrect.* Denitrogenation by mask ventilation may be more rapid with an increased baseline respiratory rate in cirrhotic patients who often present with respiratory alkalosis secondary to hyperventilation.
(B) *Incorrect.* The risk of aspiration is increased in alcoholic patients because alcohol intoxication delays gastric emptying and decreases lower esophageal sphincter tone. Aspiration risk is also increased by ascites, which mechanically increases intragastric pressure.
(C) *Correct.* While the hypoalbuminemia seen in cirrhosis results in a predictable increase in the unbound or active fraction of thiopental, the average dose of thiopental may not be different from that in nonalcoholic patients.[1] The CNS response to thiopental can be unpredictable in patients with alcoholic cirrhosis. Patients with a history of chronic alcohol abuse may exhibit tolerance or an increased sensitivity.
(D) *Incorrect.* Levels of pseudocholinesterase, the enzyme that metabolizes ester drugs such as succinylcholine and mivacurium, may be reduced by severe liver disease, and there may be a mild but clinically insignificant prolongation of succinylcholine action.
(E) *Incorrect.* Alfentanil would be an appropriate supplement, but the dose should be reduced because the elimination half-time of this hepatically cleared drug will be prolonged in a patient with cirrhosis.[1]

REASONING:

This question tests knowledge of the pathophysiology of alcoholic cirrhosis and ascites and their anesthetic implications. Choices A and D can be excluded because they suggest outcomes that may or may not occur with an alcoholic cirrhotic patient. There is no absolute contraindication to using alfentanil in a patient with liver disease, ruling out choice E. Choice B is incorrect because ascites and alcohol use clearly increase aspiration risk. C is the best choice.

REFERENCE:

1. Stoelting RK. Pharmacology and Physiology in Anesthetic Practice, 3d ed. Philadelphia, Lippincott Williams & Wilkins, 1999, pp. 282–284, 283ff, 284ff.
2. Morgan GE, Mikhail MS, Murray MJ. Clinical Anesthesiology, 3d ed. New York, McGraw-Hill, 2002, pp. 726–730.

BOOK A: **QUESTION 168**

Answer B

Clinical Anesthesia

QUESTION (Choose single best answer):

A patient being ventilated mechanically in the ICU requires wound debridement twice daily. Each of the following agents would be appropriate for induction of brief general anesthesia *except*

(A) Nitrous oxide.
(B) Etomidate.
(C) Ketamine.
(D) Methohexital.
(E) Midazolam.

CORRECT ANSWER: B

SUMMARY:

Anesthesiologists generally administer medications to induce hypnosis and amnesia, analgesia, and muscle relaxation for surgical cases. Many different anesthetic techniques can be used for the proposed procedure. The patient is being ventilated mechanically, and airway management is not a concern. We presume that the patient has reasonable hemodynamic stability. The MAC of nitrous oxide is 106 percent. This limits its effectiveness as a single agent, but it may be sufficient to induce anesthesia with supplemental narcotic administration during the brief maintenance period of anesthesia. Ketamine, methohexital, and midazolam all can provide adequate hypnosis and amnesia during the wound debridement. However, etomidate can cause adrenal suppression after even one dose, making it a poor choice for frequent induction of anesthesia in a critically ill ICU patient.[1]

EXPLANATION:

(A) *Incorrect.* Nitrous oxide typically is not used as a sole anesthetic agent because its MAC is 106 percent. However, administration of 70% nitrous oxide with supplemental narcotic as needed is a reasonable technique in this patient who requires brief periods of anesthesia for wound debridement.
(B) *Correct.* Etomidate can cause adrenal suppression after even one dose.[1] For this reason alone, frequent induction with etomidate is a poor choice in a critically ill ICU patient.
(C) *Incorrect.* Ketamine is used often for dressing changes because it provides both good analgesia and hypnosis with a rapid return to normal function.
(D) *Incorrect.* Methohexital is a short-acting barbiturate with rapid redistribution and awakening.
(E) *Incorrect.* Midazolam can be used for induction of anesthesia in this patient.

REASONING:

The key to this question is identifying the side-effect profile of etomidate and the impact of adrenal suppression in a critically ill ICU patient. Many readers may have considered nitrous oxide as the initial answer because it is used rarely as a sole anesthetic agent for induction. In this patient, however, it is a more reasonable technique than administration of etomidate. B is the best answer.

REFERENCES:

1. Wagner RL, White PF, Kan PB. Inhibition of adrenal steroidogenesis by the anesthetic etomidate. N Engl J Med 310:1415, 1984.
2 Miller RD, Miller ED, Reves JG, et al. Anesthesia, 5th ed. New York, Churchill Livingstone, 2000, pp. 216, 235–236, 244–245.
3. Morgan GE, Mikhail MS, Murray MJ. Clinical Anesthesiology, 3d ed. New York, McGraw-Hill, 2002, pp. 137–139, Chap. 8, Nonvolative Anesthetic Agents.

BOOK A:

QUESTION 169

Answer C

Cardiovascular

QUESTION (Choose single best answer):

A computer program for hemodynamic calculations has the following input values: body surface area, arterial blood pressure, heart rate, pulmonary artery occlusion pressure, pulmonary artery pressure, and cardiac output. Each of the following values can be derived with this program *except*

(A) Cardiac index.
(B) Stroke volume index.
(C) Systemic vascular resistance.
(D) Pulmonary vascular resistance.
(E) Left ventricular stroke work index.

CORRECT ANSWER: C

SUMMARY:

It is important to be able to calculate and interpret various hemodynamic variables to help guide the anesthetic care of critically ill or unstable patients. Certain parameters can be measured directly, such as heart rate, cardiac output, and blood pressure. Other variables, such as stroke volume, can be computed from these measures. SVR cannot be calculated from the available data because it requires a measure of central venous pressures.

EXPLANATION:

(A) *Incorrect.* Cardiac index = cardiac output (CO)/body surface area (BSA) (normally 2.2 to 4.2 L/min/m^2).
(B) *Incorrect.* Stroke volume index = stroke volume (SV)/BSA = (CO/heart rate)/BSA (normally 20 to 65 mL/beat/m^2).
(C) *Correct.* Systemic vascular resistance (SVR) = 80 × [mean arterial pressure (MAP) − central venous pressure (CVP)]/CO (normally 1200 to 1500 dyn · s · cm^{-5}). We are not given the CVP, so this value cannot be computed.
(D) *Incorrect.* Pulmonary vascular resistance (PVR) = 80 × [pulmonary artery pressure (PAP) − pulmonary artery occlusion pressure (PAOP)]/CO (normally 100 to 300 dyn · s · cm^{-5}).
(E) *Incorrect.* Left ventricular stroke work index − work index = 0.0136(MAP − PAOP) × stroke index (SI) (normally 45 to 60 g · m/beat/m^2).

REASONING:

This question tests knowledge of the computation of various hemodynamic variables. The reader is encouraged to review the equations for calculating these parameters.[1]

REFERENCE:

1. Barash PG, Cullen BF, Stoelting RK. Clinical Anesthesia, 4th ed. Philadelphia, Lippincott Williams & Wilkins, 2001, Table 31-4, p. 860.
2. Morgan GE, Mikhail MS, Murray MJ. Clinical Anesthesiology, 3d ed. New York, McGraw-Hill, 2002, p. 366.

BOOK A:

Answer D

OB/Regional

QUESTION 170

QUESTION (Choose single best answer):

A successful ankle block for transmetatarsal amputation of the first and second toes should include each of the following nerves *except* the

(A) Saphenous
(B) Deep peroneal
(C) Superficial peroneal
(D) Sural
(E) Tibial

CORRECT ANSWER: D

SUMMARY:

The ankle block is a simple and safe regional anesthetic technique for surgeries involving the foot. It involves blocking five nerves at the level of the ankle.[1] The saphenous nerve is a branch of the femoral nerve. The remaining nerves—deep and superficial peroneal, sural, and tibal—all derive from the sciatic nerve.

EXPLANATION:

(A) *Incorrect.* The saphenous nerve is anesthetized by infiltrating 5 mL local anesthetic around the saphenous vein as it passes anterior to the medial malleolus.[2] It supplies sensory input for the superficial component of the anteromedial foot.

(B) *Incorrect.* The deep peroneal nerve is blocked by injecting 5 mL local anesthetic lateral to the pulsation of the anterior tibial artery at the level of the skin crease on the anterior midline surface of the ankle.[2] It provides sensation to the medial half of the dorsal foot.

(C) *Incorrect.* The superficial peroneal nerve is blocked by infiltrating a ridge of local anesthetic along the skin crease between the anterior tibial artery and the lateral malleolus.[2] It provides sensation to the cutaneous portion of the dorsal foot and all the toes.

(D) *Correct.* The sural nerve provides sensation to the lateral foot, which would not be needed for surgery involving the first and second toes. It is blocked with a ridge of local anesthetic behind the lateral malleolus.[2]

(E) *Incorrect.* The tibial nerve provides sensation for the heal, the medial sole, and part of the lateral sole of the foot. It can be blocked with a fan-shaped injection of local anesthetic in a triangle bounded by the posterior tibial artery, Achilles tendon, and the tibia.[2]

REASONING:

This question tests knowledge of the anatomy and distribution of nerves anesthetized by an ankle block. This question relies on knowing the sensory component to each nerve of the foot. A thorough understanding of the anatomy is essential to derive the correct answer.

REFERENCES:

1. Schurman DJ. Angle block anesthesia for foot surgery. Anesthesiology 44:342, 1976.

2. Barash PG, Cullen BF, Stoelting RK. Clinical Anesthesia, 4th ed. Philadelphia, Lippincott Williams & Wilkins, 2001, p. 741.

3. Morgan GE, Mikhail MS, Murray MJ. Clinical Anesthesiology, 3d ed. New York, McGraw-Hill, 2002, p. 303.

BOOK A:

Answer A

Pharmacology

QUESTION 171 (OPTIONAL)

QUESTION (Choose single best answer):

Each of the following contributes to hypotension following induction of anesthesia with propofol *except*

(A) Central vagal stimulation.
(B) Decreased central sympathetic tone.
(C) Direct myocardial depression.
(D) Resetting of arterial baroreceptors.
(E) Systemic vasodilation.

CORRECT ANSWER: A

SUMMARY:

Propofol is a cardiac depressant. It decreases contractility, cardiac output, and systemic vascular resistance. The decrease in blood pressure seen at induction is probably due to myocardial depression and vasodilation (both direct vasodilation and indirectly from decreased central sympathetic output). Arterial baroreceptor function may be impaired or even reset with the use of propofol so that tachycardia does not develop to compensate for hypotension.

EXPLANATION:

(A) *Correct.* There is some controversial evidence in the literature to suggest that propofol possesses vagotonic properties and may increase central vagal stimulation. These studies mainly cite observations of bradycardia or even asystole with propofol anesthesia.[1,2] However, this evidence does not demonstrate conclusively that the etiology of these observations is a propofol-induced increase in central vagal stimulation. It has been shown recently in animal models that propofol-induced bradycardia cannot be prevented by pretreatment with atropine.[3] The decrease in heart rate that is sometimes observed with propofol may be due to decreased sympathetic cardioaccelerator tone rather than vagomimetic activity.[4] Standard anesthesia texts state that heart rate does not change significantly with an induction dose of propofol.[5] In summary, current evidence does not support the notion that hypotension after induction of anesthesia with propofol is due to central vagal stimulation.

(B) *Incorrect.* Propofol decreases central sympathetic tone.[5]

(C) *Incorrect.* Propofol causes direct myocardial depression.[5]

(D) *Incorrect.* Propofol does reset or inhibit the arterial baroreceptor response.[5]

(E) *Incorrect.* Propofol causes systemic vasodilation.[5]

REASONING:

This question tests detailed knowledge of the physiologic effects responsible for propofol-induced hypotension. The examiners are asking for the incorrect statement, which in this case is choice A. Choices B, C, and E can be eliminated easily because induction with propofol causes a drop in blood pressure by decreasing sympathetic tone resulting in systemic vasodilation and myocardial depression. This leaves only choices A and D as possibilities. Choice D is a correct statement because propofol can impair/reset the arterial baroreceptor response. Thus A is the best answer.

REFERENCES:

1. Baraka A. Severe bradycardia following propofol-suxamethonium sequence. Br J Anaesth 61:482–483, 1988.
2. Egan TD, Brock-Utne JG. Asystole after anesthesia induction with a fentanyl, propofol, and succinylcholine sequence. Anesth Analg 73:818–820, 1991.
3. Hashiba E, Hirota K, Suzuki K, Matsuki A. Effects of propofol on bronchoconstriction and bradycardia induced by vagal nerve stimulation. Acta Anaesthesiol Scand 47(9):1059–1063, 2003.
4. Krassioukov AV, Gelb AW, Weaver LC. Action of propofol on central sympathetic mechanisms controlling blood pressure. Can J Anaesth 40:761–769, 1993.
5. Miller RD, Miller ED, Reves JG, et al. Anesthesia, 5th ed. New York, Churchill Livingstone, 2000, p. 253.
6. Morgan GE, Mikhail MS, Murray MJ. Clinical Anesthesiology, 3d ed. New York, McGraw-Hill, 2002, p. 174.

BOOK A:

QUESTION 172

Answer A

OB/Regional

QUESTION (Choose single best answer):

Inhibition of labor by terbutaline causes each of the following maternal side effects *except*

(A) Hyperkalemia.
(B) Hypotension.
(C) Ventricular dysrhythmias.
(D) Hyperglycemia.
(E) Pulmonary edema.

CORRECT ANSWER: A

SUMMARY:

Terbutaline and ritrodine are beta-adrenergic agonists used to treat preterm labor. They exert their tocolytic effects by binding to uterine beta$_2$ receptors, causing cyclic AMP–mediated relaxation of uterine smooth muscle. Increased cardiac output, stroke volume, heart rate, and left ventricular ejection fraction are a result of beta$_1$-receptor activation and may result in arrhythmias, myocardial ischemia, and congestive heart failure. Other side effects include hyperglycemia, pulmonary edema, hypokalemia, anxiety, nervousness, and hypotension.

EXPLANATION:

(A) **Correct.** *Hypokalemia* is a side effect of beta-agonist therapy. This is due to insulin-mediated intracellular movement of glucose and potassium and activation of sodium/potassium ATPase in skeletal muscle cells.[1]

(B) **Incorrect.** Hypotension can occur due to beta-receptor-mediated vasodilation.

(C) **Incorrect.** Beta$_1$-receptor activation leads to increased heart rate, stroke volume, left ventricular ejection fraction, and cardiac output. This can result in dysrhythmias, including premature ventricular contractions, nodal contractions, atrial fibrillation, and myocardial ischemia.[1]

(D) **Incorrect.** Hyperglycemia occurs with beta-agonist therapy as a result of activation of hepatic phosphorylase, resulting in increased glycogen breakdown and glucose production.[1]

(E) **Incorrect.** Pulmonary edema is the most frequent serious complication of beta-agonist therapy. Although the mechanism is not clearly understood, increased fluid retention owing to beta-receptor therapy is a key component.[1] Additionally, patients at risk of cardiogenic pulmonary edema will be more likely to develop this complication when exposed to the cardiac effects of beta-adrenergic receptor stimulation.[1]

REASONING:

This question tests knowledge of the pharmacology and side effects of terbutaline. To answer this question correctly, one must know that terbutaline is a beta-adrenergic receptor agonist and recall the physiologic effects of these drugs. Choices B, C, and D are all effects of beta-agonists. Choice E occurs more commonly in pregnant patients treated with these medications. Choice A is clearly incorrect because hypokalemia is associated with beta-receptor agonists.

REFERENCES:

1. Hughes SC, Levinson G, Rosen MA. Shnider and Levinson's Anesthesia for Obstetrics, 4th ed. Philadelphia, Lippincott Williams & Wilkins, 2002, pp. 327–329.
2. Barash PG, Cullen BF, Stoelting RK. Clinical Anesthesia, 4th ed. Philadelphia, Lippincott Williams & Wilkins, 2001, Table 12-20, p. 304.
3. Morgan GE, Mikhail MS, Murray MJ. Clinical Anesthesiology, 3d ed. New York, McGraw-Hill, 2002, p. 836–37.

BOOK A:

Answer A

Pharmacology

QUESTION 173

QUESTION (Choose single best answer):

A 66-year-old man with chronic obstructive pulmonary disease (COPD) who underwent colectomy 12 hours ago has been receiving an epidural infusion of fentanyl at a rate of 100 μg/h. Which of the following is *least* likely to develop?

(A) Hypotension
(B) Nausea
(C) Pruritus
(D) Respiratory depression
(E) Urinary retention

CORRECT ANSWER: A

SUMMARY:

Epidural opiates cause many side effects. These include early respiratory depression, delayed respiratory depression, pruritus, nausea, urinary retention, sedation, and ileus. The most worrisome side effect is delayed respiratory depression, which occurs because of cephalad diffusion of opiates in cerebrospinal fluid affecting the medullary respiratory center. Hypotension is a common side effect of local anesthetics in the epidural space, not opiates.

EXPLANATION:

(A) **Correct.** Hypotension is not a common side effect of epidural opiates.
(B) **Incorrect.** Nausea, pruritus, respiratory depression, and urinary retention are all likely side effects from epidural opiates.
(C) **Incorrect.** See above.
(D) **Incorrect.** See above.
(E) **Incorrect.** See above.

REASONING:

This question test knowledge of the side effects commonly associated with epidural opioid administration. Common side effects are nausea, pruritus, respiratory depression, and urinary retention (choices B through E).[1] Hypotension is a common side effect associated with epidural administration of local anesthetics, not opiates. A is the least likely and is the best answer.

REFERENCE:

1. Barash PG, Cullen BF, Stoelting RK. Clinical Anesthesia, 4th ed. Philadelphia, Lippincott Williams & Wilkins, 2001, Table 54-8, pp. 1418–1419.
2. Morgan GE, Mikhail MS, Murray MJ. Clinical Anesthesiology, 3d ed. New York, McGraw-Hill, 2002, p. 346–347.

BOOK A:

Answer B

Clinical Anesthesia

QUESTION 174

QUESTION (Choose single best answer):

A 65-year-old man is disoriented and has a headache and nausea in the recovery room 30 minutes after transurethral resection of the prostate (TURP) with glycine irrigation performed under spinal anesthesia. Heart rate is 50 beats per minute, and blood pressure is 180/110 mm Hg. Which of the following is *least* likely?

(A) Decreased serum osmolality
(B) Serum sodium concentration of 132 mEq/L
(C) Increased serum ammonia concentration
(D) Bibasilar rales
(E) Jugular venous distension

CORRECT ANSWER: B

SUMMARY:

TURP syndrome is caused by the absorption of hypotonic irrigation solution from prostatic venous sinuses during TURP. The signs and symptoms relate to three issues: hypervolemia, hypo-osmolar hyponatremia, and chemical effects of the solute in the irrigation. Irrigation fluid dilutes blood, causing decreased serum osmolality and hyponatremia. Hypervolemia can lead to bibasilar rales and jugular venous distension. Metabolism of absorbed glycine causes hyperammonemia and hyperglycinemia. However, the neurologic symptoms described do not develop until serum sodium concentration drops closer to 120 mEq/L.

EXPLANATION:

(A) *Incorrect.* Decreased serum osmolarity is found in virtually all patients with TURP syndrome.
(B) *Correct.* It would be unlikely to observe the patient's symptoms with the mild hyponatremia of 132 mEq/L.
(C) *Incorrect.* Glycine absorption likely will result in some increase in ammonia concentration.
(D) *Incorrect.* Bibasilar rales are likely to occur with the significant volume overload associated with TURP syndrome.
(E) *Incorrect.* Jugular venous distension is likely to occur owing to the significant volume overload associated with TURP syndrome.

REASONING:

This question tests knowledge of the symptoms associated with TURP syndrome. All the choices could be found following a TURP. The patient's elevated blood pressure following spinal anesthesia suggests fluid overload, and bibasilar rales with an elevated jugular venous pressure would be quite possible. However, fluid overload alone will not result in

271

the nausea and disorientation described. These are most likely due to hyponatremia, which typically would be asymptomatic with a sodium of 132 mEq/L. The patient's sodium is likely much lower. Increased serum ammonia results from metabolism of the absorbed glycine. Thus, while all the choices might be found following a TURP, the symptoms described would likely be seen only in a patient with a more serious hyponatremia. B is the best answer.

REFERENCES:

Barash PG, Cullen BF, Stoelting RK. Clinical Anesthesia, 4th ed. Philadelphia, Lippincott Williams & Wilkins, 2001, pp. 101912-21.

Morgan GE, Mikhail MS, Murray MJ. Clinical Anesthesiology, 3d ed. New York, McGraw-Hill, 2002, p. 603.

BOOK A:

Answer E

Physiology

QUESTION 175

QUESTION (Choose single best answer):

A 70-year-old man sustains injuries to both carotid bodies during bilateral carotid endarterectomies performed 4 days apart. Two hours after the second procedure, the patient is breathing room air in the PACU. Which of the following sets of arterial blood gas values is *least* likely?

	pH	PCO$_2$ (mm Hg)	PO$_2$ (mm Hg)
(A)	7.3	50	58
(B)	7.3	50	86
(C)	7.4	40	86
(D)	7.4	42	58
(E)	7.5	32	58

CORRECT ANSWER: E

SUMMARY:

Potential postoperative problems following carotid endarterectomy (CEA) include labile blood pressure, neck hematoma causing airway compromise, stroke, myocardial infarction, and loss of carotid body function.[1] Unlike central chemoreceptors that are more sensitive to changes in PaCO$_2$, the carotid bodies are most sensitive to changes in PaO$_2$. Denervation of the carotid bodies following bilateral CEA may eliminate the ventilatory response to hypoxemia.

EXPLANATION:

(A) *Incorrect.* This ABG is possible if the patient has lost hypoxic ventilatory drive. Even with the PaO$_2$ of 58 mm Hg, the patient is hypoventilating and develops respiratory acidosis.

(B) *Incorrect.* Hypoventilation in the PACU owing to residual anesthetic effects may result in respiratory acidosis, as reflected in this ABG.

(C) *Incorrect.* This is a normal blood gas for a patient breathing room air.

(D) *Incorrect.* A patient who lacks hypoxic ventilatory drive could have this ABG. The PaO$_2$ of 58 mm Hg has not stimulated a hyperventilatory response.

(E) *Correct.* Bilateral CEA may produce complete denervation of the carotid bodies, resulting in the absence of ventilatory response to hypoxemia. A pH of 7.5 and PaCO$_2$ of 32 mm Hg result from hyperventilation, which would not occur in this patient.

REASONING:

This question tests knowledge of the physiologic changes associated with carotid body injury following CEA. A patient with injury to both carotid bodies will lack hypoxic ventilatory drive. The key to the correct answer is identifying the ABG that corresponds to the least likely clinical situation. Choice E represents an ABG from a patient who is hypoxic and hyperventilating. This is not a likely scenario following bilateral CEA. E is the best answer.

REFERENCE:

1. Stoelting RK, Miller RD. Basics of Anesthesia, 4th ed. New York, Churchill Livingstone, 2000, p. 327.
2. Morgan GE, Mikhail MS, Murray MJ. Clinical Anesthesiology, 3d ed. New York, McGraw-Hill, 2002, p. 471, 507.

ANSWERS TO
BOOK B EXAMINATION

Answer A

Equipment/Physics

QUESTION (Choose single best answer):

The need for increased doses of nondepolarizing muscle relaxants in patients with extensive burns is best explained by

(A) Increased protein binding.
(B) Hypermetabolism.
(C) Increased glomerular filtration rate.
(D) Proliferation of receptors on burned muscle.
(E) Decreased volume of distribution.

CORRECT ANSWER: A

SUMMARY:

Burn patients have a relative resistance to nondepolarizing muscle relaxants (NDMRs) because of altered protein binding and the proliferation of neuromuscular junctional and extrajunctional acetylcholine receptors. The proliferation of acetylcholine receptors occurs not on burned muscle but on viable tissue. Altered protein binding in burn patients is a consequence of decreased serum albumin immediately after injury (for up to 60 days) and increases in alpha$_1$-acid glycoprotein (AAG). The free fraction of NDMRs is reduced owing to binding with AAG. The net effect is thought to be a relative resistance to NDMRs and the requirement of a higher dose to reach clinical effect.

EXPLANATION:

(A) **Correct.** Highly protein bound drugs circulate longer in plasma and are not available to the site of action (e.g., the neuromuscular junction) as quickly as non-protein-bound drugs. In burn patients there is upregulation of alpha$_1$-acid glycoprotein (AAG) leading to higher dose requirements of drug to achieve the same clinical effect.

(B) **Incorrect.** Although burn patients exhibit hypermetabolic states, the primary effect of this change is on increased oxygen consumption and CO_2 production, leading to increased alveolar ventilation. Although there may be some effect on the rate of metabolism of drugs, the initial potency of NDMRs used in the clinical burn setting (usually as single-dose administration for intubation) is more affected by protein binding, volume of distribution, and receptor expression.

(C) **Incorrect.** While it is true that glomerular filtration rate (GFR) has been shown to rise in burn patients,[1] the effect of this on an initial bolus dose of NDMRs likely would be small. This statement assumes that the drug effect is terminated during the distribution phase because then the GFR would not contribute to an increased need for drug (at least not in a single-dose setting). However, if drug plasma levels are still effective during the elimination phase of the drug, then an increased GFR may shorten drug action.

(D) **Incorrect.** The proliferation of acetylcholine receptors in burn patients occurs not on burned muscle but in extrajunctional and junctional nondamaged tissue.

(E) **Incorrect.** The volume of distribution of drug reflects the volume of plasma that would account for the plasma concentration observed after administering a dose of drug, i.e.,

$$V_d = \frac{\text{dose}}{\text{plasma concentration}}$$

Burn patients have an increased vascular permeability owing to decreased capillary integrity (especially in the first 24 to 48 hours). However, the V_d of NDMR is unchanged or decreased.[2–5] A decreased V_d would require a smaller amount of drug to achieve the desired plasma concentration.

REASONING:

This question tests knowledge of the pathophysiology associated with burn injury and its effects on the pharmacokinetics of muscle relaxants. It is challenging because the wording used in choice D attempts to lead you down a path that is clearly wrong once the choice is examined carefully. Burned muscle tissue does not regenerate acetylcholine receptors. Rather, the sites of healthy tissue (both intra- and extrajunctional) have been correlated with increased expression of acetylcholine receptors. Choices B and C can be eliminated because the they do not significantly affect the pharmacokinetics of muscle relaxants. Choice A is the best answer because the direction of association is correct (increased protein binding leading to decreased drug potency) and the pharmacokinetics involved relate directly to drug potency. It is important to note that depolarizing muscle relaxants should not be administered to burn patients after the first 24 hours (owing to proliferation of acetylcholine receptors) because they can cause severe hyperkalemia leading to cardiac arrest. This effect is thought to peak 20 to 90 days after the injury[6–10] but has been reported to persist for up to 2 years.[8,11,12]

REFERENCES:

1. Loirat P, Rohan J, Baillet A, et al. Increased glomerular filtration rate in patients with major burns and its effect on the pharmacokinetics of tobramycin. N Engl J Med 299(17):915–919, 1978.
2. Jaede U, Sorgel F. Clinical pharmacokinetics in patients with burns. Clin Pharmacokinet 29(1):15–28, 1995.
3. Leibel WS, Martyn JA, Szyfelbein SK, Miller KW. Elevated plasma binding cannot account for the burn-related D-tubocurarine hyposensitivity. Anesthesiology 54(5):378–382, 1981.
4. Marathe PH, Dwersteg JF, Pavlin EG, et al. Effect of thermal injury on the pharmacokinetics and pharmacodynamics of atracurium in humans. Anesthesiology 70(5):752–755, 1989.
5. Martyn JA, Matteo RS, Greenblatt DJ, et al. Pharmacokinetics of D-tubocurarine in patients with thermal injury. Anesth Analg 61(3):241–246, 1982.
6. Gronert GA, Theye RA. Pathophysiology of hyperkalemia induced by succinylcholine. Anesthesiology 43(1):89–99, 1975.
7. Gronert GA, Dotin LN, Ritchey CR, Mason AD Jr. Succinylcholine-induced hyperkalemia in burned patients, part II. Anesth Analg 48(6):958–962, 1969.
8. Gronert GA. A possible mechanism of succinylcholine-induced hyperkalemia. Anesthesiology 53(4):356, 1980.
9. Schaner PJ, Brown RL, Kirksey TD, et al. Succinylcholine-induced hyperkalemia in burned patients, part I. Anesth Analg 48(5):764–770, 1969.
10. Viby-Mogensen J, Hanel HK, Hansen E, et al. Serum cholinesterase activity in burned patients. Acta Anaesthesiol Scand 9(3):159–179, 1975.
11. Martyn J, Goldhill DR, Gousouzian NG. Clinical pharmacology of muscle relaxants in patients with burns. Clin Pharmacol 26(8):680–685, 1986.
12. Martyn JA, Matteo RS, Szyfelbein SK, Kaplan RF. Unprecedented resistance to neuromuscular blocking effects of metocurine with persistence after complete recovery in a burned patient. Anesth Analg 61(7):614–617, 1982.
13. Bonate PL. Clinical pharmacology of muscle relaxants in patients with burns. Clin Pharmacokinet 5(6):548–556, 1980.
14. Morgan GE, Mikhail MS, Murray MJ. Clinical Anesthesiology, 3d ed. New York, McGraw-Hill, 2002, pp. 803, Table 9-7 (p. 190), Diseases with Altered Responses to Muscle Relaxants.

BOOK B:

Answer D

Pediatrics

QUESTION 2

QUESTION (Choose single best answer):

Which of the following parts of the infant's airway determines the appropriate diameter of a nasotracheal tube?

(A) Nares
(B) Glottis
(C) Vocal cords
(D) Cricoid cartilage
(E) Third tracheal ring

SUMMARY:

The cricoid cartilage is the narrowest portion of the infant airway and determines the appropriate diameter of a tracheal tube. This is true whether the tube is inserted orally or nasally. A tube of proper size should have a leak at 15 to 20 cm H_2O with positive-pressure ventilation. A tube that is too small may result in inadequate ventilation, whereas an oversized tube places the patient at risk for postoperative airway edema.

EXPLANATION:

(A) *Incorrect.* Although the size of the nare is an important consideration, it does not determine the appropriate size of the tracheal tube in infants.

(B) *Incorrect.* The glottis is the narrowest portion of the adult airway.

(C) *Incorrect.* The glottic opening between the vocal cords is the narrowest portion of the adult airway.

(D) *Correct.* The cricoid ring is the narrowest portion of the infant airway and determines the appropriate size of a properly placed tracheal tube.

(E) *Incorrect.* The third tracheal ring does not factor into sizing adult or pediatric tracheal tubes.

REASONING:

This question is challenging only because it describes nasotracheal intubation. It is tempting to choose A because of the perception that nasotracheal intubation requires a smaller tube. However, the nare prepped with vasoconstrictors can accommodate a tube of proper size. The risk of placing an inappropriately small tracheal tube is excessive leak and inadequate ventilation.

REFERENCE:

Stoelting RK, Miller RD. Basics of Anesthesia, 4th ed. New York, Churchill Livingstone, 2000, p. 159.

Morgan GE, Mikhail MS, Murray MJ. Clinical Anesthesiology, 3d ed. New York, McGraw-Hill, 2002, pp. 850, 861, Table 44-1 (p. 851), Characteristics of Neonates and Infants that Differentiate Them from Adult Patients.

BOOK B:

QUESTION 3

Answer C

Pharmacology

QUESTION (Choose single best answer):

Administration of 200 mEq sodium bicarbonate during cardiopulmonary resuscitation is associated with

(A) Cerebrospinal fluid (CSF) alkalosis.
(B) Hypercalcemia.
(C) Hypercarbia.
(D) Hyperkalemia.
(E) Shift of the oxyhemoglobin dissociation curve to the right.

CORRECT ANSWER: C

SUMMARY:

Administration of sodium bicarbonate is associated with CO_2 production owing to neutralization of H^+ ion, which initially produces carbonic acid. It is immediately broken down to CO_2 and water. Other effects include hypernatremia, hyperosmolality, and leftward shift of the oxyhemoglobin dissociation curve.

EXPLANATION:

(A) **Incorrect.** CO_2 produced from bicarbonate administration causes CSF acidosis from rapid passage of CO_2 across cell membranes.

(B) **Incorrect.** Alkalosis produces hypocalcemia by altering the equilibrium of ionized and bound calcium.

(C) **Correct.** The neutralization of hydrogen ion produces carbonic acid that immediately dissociates to CO_2 and water. CO_2 is eliminated in the lungs through expiration. Inadequate alveolar ventilation can result in hypercarbia.

(D) **Incorrect.** Alkalosis produces hypokalemia.

(E) **Incorrect.** Sodium bicarbonate adminstration produces alkalosis, resulting in a leftward shift of oxyhemoglobin curve.

REASONING:

This question is challenging because two choices, A and C, seem like plausibly correct choices. Most readers recognize that sodium bicarbonate administration causes an elevation in serum bicarbonate, leading to alkalosis. Most readers also recognize that sodium bicarbonate adminstration is associated with a transient hypercarbia. The key to this question is that choice A refers to CSF alkalosis, not serum blood levels. C is the best answer.

REFERENCE:

Barash PG, Cullen BF, Stoelting RK. Clinical Anesthesia, 4th ed. Philadelphia, Lippincott Williams & Wilkins, 2001, p. 167–168.

Morgan GE, Mikhail MS, Murray MJ. Clinical Anesthesiology, 3d ed. New York, McGraw-Hill, 2002, p. 924.

BOOK B:

Answer C

Pharmacology

QUESTION 4

QUESTION (Choose single best answer):

When compared with diazepam, midazolam

(A) Metabolites contribute more significantly to the sedative effect.
(B) Elimination is less dependent on hepatic metabolism.
(C) Has more predictable action after intramuscular administration.
(D) Produces less respiratory depression.
(E) Produces less hypotension during induction of anesthesia with opioids.

CORRECT ANSWER: C

SUMMARY:

The differences between midazolam and diazepam are tested frequently on board examinations. These drugs differ primarily in onset and duration of action, route of administration, extent of biotransformation to active metabolites, and suitability for use in the intraoperative setting. Midazolam is a highly protein bound benzodiazepine that is suitable for intravenous, oral, and intramuscular administration. It is associated with rapid onset of action and elimination, lack of active metabolites, and significant respiratory depression at higher dosages, especially in elderly patients. Diazepam is suitable for oral and intravenous administration but not for intramuscular usage owing to pain at the site of injection and unreliability of action when given via the intramuscular route. Diazepam has active metabolites that prolong its duration of action. The duration of action of both diazepam and midazolam is dependent on hepatic clearance.

EXPLANATION:

(A) **Incorrect.** Diazepam metabolites contribute more significantly to the sedative effect. Midazolam has virtually no active metabolites.[1]

(B) *Incorrect.* Both midazolam and diazepam are dependent on hepatic metabolism for clearance. They both undergo oxidation and conjugation reactions in the liver prior to clearance. These reactions are affected most commonly by age, cirrhosis, and coadministration of other drugs (especially those metabolized by the cytochrome P450 enzyme system).

(C) *Correct.* Midazolam has a much more reliable onset and action when given intramuscularly than diazepam. Diazepam is also painful on injection.

(D) *Incorrect.* Midazolam is associated with greater respiratory depression because of increased potency of the drug compared with diazepam. After initial Food and Drug Administration (FDA) approval of midazolam, there were deaths related to inadvertent overdosing that led to fatal respiratory depression. A decrease in the dosing recommendations as well as unit repackaging ensued.

(E) *Incorrect.* Benzodiazepines and high-dose narcotics have been reported to produce hypotension during induction for coronary bypass surgery.[2] A study by Liang and colleagues found no significant differences in hemodynamic changes associated with induction of anesthesia with fentanyl (5 μg/kg) and midazolam (0.3 mg/kg) versus fentanyl (5 μg/kg) and diazepam (0.3 mg/kg).[3]

REASONING:

This is a somewhat challenging question that reflects the often-tested pharmacodynamic and pharmacokinetic comparisons between midazolam and diazepam. The reader should ensure that these differences are understood clearly. Choice D can be eliminated with knowledge of midazolam's sixfold increased intrinsic potency compared with diazepam.[4] One might also have used this knowledge to exclude choice E. Knowledge of the Liang study similarly would have excluded choice E. Similarly, choice A can be eliminated if the reader recalls that diazepam has two active metabolites, whereas midazolam does not have any. Choice B is incorrect because all benzodiazepines are dependent on hepatic clearance for elimination. This leaves choice C, which makes empirical sense because diazepam is not given intramuscularly in the clinical setting.

REFERENCES:

1. Miller RD, Miller ED, Reves JG, et al, Anesthesia, 5th ed. New York, Churchill Livingstone, 2000, pp. 229–236.

2. Tuman KJ, McCarthy RJ, el-Ganzouri AR, et al. Sufentanil-midazolam anesthesia for coronary artery surgery. J Cardiothorac Anesth 4(3):308–313, 1990.

3. Liang SW. [Studies of midazolam, diazepam and thiopentone on respiratory and cardiovascular function during induction anesthesia.] Zhonghua Wai Ke Za Zhi 29(3):161–164, 205, 1991.

4. Mould DR, DeFeo TM, Reele S, et al. Simultaneous modeling of the pharmacokinetics and pharmacodynamics of midazolam and diazepam. Clin Pharmacol Ther 58(1):35–43, 1995.

5. Buhrer M, Maitre PO, Crevoisier C, Stanski DR. Electroencephalographic effects of benzodiazepines: II. Pharmacodynamic modeling of the electroencephalographic effects of midazolam and diazepam. Clin Pharmacol Ther 48(5):555–567, 1990.

6. Morgan GE, Mikhail MS, Murray MJ. Clinical Anesthesiology, 3d ed. New York, McGraw-Hill, 2002, pp. 160–164.

BOOK B:

QUESTION 5

Answer A

Pharmacology

QUESTION (Choose single best answer):

Which of the following statements concerning a patient who has been receiving nitroprusside for several days is true?

(A) Biotransformation of cyanide requires a sulfur donor.
(B) Formation of methemoglobin increases cyanide toxicity.
(C) Increased serum thiocyanate concentrations are innocuous.
(D) Mixed venous P_{O_2} decreases as cyanide toxicity develops.
(E) Serum thiocyanate concentrations reflect the degree of cyanide toxicity.

CORRECT ANSWER: A

SUMMARY:

Sodium nitroprusside (SNP) is metabolized to cyanide ions, which can combine with methemoglobin, thiosulfate, or cytochrome oxidase. It is the interaction with cytochrome oxidase that interrupts cellular respiration. This leads to anerobic respiration and accumulation of lactic acid, acidosis, and increased mixed venous oxygen owing to a cellular inability to use oxygen. Untreated, this process eventually causes cell death. Toxic blood cyanide levels (>100 mg/dL) are associated with greater than 1 mg/kg SNP infused over 2 hours or more then 0.5 mg/kg per hour administered within 24 hours.[1]

EXPLANATION:

(A) *Correct.* Cyanide ions are metabolized by rhodanase enzyme present in liver and kidney to produce thiocyanate. Rhodanase requires thiosulfate ions as sulfur donors to catalyse this reaction.

(B) *Incorrect.* The nitroprusside moiety breaks down to yield five cyanide radicals and one NO molecule. These cyanide radicals can be cleared by one of the three mechanisms. CN^- can combine with methhemoglobin to give cyanomethemoglobin. Therefore, formation of methemoglobin does not increase cyanide toxicity. On the contrary, it leads to safe elimination of cyanide.

(C) *Incorrect.* Elevated thiocyanate levels (5 to 10 mg/dL) can cause central nervous system (CNS) abnormalities.[1]

(D) *Incorrect.* Mixed venous P_{O_2} increases because CN^- prevents utilization of oxygen as the final electron acceptor in the electron transport pathway involved with cellular respiration.

(E) *Incorrect.* Thiocyanate is cleared by the kidney. Its accumulation in renal failure produces toxicity characterized by nausea, muscle weakness, altered mental state, and thyroid dysfunction. Kidney or liver disease does not increase the likelihood of cyanide toxicity.

REASONING:

A commonly tested complication to chronic SNP infusion is the potential for toxicity related to cyanide and thiocyanate. It should be noted that toxicity is unlikely if a constant-rate infusion is kept below 0.5 μg/kg per minute (for chronic infusion, i.e., >3 hours). For infusions of short duration, the dose can go up to 8 to 10 μg/kg per minute. Cyanide toxicity occurs by interfering with mitochondrial respiration. This produces acidosis, increased mixed venous oxygen saturation, and ultimately, death. Increasing dose requirements to achieve pharmacologic effect (tachyphalaxis) may be the first clue to the onset of cyanide toxicity. Treatment consists of termination of the SNP infusion, ventilation with 100% oxygen, and infusion of thiosulfate (as a sulfur donor) and sodium nitrate (to produce methhemoglobin). Administration of hydroxocobalamine instead of thiosulfate is recommended in patients with coexisting renal failure.[1]

REFERENCES:

1. Barash PG, Cullen BF, Stoelting RK. Clinical Anesthesia, 4th ed. Philadelphia, Lippincott Williams & Wilkins, 2001, pp. 773–775, Fig. 28-13.
2. Stoelting RK. Pharmacology and Physiology in Anesthetic Practice, 3d ed. Philadelphia, Lippincott Williams & Wilkins, 1999, p. 316.
3. Morgan GE, Mikhail MS, Murray MJ. Clinical Anesthesiology, 3d ed. New York, McGraw-Hill, 2002, p. 226.

Answer D

OB/Regional

QUESTION (Choose single best answer):

Which of the following increases the cephalad spread of hyperbaric intrathecal local anesthetics?

(A) Cephalad-directed needle bevel
(B) Coughing
(C) Lithotomy position
(D) Obesity
(E) Rapid injection

CORRECT ANSWER: D

SUMMARY:

Hyperbaric local anesthetic solutions are by definition denser than cerebrospinal fluid (CSF), and their distribution therefore is governed largely by gravity. Patient position is one of the most important factors in the spread of these agents, especially the Trendelenburg, lateral, and jackknife positions. Factors that affect the spread of local anesthetics include patient age, patient height, anatomic configuration of the spinal column, site of injection, direction of the needle during injection, volume and density of CSF, dosage of anesthetic, and volume of anesthetic solution. Factors that have been shown to have limited clinical importance include gender, direction of the needle bevel, turbulence, composition of CSF, CSF pressure, concentration of local anesthetic used, CSF circulation, and addition of vasoconstrictors.

EXPLANATION:

(A) ***Incorrect.*** When studied, the direction of the needle bevel had no effect on the distribution of local anesthetic in the CSF. When a solution is injected through a standard beveled lumbar puncture needle, the solution exits in a straight line regardless of the needle bevel direction. Exceptions to this may be the Whitticare and Tuohy needles, which have different bevel openings, but the question does not specifically ask about these types of needles.[1]

(B) ***Incorrect.*** Although CSF pressure increases with coughing, studies demonstrate that it does not have an effect on the spread of local anesthetic.[1]

(C) ***Incorrect.*** Although other patient positions have a significant effect on spread of hyperbaric local anesthetics, lithotomy position does not. Lithotomy position may remove the pooling effect of the lumbar lordosis on local anesthetic distribution, but the thoracic kyphosis decreases its cephalad spread.[2]

(D) ***Correct.*** Weight does not have an effect on local anesthetic spread in nonobese adults.[1] However, magnetic resonance imaging (MRI) data indicate that obese patients have substantially less CSF volume.[3] Decreased CSF volume causes higher peak block height with hyperbaric anesthetics.[3]

(E) ***Incorrect.*** When studied, the level of sensory anesthesia was the same with varying injection rates up to 1 mL/s.[1]

REASONING:

This question had many possible choices, including some that are intuitively correct but have been refuted when studied. Since hyperbaric solutions will follow gravity, choices A and C could be eliminated. Choices B and E are controversial at best and refuted in many studies. D is the answer that has the most effect on CSF volume and therefore block height, so it is the best answer.

REFERENCES:

1. Greene NM. Distribution of local anesthetic solutions within the subarachnoid space. Anesth Analg 97:715–729, 1985.
2. Barash PG, Cullen BF, Stoelting RK. Clinical Anesthesia, 4th ed. Philadelphia, Lippincott Williams & Wilkins, 2001, pp. 697–700.
3. Liu SS, McDonald SB. Current issues in spinal anesthesia. Anesthesiology 94:888–906, 2001.
4. Morgan GE, Mikhail MS, Murray MJ. Clinical Anesthesiology, 3d ed. New York, McGraw-Hill, 2002, pp. 267–268, Table 16-3 (p. 267), Factors Affecting the Level of Spinal Anesthesia.

BOOK B:

QUESTION 7

Answer B

Pharmacology

QUESTION (Choose single best answer):

Compared with a patient without liver disease, a patient with cirrhosis will have

(A) Greater accumulation of vecuronium with infusion.
(B) Increased unbound plasma vecuronium concentration.
(C) More frequent occurrence of phase II block after succinylcholine administration.
(D) Prolonged elimination half-life of atracurium.
(E) Unchanged volume of distribution for pancuronium.

CORRECT ANSWER: B

SUMMARY:

Vecuronium is metabolized by liver only to a limited extent. It is cleared largely by biliary excretion (75 percent) and to a small extent by renal excretion (25 percent). Muscle relaxants are water-soluble drugs with increased volume of distribution in disease states such as liver or renal failure. Multiple factors affect dose and duration of action of neuromuscular blocking agents.

EXPLANATION:

(A) *Incorrect.* Although vecuronium depends largely on biliary excretion, its action usually is not prolonged significantly in cirrhosis unless large amounts (>0.15 mg/kg) are given.
(B) *Correct.* Vecuronium exhibits a moderate to high protein binding capacity of 60 to 80 percent. Cirrhosis usually is accompanied by hypoalbuminemia, leading to increased plasma concentration of the unbound drug.
(C) *Incorrect.* Decreased levels of pseudocholinesterase that occur in liver disorders produce prolonged phase I block.
(D) *Incorrect.* Pancuronium undergoes limited deacetylation by the liver and is cleared primarily through renal excretion (40 percent). Prolonged elimination of pancuronium is seen most often in patients with renal failure.
(E) *Incorrect.* Liver failure produces increased volume of distribution for water-soluble drugs such as pancuronium. Thus there is a need for larger initial dose and less frequent maintenance doses in these patients.

REASONING:

This question is challenging because two choices, A and B, are plausibly correct. Greater drug accumulation plausibly can occur in patients with impaired hepatic elimination. However, the high protein binding capacity of vecuronium, coupled with the knowledge that the duration of action is usually not significantly prolonged in cirrhotic patients, makes B the best answer.[1]

REFERENCE:

1. Barash PG, Cullen BF, Stoelting RK. Clinical Anesthesia, 4th ed. Philadelphia, Lippincott Williams & Wilkins, 2001, pp. 1094–1095.
2. Morgan GE, Mikhail MS, Murray MJ. Clinical Anesthesiology, 3d ed. New York, McGraw-Hill, 2002, pp. 189, 195.

Answer E

Pharmacology

QUESTION (Choose single best answer):

Intrathecally administered opioids exert their analgesic effects primarily in the

(A) Brain stem.
(B) Fourth ventricle.
(C) Spinal nerve roots.
(D) Spinothalamic tracts.
(E) Substantia gelatinosa.

CORRECT ANSWER: E

SUMMARY:

Opioids are administered into either the intrathecal or epidural space to control acute postoperative pain for many surgical procedures. The main advantage of neuraxial opioids is placement of drug near its spinal site of action, thereby avoiding supraspinally mediated side effects such as sedation and respiratory depression. Neuraxial opioids act primarily in the substantia gelatinosa or Rexed's lamina II in the dorsal horn of the spinal cord. The high density of opioid receptors and their role in modulating neuronal pain pathways make these areas the most effective in producing analgesia.

EXPLANATION:

(A) *Incorrect.* See above.
(B) *Incorrect.* See above.
(C) *Incorrect.* See above.
(D) *Incorrect.* See above.
(E) *Correct.* Opioid receptors are found in many places other than the substantia gelatinosa. These other locations include the periaqueductal gray area of the brain stem and peripheral nerve fibers. However, the primary site of action for neuraxial opioids is the substantia gelatinosa because of its high density of opioid receptors and the role of these receptors in modulating neuronal pain pathways.

REASONING:

The key to answering this question is not focusing on where opiate receptors are located because they are found throughout the CNS. Rather, the reader should focus on knowing the primary site of action for neuraxial opioids, namely, the substantia gelatinosa. Analgesic effects are produced here because of the high density of opioid receptors at this location and the role of these receptors in modulating pain pathways. The brain stem and fourth ventricle are the site of action for side effects such as delayed respiratory depression. Choices A and B therefore can be eliminated. The best answer is E.

REFERENCES:

Stoelting RK, Miller RD. Basics of Anesthesia, 4th ed. New York, Churchill Livingstone, 2000, pp. 429–430.

Miller RD, Miller ED, Reves JG, et al. Anesthesia, 5th ed. New York, Churchill Livingstone, 2000, pp. 280–283.

Morgan GE, Mikhail MS, Murray MJ. Clinical Anesthesiology, 3d ed. New York, McGraw-Hill, 2002, pp. 164, 346–347.

Answer D

Clinical Anesthesia

QUESTION (Choose single best answer):

During laser excision of vocal cord polyps in a 5-year-old boy, dark smoke suddenly appears in the surgical field. The trachea is intubated, and anesthesia is being maintained with halothane, nitrous oxide, and oxygen. The most appropriate initial step is to

(A) Change from oxygen and nitrous oxide to air.
(B) Fill the oropharnyx with water.
(C) Instill water into the endotracheal tube.
(D) Remove the endotracheal tube.
(E) Ventilate with carbon dioxide.

CORRECT ANSWER: D

SUMMARY:

Airway fire is a dreaded complication of laser airway surgery. Methods to prevent fire include (1) using non-PVC tubes such as specially designed endotracheal tubes for laser surgery, (2) filling the cuff with colored saline for use as a heat sink or marker if the cuff is ruptured, (3) ventilating with blended air and oxygen at low concentrations or a mixture of helium and oxygen, or (4) using an anesthetic technique that does not require endotracheal intubation.[1] While these methods can help to prevent fire, no method is 100 percent effective, and proper management of this crisis hopefully will lead to a favorable outcome. First, remove the source by turning off the laser. Discontinue ventilation, and extubate the trachea. Turn off all combustible gases (nitrous oxide and oxygen). Water may be used to extinguish flaming debris, and then oxygen may be administered by mask.[2]

EXPLANATION:

(A) *Incorrect.* Although combustible gases eventually should be switched over to air, it is imperative to discontinue ventilation first. Changing gases does not occur immediately, so continuing to ventilate the lungs will deliver oxygen and nitrous oxide that is already in the breathing circuit.
(B) *Incorrect.* Most airway fires should extinguish with removal of the laser and stopping ventilation. A persistent fire may require flushing water in the oropharynx but not as the initial step.
(C) *Incorrect.* The same reasoning as choice B above applies. The endotracheal tube should be removed with discontinuation of ventilation to prevent the "blowtorch effect."
(D) *Correct.* This is the most appropriate initial step, along with discontinuing ventilation.
(E) *Incorrect.* Continuing to ventilate with CO_2 will still deliver combustible gases (oxygen and nitrous oxide) already present in the circuit.

REASONING:

This is a difficult question. It is easy to narrow down the choices to A or D. The key is the *initial step*. Published protocols describe the first step as discontinuing ventilation and extubating the trachea.[2] Choice A does not mention stopping ventilation, so D is the best answer.

REFERENCES:

1. Barash PG, Cullen BF, Stoelting RK. Clinical Anesthesia, 4th ed. Philadelphia, Lippincott Williams & Wilkins, 2001, pp. 936–938.
2. Stoelting RK, Miller RD. Basics of Anesthesia, 4th ed. New York, Churchill Livingstone, 2000, p. 351 (airway fire protocol).
3. Morgan GE, Mikhail MS, Murray MJ. Clinical Anesthesiology, 3d ed. New York, McGraw-Hill, 2002, pp. 773–774, Table 39-3 (p. 774), Airway Fire Protocol.

Answer E

Neuroanesthesia

QUESTION (Choose single best answer):

During craniotomy in the sitting position, end-tidal carbon dioxide tension suddenly decreases. Ventilatory excursion of the chest is normal. Further evaluation is most likely to show a decrease in

(A) Alveolar-to-arterial oxygen tension difference.
(B) Alveolar-to-arterial carbon dioxide tension difference.
(C) Dead space ventilation.
(D) Pulmonary artery pressure.
(E) Pulmonary artery occlusion pressure.

CORRECT ANSWER: E

SUMMARY:

The incidence of air embolism in patients undergoing surgery in the sitting position averages 40 to 45 percent.[1] Because of the 20 to 30 percent population incidence of patent foramen ovale, the calculated risk of paradoxical air embolism in the sitting position reaches 5 to 10 percent.[1] Clinical signs of air embolism include a decrease in ET_{CO_2} and a decrease in Sp_{O_2} owing to increased dead space ventilation (increased A–a gradient for O_2 and CO_2). A large volume of air in the right ventricle can lead to right ventricular outflow tract obstruction and increased pulmonary artery pressures. Right ventricular outflow tract obstruction will lead to decreased left ventricular preload and decreased pulmonary artery occlusion pressure (PAOP).

EXPLANATION:

(A) *Incorrect.* There is an increase in the A–a O_2 gradient.
(B) *Incorrect.* There is an increase in the A–a CO_2 gradient.
(C) *Incorrect.* Dead space ventilation increases.
(D) *Incorrect.* The pulmonary artery pressure is increased with air embolism.
(E) *Correct.* Right ventricular outflow tract obstruction will lead to decreased left ventricular preload, resulting in a decreased PAOP.

REASONING:

This question tests knowledge of the signs of venous air embolism (VAE) in a patient undergoing craniotomy in the sitting position. VAE can occur anytime the surgical area is above the level of the heart and there are large venous sinuses or plexuses that can entrain air. Clinical signs of VAE under anesthesia depend on the amount and rate of entrainment and the preexisting cardiopulmonary derangement. Signs can range from subtle to catastrophic cardiorespiratory collapse. It is common to see a decrease in ET_{CO_2} and Sp_{O_2} in VAE. Rapid sudden rise in the end-tidal nitrogen concentration is also seen. Hypotension often can present as the first sign. Right ventricular outflow tract and pulmonary arterial obstruction leads to increased pulmonary artery pressure, right ventricular strain and failure, and cardiovascular collapse. The key to this question is understanding that right ventricular outflow tract obstruction leads to decreased left ventricular preload, reflected by a decreased PAOP. E is the single best answer.

REFERENCE:

1. Barash PG, Cullen BF, Stoelting RK. Clinical Anesthesia, 4th ed. Philadelphia, Lippincott Williams & Wilkins, 2001, p. 766.
2. Morgan GE, Mikhail MS, Murray MJ. Clinical Anesthesiology, 3d ed. New York, McGraw-Hill, 2002, pp. 574–575.

Answer A

OB/Regional

QUESTION (Choose single best answer):

Which of the following is a cardiorespiratory effect of epidural block to a T4 sensory level?

(A) Decreased expiratory reserve volume
(B) Decreased tidal volume
(C) Increased circulating catecholamine concentrations
(D) Increased heart rate
(E) Unchanged vital capacity

CORRECT ANSWER: A

SUMMARY:

Epidural anesthesia results in blockade of sympathetic fibers two to six levels above the sensory level, resulting in decreased heart rate, cardiac output, and blood pressure. In healthy individuals, respiratory effects of neuraxial blockade are relatively minimal. Tidal volume, minute ventilation, dead space, arterial blood gas tensions, and shunt fraction are minimally affected.[1] Sensory levels affecting abdominal and intercostal musculature can have an effect on respiratory function by decreasing active exhalation and therefore decreasing expiratory reserve volume (ERV). Of note is the fact that apnea associated with neuraxial block is due to hypoperfusion of the brain stem respiratory centers rather than diaphragmatic or phrenic nerve paralysis.

EXPLANATION:

(A) *Correct.* Epidural blockade with a T4 sensory level is associated with abdominal and intercostal muscle paralysis, which can impair active exhalation and therefore decrease expiratory reserve volume (ERV).
(B) *Incorrect.* Tidal volume remains unchanged.
(C) *Incorrect.* Epidural anesthesia is associated with blockade of sensory afferent fibers associated with the stress response to surgery, and therefore, levels of catecholamines are reduced.
(D) *Incorrect.* Because of the differential blockade of nerve fibers associated with neuraxial anesthesia, the sympathetic fibers two to six levels above the sensory level will be affected. A T4 sensory level will be associated with blockade of the cardioaccelerator fibers at T1–4 and will result in decreased heart rate.[2]
(E) *Incorrect.* Vital capacity includes expiratory reserve volume. Since the ERV is decreased, vital capacity must decrease.[2]

REASONING:

The key concepts for answering this question involve understanding differential blockade, the components of pulmonary volumes and capacities, and the physiologic effects of neuraxial blockade. Since ERV is a component of vital capacity, choice E can be eliminated. Knowledge of the effects of sympathetic blockade eliminates choices C and D, and understanding that unless the brain stem is hypoperfused with an unusually high block, the minute ventilation should remain unchanged eliminates choice B.

REFERENCES:

1. Barash PG, Cullen BF, Stoelting RK. Clinical Anesthesia, 4th ed. Philadelphia, Lippincott Williams & Wilkins, 2001, pp. 706–707.
2 Miller RD, ed. Anesthesia, 5th ed. New York, Churchill Livingstone, 2001, p. 1497.
3. Morgan GE, Mikhail MS, Murray MJ. Clinical Anesthesiology, 3d ed. New York, McGraw-Hill, 2002, pp. 260–261, 489, Fig. 22-5 (p. 484), Spirogram Showing Static Lung Volumes.

Answer E

Physiology

QUESTION (Choose single best answer)

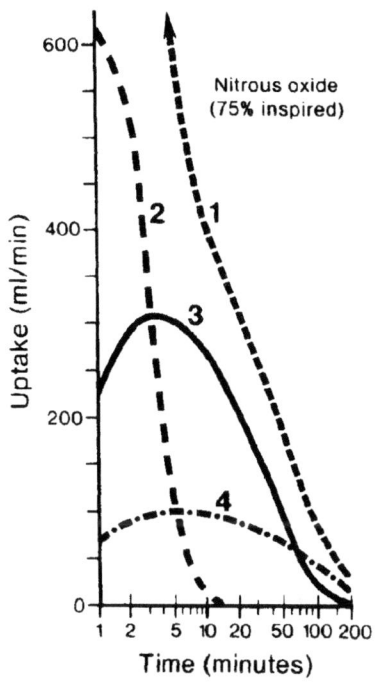

The figure above describes the uptake of nitrous oxide 75% by individual tissue groups (VRG = vessel-rich group, MG = muscle group, FG = fat group) and their sum (total uptake, TU). Which set of labels accurately describes the curves?

	1	2	3	4
(A)	MG	FG	VRG	TU
(B)	VRG	MG	FG	TU
(C)	FG	MG	TU	VRG
(D)	TU	FG	MG	VRG
(E)	TU	VRG	MG	FG

CORRECT ANSWER: E

SUMMARY:

The uptake of inhaled anesthetics by tissues is influenced by blood gas solubility, blood flow, and the partial pressure difference (arterial and venous blood). The vessel-rich group (VRG) has a rapid uptake and limited capacity, so it gets saturated quickly (curve 2). The muscle group has less blood supply but greater capacity, so it can have continued uptake for hours (curve 3). The fat group has poor blood supply but enormous capacity for gases with increased lipid solubility. Since fat can have prolonged uptake (days), total uptake by the body will continue, albeit at a lower rate.

EXPLANATION:

(A) *Incorrect.* For all inhaled anesthetics, greatest uptake in the initial period occurs in the VRG group. The VRG organs, such as the brain, heart, kidney, liver, and endocrine system, have limited capacity and are saturated rapidly, and uptake decreases.

(B) *Incorrect.* The muscle group has smaller blood supply and huge capacity and continues to take up anesthetic for hours.

(C) *Incorrect.* The fat group has poor blood supply and the greatest capacity. It will have continued uptake for days (except for N_2O).

(D) *Incorrect.* See above.

(E) *Correct.* See above.

REASONING:

This is a challenging question that tests knowledge of uptake and distribution of inhaled anesthetics. Curve 2 fits the description of the VRG, and only answer E has curve 2 in the correct order. By this reasoning, the reader can disregard all other answers. E is the best answer.

REFERENCE:

Barash PG, Cullen BF, Stoelting RK. Clinical Anesthesia, 4th ed. Philadelphia, Lippincott Williams & Wilkins, 2001, pp. 380–381.

Morgan GE, Mikhail MS, Murray MJ. Clinical Anesthesiology, 3d ed. New York, McGraw-Hill, 2002, pp. 129–130.

BOOK B:

QUESTION 13

Answer B

OB/Regional

QUESTION (Choose single best answer):

A 67-year-old man undergoes spinal anesthesia with hyperbaric tetracaine 10 mg for transurethral resection of the prostate (TURP). At the end of the 50-minute procedure, the level of anesthesia is T6, and blood pressure is 120/70 mm Hg. Within 2 minutes of transfer to a stretcher, the patient has nausea, and his blood pressure decreases to 76/42 mm Hg. Which of the following is the most likely cause of the acute hypotension?

(A) Acute congestive heart failure.

(B) Decreased venous return.

(C) Dilutional hyponatremia.

(D) Progression of sympathetic block.

(E) Unrecognized bladder perforation.

CORRECT ANSWER: B

SUMMARY:

Transurethral resection of the prostate (TURP) can be associated with excessive fluid absorption and subsequent fluid overload. The resulting clinical signs and symptoms are due to hyponatremia and increased intravascular volume and are collectively termed TURP syndrome. This syndrome is characterized clinically by restlessness, confusion, nausea, vomiting, lethargy, hypertension, bradycardia, tachypnea, and seizures. This constellation of symptoms is difficult to assess in a patient under general anesthesia. For this reason, regional techniques, especially spinal anesthesia, are popular for this procedure. While spinal block is considered preferable to general anesthesia for TURP, the patient is still vulnerable to its cardiovascular effects. These include decreased arterial vascular sympathetic tone, decreased venous return, and decreased cardiac output, and they can be exacerbated by changes in position during the procedure. When complications occur, the astute clinician must be able to differentiate between complications attributable to the procedure and those attributable to the anesthetic technique.

EXPLANATION:

(A) **Incorrect.** Acute congestive heart failure, presumably owing to fluid overload, is unlikely in this case because the patient did not exhibit any of the symptoms of the TURP syndrome prior to his hemodynamic instability.

(B) **Correct.** Spinal anesthesia results in decreased venous return. The position commonly used for TURP is lithotomy with Trendelenburg, which facilitates venous return.[1] When the patient was transferred out of this position and his legs were placed in a dependent position, venous return was decreased. Combined with the sympathectomy from the spinal block, this change in position resulted in severe hypotension.

(C) **Incorrect.** Dilutional hyponatremia occurs following TURP owing to excessive fluid absorption. It causes many of the clinical symptoms associated with TURP syndrome, including lethargy, confusion, and seizures. TURP syndrome is also associated with hypertension, which is not seen in this situation, so it is unlikely.

(D) **Incorrect.** Progression of sympathetic block is unlikely in this situation because the patient was hemodynamically stable until movement to the stretcher. While tetracaine is a local anesthetic with a long duration of action, it is likely that the block is stable or even receding after a 50-minute procedure.

(E) **Incorrect.** Bladder perforation is a complication of TURP. It manifests as abdominal pain, commonly referred to the shoulder, even in patients with adequate neuraxial blockade. This pain tends to have a temporal relationship to the perforation and occurs during the procedure.

REASONING:

The key to this question is the timing of this patient's hypotension. It occurs after the procedure and is associated with moving to the stretcher. It is important to know the signs and symptoms of TURP syndrome to recognize that this patient does not appear to have this condition. Therefore, choices A and C can be eliminated. The timing of the hypotension eliminates choices C and D. Lack of abdominal pain makes choice E unlikely. The best answer is B.

REFERENCES:

1. Miller RD, Miller ED, Reves JG, et al. Anesthesia, 5th ed. New York, Churchill Livingstone, 2000. pp. 1498–1505, 1947–1949.

2. Barash PG, Cullen BF, Stoelting RK. Clinical Anesthesia, 4th ed. Philadelphia, Lippincott Williams & Wilkins, 2001, pp. 1019–1021.

3. Morgan GE, Mikhail MS, Murray MJ. Clinical Anesthesiology, 3d ed. New York, McGraw-Hill, 2002, pp. 693–696, Fig. 33-2 (pp. 266–268), Manifestations of the TURP Syndrome.

BOOK B: **QUESTION 14**

Answer A

OB/Regional

QUESTION (Choose single best answer):

A 26-year-old woman has persistent uterine bleeding following a normal spontaneous delivery without anesthesia. The uterus is firm on manual examination. Which of the following anesthetics is most appropriate for manual extraction of the placenta?

(A) Halothane
(B) Pudendal block with lidocaine
(C) Subarachnoid tetracaine
(D) Thiopental
(E) Vecuronium

CORRECT ANSWER: A

SUMMARY:

Retained products of conception that require manual extraction are a common cause of postpartum hemorrhage. An important distinction is whether the patient requires analgesia and/or uterine relaxation. If the patient has a functioning epidural or spinal block, this may be adequate for manual extraction if the uterus is not contracted. If the uterus has contracted, it will be virtually impossible for the obstetrician to extract the placenta without relaxation. Classically, this has been done with volatile anesthetic agents, frequently requiring induction of general anesthesia and endotracheal intubation for airway protection. More recently, nitroglycerin (intravenous or sublingual) has been used with great success.[1] Hypotension with nitroglycerin has not been a clinically significant problem, and the risk of hypotension is outweighed by the advantages of not requiring an anesthetic machine, protection of airway reflexes, avoidance of general anesthesia, and the short duration of action.[1]

EXPLANATION:

(A) **Correct.** The question mentions that the uterus is firm and that manual extraction of the placenta is required. This cannot be accomplished without uterine relaxation, and halothane is the only agent among the choices that will provide uterine relaxation.

(B) **Incorrect.** Pudendal block will anesthetize the somatic nerves associated with the pain of the second stage of labor but will not relax the uterus.

(C) **Incorrect.** Subarachnoid tetracaine will provide spinal anesthesia, which does not relax the uterus. Of note, tetracaine will have a prolonged onset and long duration of action in this patient who is bleeding and has the potential for hemodynamic instability. Thus it would not be a preferable agent for spinal anesthesia.

(D) **Incorrect.** Thiopental will induce general anesthesia but will not provide uterine relaxation.

(E) **Incorrect.** Vecuronium is a nondepolarizing muscle relaxant. It will not relax the uterus, and its administration to this patient would result in a paralyzed, awake patient with an unprotected airway.

REASONING:

This question is straightforward, provided that one knows that the patient and obstetrician require uterine relaxation for manual extraction of the placenta. The only agent among the list of choices that provides uterine relaxation is halothane. Current practice is to use nitroglycerin for this procedure, but at the time the test question was written, it may not have been in widespread use.

REFERENCES:

1. Riley ET, Flanagan B, Cohen SE, Chitkara U. Intravenous nitroglycerin: A potent uterine relaxant for emergency obstetric procedures. Review of literature and report of three cases. Int J Obst Anesth 5:264–268, 1996.

2. Hughes SC, Levinson G, Rosen MA. Shnider and Levinson's Anesthesia for Obstetrics, 4th ed. Philadelphia, Lippincott Williams & Wilkins, 2002, p. 367.

3. Morgan GE, Mikhail MS, Murray MJ. Clinical Anesthesiology, 3d ed. New York, McGraw-Hill, 2002, p. 840.

Answers B

Physiology

QUESTION (Choose single best answer):

Compared with intermittent positive-pressure ventilation (IPPV), intermittent mandatory ventilation (IMV)

(A) Better maintains cardiac output.
(B) Provides less than full mechanical ventilatory support.
(C) Requires a greater level of sedation.
(D) Requires a higher F_{IO_2}.
(E) Requires a lower inspiratory flow rate.

CORRECT ANSWER: B

SUMMARY:

IPPV is a mode of ventilation often referred to as continuous mandatory ventilation (CMV) in which a set number of breaths is delivered per minute, and the patient's spontaneous efforts are not allowed. It therefore will provide full ventilatory support. In contrast, IMV provides a set number of breaths per minute but allows the patient to take spontaneous unassisted breaths between ventilatory breaths and thus provides less than full ventilatory support. IPPV is the ventilatory mode most anesthesiologists use in the operating room with a paralyzed patient.

EXPLANATION:

(A) **Unknown.** The evidence supporting this choice is controversial. Downs and colleagues found that patients ventilated with IPPV had decreased atrial filling pressures and cardiac output. Patients ventilated with IMV maintained negative intrapleural pressures, atrial filling pressures, and cardiac output. The authors conclude that IMV may better maintain cardiopulmonary function.[1] Other studies found patients with poor ventricular function show decreased cardiac output when changed from CMV to IMV.[3]

(B) **Correct.** The difference between IPPV and IMV is that IMV allows the patient to breath spontaneously in an unassisted, unsynchronized manner in between the machine-delivered breaths. In IPPV, the patient's efforts are met with closed valves.

(C) **Incorrect.** Because IPPV does not allow for the patient's spontaneous efforts, it is more appropriate for the patient to be more deeply sedated so that spontaneous breathing is avoided. IMV allows spontaneous breaths and thus requires less sedation relative to IPPV.

(D) **Incorrect.** Any level of F_{IO_2} can be used with either setting, and flow rates do not differ.

(E) **Incorrect.** See above.

REASONING:

This question tests knowledge of two different modes of ventilation: IMV and IPPV. IPPV is often used now as a generic term but was defined as ventilation with positive inspiratory pressure and zero expiratory pressure. It is the mode used in the operating room with a primitive ventilator in the paralyzed patient. IMV was a step forward from the primitive IPPV (not to be confused with pressure-control ventilation or pressure-support ventilation) in that it allowed the patient to breathe spontaneously between breaths so that the patient did not have to be sedated or paralyzed. Evidence supporting choice A is controversial. On an actual examination, we would choose B because this is clearly correct and undisputed fact.

REFERENCES:

1. Downs JB, Douglas ME, Sanfelippo PM, et al. Ventilatory pattern, intrapleural pressure, and cardiac output. Anesth Analg 56:88–96, 1977.
2. Barash PG, Cullen BF, Stoelting RK. Clinical Anesthesia, 3d ed. Philadelphia, Lippincot-Raven, 1997, p. 1373.
3. Mathru M, Rao TL, El-Etr AA, et al. Hemodynamic response to changes in ventilatory patterns in patients with normal and poor left ventricular reserve. Crit Care Med 10:423–426, 1982.
4. Morgan GE, Mikhail MS, Murray MJ. Clinical Anesthesiology, 3d ed. New York, McGraw-Hill, 2002, pp. 809–811.

BOOK B:

Answer D

Neuroanesthesia

QUESTION 16

QUESTION (Choose single best answer):

Which of the following findings would be considered normal in the electroencephalogram of an adult?

(A) Decreased frequency during induction with halogenated anesthetics.
(B) Decreased frequency in frontal areas with administration of nitrous oxide 50%.
(C) Dominance of beta rhythm at 20 to 30 Hz during the awake relaxed state.
(D) Electrical silence with administration of isoflurane 2.5 MAC.
(E) The presence of burst suppression during natural sleep.

CORRECT ANSWER: D

SUMMARY:

Isoflurane normally produces an isoelectric electroencephalogram at high clinical doses of 1 to 2 MAC and therefore would be expected to produce electrical silence at 2.5 MAC. Electrical silence also may be produced by severe hypoxia, hypothermia, brain death, and intravenous induction agents such as etomidate, propofol, and barbiturates in high doses.[1] Other volatile anesthetics such as desflurane and enflurane can produce burst suppression but not electrical silence.

EXPLANATION:

(A) **Incorrect.** Halogenated anesthetics cause increased frequency during induction in a biphasic pattern followed by depression with deep levels of anesthesia.
(B) **Incorrect.** Nitrous oxide produces increased frequency at 30% to 70% concentration.[1]
(C) **Incorrect.** The awake relaxed state produces predominance of alpha rhythm (8 to 13 Hz) on electroencephalogram. Beta activity (>13 Hz) is associated with mental activity in the awake person or light anesthesia.[1]
(D) **Correct.** Isoflurane produces electrical silence at high clinical doses of 1 to 2 MAC.
(E) **Incorrect.** Burst suppression does not occur during natural sleep and is produced by deep levels of anesthesia and pathologic states of brain injury.

REASONING:

This is a difficult question that tests knowledge of the physiologic properties of anesthetic agents on the electroencephalogram. Choices C and E require familiarity with normal EEG patterns. Nitrous oxide and subanesthetic concentrations of volatile agents increase frequency, so A and B are incorrect. D should stand out as the only choice that is definitely correct.

REFERENCE:

1. Barash PG, Cullen BF, Stoelting RK. Clinical Anesthesia, 4th ed. Philadelphia, Lippincott Williams & Wilkins, 2001, pp. 636, 708–710.
Morgan GE, Mikhail MS, Murray MJ. Clinical Anesthesiology, 3d ed. New York, McGraw-Hill, 2002, pp. 562–564, Table 25-2 (p. 563), Electroencephalographic Changes during Anesthesia.

Answer B

Equipment/Physics

QUESTION (Choose single best answer):

Proper zeroing of an arterial pressure transducer attached to a supine anesthetized patient is best accomplished by

(A) Continuous flow of fluid through the intravascular catheter.
(B) Opening the system to air at heart level.
(C) Placement of the transducer diaphragm at heart level.
(D) Proper damping of the transducer system.
(E) Zeroing the transducer during the expiration phase of mechanical ventilation.

CORRECT ANSWER: B

SUMMARY:

Arterial blood pressure monitoring requires proper zeroing and leveling to obtain accurate values. Zeroing is accomplished by opening the stopcock at the transducer, exposing it to atmospheric pressure, and pressing the zero pressure button on the transducer. Moving the transducer to the desired zero reference point, typically at the uppermost aspect of the left ventricle, is leveling the transducer. These two procedures can be accomplished in one step, allowing for accurate blood pressure measurements. (See also Question 61, Book B.)

EXPLANATION:

(A) *Incorrect.* *Zero reference point* is defined as atmospheric pressure, not a continuous flow of fluid through the catheter.
(B) *Correct.* This accomplishes both zeroing and leveling of the transducer to allow for accurate measurements.
(C) *Incorrect.* Placement of the transducer at the heart levels the transducer but fails to zero it to atmospheric pressure.
(D) *Incorrect.* The damping coefficient is a measure of how long it takes an oscillating system to come to rest, which is important for accurate measurements but is not involved in the zeroing procedure.
(E) *Incorrect.* Ventilation has no effect on zeroing. This is so because the arterial pressure is not being measured during zeroing—the atmospheric pressure is.

REASONING:

This question tests knowledge of proper zeroing and leveling of a catheter-fluid arterial pressure transducer system. Answers A, D, and E can be eliminated because they are clearly not involved in the zeroing process. Answer C is tempting because proper leveling does require placement of the transducer at the level of the desired reference point. However, on closer inspection, answer C neglects to zero the transducer to atmospheric pressure. Answer B does zero the transducer to atmospheric pressure and is the correct answer.

REFERENCE:

Miller RD, Miller ED, Reves JG, et al. Anesthesia, 5th ed. New York, Churchill Livingstone, 2000, pp. 1136–1137.
Morgan GE, Mikhail MS, Murray MJ. Clinical Anesthesiology, 3d ed. New York, McGraw-Hill, 2002, pp. 94–95.

QUESTION (Choose single best answer):

A 1-month-old infant becomes hypoxemic faster during apnea than an adult. Which of the following is the primary cause of this difference?

(A) Functional residual capacity in an infant is half that of an adult.
(B) Metabolic rate in an infant is twice that of an adult.
(C) Resting Pao_2 in an infant is lower than that in an adult.
(D) The number of alveoli in an infant is 12 percent the number in an adult.
(E) The hemoglobin dissociation curve in an infant is shifted to the right.

CORRECT ANSWER: B

SUMMARY:

Neonates and infants desaturate faster than adults for a number of reasons. Most important, the oxygen consumption $\dot{V}o_2$ in an infant is 7 to 9 mL/kg per minute compared with 3 mL/kg per minute in an adult.[1] Infants increase their minute ventilation in order to meet this demand. The resulting minute ventilation (MV)–functional residual capacity (FRC) ratio in infants is 5:1, whereas it is only 1.5:1 in adults.[1] Other factors that contribute to rapid desaturation in neonates include a high closing volume and a pliable rib cage.[1]

EXPLANATION:

(A) *Incorrect.* FRC in the adult is 30 mL/kg. Infants may have a slightly reduced FRC of 27 to 30 mL/kg.[1] Other sources report the FRC in infants to be as low as 25 mL/kg but not half the adult value.[2]
(B) *Correct.* Oxygen consumption and metabolic rate in a 1-month-old infant are twice those of an adult.
(C) *Incorrect.* Pao_2 increases to childhood levels several days after birth.[2] Resting Pao_2 in an infant may be lower than the adult value, but this is not the primary cause for rapid desaturation.
(D) *Incorrect.* Although infants have a smaller number of alveoli compared with adults, this is not the primary reason for their propensity to desaturate rapidly. During the first 8 years of life, the number of alveoli rapidly increases to the adult level.[3]
(E) *Incorrect.* The oxyhemoglobin dissociation curve is shifted to the left in neonates owing to HbF.[2]

REASONING:

The key to answering this question correctly is identifying the *primary cause* for rapid desaturation. Choices C and D can be misleading because, while they may be true, they are not the primary cause. The higher ratio of minute ventilation to FRC in infants is an important cause of rapid desaturation, but FRC alone does not differ enough from adult values to account for the more rapid desaturation in infants. The best answer is B.

REFERENCES:

1. Barash PG, Cullen BF, Stoelting RK. Clinical Anesthesia, 4th ed. Philadelphia, Lippincott Williams & Wilkins, 2001, pp. 1095–1096.
2. Stoelting RK, Miller RD. Basics of Anesthesia, 4th ed. New York, Churchill Livingstone, 2000, pp. 381–382.
3. Gregory GA. Pediatric Anesthesia, 4th ed. New York, Churchill Livingstone, 2002, p. 423.
4. Morgan GE, Mikhail MS, Murray MJ. Clinical Anesthesiology, 3d ed. New York, McGraw-Hill, 2002, pp. 850–851, Table 44-1 (p. 851), Characteristics of Neonates and Infants that Differentiate Them from Adult Patients.

Answer B

Clinical Anesthesia

QUESTION (Choose single best answer):

During extracorporeal shock wave lithotripsy, the shock wave should be synchronized with

(A) The P wave of the ECG.
(B) The R wave of the ECG.
(C) The T wave of the ECG.
(D) Peak inspiration.
(E) End expiration.

CORRECT ANSWER: B

SUMMARY:

Extracorporeal shock wave lithotripsy (ESWL) is used for the disintegration of renal or upper ureteral calculi. These shock waves can cause several complications, including local tissue injury and cardiac arrhythmias. During ESWL, shock waves cause mechanical stress on the heart, which can induce arrhythmias. The frequency of arrhythmias can be minimized by synchronizing the shock wave with the refractory period of the cardiac cycle or R wave on the electrocardiogram (ECG). Even with synchronization, shock waves induce arrhythmias in roughly 10 percent of patients undergoing ESWL.

EXPLANATION:

(A) *Incorrect.* The P wave on the ECG does not correspond with the ventricular refractory period of the cardiac cycle, and more arrhythmias will be induced if ESWL is employed during this period.
(B) *Correct.* Shock waves are timed to occur 20 ms after the R wave on the ECG, which corresponds to the refractory period of the ventricles.
(C) *Incorrect.* The T wave on the ECG does not correspond with the ventricular refractory period of the cardiac cycle, and more arrhythmias will be induced if ESWL is employed during this period.
(D) *Incorrect.* Tissue damage will occur if the lungs are within the path of the shock wave because of the air-tissue interface. However, the lungs are typically not in the path of the shock wave regardless of where they are in the ventilatory cycle. This is corroborated by the fact that patients who are breathing spontaneously after undergoing regional anesthesia have been treated safely and effectively with ESWL.
(E) *Incorrect.* See above.

REASONING:

The key to answering this question is the knowledge that arrhythmias are a common occurrence during ESWL and can be minimized by proper timing with the cardiac cycle. Choices A and C can be eliminated because these are not the refractory period of the ventricles. Choices D and E can be eliminated by knowing that regional anesthesia can be used successfully for ESWL in spontaneously breathing patients. This leaves B as the best answer.

REFERENCE:

Miller RD, Miller ED, Reves JG, et al. *Anesthesia,* 5th ed. New York, Churchill Livingstone, 2000, pp. 1950–1952.
Morgan GE, Mikhail MS, Murray MJ. Clinical Anesthesiology, 3d ed. New York, McGraw-Hill, 2002, pp. 697–699.

Answer E

Cardiovascular

QUESTION (Choose single best answer)

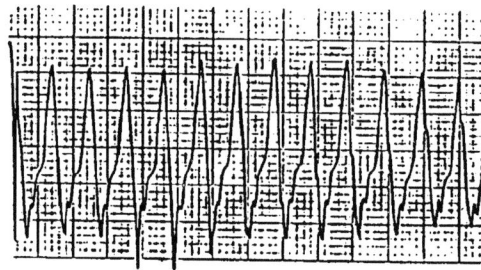

The cardiac rhythm illustrated above appeared suddenly in an anesthetized patient. The most appropriate management is

(A) Administration of adenosine.
(B) Administration of digoxin.
(C) Administration of epinephrine.
(D) Overdrive pacing.
(E) Synchronous cardioversion.

CORRECT ANSWER: E

SUMMARY:

The ECG is consistent with ventricular tachycardia (VT). Treatment of the arrhythmia depends on the patient's hemodynamic state. Pulseless VT or ventricular fibrillation is treated with immediate defibrillation. Stable, monomorphic VT is treated with synchronized cardioversion or with drugs such as amiodarone, lidocaine, sotolol, or procainamide.

EXPLANATION:

(A) *Incorrect.* Adenosine is used in the treatment of supraventricular tachycardia (SVT) and narrow- and wide-complex tachycardia of supraventricular origin. Adenosine also helps differentiate between wide-complex tachycardia of supraventricular and ventricular origin.
(B) *Incorrect.* Digoxin has no place in the acute management of an unstable patient.
(C) *Incorrect.* Epinephrine is second-line drug in pulseless VT or ventircular fibrillation.
(D) *Incorrect.* Overdrive pacing describes a method of controlling certain tachycardias and arrythmias by electrically pacing the heart at a rate that exceeds the patient's intrinsic rhythm. This treatment is not indicated for VT. Patients with a prolonged QT interval may benefit from overdrive pacing in addition to correcting electrolytes and administration of magnesium, isopreterenol, phenytoin, or lidocaine.
(E) *Correct.* Given the case scenario and the available answer choices, we assume stable, monomorphic VT and unknown cardiac function. The treatment is synchronized cardioversion.

REASONING:

This question tests knowledge of the diagnosis and treatment of ventricular tachycardia. The ECG tracing should be recognized immediately. The most appropriate management of the arrythmia depends on the hemodynamic response of the patient. Since we are not certain of the patient's hemodynamic status, conservative treatment mandates synchronized cardioversion. Given the available choices, the best answer is E.

REFERENCE:

Arrhythmia and Their Treatment: ACLS—The Reference Textbook (70-2500). Chicago, American Heart Assocation.

Morgan GE, Mikhail MS, Murray MJ. Clinical Anesthesiology, 3d ed. New York, McGraw-Hill, 2002, p. 922.

BOOK B:

Answer B

Clinical Anesthesia

QUESTION 21

QUESTION (Choose single best answer):

Which of the following statements concerning hyperkalemia after succinylcholine administration to a patient with a spinal cord injury is true?

(A) It is unlikely to occur if the lesion is located below T6.
(B) It is unlikely to occur within 24 hours of the injury.
(C) It is unlikely to occur more than 60 days after the initial injury.
(D) It is prevented by pretreatment with small doses of a nondepolarizing agent.
(E) It is decreased in magnitude by pretreatment with calcium chloride.

CORRECT ANSWER: B

SUMMARY:

Succinylcholine normally raises serum potassium levels by 0.5 mEq/L. In skeletal muscle injuries or atrophy caused by spinal cord injury, there is upregulation of immature acetylcholine receptors outside the neuromuscular junction. Widespread depolarization of these receptors can result in life-threatening potassium levels, causing irreversible cardiac arrest and dysrhythmias. This process peaks 7 to 10 days after spinal cord injury. Administration of succinylcholine is unlikely to cause hyperkalemia during the first 24 hours after an injury but should be avoided after that time. Although the risk of hyperkalemia probably decreases after 6 months, the use of nondepolarizing muscle relaxants is preferred.[1]

EXPLANATION:

(A) *Incorrect.* Injuries below T1 and above L4 result in paraplegia, which places patients at risk for succinylcholine-induced hyperkalemia.
(B) *Correct.* Succinylcholine-induced hyperkalemia is unlikely to occur within 24 hours of a spinal cord injury.
(C) *Incorrect.* While most sources report that the risk of hyperkalemia after a spinal cord injury probably decreases after 6 months, the true duration is unknown. The use of a nondepolarizing muscle relaxant is preferred even in injuries that have occurred more than 6 months ago.
(D) *Incorrect.* Life-threatening hyperkalemia after succinylcholine administration is not reliably prevented by pretreatment with a nondepolarizing muscle relaxant.
(E) *Incorrect.* Hyperkalemia is not decreased in magnitude by pretreatment with calcium chloride. The cardiac arrest that can occur with succinylcholine-induced hyperkalemia after a spinal cord injury may be refractory to normal cardiopulmonary resuscitation, including treatment with calcium chloride.

REASONING:

Choice B is clearly correct. The risk of a hyperkalemic response peaks at 7 to 10 days after an injury, yet it is considered safe to administer succinylcholine to a normokalemic patient within 24 hours of a spinal cord injury. Choices A, D, and E are clearly incorrect. Choice C is likely, but since succinylcholine administration is not recommended even more than 6 months after a spinal cord injury, B is the best answer.

REFERENCES:

1. Barash PG, Cullen BF, Stoelting RK. Clinical Anesthesia, 4th ed. Philadelphia, Lippincott Williams & Wilkins, 2001, p. 1268.
2. Stoelting RK, Miller RD. Basics of Anesthesia, 4th ed. New York, Churchill Livingstone, 2000, pp. 94–95.
3. Morgan GE, Mikhail MS, Murray MJ. Clinical Anesthesiology, 3d ed. New York, McGraw-Hill, 2002, pp. 186–187, 189, 589–590, 798.

BOOK B:

Answer E

Physiology

QUESTION 22

QUESTION (Choose single best answer):

The severity of chronic bronchitis is best assessed by measuring

(A) Tidal volume.
(B) Carbon dioxide diffusing capacity.
(C) Sputum production over 24 hours.
(D) Forced vital capacity.
(E) Arterial blood gases.

CORRECT ANSWER: E

SUMMARY:

Chronic bronchitis is characterized clinically by a productive cough present for 3 consecutive months for at least 2 consecutive years. Hypertrophy of the bronchial mucus glands results in increased airway secretions. Patients with chronic bronchitis develop hypercarbia and hypoxemia earlier than patients with emphysema and are predisposed to early cor pulmonale.[1] Therefore, preoperative assessment of patients with chronic bronchitis should include an arterial blood gas sample if the severity of the disease is in question.

EXPLANATION:

(A) *Incorrect.* Residual volume may be increased, but tidal volume remains near normal in patients with chronic bronchitis.
(B) *Incorrect.* Restrictive lung disease such as pulmonary fibrosis can result in decreased carbon dioxide diffusion capacity. DLco tends to be normal in obstructive lung disease.
(C) *Incorrect.* Patients with chronic bronchitis produce copious amounts of sputum owing to hypertrophy of mucus glands. However, measuring 24-hour sputum production is not an accurate assessment of disease severity.
(D) *Incorrect.* While patients with chronic obstructive pulmonary disease (COPD) can have a decreased FEV_1/FVC ratio on pulmonary function tests, measuring FVC alone is not the best assessment of severity.
(E) *Correct.* Arterial blood gas sampling is the best assessment of disease severity. Patients with chronic bronchitis are at risk for hypoxemia and hypercarbia earlier than patients with emphysema. Chronic hypoxemia eventually can lead to right ventricular failure or cor pulmonale.

REASONING:

The key to this question is to remember the progression of chronic bronchitis. Think of the "blue bloater." The most severe result of chronic bronchitis is the development of cor pulmonale that carries a high mortality rate. The greatest risk factors for the development of this condition, hypoxemia and hypercarbia, can be detected by arterial blood gases.

REFERENCE:

1. Stoelting RK, Miller RD. Basics of Anesthesia, 4th ed. New York, Churchill Livingstone, 2000, p. 279, Table 19-2 (comparative features of COPD).
2. Morgan GE, Mikhail MS, Murray MJ. Clinical Anesthesiology, 3d ed. New York, McGraw-Hill, 2002, pp. 516–519, Table 23-3 (p. 516), Signs and Symptoms of COPD.

BOOK B:

Answer B

Pediatrics

QUESTION 23

QUESTION (Choose single best answer):

An 8-kg 1-year-old boy is scheduled for a bilateral inguinal hernia repair. If regional anesthesia is to be used for postoperative analgesia, which of the following statements is true?

(A) Caudal administration of 0.25% bupivacaine will provide analgesia without evidence of motor block.
(B) Caudal administration of 0.125% bupivacaine is as effective as caudal administration of 0.25% bupivacaine.
(C) Caudal analgesia is more difficult to achieve in young children than in adults.
(D) The recommended volume of local anesthetic used for caudal analgesia in children is 3 mL per year of age.
(E) The volume of 0.25% bupivacaine required for bilateral ilioinguinal and iliohypogastric nerve blocks would be too large.

CORRECT ANSWER: B

SUMMARY:

Caudal anesthesia can provide effective postoperative analgesia for pediatric patients undergoing inguinal hernia repair. Bupivacaine 0.125% is as effective as 0.25% in providing postoperative analgesia and produces less motor block.[1] The caudal space is accessed via the sacral hiatus and is typically easier to identify in children than adults. Potential complications include spinal, intravenous, or interosseous injection, but the overall rate is low. Other side effects include residual motor block and urinary retention in the early postoperative period.

EXPLANATION:

(A) **Incorrect.** Bupivacaine caudal anesthesia is associated with motor blockade. A retrospective study of 750 consecutive patients reported the incidence to be 54 percent.[2] Another study demonstrated that motor block with bupivacaine increases with higher concentration.[3]
(B) **Correct.** A study of 105 infants and children who received caudal anesthesia for postoperative pain control found that 0.125% bupivacaine was as effective as 0.25% with significantly less motor blockade.[1] In a recent study comparing pain scores and oral analgesic administration postoperatively, there was no significant difference between patients who received caudal analgesia using 0.125% versus 0.25% bupivacaine in combination with fentanyl.[4]
(C) **Incorrect.** Caudal analgesia is easier to achieve in young children than in adults. Calcification of the sacrococcygeal ligament in adults can make identification of the caudal space more difficult.
(D) **Incorrect.** Recommended volumes of local anesthetic used for caudal analgesia are based on weight (0.5 to 1 mL/kg), not age.
(E) **Incorrect.** Bilateral ilioinguinal and iliohypogastric nerve blocks also can provide postoperative analgesia following hernia repair. These blocks can be performed safely with a volume of local anesthetic under the toxic bupivacaine dose.

REASONING:

This question tests knowledge of regional anesthesia for postoperative analgesia in children. This question is challenging because there is some conflict in the literature regarding the optimal bupivacaine dose for intraoperative caudal anesthesia. However, since the question concerns postoperative analgesia, B is the best answer.

REFERENCES:

1. Wolf AR, Valley RD, Fear DW, et al. Bupivacaine for caudal analgesia in infants and children: The optimal effective concentration. Anesthesiology 69(1):102–106, 1988.
2. Dalens B, Hasnaoui A. Caudal anesthesia in pediatric surgery: Success rate and adverse effects in 750 consecutive patients. Anesth Analg 68(2):83–89, 1989.
3. Gunter JB, Dunn CM, Bennie JB, et al. Optimum concentration of bupivacaine for combined caudal-general anesthesia in children. Anesthesiology 75(1):57–61, 1991.
4. Joshi W, Connelly NR, Dwyer M, et al. A comparison of two concentrations of bupivacaine and adrenaline with and without fentanyl in paediatric inguinal herniorrhaphy. Paediatr Anaesth 9(4):317–320, 1999.
5. Morgan GE, Mikhail MS, Murray MJ. Clinical Anesthesiology, 3d ed. New York, McGraw-Hill, 2002, pp. 273–274.

BOOK B:

Answer A

Clinical Anesthesia

QUESTION 24

QUESTION (Choose single best answer):

After inserting a left-sided double-lumen endotracheal tube, both cuffs are inflated. When the right (tracheal) lumen is clamped, breath sounds are heard only in the lower right lung field. When the left (bronchial) lumen is clamped, breath sounds are heard over the entire left lung field. Where is the tube positioned?

(A) Tracheal orifice above the carina and bronchial limb in the right bronchus.
(B) Tracheal orifice above the carina and bronchial limb in the left bronchus.
(C) Tracheal orifice and bronchial limb both above the carina.
(D) Tracheal cuff and bronchial limb both in the right bronchus.
(E) Tracheal orifice and bronchial limb both in the left bronchus.

CORRECT ANSWER: A

SUMMARY:

Double-lumen endotracheal tubes (DLTs) are used for single-lung ventilation or isolation of the two lungs. DLTs are designed specifically for either the right or left lung because there are anatomic differences between the two sides. Some differences include (1) the right mainstem takes off at a smaller angle than the left mainstem, (2) there are three branches of the right mainstem bronchus and two branches of the left mainstem bronchus, and (3) the takeoff of the right upper lobe bronchus is closer to the carina than the first branch of the left mainstem. Right-sided DLTs have an orifice in the bronchial cuff that allows for ventilation of the right upper lobe when positioned in the right main bronchus. Left-sided DLTs do not have such an orifice. (See also Question 33, Book B, for indications of single-lung ventilation.)

EXPLANATION:

(A) **Correct.** This is the wrong way to position a left-sided double-lumen tube, but it does satisfy the clinical description. Clamping the left (bronchial) lumen will insufflate air into the left lung, whereas clamping the right (tracheal) lumen will insufflate air into the right lower field because the right upper lobe bronchus is occluded by the bronchial cuff.

(B) **Incorrect.** This is how a left-sided double-lumen tube *should* be positioned: bronchial lumen and cuff in the left main bronchus and tracheal orifice and cuff in the trachea above the carina. However, this configuration does not satisfy the clinical description.

(C) **Incorrect.** Positioning both the tracheal orifice and the bronchial limb above the carina is no different from having a single-lumen endotracheal tube. You should not hear any difference in breath sounds by clamping either lumen.

(D) **Incorrect.** Positioning both the tracheal cuff and the bronchial limb in the right bronchus would be similar to inserting a single-lumen endotracheal tube into the right mainstem bronchus. No air should be entering the left lung.

(E) **Incorrect.** Positioning both the tracheal orifice and the bronchial limb in the left bronchus is similar to inserting a single-lumen endotracheal tube into the left mainstem bronchus. The only difference would be that the tracheal cuff might not be deep enough in the left bronchus to prevent air from escaping to the right lung.

REASONING:

This question tests knowledge of the differences between right and left lung anatomy and the design of right- and left-sided endotracheal tubes. With this knowledge, the reader should be able to determine that choice A, albeit malpositioned, is the only configuration that would satisfy the clinical description.

REFERENCE:

Barash PG, Cullen BF, Stoelting RK. Clinical Anesthesia, 4th ed. Philadelphia, Lippincott Williams & Wilkins, 2001, pp. 824–826.

Morgan GE, Mikhail MS, Murray MJ. Clinical Anesthesiology, 3d ed. New York, McGraw-Hill, 2002, pp. 529–533, Fig. 24-6 (p. 531).

BOOK B:

Answer B

Clinical Anesthesia

QUESTION 25

QUESTION (Choose single best answer):

A 27-year-old man with type 1 von Willebrand's disease requires internal fixation of an open fracture of the femur. Prothrombin time, partial thromboplastin time, and platelet count are normal. During surgery, there is significant oozing from the wound, and the surgeon notes poor clot quality. The most appropriate therapy at this time is administration of

(A) Cryoprecipitate.
(B) Desmopressin.
(C) Fresh frozen plasma.
(D) Lyophilized factor VII concentrate.
(E) Platelets.

CORRECT ANSWER: B

SUMMARY:

von Willebrand's Disease (vWD) occurs in approximately 0.1 percent of patients. It is caused by a defective or diminished level of von Willebrand's factor (vWF), a carrier for factor VIII and promoter of platelet aggregation and adherence. In type 1 disease (70 to 80 percent of vWD), levels of normal vWF are decreased. Patients have a prolonged bleeding time, low vWF levels, decreased factor VIII activity, but normal PT, PTT, and platelet counts. Desmopressin promotes the release of vWF and can increase vWF concentration two- to fivefold in most patients.[1] It is the first-line therapy for type 1 and 2A disease but should not be given to patients with type 2B disease because it can cause thrombocytopenia in these patients.[2] Cryoprecipitate, which contains vWF and factor VIII, is given for urgent correction of this disorder. Currently, virus-inactivated factor VIII concentrate containing VIII and vWF is preferred over cryoprecipitate, which is pooled from many donors and carries an infectious risk.[1]

EXPLANATION:

(A) **Incorrect.** The patient in the question is oozing from his wound and requires increased plasma concentrations of vWF and factor VIII. This can be accomplished effectively and without infectious risk by administration of desmopressin in most patients with type 1 disease. If there were hemodynamically significant hemorrhage and cryoprecipitate were immediately available, it could be administered for urgent correction of this disorder.

(B) **Correct.** Desmopressin promotes the release of vWF.[1] Even though it does not reach peak effect until after 30 minutes, it has been reported to stop bleeding promptly in vWD patients during surgery.[3] It is often administered prior to surgery in patients with type 1 disease to minimize intraoperative coagulopathy. In this scenario, there does not appear to be catastrophic bleeding. It is reasonable first to attempt to correct the coagulopathy with administration of desmopressin. If poor clot quality persists or bleeding becomes ominous, urgent correction can be achieved by administration of cryoprecipitate.

(C) **Incorrect.** Fresh frozen plasma contains all the plasma proteins, including clotting factors. It is indicated for the immediate reversal of warfarin therapy, treatment of specific factor deficiencies for which factor concentrates are not available, or treatment of coagulopathies owing to liver failure.

(D) **Incorrect.** Factor VII is not deficient in vWD.

(E) **Incorrect.** Platelets counts are normal in vWD.

REASONING:

This question tests knowledge of the pathophysiology and treatment of vWD. Choices C, D, and E are clearly incorrect because they are not therapies used to treat vWD. Choice B is a first-line therapy for type 1 vWD and ideally should be given 30 minutes prior to incision. This patient's bleeding does not appear catastrophic. Desmopressin has been shown to stop surgical bleeding quickly and is a reasonable first-line therapy in this setting. If bleeding were catastrophic, cryoprecipitate would be a preferred first-line therapy if it were immediately available.

REFERENCES:

1. Barash PG, Cullen BF, Stoelting RK. Clinical Anesthesia, 4th ed. Philadelphia, Lippincott Williams & Wilkins, 2001, pp. 224–226

2. Mannucci PM, Lombardi R, Bader R, et al. Heterogeneity of type I von Willebrand disease: Evidence for a subgroup with an abnormal von Willebrand factor. Blood 66(4):796–802, 1985.

3. Mariana G, Ciavarella N, Mazzucconi MG, et al. Evaluation of the effectiveness of DDAVP in surgery and in bleeding episodes in haemophilia and von Willebrand's disease: A study on 43 patients. Clin Lab Haematol 6(3):229–238, 1984.

4. Stoetling RK, Dierdorf SF. Anesthesia and Co-Existing Disease, 4th ed. New York, Churchill Livingstone, 2002, pp. 492–493.

5. Morgan GE, Mikhail MS, Murray MJ. Clinical Anesthesiology, 3d ed. New York, McGraw-Hill, 2002, pp. 635, 721–722.

BOOK B:

Answer E

Clinical Anesthesia

QUESTION 26

QUESTION (Choose single best answer):

A 30-year-old man is brought to the emergency department after being rescued from a house fire. With the trachea intubated and FIO_2 at 1.0, arterial blood gas values are PaO_2 495 mm Hg, $PaCO_2$ 28 mm Hg, and pH 7.28. Hemoglobin saturation measured by co-oximeter is 50 percent. The most appropriate next step is to

(A) Add positive end-expiratory pressure (PEEP).
(B) Add *n*-acetylcysteine to the inhaled gases.
(C) Administer sodium bicarbonate intravenously.
(D) Transfuse 2 units of packed red blood cells.
(E) Transfer to a hyperbaric chamber.

CORRECT ANSWER: E

SUMMARY:

Carbon monoxide (CO) poisoning is an early and major cause of mortality in smoke inhalation. CO causes tissue hypoxia because it has 200 times the affinity of oxygen for hemoglobin and shifts the oxygen dissociation curve to the left, decreasing the release of oxygen to tissues. CO poisoning should be suspected when pulse oximetry readings are normal and a co-oximeter indicates low oxygen saturation. Arterial blood gas will reveal a normal P_{O_2}, a P_{CO_2} that is reduced by hyperventilation, and a lactic acidosis from anaerobic metabolism. The principal treatment is terminating the patient's exposure to CO and administering 100% high-flow normobaric oxygen. Oxygen shortens the carboxyhemoglobin half-life from 4 to 6 hours (room air) to 60 to 80 minutes. A hyperbaric chamber is useful for severe cases and can decrease the carboxyhemoglobin half-life to 15 to 30 minutes.[1]

EXPLANATION:

(A) *Incorrect.* Adding PEEP will not increase the displacement of carbon monoxide from hemoglobin.

(B) *Incorrect.* *N*-Acetylcysteine (Mucomyst) is a mucolytic agent used in patients with viscous secretions. It also replenishes glutathione and is used to treat acetaminophen toxicity but is not a recommended therapy for carbon monoxide poisoning.

(C) *Incorrect.* Sodium bicarbonate may ameliorate the metabolic acidosis caused by anaerobic metabolism but would not treat the underlying cause: impaired oxidative metabolism caused by severe CO poisoning.

(D) *Incorrect.* Transfusion therapy is a reported treatment method for carbon monoxide poisoning in some anesthesia texts[2] and is commented on in the literature through sporadic case reports.[3,4] However, a current review of the literature does not reveal definitive data to support this practice.

(E) *Correct.* The treatment for CO poisoning is 100% oxygen, which displaces carbon monoxide from the hemoglobin molecule, significantly shortening the half-life of carboxyhemoglobin. Even greater levels of oxygen may be delivered to the blood in a hyperbaric chamber to facilitate the displacement of CO from hemoglobin. Suggested indications for hyperbaric oxygen include (1) coma, (2) any period of unconsciousness, (3) carboxyhemoglobin level greater than 40 percent, (4) pregnancy and carboxyhemoglobin level greater than 15 percent, (5) signs of cardiac ischemia or arrhythmia, (6) history of ischemic heart disease and carboxyhemoglobin level greater than 20 percent, (7) recurrent symptoms for up to 3 weeks, and (8) symptoms that do not resolve with normobaric oxygen after 4 to 6 hours.[5]

REASONING:

This patient is suffering from carbon monoxide poisoning secondary to smoke inhalation. He is already intubated (presumably owing to airway swelling and risk of acute airway compromise) and on an F_{IO_2} of 1.0, the best immediate treatment for carbon monoxide poisoning. We are not given adequate information to determine if the patient meets recommended criteria for hyperbaric oxygen therapy. Indeed, there are risks associated with hyperbaric oxygen, including transport of the patient to the treatment site, hyperoxic seizures, and barotrauma.[6] However, of all the listed options, only choice E is a well-studied and efficacious treatment for carbon monoxide poisoning.

REFERENCES:

1. Pace N, Strajman E, Walker EL. Acceleration of carbon monoxide elimination in man by high pressure oxygen. Science 111:652–654, 1950.

2. Barash PG, Cullen BF, Stoelting RK. Clinical Anesthesia, 4th ed. Philadelphia, Lippincott Williams & Wilkins, 2001, pp. 1275, 1480.

3. Ireland BJ. A case of carbon monoxide poisoning treated by replacement blood transfusion. Med J Aust 1(10):331–332, 1952 (publication unavailable and not reviewed).

4. Radevich OL. Use of exchange blood transfusion in carbon monoxide poisoning. Vrach Delo 1:139–140, 1967 (publication unavailable and not reviewed).

5. Myers RAM, Thom SR. Carbon monoxide and cyanide poisoning. In Kindwall EP, ed. Hyperbaric Medicine Practice. Flagstaff, AZ, Best Publishing, 1994, p. 357.

6. Weaver LK, Hopkins RO, Chan KJ, et al. Hyperbaric oxygen for acute carbon monoxide poisoning. N Engl J Med 347(14):1057–1067, 2002.

7. Morgan GE, Mikhail MS, Murray MJ. Clinical Anesthesiology, 3d ed. New York, McGraw-Hill, 2002, pp. 801–802, 974–975.

BOOK B:

QUESTION 27

Answer A

Physiology

QUESTION (Choose single best answer):

A 60-kg 45-year-old woman who takes digoxin for atrial fibrillation receives furosemide 40 mg and mannitol 60 g during resection of a supratentorial meningioma. After initiation of hyperventilation to decrease $Paco_2$ from 35 to 20 mm Hg, multifocal premature ventricular contractions are noted on the ECG. The most likely cause is

(A) Acute hypokalemia.
(B) Cerebral ischemia.
(C) Impending herniation of the brain stem.
(D) Paradoxical air embolism.
(E) Surgical manipulation of the meningioma.

CORRECT ANSWER: A

SUMMARY:

Acute hypokalemia can be caused by loss of total-body potassium stores or a shift into the intracellular space. Most people are asymptomatic until levels decline below 3 mEq/L. Cardiovascular signs of hypokalemia include ECG changes, arrhythmias, labile blood pressure owing to autonomic dysfunction, and decreased myocardial contractility. Hypokalemia can exacerbate digoxin toxicity.

EXPLANATION:

(A) **Correct.** Diuretics increase the renal loss of potassium. Hyperventilation with its attendant alkalosis causes an intracellular shift of potassium. Hypokalemia and hypercalcemia can interact with digoxin to produce toxicity.

(B) **Incorrect.** Arrhythmias are unlikely to be the initial and only signs in focal or global cerebral ischemia. Brain death in later stages can produce arrhythmia secondary to massive sympathetic outflow.

(C) **Incorrect.** Raised intracranial pressure (ICP) and impending herniation are unlikely in a patient with open dura. Bradycardia and hypertension are the classic signs of impending herniation.

(D) **Incorrect.** Paradoxical air embolus can produce stroke and myocardial or other visceral ischemia. It is associated with other signs of air embolus. Coronary air will manifest as ST-T-wave changes in inferior leads (right coronary territory), and there can be various arrhythmias.

(E) **Incorrect.** Surgical manipulation of the brain stem area is more likely to produce cardiovascular changes. This meningioma is supratentorial.

REASONING:

This question tests knowledge of the causes and effects of hypokalemia and its drug interaction with digoxin. Considering all the changes occurring in the patient—diuresis, acute respiratory alkalosis, and preexisting digoxin therapy—acute hypokalemia is highest on the differential diagnosis as the etiology of the premature ventricular contractions (PVCs). Although choices B and D can produce arrhythmias, they are unlikely in the absence of other signs.

REFERENCE:

Barash PG, Cullen BF, Stoelting RK. Clinical Anesthesia, 4th ed. Philadelphia, Lippincott Williams & Wilkins, 2001, p. 907.

Morgan GE, Mikhail MS, Murray MJ. Clinical Anesthesiology, 3d ed. New York, McGraw-Hill, 2002, pp. 613–615.

BOOK B: **QUESTION 28**

Answer D

Neuroanesthesia

QUESTION (Choose single best answer):

A 50-year-old woman with subarachnoid hemorrhage and left hemiparesis undergoes clipping of a right cerebral aneurysm. On the second postoperative day, mental status deteriorates. Blood pressure is 110/70 mm Hg. A cerebral angiogram shows vasospasm. The most appropriate management is to

(A) Administer dexamethasone.
(B) Administer mannitol.
(C) Administer phentolamine.
(D) Expand intravascular volume.
(E) Intubate and hyperventilate to a $Paco_2$ of 28 mm Hg.

CORRECT ANSWER: D

SUMMARY:

Cerebral vasospasm is a complication of subarachnoid hemorrhage (SAH) that can be detected on angiogram in up to 70 percent of patients.[1] The peak incidence of vasospasm after SAH is 6 to 7 days.[2] The cornerstone of treatment is "triple H" therapy: hypervolemia, hypertension, and hemodilution. The goal is to increase cerebral blood flow. Patients with SAH receive calcium channel blockers (e.g., nimodipine or nicardipine) to prevent vasospasm.

EXPLANATION:

(A) *Incorrect.* Corticosteroids are used to reduce cerebral edema, not to increase blood flow.
(B) *Incorrect.* Mannitol can transiently increase cerebral blood flow as an osmotic agent, but it promotes diuresis, with the end result being hypovolemia.
(C) *Incorrect.* Phentolamine is an alpha-blocker that can dilate blood vessels but leads to an overall reduction in blood pressure, which decreases cerebral perfusion.
(D) *Correct.* Expanding intravascular volume, hypervolemia, is one of the mainstays of treatment of cerebral vasospasm.
(E) *Incorrect.* Hyperventilation to decrease $Paco_2$ is an intervention that results in decreased cerebral blood flow.

REASONING:

This question tests knowledge of the treatment of cerebral vasospasm after SAH. Most of the available answer choices are more appropriate for treatment of increased intracranial pressure. "Triple H" therapy is designed to overcome the resistance from vasospasm and increase perfusion to the brain. Expanding the intravascular volume can produce hypervolemia and also can provide beneficial hemodilution of the circulating blood.

REFERENCES:

1. Barash PG, Cullen BF, Stoelting RK. Clinical Anesthesia, 4th ed. Philadelphia, Lippincott Williams & Wilkins, 2001, pp. 770–771.
2. Kassell NF, Torner JC, Haley EC Jr, et al. The International Cooperative Study on the Timing of Aneurysm Surgery: 1. Overall management results. J Neurosurg 73(1):18–36, 1990.
3. Morgan GE, Mikhail MS, Murray MJ. Clinical Anesthesiology, 3d ed. New York, McGraw-Hill, 2002, pp. 578–579.

BOOK B:

Answer B

Neuroanesthesia

QUESTION 29

QUESTION (Choose single best answer):

Which of the following statements concerning cerebral blood flow (CBF) during anesthesia is true?

(A) CBF changes minimally when $Paco_2$ increases from 30 to 40 mm Hg.
(B) CBF changes minimally when Po_2 decreases from 160 to 100 mm Hg.
(C) CBF is autoregulated when mean arterial pressure (MAP) is 40 mm Hg.
(D) CBF is coupled to cerebral metabolism during isoflurane anesthesia.
(E) CBF is unaffected by 1.2% isoflurane at a $Paco_2$ of 40 mm Hg.

CORRECT ANSWER: B

SUMMARY:

Coupling of cerebral blood flow (CBF) and cerebral metabolic rate (CMR) describes the parallel adjustment of CBF to meet the needs of CMR. In a normotensive adult, CBF is kept nearly constant between mean arterial blood pressures (MAP) of 50 to 150 mm Hg. This autoregulation curve can be shifted to the right in patients with chronic hypertension. Outside these limits, CBF becomes pressure-dependent. Whereas CBF increases significantly only when Pao_2 drops below 50 mm Hg, CBF changes proportionately with $Paco_2$ of between 20 and 80 mm Hg.

EXPLANATION:

(A) *Incorrect.* A 33 percent increase of $Paco_2$ from 30 to 40 mm Hg results in a more than minimal proportionate increase of CBF.
(B) *Correct.* CBF does not change significantly with Po_2 in the range of 160 to 100 mm Hg. Hypoxemia with a Pao_2 of less than 50 mm Hg will increase CBF. Hyperoxemia may minimally decrease CBF, but CBF remains relatively constant with Pao_2 from 50 to 175 mm Hg.
(C) *Incorrect.* At 40 mm Hg, CBF is not autoregulated; i.e., the brain depends on MAP to maintain perfusion.
(D) *Incorrect.* Inhalational agents tend to increase CBF in a dose-dependent manner. Isoflurane is also a potent inhibitor of CMR. The net effect is an increase in the CBF/CMR ratio.[1]
(E) *Incorrect.* CBF is increased by 1.2% isoflurane at a $Paco_2$ of 40 mm Hg. As with sevoflurane and desflurane, increases in CBF may be prevented by simultaneous hyperventilation. This is in contrast to halothane or enflurane, for which hyperventilation must be initiated prior to use.

REASONING:

Important concepts for answering this question include an understanding of factors that affect cerebral blood flow. The reader should be able to rule out choice A because 33 percent is more than a minimal change. Because 40 mm Hg is out of the range of normal autoregulation, choice C also can be eliminated. Knowledge that a Pa_{CO_2} of 40 mm Hg is not enough to abolish the increase in CBF with isoflurane helps to rule out choice E. Choice D is controversial depending on how "coupling" is interpreted. A strict interpretation is that CBF should increase with CMR. A looser interpretation is that the relationship is still "coupled" just in a new, "redefined" manner such that the CBF/CMR ratio is higher. Regardless of the ambiguity, B is clearly correct because there is only minimal change in CBF in that range of Pa_{O_2}.

REFERENCE:

1. Miller RD, Miller ED, Reves JG, et al. Anesthesia, 5th ed. New York, Churchill Livingstone, 2000, p. 706.
2. Morgan GE, Mikhail MS, Murray MJ. Clinical Anesthesiology, 3d ed. New York, McGraw-Hill, 2002, pp. 552–558.

BOOK B:

QUESTION 30

Answer C

Pharmacology

QUESTION (Choose single best answer):

Which of the following drugs is contraindicated in patients with Parkinson's disease?

(A) Atropine
(B) Dopamine
(C) Droperidol
(D) Fentanyl
(E) Isoflurane

CORRECT ANSWER: C

SUMMARY:

Parkinson's disease is a neurologic disorder characterized by dyskinetic movements, gait disorders, and abnormal facial expression. The disease process is largely due to progressive depletion of dopamine in the substantia nigra of the midbrain. Medications that worsen the clinical effect of dopamine depletion or worsen the symptoms associated with Parkinson's would be relatively contraindicated. Droperidol may worsen dyskinetic movements in Parkinson's patients by blocking dopamine receptors. Other medications that should be avoided in Parkinson's patients include phenothiazines (e.g., thorazine, compazine, and promethazine) and metoclopramide.

EXPLANATION:

(A) *Incorrect.* Atropine is an antimuscarinic that counteracts the effect of vagus nerve stimulation. Effects of atropine include increased heart rate, decreased mucus production and secretion, increased blood pressure, pupilary dilation, decreased intestinal motility, and urinary retention. None of these effects would be particularly problematic in Parkinson's patients.

(B) *Incorrect.* Dopamine is the neurotransmitter that is depleted in Parkinson's patients. Levodopa is the most common drug used to treat Parkinson's disease. It is converted to dopamine in vivo and exerts its clinical effect in that form. Therefore, dopamine would not be contraindicated in Parkinson's patients.

(C) *Correct.* Droperidol is a butyrophenone (of the same class as the antipsychotic drug haloperidol) that acts by blocking dopamine receptors. Since Parkinson's patients already have depleted dopamine, administration of droperidol is relatively contraindicated in Parkinson's patients and can worsen the symptoms associated with the disease.

(D) *Incorrect.* Fentanyl is a rapidly acting opioid that blocks mu opioid receptors and interferes with substance P in the spinal cord. Mu receptors are not involved in the Parkinson's disease process.

(E) *Incorrect.* Isoflurane is a halogenated hydrocarbon that is not known to have an effect on dopamine transmission in the central nervous system.

REASONING:

This question tests knowledge of basic pharmacology and pathophysiology of Parkinson's disease. Choices A, D, and E are incorrect because these drugs do not exert their effects on dopaminergic neurons. Choice B is incorrect because drugs that are converted to dopamine are used to treat Parkinson's disease, and dopamine is known to improve symptoms in Parkinson's patients. Choice C is the only agent that interferes directly with dopaminergic neurons in a manner that would worsen rather than improve symptoms.

REFERENCE:

Barash PG, Cullen BF, Stoelting RK. Clinical Anesthesia, 4th ed. Philadelphia, Lippincott Williams & Wilkins, 2001, pp. 501–502.

Morgan GE, Mikhail MS, Murray MJ. Clinical Anesthesiology, 3d ed. New York, McGraw-Hill, 2002, pp. 586–587.

BOOK B: **QUESTION 31**

Answer D

Clinical Anesthesia

QUESTION (Choose single best answer):

A 70-kg patient with no acute bleeding has a preoperative platelet count of 40,000/mm^3. Following preoperative transfusion of platelets 10 units, the predicted platelet count would be

(A) 50,000/mm^3.
(B) 80,000/mm^3.
(C) 90,000/mm^3.
(D) 140,000/mm^3.
(E) 190,000/mm^3.

CORRECT ANSWER: D

SUMMARY:

Platelets are an essential part of the hemostatic mechanism that includes the various coagulation factors. In general, platelet transfusions are not necessary for patients without bleeding until the platelet count reaches 10,000 to 20,000/mm^3, below which there is an increased risk of spontaneous hemorrhage. For patients undergoing surgery, platelet counts less than 50,000/mm^3 are associated with increased surgical blood loss. However, the threshold for transfusion should take into consideration the type of surgery, probability of blood loss, number and function of platelets, and etiology of the thrombocytopenia and/or platelet dysfunction. Platelet concentrates are prepared from a single unit of whole blood, whereas an apheresis unit is equivalent to 6 to 8 standard units in a concentrated lower-volume unit.

EXPLANATION:

(A) *Incorrect.* 50,000/mm^3 is much lower than would be expected.
(B) *Incorrect.* 80,000/mm^3 is lower than what would be expected.
(C) *Incorrect.* 90,000/mm^3 is lower than expected but not impossible.

(D) **Correct.** For a 70-kg adult, 1 unit of platelet concentrate will increase the platelet count by 7000 to 10,000/mm³ under ideal circumstances.[3] Therefore, with a starting platelet count of 40,000/mm³, a transfusion of 10 units would raise the count by 70,000 to 100,000/mm³ to 110,000 to 140,000/mm³. Thus 140,000/mm³ is the upper limit of what would be expected.

(E) **Incorrect.** 190,000/mm³ much greater than would be expected.

REASONING:

The key concept for answering this question is knowing how much the platelet count would rise with a transfusion of a given number of units of platelets. This would be a straightforward question if it were not for the fact that different texts give different estimates for the expected results. For adults, Miller gives a range of 7000 to 10,000/mm³ per unit increase.[3] For children, 0.1 to 0.3 unit/kg of body weight should raise the platelet count by 20,000 to 70,000/mm³.[1] Alternatively, 10 mL/kg of platelet concentrate will raise count by 50,000/mm³.[2] In practice, each patient may respond differently depending on the etiology of the thrombocytopenia (e.g., splenomegaly, autoimmune destruction, and bleeding) and whether there is ongoing bleeding. In practice, one should assume the worst outcome and correlate with clinical signs (e.g., ongoing coagulopathy or bleeding) and/or laboratory tests (e.g., coagulation tests or platelet count). For purposes of this examination, choice D should be correct under optimal circumstances.

REFERENCES:

1. Cote CJ. A Practice of Anesthesia for Infants and Children, 3d ed. Philadelphia, Saunders, 2001, pp. 238–239.
2. Sidberry GK, Iannone R. Harriet Lane Handbook, 15th ed. St Louis, Mosby, 2000, pp. 320–321.
3. Miller RD, Miller ED, Reves JG, et al. Anesthesia, 5th ed. New York, Churchill Livingstone, 2000, pp. 1636–1637.
4. Morgan GE, Mikhail MS, Murray MJ. Clinical Anesthesiology, 3d ed. New York, McGraw-Hill, 2002, pp. 635–636.

BOOK B:

Answer B

Cardiovascular

QUESTION 32

QUESTION (Choose single best answer):

Two hours after coronary artery bypass grafting, a 60-year-old man has a heart rate of 140 beats per minute and a blood pressure of 80/60 mm Hg. Cardiac index is 1.5 L/min/m². Central venous pressure is 23 mm Hg, with large *a* waves in the right atrial pressure tracing. A pulsus paradoxus of 6 mm Hg is noted. Which of the following is the most likely diagnosis?

(A) Atrial flutter
(B) Cardiac tamponade
(C) Hypovolemia
(D) Junctional tachycardia
(E) Tension pneumothorax

CORRECT ANSWER: B

SUMMARY:

The usual suspects for postoperative hypotension and tachycardia in cardiac surgery patients include bleeding, hypovolemia, cardiac tamponade, and ventricular dysfunction. This patient presents with classic signs of cardiac tamponade. Tamponade is characterized by tachycardia, hypotension, increased central venous pressure (CVP), pulsus paradoxus, and equalization of diastolic pressures across the chambers of the heart. Cardiac tamponade impairs the diastolic filling of the heart and eventually leads to cardiovascular collapse.

EXPLANATION:

(A) *Incorrect.* Atrial flutter with fast ventricular response could lead to hypotension from impaired filling of the heart but will not have pulsus paradoxus or increased CVP. Flutter waves usually are seen on ECG.

(B) *Correct.* In the postoperative period, cardiac patients can have tamponade from loculated clot within the open pericardium. In this case the diastolic pressure equalization is not seen.

(C) *Incorrect.* Hypovolemia can cause tachycardia and hypotension, but the CVP would below normal and without evidence of pulsus paradoxus.

(D) *Incorrect.* Junctional tachycardia can give rise to hypotension and tachycardia. It can produce large *a* waves from atrioventricular (AV) dissociation. But the CVP should be in the normal range. It can be diagnosed by ECG and treated with atropine to increase the sinus rate.

(E) *Incorrect.* Besides hypotension and tachycardia, other signs of tension pneumothorax include elevated airway pressure, hypoxia, and mediastinal shift.

REASONING:

There are numerous confounding events that can cause postoperative hypotension in the cardiac surgical patient. It is important to distinguish between the surgical and medical causes. Presence of high CVP in the postoperative cardiac patient, along with tachycardia and hypotension, should place tamponade highest on the differential diagnosis.

REFERENCE:

Stoelting RK, Miller RD. Basics of Anesthesia, 4th ed. New York, Churchill Livingstone, 2000, pp. 108–109.

Morgan GE, Mikhail MS, Murray MJ. Clinical Anesthesiology, 3d ed. New York, McGraw-Hill, 2002, pp. 464–465.

BOOK B:

QUESTION 33

Answer C

Clinical Anesthesia

QUESTION (Choose single best answer):

Which of the following is the strongest indication for one-lung ventilation?

(A) Descending thoracic aortic aneurysm
(B) Esophageal resection
(C) Lobectomy for lung abcess
(D) Lobectomy for tumor
(E) Pneumonectomy for tumor

CORRECT ANSWER: C

SUMMARY:

Separation of the two-lungs and/or one-lung ventilation involves placing double-lumen endotracheal tubes or bronchial blockers. Both techniques require skill and special equipment to perform successfully. Absolute indications for one-lung ventilation include isolation of one lung to prevent infection or blood from spilling into the other lung, as in cases of abscess or hemorrhage; to control the distribution of ventilation, as in cases of bronchopleural fistula or unilateral lung disease; and to enable unilateral bronchial lavage.[1] Relative indications mainly encompass optimization of surgical exposure for thoracic procedures such as thoracic aortic aneurysm, pneumonectomy, thoracic spine surgery, or esophageal surgery.

EXPLANATION:

(A) *Incorrect.* Surgical exposure for repair of descending thoracic aortic aneurysm is a *relative* indication for one-lung ventilation.

(B) *Incorrect.* Surgical exposure for esophageal resection is a *relative* indication for one-lung ventilation.

(C) *Correct.* Isolation of the lungs to prevent contamination of lung abscess into the contralateral lung is an *absolute* indication for one-lung ventilation.

(D) *Incorrect.* Surgical exposure for lobectomy for tumor resection is a *relative* indication for one-lung ventilation.

(E) *Incorrect.* Surgical exposure for pneumonectomy for tumor is a *relative* indication for one-lung ventilation.

REASONING:

This question tests knowledge of the relative and absolute indications for one-lung ventilation. Choices A, B, D, and E are all relative indications because their main purpose for one-lung ventilation is to optimize surgical exposure. Choice C is the only situation where isolation of one lung may protect the other, presumably healthier lung from being infected if the abscess should rupture.

REFERENCES:

1. Barash PG, Cullen BF, Stoelting RK. Clinical Anesthesia, 4th ed. Philadelphia, Lippincott Williams & Wilkins, 2001, p. 824, Table 30-2.

2. Miller RD, Miller ED, Reves JG, et al. Anesthesia, 5th ed. New York, Churchill Livingstone, 2000, p. 1690.

3. Morgan GE, Mikhail MS, Murray MJ. Clinical Anesthesiology, 3d ed. New York, McGraw-Hill, 2002, p. 529.

BOOK B:

Answer C

Clinical Anesthesia

QUESTION 34

QUESTION (Choose single best answer):

In a 65-year-old man, which of the following findings on preoperative pulmonary function testing is associated with the highest risk for respiratory insufficiency following pneumonectomy?

(A) Maximum voluntary ventilation at 65 percent of predicted
(B) Mean pulmonary artery pressure of 28 mm Hg
(C) Predicted postoperative forced expiratory volume in 1 second (FEV_1) of 800 mL
(D) Residual-volume-to-total-lung-capacity (RV/TLC) ratio of 0.35
(E) Vital capacity of 3 L

CORRECT ANSWER: C

SUMMARY:

Candidates for pneumonectomy are selected based on anatomic staging and postoperative risk of the pulmonary tumor resection. The extent of lung impairment preoperatively correlates with postoperative mortality and morbidity. Spirometry is one of many pulmonary function tests (PFTs), and it can assess a patient's vital capacity, forced vital capacity, and forced expiratory volume over a time interval. A preoperative FEV_1 of less than 1 L is associated with 20 to 45 percent mortality. Other predictors of poor postoperative respiratory function include a maximum voluntary ventilation (MVV) less than 50 percent, RV/TLC ratio >0.5, and vital capacity <2L.

EXPLANATION:

(A) *Incorrect.* MVV is effort-dependent and is the largest volume of gas that can be inspired in 1 minute. MVV reflects the endurance of the muscles of respiration. A typical MVV of a healthy adult is 170 L/min. An MVV of less than 50 percent predicted, not 65 percent, generally is considered high risk.[1]

(B) *Incorrect.* Postoperative stress on the remaining pulmonary vasculature and right ventricle may occur after pneumonectomy owing to increased pulmonary vascular resistance from the reduced pulmonary vascular bed.[1] This postresection pulmonary physiology can be simulated by using a special pulmonary artery catheter to occlude the pulmonary artery of the lung that will be resected. The patient may not be able to tolerate pneumonectomy if the mean pulmonary artery pressure (PAP) rises greater than 40 mm Hg, Pa_{O_2} is less than 60 mm Hg, or Pa_{CO_2} is greater than 45 mm Hg with this maneuver.[1] Although not specifically mentioned, we assume the reported PAP was measured during a unilateral pulmonary artery occlusion test.

(C) *Correct.* A postoperative predicted FEV_1 of less than 1000 mL is associated with a 20 to 45 percent mortality.[1]

(D) *Incorrect.* A normal RV/TLC ratio is 0.20 to 0.25. An RV/TLC ratio of 0.4 or less is associated with only 7 percent mortality. An RV/TLC ratio of 0.5 is generally considered high risk.

(E) *Incorrect.* A vital capacity of three times the tidal volume is required for an effective cough. Normal vital capacity is about 60 mL/kg or about 4200 mL for the average adult. A vital capacity of less than 2 L is predictive of increased postoperative mortality and morbidity following pneumonectomy.

REASONING:

This question tests knowledge of the role of preoperative pulmonary function testing in assessing postoperative function after lung resection. These tests and the associated clinical assessment algorithm should be reviewed carefully by the reader.[1] The general approach is to begin with studies of whole-lung function (FVC, FEV_1, VC, etc.) and progress to split-lung function testing and even pulmonary artery occlusion testing if indicated. Of the available choices in this answer, choice C is associated with the highest postoperative mortality.

REFERENCE:

1. Barash PG, Cullen BF, Stoelting RK. Clinical Anesthesia, 4th ed. Philadelphia, Lippincott Williams & Wilkins, 2001, pp. 814–816, Fig. 30-3.
2. Morgan GE, Mikhail MS, Murray MJ. Clinical Anesthesiology, 3d ed. New York, McGraw-Hill, 2002, pp. 535–536.

BOOK B: **QUESTION 35**

Answer C

Clinical Anesthesia

QUESTION (Choose single best answer):

During transurethral resection of the prostate (TURP), intravascular absorption of glycine irrigant most commonly produces

(A) Alkalosis.
(B) Hemolysis.
(C) Hypertension.
(D) Tachycardia.
(E) Wheezing.

CORRECT ANSWER: C

SUMMARY:

Continuous irrigation is used during a transurethral resection of the prostate (TURP) to facilitate visualization and removal of excised tissue. Ideal irrigants are nonhemolytic, nonionized, and isotonic. Systemic absorption of this irrigant occurs through venous sinuses that are exposed during resection of the prostate tissue. Excessive absorption of irrigant fluid (at least 2 L) may lead to intravascular fluid overload, water intoxication, and solute toxicity. The average absorption of irrigant during resection of the prostate is 20 mL/min.[1] The absorption rate of irrigant depends on resection time (ideally less than 1 hour), number of exposed venous sinuses, and hydrostatic pressure of the irrigation fluid (ideally more than 30 cm above the operating table initially and less than 15 cm near conclusion of the procedure).[1] The typical progression of TURP syndrome begins with acute volume overload, resulting in intial hypertension and bradycardia. Continued absorption eventually will lead to left-sided heart failure, pulmonary edema, and cardiovascular collapse. Dilutional hyponatremia can ensue, resulting in cerebral and neuronal edema, restlessness, and confusion that eventually progress to loss of consciousness and seizures. Blindness is a side effect that is specific to glycine irrigant. Glycine is metabolized in the liver to ammonia and glyoxylic acid. Excessive absorption of glycine can lead to encephalopathy from hyperammonemia. (See also Question 140, Book A.)

EXPLANATION:

(A) *Incorrect.* Alkalosis is not commonly associated with glycine absorption during TURP.

(B) *Incorrect.* Glycine can be used as an irrigant because it is only mildly hypotonic compared with normal plasma osmolality. Hemolysis is less likely to occur.

(C) *Correct.* Volume overload from TURP syndrome initially causes hypertension.

(D) *Incorrect.* Volume overload causes a compensatory bradycardia, not tachycardia. Increased volume sensed by baroreceptors in the carotid sinus and aortic arch cause an increase in vagal tone. Increased vagal tone produces a relative vasodilation and slower heart rate in an attempt to decrease blood pressure.

(E) *Incorrect.* Wheezes on auscultation of the lungs are a sign of "dry" breath sounds and are indicative of airway obstruction. Rales or crackles are caused by excessive fluid in the airway and are more indicative of pulmonary edema. While pulmonary edema can result from excessive irrigant absorption, it does not occur before hypertension.

REASONING:

This question tests knowledge of TURP syndrome and the side effects that can develop from excessive absorption of irrigant solutions. It is important to remember the main pathophysiology of TURP syndrome is fluid overload. Acute volume overload, first and foremost, results in hypertension and bradycardia. Other side effects can occur later and are less common.

REFERENCE:

1. Barash PG, Cullen BF, Stoelting RK. Clinical Anesthesia, 4th ed. Philadelphia, Lippincott Williams & Wilkins, 2001, pp. 1019–1021.
2. Morgan GE, Mikhail MS, Murray MJ. Clinical Anesthesiology, 3d ed. New York, McGraw-Hill, 2002, pp. 695–697.

Answer D

Pediatrics

QUESTION (Choose single best answer):

A 2.2-kg, 6-hour-old neonate is to undergo gastrostomy followed by repair of a tracheo-esophageal fistula. During induction with halothane, air, and oxygen, the abdomen becomes distended. Appropriate management is to

(A) Intubate and assist spontaneous ventilation.
(B) Intubate and control ventilation.
(C) Insert an orogastric tube.
(D) Allow the patient to breathe spontaneously by mask until gastrostomy.
(E) Control ventilation by mask until gastrostomy.

CORRECT ANSWER: D

SUMMARY:

The most common form of tracheoesophageal fistula (TEF) is a blind-ending upper esophagus with a fistula connecting the trachea to the lower esophagus. These patients require frequent suctioning of oral secretions. Proper management includes avoiding positive-pressure ventilation prior to proper placement of an endotracheal tube. A gastrostomy tube and central venous line may be placed under local anesthesia as a first-stage operation to allow the patient to grow until a complete repair can be performed.[1]

EXPLANATION:

(A) *Incorrect.* Ideally, intubation should be performed under controlled circumstances with a gastrostomy tube open to vent the stomach.
(B) *Incorrect.* Controlled ventilation without a gastrostomy tube may cause significant gastric distension.
(C) *Incorrect.* Placing an orogastric tube is impossible in the most common form of TEF because the upper esophagus ends as a blind pouch.[1]
(D) *Correct.* Proper management of a patient with a TEF involves maintaining spontaneous ventilation as long as possible until intubation. Once a gastrostomy tube is placed, the patient can be intubated under controlled circumstances.
(E) *Incorrect.* Positive-pressure ventilation by mask is likely to cause gastric distension in a patient with TEF without a gastrostomy tube. Patients may safely undergo inhalation induction with a gastrostomy tube venting the stomach.[1]

REASONING:

Appropriate management of patients with TEF includes avoiding gastric distension and careful, accurate endotracheal intubation. In some patients, TEF repair may be performed following a first-stage gastrostomy tube placement under local anesthesia.[1] Placing a gastrostomy tube facilitates rehydration and growth of the patient, and it can be used later as a vent for the stomach during anesthetic induction for later surgery.

REFERENCE:

1. Cote CJ. A Practice of Anesthesia for Infants and Children, 3d ed. Philadelphia, Saunders, 2001, pp. 302–303.
2. Morgan GE, Mikhail MS, Murray MJ. Clinical Anesthesiology, 3d ed. New York, McGraw-Hill, 2002, pp. 865–866.

Answer A

Equipment/Physics

QUESTION (Choose single best answer):

Which of the following is an advantage of a circle system over a Mapleson D system?

(A) Better anesthetic conservation
(B) Lower dead space
(C) Lower circuit resistance
(D) More efficient scavenging
(E) More rapid changes in inspired gas concentration

CORRECT ANSWER: A

SUMMARY:

The circle system used in anesthesia has several advantages over Mapleson D circuits. Because of the unidirectional intake and outflow valves, the dead space in a circle system includes only the tubing distal to the Y-piece where inspiratory and expiratory gases mix. Therefore, the length of the breathing tube proximal to the Y-piece in a circle system does not add to the circuit dead space. This is not true for Mapleson D circuits, where tubing length adds to dead space. Other advantages of the circle system over the Mapleson D circuit are (1) greater preservation of anesthetic gases, (2) conservation of airway heat and humidity, and (3) more reliable scavenging. The Mapleson D circuit is efficient during controlled (versus spontaneous) ventilation, is lightweight, and allows more rapid adjustments of inspired gas concentrations. However, it is associated with variable control of anesthetic depth, inability to conserve heat and humidity, and variable scavenging of anesthetic gases.

EXPLANATION:

(A) **Correct.** Anesthetic gases are conserved in a circle system because they are rebreathed after being exhaled (e.g., closed-circuit anesthesia). This is not true with Mapleson D circuits, where expired gases are primarily wasted.
(B) **Incorrect.** Although tubing length does contribute to dead space in Mapleson D circuits (unlike circle systems), this is a poor choice because tubing length is not specified in the question.
(C) **Incorrect.** Resistance is higher in circle systems than in Mapleson D circuits.
(D) **Incorrect.** Mapleson D circuits have variable scavenging capabilities and are not as effective as circle systems in scavenging waste gases.
(E) **Incorrect.** Mapleson D circuits have the advantage here—they are better at making rapid changes in inspired gas concentrations because there is little to no mixing of inspired and expired gases.

REASONING:

This question tests fairly specific knowledge of the circle system (the circuits on most modern anesthesia machines) and the Mapleson D circuit. Choices C and E can be eliminated immediately with knowledge that these options actually are advantages of the Mapleson D circuit compared with the circle system. Choice B is very tempting and is correct if a Mapleson D circuit with significant tubing length is used for the comparison. However, tubing length is not specified, and this makes B a poor choice. The same is true of choice D because scavenging is variable with Mapleson D circuits. This leaves choice A, which is true for all Mapleson D circuits—there is little conservation of anesthetic because exhaled gases go out into the environment.

REFERENCE:

Barash PG, Cullen BF, Stoelting RK. Clinical Anesthesia, 4th ed. Philadelphia, Lippincott Williams & Wilkins, 2001, pp. 580–582.

Morgan GE, Mikhail MS, Murray MJ. Clinical Anesthesiology, 3d ed. New York, McGraw-Hill, 2002, pp. 29–36, Table 3-2 (p. 33).

BOOK B:

Answer C

Neuroanesthesia

QUESTION 38

QUESTION (Choose single best answer):

A 27-year-old man with a 1-month history of quadriplegia at a C6 level is given general anesthesia for cystoscopy. During the cystoscopy, blood pressure suddenly increases to 220/120 mm Hg. Further evaluation is most likely to show

(A) Atrial fibrillation (ventricular rate 100 beats per minute).
(B) Paroxysmal atrial tachycardia (160 beats per minute).
(C) Sinus bradycardia.
(D) Piloerection above the level of C6.
(E) Sweating above the level of C6.

CORRECT ANSWER: C

SUMMARY:

Patients with spinal cord transection at T6 and above are at risk for autonomic hyperreflexia. Stimulation below the level of the transection, typically distension of viscera or surgery, can cause unopposed reflex sympathetic discharge. The patient develops hypertension and vasoconstriction below the injury level. Vasodilation occurs above the injury level. Bradycardia occurs via vagal reflexes. Autonomic hyperreflexia can be prevented by regional and deep general anesthesia. Besides providing adequate analgesia, treatment consists of ganglionic blockade, alpha-blockade, or administration of direct vasodilating agents.

EXPLANATION:

(A) *Incorrect.* Arrythmias may occur, but the patient is most likely to have sinus bradycardia via vagal baroreceptor stimulation.
(B) *Incorrect.* See above.
(C) *Correct.* Baroreceptors in the aortic arch and carotid sinus sense the increased pressure, producing an increase in vagal tone. This causes bradycardia.
(D) *Incorrect.* Piloerection is sympathetically mediated; thus it will not occur above the level of cord transection. Piloerection may be present below the transection.
(E) *Incorrect.* Sweating is sympathetically mediated. The patient will be flushed above the level of transection but will not be sweating.

REASONING:

This question tests knowledge of the signs and symptoms of autonomic hyperreflexia and knowing which physiologic responses are sympathetically versus parasympathetically mediated. Below the level of the transection, sympathetic tone predominates because there is no opposing tone coming from higher centers (the pathway is transected). Above the transection, there is opposing tone, leading to a predominance of parasympathetic control. Piloerection and sweating are both sympathetic responses, and they will not predominate above the cord injury. The first three choices are all possibilities. However, the most likely is a straightforward sinus bradycardia. C is the single best answer.

REFERENCE:

Barash PG, Cullen BF, Stoelting RK. Clinical Anesthesia, 4th ed. Philadelphia, Lippincott Williams & Wilkins, 2001, pp. 1109–1110.

Morgan GE, Mikhail MS, Murray MJ. Clinical Anesthesiology, 3d ed. New York, McGraw-Hill, 2002, p. 590.

Answer D

Cardiovascular

QUESTION (Choose single best answer):

Which of the following is the primary factor regulating normal coronary blood flow?

(A) Aortic diastolic pressure
(B) Coronary perfusion pressure
(C) Heart rate
(D) Myocardial oxygen consumption
(E) Systolic wall tension

CORRECT ANSWER: D

SUMMARY:

Within the ranges of normal coronary perfusion pressure (50 to 120 mm Hg), coronary blood flow is a function of coronary arterial tone and is regulated primarily by myocardial metabolic needs (i.e., myocardial oxygen consumption). This is in contrast to the primary determinant of coronary blood flow at elevated perfusion pressures (>120 mm Hg). At higher pressures, coronary blood flow depends primarily on coronary perfusion pressure (equal to aortic diastolic pressure minus left ventricular end-diastolic pressure [LVEDP]). This question asks you to distinguish these two scenarios and presents you with options for both.

EXPLANATION:

(A) *Incorrect.* Although aortic diastolic pressure is the primary determinant of perfusion pressure (coronary perfusion pressure = aortic diastolic pressure − LVEDP), perfusion pressure does not dictate blood flow under normal conditions.
(B) *Incorrect.* Perfusion pressure is not the primary determinant of coronary blood flow under normal conditions.
(C) *Incorrect.* Although heart rate is a component of myocardial oxygen demand, it does not directly cause changes in arteriolar tone.
(D) *Correct.* Myocardial oxygen consumption determines myocardial metabolic needs, which, in turn, regulate coronary arteriolar tone at normal perfusion pressures. Thus the demand of the heart itself plays a large part in determining vascular tone and coronary blood flow.
(E) *Incorrect.* Systolic wall tension is not the primary determinant, although it may contribute to smaller changes in coronary blood flow.

REASONING:

This question tests knowledge of coronary autoregulation and the determinants of coronary arterial blood flow at normal and high systemic arterial pressures. Under normal conditions, myocardial oxygen demand (and thus metabolism) dictates coronary arteriolar tone, whereas at high pressures it is perfusion pressure that determines coronary artery tone. Choice A, aortic diastolic pressure, is the primary determinant of coronary perfusion pressure (choice B) and contributes largely to coronary blood flow, but only at very high pressures. You can eliminate choices C and E because they do not play a major role in determining coronary blood flow or perfusion pressure. This leaves choice D, which is the primary determinant of coronary blood flow under normal physiologic conditions.

REFERENCE:

Barash PG, Cullen BF, Stoelting RK. Clinical Anesthesia, 4th ed. Philadelphia, Lippincott Williams & Wilkins, 2001, pp. 866–867.
Morgan GE, Mikhail MS, Murray MJ. Clinical Anesthesiology, 3d ed. New York, McGraw-Hill, 2002, pp. 376–379.

Answer D

Equipment/Physics

QUESTION (Choose single best answer):

Which of the following statements concerning pressure support ventilation is true?

(A) Continuous positive airway pressure is provided during inspiration and expiration.
(B) Delivered tidal volume remains the same with decreasing lung compliance.
(C) Inspiratory effort of less than -2 cm H_2O is not assisted.
(D) The overall work of breathing decreases when weaning from mechanical ventilation.
(E) The patient will need more sedation than during intermittent mandatory ventilation.

CORRECT ANSWER: D

SUMMARY:

During pressure-support ventilation, the spontaneously breathing patient initiates a breath, thereby generating a transient negative deviation of pressure from the baseline. The ventilator then delivers a constant preset pressure until inspiratory flow reaches a predetermined level, at which point the ventilator pressure returns to baseline. By assisting the patient's spontaneous efforts, pressure-support ventilation decreases the work of breathing.

EXPLANATION:

(A) *Incorrect.* Airway pressure at the initiation of inspiration may be negative before the ventilator assists the breath. In addition, if there is no positive end-expiratory pressure (PEEP) added, pressure-support ventilation does not deliver continuous positive airway pressure during exhalation.
(B) *Incorrect.* Pressure-support ventilation delivers a constant inspiratory pressure. Less compliant lungs therefore will receive lower inspiratory volumes.
(C) *Incorrect.* An inspiratory effort of less than -2 cm H_2O may be assisted depending on the sensitivity settings on the ventilator.
(D) *Correct.* During weaning from mechanical ventilation, pressure-support ventilation decreases the overall work of breathing.
(E) *Incorrect.* Pressure-support ventilation is well tolerated by the patient and requires relatively little sedation.

REASONING:

Pressure-support ventilation is a mode of assisting and augmenting ventilation in the spontaneously breathing patient and thus is not appropriate for full ventilatory support. During pressure-support ventilation, the ventilator detects the patient's inspiratory effort that produces a negative deviation of proximal airway pressure from baseline. The ventilator sensitivity can be adjusted to detect larger or smaller patient efforts. The patient therefore determines the number of breaths per minute. Once activated by the patient's effort, the ventilator augments the patient's breath by providing a constant amount of proximal airway pressure until the inspiratory flow rate drops to 25 percent of the maximal inspiratory flow rate.[1] The ventilator then allows the pressure to return to baseline. The baseline pressure may either be zero or a preselected PEEP set independently. D is the best answer.

REFERENCES:

1. Marino P: The ICU Book, 2d ed. Baltimore, Williams & Wilkins, 1998, p. 440.
2. Barash PG, Cullen BF, Stoelting RK. Clinical Anesthesia, 4th ed. Philadelphia, Lippincott Williams & Wilkins, 2001, p. 1470.
3. Morgan GE, Mikhail MS, Murray MJ. Clinical Anesthesiology, 3d ed. New York, McGraw-Hill, 2002, p. 811.

Answer D

Pharmacology

QUESTION (Choose single best answer):

If administered epidurally in equipotent doses, which of the following opioids will produce analgesia over the greatest number of dermatomes?

(A) Fentanyl
(B) Hydromorphone
(C) Meperidine
(D) Morphine
(E) Sufentanil

CORRECT ANSWER: D

SUMMARY:

The onset and migration of epidurally administered opioids depend on the density, pK$_a$, molecular weight, protein binding, and lipid solubility of the drug. Of these, lipid solubility is the most influential factor controlling drug onset and degree of dermatomal spread. Highly lipid-soluble (thus hydrophobic) drugs such as sufentanil and fentanyl have relatively low dermatomal spread rostrally because of binding to lipophilic structures within the spinal cord that prevent spread. They will therefore not induce analgesia across as many dermatomes as lipid-insoluble or hydrophobic drugs such as morphine and hydromorphone. Morphine is slightly more hydrophilic than hydromorphone and is associated with the highest degree of rostral spread. Unfortunately, this also can lead to undesirable respiratory depression.

EXPLANATION:

(A) *Incorrect.* Fentanyl is highly lipophilic and associated with a low degree of rostral dermatomal spread.
(B) *Incorrect.* Hydromorphone, although relatively hydrophilic, is not as hydrophilic as morphine.
(C) *Incorrect.* Meperidine is not as hydrophilic as morphine.
(D) *Correct.* Morphine is the most hydrophilic and lipid-insoluble drug listed and is associated with the greatest degree of dermatomal spread.
(E) *Incorrect.* Sufentanil is the most lipophilic drug listed and will lead to the least dermatomal spread.

REASONING:

This question tests knowledge of opioids and their spread in the epidural space. Knowing that lipid-soluble drugs are associated with a small amount of rostral spread can assist the reader in eliminating fentanyl and sufentanil because these are highly lipophilic drugs. Although meperidine is not particularly lipid-soluble, it is less hydrophilic than morphine and dilaudid and can be eliminated. This leaves morphine and hydromorphone (which makes sense because these are the two most commonly administered epidural opioids in clinical practice). Morphine is just slightly more hydrophilic than hydromorphone (relative lipid solubility is 1 for morphine and 1.5 for hydromorphone). This makes morphine, choice D, the best answer.

REFERENCES:

Barash PG, Cullen BF, Stoelting RK. Clinical Anesthesia, 4th ed. Philadelphia, Lippincott Williams & Wilkins, 2001, pp. 1417–1422.

Wagemans MFM, Zuurmond WWA, de Lange JJ. Long-term spinal opioid therapy in terminally ill cancer pain patients. Oncologist 2:70–75, 1997.

Morgan GE, Mikhail MS, Murray MJ. Clinical Anesthesiology, 3d ed. New York, McGraw-Hill, 2002, p. 347, Table 18-14.

QUESTION (Choose single best answer):

Which of the following is decreased by alkalinization of a 1.5% lidocaine solution?

(A) Concentration of free base
(B) Dose required for anesthesia
(C) Duration of anesthesia
(D) Intracellular concentration of ionized lidocaine
(E) Time to onset of anesthesia

CORRECT ANSWER: E

SUMMARY:

Alkalinization of local anesthetic solutions has been used to hasten the onset of anesthesia for more than a century.[1] There are many likely reasons why alkalinization affects local anesthetic activity. Prepackaged local anesthetic solutions typically are acidotic, especially when they contain additional epinephrine. Alkalinizing these solutions increases the lipid-soluble neutral form of local anesthetic in solution that can cross into the neuronal cytoplasm to achieve effect.[2] Alkalinization also may potentiate the vasoconstrictive effects of epinephrine in situ. Alkalinization of the local neuronal environment also can inhibit neuronal impulse conduction.[3]

EXPLANATION:

(A) *Incorrect.* The concentration of free base would increase with alkalinization of lidocaine.
(B) *Incorrect.* Addition of alkalinizing agents such as bicarbonate does not affect the dose of anesthetic required for adequate analgesia because it does not alter the drug potency or duration of action.
(C) *Incorrect.* The duration of action of local anesthetics depends primarily on protein binding, tissue vascularity, use of vasoconstricting agents such as epinephrine, and the rate of drug elimination. None of these is altered by alkalinization.
(D) *Incorrect.* Alkalinization of lidocaine increases the intracellular concentration of its lipid-soluble neutral form (un-ionized). Once inside the cell, the neutral form will reach an equilibrium with the ionized form, which is the form that binds to the receptor within the sodium channel.
(E) *Correct.* Time to onset of lidocaine (and other local anesthetics) is reduced with the addition of bicarbonate. See above.

REASONING:

This question tests knowledge of the effects of alkalinization on the pharmacology of local anesthetic agents. Choice A can be eliminated easily because the base concentration would increase with alkalinization. Choices B and C can be eliminated because alkalinization does not affect potency or duration of action. Choice D is challenging and requires an understanding of the relationship between the degree of un-ionized fraction of drug and ease of movement across the cell membrane. Since it is primarily un-ionized drug that crosses the cell membrane, choice D does not make sense. E is the best choice because bicarbonate is the agent of choice for speeding onset of local anesthetics.

REFERENCES:

1. Curatolo M, Petersen-Felix S, Arendt-Nielsen L, et al. Adding sodium bicarbonate to lidocaine enhances the depth of epidural blockade. Anesth Analg 86(2):341–347, 1998.

2. Barash PG, Cullen BF, Stoelting RK. Clinical Anesthesia, 4th ed. Philadelphia, Lippincott Williams & Wilkins, 2001, pp. 455–456.

3. Wong K, Strichartz GR, Raymond SA. On the mechanisms of potentiation of local anesthetics by bicarbonate buffer: Drug structure-activity studies on isolated peripheral nerve. Anesth Analg 76(1):131–143, 1993.

4. Morgan GE, Mikhail MS, Murray MJ. Clinical Anesthesiology, 3d ed. New York, McGraw-Hill, 2002, pp. 234–238.

BOOK B:

Answer D

Pharmacology

QUESTION 43

QUESTION (Choose single best answer):

Cyanide toxicity from nitroprusside is unlikely in patients with renal dysfunction because

(A) Renal excretion of thiosulfate is decreased.
(B) Metabolic acidosis inactivates cyanide.
(C) Anemia inhibits breakdown of nitroprusside by oxyhemoglobin.
(D) Thiocyanate is formed in the liver.
(E) The dose of nitroprusside necessary to lower blood pressure is greatly decreased.

CORRECT ANSWER: D

SUMMARY:

Sodium nitroprusside (SNP) is a potent arteriolar and venous smooth muscle dilator that is used commonly as a hypotensive agent. Its mechanism of action involves the formation of nitric oxide. Metabolism of SNP produces potentially toxic compounds, including methemoglobin, thiocyanate, and cyanide.[1] Patients with renal dysfunction accumulate thiocyanate but are not at increased risk for cyanide toxicity.

EXPLANATION:

(A) *Incorrect.* Renal excretion of thiocyanate is decreased, not thiosulfate.
(B) *Incorrect.* Cyanide toxicity produces metabolic acidosis from its interaction with cytochrome oxidase enzymes and impairment of oxidative metabolism.
(C) *Incorrect.* SNP receives an electron from oxyhemoglobin inside red blood cells to produce methemoglobin and cyanide ions. Anemia is characterized by fewer red blood cells, but it does not inhibit the breakdown of SNP.
(D) *Correct.* Thiocyanate is formed in the liver by thiosulfate and cyanide ion in a reaction catalyzed by the enzyme rhodanase and vitamin B_{12}. Thiocyanate accumulates in patients with renal dysfunction because it is cleared primarily by the kidney.[2]
(E) *Incorrect.* The dose of SNP necessary to lower blood pressure is not decreased. In fact, patients with renal failure and hypertension may require higher doses of SNP if they develop tolerance to the hypotensive effect. Tachyphylaxis or acute tolerance to SNP may be an early sign of cyanide toxicity.

REASONING:

Unfortunately, this question is somewhat confusing because it indirectly implies that cyanide toxicity is less likely with renal dysfunction than in the absence of renal dysfunction, which clearly is not true. Indeed, these patients may need increased doses of SNP for blood pressure control, placing them at potentially increased risk for cyanide toxicity. Setting aside these concerns, the major difference with exposure to SNP in patients with renal failure is that they do not clear thiocyanate as well as patients with normal renal function and have an increased risk for thiocyanate toxicity. Thiocyanate toxicity can result in seizures and coma when it reaches plasma levels exceeding 60 mg/L.[1] The statement that most correctly articulates the differences in SNP toxicity in patients with renal dysfunction is D.

REFERENCES:

1. Friederich JA, Butterworth JF 4th. Nitroprusside: Twenty years and counting. Anesth Analg 81(1):152–162, 1995.
2. Barash PG, Cullen BF, Stoelting RK. Clinical Anesthesia, 4th ed. Philadelphia, Lippincott Williams & Wilkins, 2001, p. 773.
3. Morgan GE, Mikhail MS, Murray MJ. Clinical Anesthesiology, 3d ed. New York, McGraw-Hill, 2002, pp. 224, 225–227, Fig. 13-2, The Metabolism of Sodium Nitroprusside.

BOOK B:

Answer D

OB/Regional

QUESTION 44

QUESTION (Choose single best answer):

Twelve hours after an uneventful hysterectomy with lidocaine epidural anesthesia, a 70-year-old woman has partial paralysis of the lower extremities. She is receiving morphine 0.5 mg/h through an epidural catheter and is pain-free. On examination, definite motor loss is noted in the lower extremities, but no other deficits are apparent. The most appropriate action at this time is to

(A) Administer naloxone.
(B) Substitute fentanyl for morphine infusion.
(C) Remove the epidural catheter.
(D) Obtain magnetic resonance imaging (MRI) of the lumbar spine.
(E) Reassure the patient.

CORRECT ANSWER: D

SUMMARY:

Rare but potentially devastating neurologic complications associated with epidural anesthesia include epidural abscess or hematoma. Epidural hematomas can be associated with placement or removal of an epidural catheter and are seen most commonly in patients with a known coagulopathy, either drug-induced or owing to a disease process. The symptoms of abscess or hematoma include sharp back or leg pain with progression to numbness, motor weakness, or sphincter dysfunction. It is important to note that local anesthetics or narcotics being infused through the catheter may mask these symptoms. When this complication is suspected, immediate action must be taken. Neurologic imaging, preferably MRI, should be done to obtain a diagnosis. The treatment is surgical decompression.

EXPLANATION:

(A) *Incorrect.* The neurologic symptoms are not a result of morphine and would not be reversed by naloxone.
(B) *Incorrect.* Epidural narcotics do not cause motor blockade and are not likely to be responsible for the symptoms in this patient. Changing from morphine to fentanyl will not correct the problem.
(C) *Incorrect.* Removal of the catheter has been associated with epidural hematoma in patients with coagulopathy. The question states that the procedure was uneventful and does not mention any reason for the patient to be coagulopathic. However, it would be best to do further testing such as MRI and coagulation studies prior to removing the catheter.
(D) *Correct.* The patient has an unexplained neurologic deficit after epidural blockade. She should have an MRI to rule out the worst-case scenario, which would be epidural hematoma or abscess. It is important to note that the patient likely does not have pain associated with her symptoms because of the epidural morphine she is receiving.

(E) *Incorrect.* While every effort should be made to communicate with this patient and provide reassurance, this should be done *in addition* to determining the diagnosis. Reassurance and no action in this case could have devastating consequences.

REASONING:

This patient has motor blockade after a seemingly uneventful epidural anesthetic and surgical procedure. She is only receiving epidural morphine and no local anesthetic. This should provide analgesia without motor blockade. Twelve hours have passed since she received epidural lidocaine, which normally lasts 2 to 3 hours. Given the clinical situation, one must rule out a neurologic complication and obtain a spine MRI, which makes D the best answer.

REFERENCES:

Barash PG, Cullen BF, Stoelting RK. Clinical Anesthesia, 4th ed. Philadelphia, Lippincott Williams & Wilkins, 2001, p. 709.

Rainov NG, Heidecke V, Burkert WL. Epidural hematoma: Report of a case and review of the literature. Neurosurg Rev 18(1):53–60, 1995.

Morgan GE, Mikhail MS, Murray MJ. Clinical Anesthesiology, 3d ed. New York, McGraw-Hill, 2002, p. 279

BOOK B:

QUESTION 45

Answer A

Equipment/Physics

QUESTION (Choose single best answer):

Equipment that is attached to a patient should have leakage current no greater than

(A) 10 μA.
(B) 100 μA.
(C) 1 mA.
(D) 10 mA.
(E) 100 mA.

CORRECT ANSWER: A

SUMMARY:

Leakage current is current that leaks out of electrical equipment as a result of contact between internal electrical equipment and capacitance coupling or insulation that is defective. The threshold for causing ventricular fibrillation in a patient owing to transcutaneous electrical shock is approximately 100 mA. The maximum leakage current allowed in the operating room equipment is 10 μA. It should be noted that current that is delivered directly to the heart through low-impedance tissues (i.e., directly to the myocardium or through blood) can cause cardiac arrest with much smaller current (100 μA).

EXPLANATION:

(A) *Correct.* 10 μA is the maximum allowable leakage current because it is well below the level that can induce ventricular fibrillation if delivered in the form of microshock.

(B) *Incorrect.* 100 μA is the level at which microshock can induce ventricular fibrillation.

(C) *Incorrect.* 1 mA is 10 times the current that can induce ventricular fibrillation in the setting of microshock.

(D) *Incorrect.* 10 mA is 100 times the current that can induce ventricular fibrillation in the setting of microshock.

(E) *Incorrect.* 100 mA is 1000 times the current that can induce ventricular fibrillation in the setting of microshock.

REASONING:

This question tests knowledge of microshock and macroshock. In general terms, 100 μA is the minimum level of electric shock associated with potentially fatal arrythmias. Even if the reader did not know that the current standard leakage limit is less than 10 μA,[1] one might reason that a safe cutoff for electrical equipment would provide a margin of safety of either 1/10 or 1/100 that value. Given that 1 μA is not an option, your best choice is 10 μA. A is the single best answer.

REFERENCE:

1. Barash PG, Cullen BF, Stoelting RK. Clinical Anesthesia, 4th ed. Philadelphia, Lippincott Williams & Wilkins, 2001, pp. 155–157.
2. Morgan GE, Mikhail MS, Murray MJ. Clinical Anesthesiology, 3d ed. New York, McGraw-Hill, 2002, p. 21.

BOOK B:

Answer C

Basic Science

QUESTION 46

QUESTION (Choose single best answer):

When the inspired gas is changed from air to 20% oxygen and 80% nitrous oxide, Pao_2 increases because

(A) Increased pulmonary artery pressure perfuses alveoli that previously enhanced dead space.
(B) Nitrous oxide stimulates the respiratory center.
(C) Rapid absorption of nitrous oxide increases alveolar oxygen concentration.
(D) Replacement of nitrogen by nitrous oxide expands atelectatic alveoli.
(E) Respiratory depression from nitrous oxide shifts the oxyhemoglobin dissociation curve.

CORRECT ANSWER: C

SUMMARY:

The addition of inspired nitrous oxide can increase the alveolar partial pressure of other gases. This observation is explained by the concentrating effect—one of two components that describe the concentration effect.[1] The initial alveolar gas (i.e., air) consists of 21% oxygen. The new gas mixture consists of 20% oxygen and 80% nitrous oxide. Because nitrous oxide is more diffusible than oxygen, it will be absorbed more quickly from the alveolus. Theoretically, if half the nitrous oxide were absorbed rapidly, this would leave 20 parts oxygen and 40 parts nitrous oxide, approximately 20/60, or 33%, oxygen. A higher Fio_2 will lead to increased Pao_2.

EXPLANATION:

(A) *Incorrect.* Pulmonary artery resistance is increased slightly by administration of N_2O. This results in constriction of the pulmonary vasculature that would have the opposite effect on dead space (leading to decreased perfusion of ventilated lung).
(B) *Incorrect.* N_2O may cause an increase in respiratory rate, but it also decreases tidal volume, resulting in minute ventilation that is essentially unchanged.
(C) *Correct.* This describes the concentrating effect of N_2O on Pao_2 (alveolar partial pressure of oxygen). When alveolar oxygen concentration rises, the Pao_2 also increases. Please note that the second-gas effect is a special instance of the concentrating effect that describes administration of nitrous oxide in conjunction with a potent inhalational anesthetic.[1] Technically, this question does not describe the second-gas effect.
(D) *Incorrect.* Nitrous oxide does not expand atelectatic alveoli.
(E) *Incorrect.* Administration of N_2O does not shift the oxyhemoglobin dissociation curve.

REASONING:

This question tests knowledge of the concentrating effect of nitrous oxide on alveolar gases. Choices D and E are eliminated easily because the physiology described is not associated with administration of N_2O. Choice A can be eliminated by knowing that N_2O is associated with constriction of pulmonary vessels. Choice E is not a good answer because N_2O has little effect on the oxyhemoglobin dissociation curve. The best answer is C.

REFERENCE:

1. Barash PG, Cullen BF, Stoelting RK. Clinical Anesthesia, 4th ed. Philadelphia, Lippincott Williams & Wilkins, 2001, p. 384.
2. Morgan GE, Mikhail MS, Murray MJ. Clinical Anesthesiology, 3d ed. New York, McGraw-Hill, 2002, pp. 131–132.

BOOK B:

Answer B

Pharmacology

QUESTION 47

QUESTION (Choose single best answer):

Which of the following characteristics of local anesthetics is associated with long duration of action?

(A) High degree of lipid solubility
(B) High degree of protein binding
(C) High molecular weight
(D) High pK_a
(E) Presence of ester linkage

CORRECT ANSWER: B

SUMMARY:

The duration of action of local anesthetics is predominantly affected by the degree of protein binding of drug (the higher the proportion of protein-bound drug, the longer is the duration of action). Protein binding is a key factor determining duration of action because more prominent binding to membrane proteins near the sodium channel of nerves is thought to result in a longer mean residence time of the drug at the site of action. The most protein-bound local anesthetics are bupivicaine (95 percent), ropivacaine (94 percent), and etidocaine (95 percent).[1] Other factors influencing the duration of action of local anesthetics include dose (directly related), degree of tissue vascularity (inversely related), use of epinephrine (directly related), and rate of elimination (inversely related).

EXPLANATION:

(A) *Incorrect.* The degree of lipid solubility determines potency of local anesthetics because lipid-soluble drugs insert more easily into nerve cell membranes.
(B) *Correct.* Duration of action of local anesthetics is determined primarily by the degree of protein binding of the drug.
(C) *Incorrect.* Molecular weight does not affect duration of action.
(D) *Incorrect.* The pK_a of the drug relates to its speed of onset, not its duration of action.
(E) *Incorrect.* Ester linkages are found in ester-type local anesthetics (e.g., procaine, tetracaine, and chlorprocaine). These drugs are metabolized by plasma pseudo-cholinesterases and, as a group, have a shorter duration of action than amides. However, protein binding is the stronger determinant of duration of action.

REASONING:

This question tests knowledge of local anesthetic pharmacokinetics. Choices A and D can be eliminated by knowing that these properties determine onset, not duration of action, of local anesthetics. Choice D is incorrect because molecular weight is not a pharmaco-kinetic property of these drugs. Choice E is tempting because it does refer to a category of local anesthetics that are associated with a shorter duration of action. However, the degree of protein binding is the most influential factor even within these two categories of drugs (both esters and amides), and thus B is the best answer.

REFERENCE:

1. Stoelting RK. Pharmacology and Physiology in Anesthetic Practice, 3d ed. Philadelphia, Lippincott Williams & Wilkins, 1999, p. 160, Table 7-1.
2. Morgan GE, Mikhail MS, Murray MJ. Clinical Anesthesiology, 3d ed. New York, McGraw-Hill, 2002, p. 235.

BOOK B:

Answer B

Pharmacology

QUESTION 48

QUESTION (Choose single best answer):

Which of the following drugs used to produce or reverse muscle relaxation has the greatest prolongation of action in a patient with end-stage renal disease?

(A) Atracurium
(B) Neostigmine
(C) Pancuronium
(D) Succinylcholine
(E) Vecuronium

CORRECT ANSWER: B

SUMMARY:

Most neuromuscular blocking drugs are associated with some degree of renal elimination. Among the nondepolarizing muscle relaxants, pancuronium is associated with the highest degree of renal excretion (up to 60 percent) and should be avoided in patients with renal failure. Atracurium and cisatracurium are metabolized by nonspecific plasma esterases and degradation via Hoffmann elimination. These elimination pathways are independent of renal function. Succinylcholine is metabolized by pseudocholinesterases that can be decreased (but not profoundly) in the setting of renal failure. They have a minimal effect on duration of action. Neostigmine is associated with a 50 to 55 percent renal clearance, and the duration of action is increased two- to threefold in the setting of renal failure.[1] Vecuronium is eliminated predominately by the liver but does have about 30 percent renal excretion. An intubating dose of vecuronium has approximately 50 percent prolonged duration of action in the setting of end-stage renal disease.[2]

EXPLANATION:

(A) **Incorrect.** Atracurium is metabolized by nonspecific plasma esterases and by Hoffmann degradation. Both are not influenced by renal function.

(B) **Correct.** The duration of action of neostigmine may be increased two- to threefold in the setting of renal failure because renal elimination accounts for approximately 50 to 55 percent of its clearance. In comparing the duration of action of neostigmine with that of nondepolarizing agents (NDMRs), Stoelting states that the duration of action is as long as, if not longer than, that of NDMRs, making the occurrence of recurarization unlikely.[1] The dosage of anticholinesterases does not have to be altered in patients with reduced renal.[2]

(C) **Incorrect.** Although the duration of action of pancuronium is increased in the setting of renal failure, the extent of this change is less than with the anti-cholinesterase drugs (e.g., neostigmine, edrophonium, and pyridostigmine).[3–5]

(D) *Incorrect.* There is minimally significant prolongation of action with succinyl-choline in the setting of renal failure.

(E) *Incorrect.* Vecuronium is metabolized primarily by the liver and has only about 30 percent renal excretion. Its duration of action is prolonged in end-stage renal disease, but not to the extent of neostigmine.

REASONING:

This question tests knowledge of the elimination pathways of common anesthetic agents. Choices A, D, and E can be eliminated immediately because these drugs are not eliminated primarily by the kidney. The duration of action for both pancuronium and neostigmine is prolonged in renal failure, and therefore, both could be appropriate choices. However, the extent of the increase in duration of action is higher with anticholinesterase drugs than with neuromuscular blocking drugs, including pancuronium. The single best answer is B.

REFERENCES:

1. Stoelting, RK. Pharmacology and Physiology in Anesthetic Practice, 3d ed. Philadelphia, Lippincott Williams & Wilkins, 1999, pp. 203, 226–228, Table 9-1.

2. Barash PG, Cullen BF, Stoelting RK. Clinical Anesthesia, 4th ed. Philadelphia, Lippincott Williams & Wilkins, 2001, pp. 1012–1014.

3. Cronnelly R, Stanski DR, Miller RD, et al. Renal function and the pharmacokinetics of neostigmine in anesthetized man. Anesthesiology 51(3):222–226, 1979.

4. Cronnelly R, Stanski DR, Miller RD, Sheiner LB. Pyridostigmine kinetics with and without renal function. Clin Pharmacol Ther 28(1):78–81, 1980.

5. Morris RB, Cronnelly R, Miller RD, et al. Pharmacokinetics of edrophonium in anephric and renal transplant patients. Br J Anaesth 53(12):1311–1314, 1981.

6. Morgan GE, Mikhail MS, Murray MJ. Clinical Anesthesiology, 3d ed. New York, McGraw-Hill, 2002, pp. 194–195.

BOOK B:

QUESTION 49

Answer B

Neuroanesthesia

QUESTION (Choose single best answer):

In a patient with chronic congestive heart failure, the safest pharmacologic approach to brain swelling during a craniotomy is

(A) Dexamethasone.
(B) Furosemide.
(C) Mannitol.
(D) Thiopental.
(E) Urea.

CORRECT ANSWER: B

SUMMARY:

Treatment of intracranial hypertension is directed at decreasing the volume in one of the following components of the cranial compartment: brain, blood, or cerebrospinal fluid (CSF). Common pharmacologic therapies include osmotic diuretics such as mannitol and urea, diuretics such as furosemide, and corticosteroids. Barbiturates such as thiopental can be used to achieve burst suppression on the electroencephalogram (EEG), but there is controversy over whether this changes outcome.[1] Nonpharmacologic treatment of increased intracranial pressure (ICP) includes proper positioning, hypothermia, sedation, hyperventilation, and surgical decompression and/or drainage of CSF.

EXPLANATION:

(A) *Incorrect.* Dexamethasone, a glucocorticoid, is effective in treating intracranial hypertension from vasogenic edema owing to tumor or abcess. It has not been shown to have any benefit in cerebral edema owing to head trauma.[1] It also has little effect on the cardiovascular system but can cause hyperglycemia that might worsen clinical outcome in the setting of ischemic brain injury if left untreated.[2]

(B) **Correct.** Furosemide, a loop diuretic, decreases intracranial water and decreases CSF formation. It may benefit the patient with congestive heart failure (CHF) by lowering preload through diuresis but also may result in electrolyte abnormalities.

(C) *Incorrect.* Mannitol, an osmotic diuretic, lowers ICP by extracting water from the intracranial compartment into the intravascular space. This may result in acute fluid overload and pulmonary edema in a patient with CHF.

(D) *Incorrect.* Thiopental, a barbiturate, can decrease cerebral blood flow and therefore ICP. It also can be used to achieve burst-suppression coma as a last resort for treatment of intracranial hypertension.[1] However, it may cause direct myocardial depression and should not be used in a patient with CHF.

(E) *Incorrect.* Urea is an osmotic diuretic with the same mechanism and contraindications for use as mannitol.[3]

REASONING:

This is a challenging question that tests knowledge of the pathophysiology of intracranial hypertension and congestive heart failure. Choices C and E can be ruled out easily because the mechanism of osmotic diuresis can result in fluid overload. Choice D also can be eliminated because thiopental is not a first-line agent to treat intracranial hypertension and can cause hypotension and decreased cardiac output. Differentiating between choices A and B is difficult because while furosemide can be used to treat intracranial hypertension as well as congestive heart failure, it is not without potentially harmful side effects. Dexamethasone is not effective in treating all causes of intracranial hypertension and has a slow time to onset. Although it has no adverse cardiovascular side effects, it can lead to hyperglycemia that can worsen ischemic brain injury.[4] In this patient, prompt treatment of the brain swelling during craniotomy is required, and furosemide will achieve the effect in an expedient and safe manner. Indeed, the associated diuresis provides additional therapeutic benefit in this patient with congestive heart failure. B is the best answer.

REFERENCES:

1. Cottrell JE, Smith JS. Anesthesia and Neurosurgery, 4th ed. St Louis, Mosby, 2001, pp. 210–211.
2. Pasternak JJ, McGregor DG, Lanier WL. Effect of single-dose dexamethasone on blood glucose concentration in patients undergoing craniotomy. Neurosurg Anesthesiol 16(2):122–125, 2004.
3. Hardman JG, Limbird LE, Goodman AG. Goodman and Gilman's The Pharmacologic Basis of Therapeutics, 10th ed. New York, McGraw-Hill, 2001, pp. 767–769.
4. Barash PG, Cullen BF, Stoelting RK. Clinical Anesthesia, 4th ed. Philadelphia, Lippincott Williams & Wilkins, 2001, p. 940.
5. Morgan GE, Mikhail MS, Murray MJ. Clinical Anesthesiology, 3d ed. New York, McGraw-Hill, 2002, pp. 156–159, 568–569.

BOOK B: **QUESTION 50**

Answer A

Clinical Anesthesia

QUESTION (Choose single best answer):

In clinical anesthesia practice, the term *informed consent* is best described as a legal concept in which patients

(A) Agree to anesthesia care based on full disclosure of the facts needed to make the decision intelligently.

(B) Are told of all possible risks of anesthesia and anesthetic procedures.

(C) Delegate all decisions regarding anesthesia care to the anesthesiologist.

(D) Release the physicians from liability.

(E) Sign global consent forms for surgical procedures that cover the administration of anesthesia care.

SUMMARY:

On establishing a doctor-patient relationship, an anesthesiologist assumes the general responsibilities that all physicians have in the care of patients. Among these are obtaining informed consent and adherence to a standard of care while providing treatment to the patient. Informed consent may be written, verbal, or implied, with the main objective that the patient is provided a fair and reasonable account of the proposed procedure. Disclosure of all possible risks is unrealistic, and the guideline requires discussion within the scope of reasonable risk for the individual patient. Anesthetic procedures are distinct from surgical procedures and therefore cannot be covered under surgical consent. With the exception of individuals who are unconscious or unable to consent, treatment of patients without informed consent places the anesthesiologist at risk for criminal battery charges. An anesthesiologist still can be held liable in a malpractice suit if breach of duty, reasonable causation, or damage occur during anesthetic care.

EXPLANATION:

(A) **Correct.** See above.
(B) **Incorrect.** Discussion of *all* possible risks of anesthesia to a layperson is often not feasible, and in certain instances, some risks are not foreseeable.
(C) **Incorrect.** Part of informed consent is to assist patients in making intelligent decisions when given the pertinent information. The patient still makes decision regarding his or her anesthetic care. Once the patient is sedated or unconscious, it is the anesthesiologist's responsibility to act within the reasonable scope of the patient wishes.
(D) **Incorrect.** See above.
(E) **Incorrect.** See above.

REASONING:

This question tests knowledge of informed consent. The reader should be able to identify the correct answer even without detailed knowledge of the legal definition. Phrases such as *all possible risks, global consent,* and *all decisions* should be viewed with the suspicion usually placed on all such absolute and inclusionary phrasing. A is the best answer.

REFERENCE:

Barash PG, Cullen BF, Stoelting RK. Clinical Anesthesia, 4th ed. Philadelphia, Lippincott Williams & Wilkins, 2001, pp. 93–95.
Morgan GE, Mikhail MS, Murray MJ. Clinical Anesthesiology, 3d ed. New York, McGraw-Hill, 2002, pp. 8–9.

BOOK B: **QUESTION 51**

Answer C

OB/Regional

QUESTION (Choose single best answer):

The low fetal/maternal plasma ratio of bupivicaine compared with lidocaine is due to

(A) Fetal tissue binding.
(B) Fetal plasma protein binding.
(C) Maternal plasma protein binding.
(D) Ionization in maternal blood.
(E) Ionization in fetal blood.

CORRECT ANSWER: C

SUMMARY:

Fetal plasma drug concentration depends on delivery of drug to the placenta via the uterine artery, transfer of drug across the placenta, and fetal uptake. Assuming constant uterine artery blood flow, transfer of free drug (i.e., not protein-bound) from the maternal to fetal circulation can be described by the Fick equation, that is,

$$\frac{\Delta q}{\Delta t} = \frac{KA(C_m - C_f)}{X}$$

where $\Delta q/\Delta t$ represents rate of transfer of the drug, A is the surface area of the membrane, C_m is the maternal drug concentration, C_f is the fetal drug concentration, X is the thickness of the membrane, and K is a diffusion constant determined by drug properties such as molecular weight, lipid solubility, degree of ionization, and spatial configuration. Simply put, the surface area and membrane thickness will remain constant, so nonionized, lipid-soluble, non-protein-bound drugs will cross the placenta more readily. Bupivicaine is highly protein bound and therefore does not cross the placenta as easily as lidocaine. (See also Question 102, Book B.)

EXPLANATION:

(A) *Incorrect.* Local anesthetics have limited fetal tissue binding.

(B) *Incorrect.* Fetal plasma protein binding is less than maternal for both lidocaine and bupivicaine and therefore would facilitate transfer from the fetal circulation to maternal circulation.[1]

(C) *Correct.* Bupivicaine is approximately 95 percent protein bound compared with lidocaine, which is approximately 50 percent protein bound.[1]

(D) *Incorrect.* Both lidocaine and bupivicaine are weak bases. The pK_a of lidocaine is 7.8, and the pK_a of bupivicaine is 8.1. However, only the non-protein-bound free drug is available for ionization, which is significantly less with bupivicaine than with lidocaine. The difference in pK_a is not enough to compensate for the high protein binding of bupivicaine.

(E) *Incorrect.* Ionization in fetal blood occurs when fetal acidosis is present. The difference in pH between the maternal and fetal circulations causes increased concentration of the ionized form of the local anesthetic and impedes transfer. This question does not refer to the acidotic fetus.

REASONING:

To answer this question, one must know that placental transfer of local anesthetic occurs when the drug is small, nonionized, and non-protein-bound. Bupivicaine is the most protein bound of the local anesthetics in common obstetrical practice.[1] Choice A refers to fetal tissue binding, which is not a significant property of local anesthetics. Choice B can be eliminated because fetal protein binding would cause a high fetal-to-maternal plasma concentration ratio. Choice E can be eliminated because the question does not refer to the acidotic fetus. Differentiating between choices C and D is difficult because the difference in pK_a between lidocaine and bupivicaine actually would result in more un-ionized form of bupivicaine, which intuitively would lead to more placental transfer. However, the important concept is that bupivicaine is so highly protein bound that the amount of free, nonionized drug available for transfer across the placenta is less than lidocaine. C is the best answer.

REFERENCE:

1. Hughes SC, Levinson G, Rosen MA. Shnider and Levinson's Anesthesia for Obstetrics, 4th ed. Philadelphia, Lippincott Williams & Wilkins, 2002, pp. 62–64.
2. Morgan GE, Mikhail MS, Murray MJ. Clinical Anesthesiology, 3d ed. New York, McGraw-Hill, 2002, pp. 233–241, 808–811, Table 14-1 (pp. 236–237), Physicochemical Properties of Local Anesthetics.

Answer B

Clinical Anesthesia

QUESTION (Choose single best answer):

A previously healthy 28-year-old man is admitted to the emergency department with a probable opioid overdose. Arterial blood gas values are Pa_{O_2} 49 mm Hg, Pa_{CO_2} 76 mm Hg, and pH 7.12 while breathing room air. Which of the following statements is true?

(A) Aspiration of gastric contents must have occurred.
(B) Hypoventilation alone can explain the acidosis and hypoxemia.
(C) The hypoxemia probably is due to noncardiogenic pulmonary edema.
(D) Naloxone should be administered only if the patient is normothermic.
(E) Pure oxygen is contraindicated.

CORRECT ANSWER: B

SUMMARY:

Acute respiratory acidosis may take time to correct because of delayed renal compensation. These arterial blood gas values demonstrate a pure respiratory acidosis, as approximated by the decrease in pH of 0.08 unit for every 10 mm Hg increase in Pa_{CO_2} above 40 mm Hg. It is important to ensure adequate oxygenation in this patient with impaired ventilation. If an opioid overdose is suspected, naloxone should be administered to antagonize its effect and possibly circumvent tracheal intubation and mechanical ventilation.

EXPLANATION:

(A) *Incorrect.* Significant gastric aspiration can result in hypoxia secondary to pulmonary shunting, along with pulmonary edema, pulmonary hypertension, and hypercapnia. Physical findings such as wheezing, tachycardia, and tachypnea also would be expected to occur with such a significant acidosis. Although this choice is possible, the absence of these findings makes it less likely to be correct.

(B) *Correct.* Acute respiratory acidosis due to hypoventilation may be extreme owing to the limited buffering capacity of hemoglobin and exchange of extracellular H^+ ion for intracellular cations. Renal compensatory response is slow, requiring days to achieve an effect. In general, every 10 mm Hg increase in Pa_{CO_2} yields a corresponding decrease in pH of 0.08 in the setting of acute respiratory acidosis.

(C) *Incorrect.* Noncardiogenic pulmonary edema reflects disruption of the alveolar/capillary membrane in the setting of nonelevated (<18 mm Hg) PAOP and results in shunting and hypoxemia. Noncardiogenic pulmonary edema can be seen after neurologic injury (neurogenic pulmonary edema), in transfusion-related acute lung injury (TRALI), or even after vigorous inspiration against a closed glottis (negative-pressure pulmonary edema). This patient was previously healthy, and there is no indication that these injuries have occurred.

(D) *Incorrect.* Hypothermia is not a contraindication to naloxone administration. There is no indication in this scenario that the respiratory acidosis is due to hypothermia.

(E) *Incorrect.* Tissue hypoxia can be significant in severe acidosis. Cardiovascular function and response to catecholamines are already compromised. Adequate oxygenation is essential for a hypoxic patient, and delivery of 100% oxygen is important for the patient's treatment.

REASONING:

This question tests knowledge of interpretation of arterial blood gas analyses. One always should be wary of obligatory statements such as "must have occurred" or inclusionary

333

statements such as "hypoventilation alone can explain. . . ." In this case, choice A can be excluded easily because aspiration of gastric contents cannot be diagnosed definitively solely from blood gas analysis. Choices C, D, and E reasonably can be excluded with a basic understanding of the principles of blood gas interpretation. The reader should take a moment to ensure a thorough understanding of acid-base interpretation and treatment.[1] The best answer is B.

REFERENCE:

1. Barash PG, Cullen BF, Stoelting RK. Clinical Anesthesia, 4th ed. Philadelphia, Lippincott Williams & Wilkins, 2001, pp. 165–170.
2. Morgan GE, Mikhail MS, Murray MJ. Clinical Anesthesiology, 3d ed. New York, McGraw-Hill, 2002, pp. 252, 652.

BOOK B: **QUESTION 53**

Answer A

Cardiovascular

QUESTION (Choose single best answer):

In which of following clinical circumstances does downregulation of beta-adrenergic receptors occur?

(A) Chronic congestive heart failure
(B) Hypothyroidism
(C) Long-term clonidine administration
(D) Long-term metoprolol administration
(E) Stable angina

CORRECT ANSWER: A

SUMMARY:

Beta-receptor downregulation is associated with any condition that chronically elevates circulating catecholamines. Beta-receptor downregulation is an established finding in patients with chronic congestive heart failure.[1] There is some evidence in animal models that associates beta-receptor downregulation with hypothyroidism.[2,3] However, this observation does not appear to have been corroborated yet in humans.

EXPLANATION:

(A) **Correct.** Patients with heart failure have a markedly decreased myocardial beta-adrenergic receptor density and response to beta-adrenergic agonists.[1] The downregulation of beta-adrenergic receptors is attributed to increased norepinephrine levels in the failing heart.[1]
(B) **Incorrect.** There is some animal data to suggest an association of beta-receptor downregulation and hypothyroidism, but this has not yet been proven in humans.
(C) **Incorrect.** Reduction of central sympathetic outflow by clonidine causes upregulation of beta-adrenoreceptors.[4]
(D) **Incorrect.** Long-term metoprolol administration results in upregulation of receptors.[5]
(E) **Incorrect.** Stable angina would not be expected to lead to adrenoreceptor downregulation.

REASONING:

This is a question tests knowledge of beta-receptor physiology and its clinical implications. There is an inverse relationship between receptor density and the level of circulating catecholamines. The question is made somewhat more challenging by animal data that imply an association between hypothyroidism and downregulation of beta-adrenergic receptors. However, choice A is clearly a well-known association with CHF and is the best answer.

REFERENCES:

1. Braunwald D, Zipes P. Heart Disease: A Textbook of Cardiovascular Medicine, 6th ed. Philadelphia, Saunders, 2001, p. 522.
2. Germack R, Starzec A, Perret GY. Regulation of beta$_1$- and beta$_3$-adrenergic agonist-stimulated lipolytic response in hyperthyroid and hypothyroid rat white adipocytes. Br J Pharmacol 129(3):448–456, 2000.
3. Rubio A, Raasmaja A, Maia AL, et al. Effects of thyroid hormone on norepinephrine signaling in brown adipose tissue: I. Beta$_1$- and beta$_2$-adrenergic receptors and cyclic adenosine 3',5'-monophosphate generation. Endocrinology 136(8):3267–3276, 1995.
4. Zoukos Y, Thomaides T, Pavitt DV, et al. Beta-adrenoceptor expression on circulating mononuclear cells of idiopathic Parkinson's disease and autonomic failure patients before and after reduction of central sympathetic outflow by clonidine. Neurology 43(6):1181–1187, 1993.
5. Heilbrunn SM, Shah P, Bristow MR, et al. Increased beta-receptor density and improved hemodynamic response to catecholamine stimulation during long-term metoprolol therapy in heart failure from dilated cardiomyopathy. Circulation 79(3):483–490, 1989.
6. Miller RD, Miller ED, Reves JG, et al. Anesthesia, 5th ed. New York, Churchill Livingstone, 2000, p. 544.

BOOK B:

Answer E

Clinical Anesthesia

QUESTION 54

QUESTION (Choose single best answer):

Which of the following is the most likely cause of apnea occurring after a retrobulbar block?

(A) Epidural injection
(B) Increased intracranial pressure
(C) Oculopontine reflex
(D) Ophthalmic artery injection
(E) Subarachnoid injection

CORRECT ANSWER: E

SUMMARY:

Retrobulbar block for eye surgery involves the injection of local anesthetic into the muscle cone behind the globe. The most common complication is retrobulbar hemorrhage secondary to vessel puncture. The postretrobulbar apnea syndrome *is due to infiltration of local anesthetic into the cerebrospinal fluid (CSF) probably from penetration of the meningeal sheaths that encase the optic nerve. Besides apnea, signs of CSF infiltration may include shivering, paraplegia (hemi- or quadroplegia), hyperreflexia, and cranial nerve blockade.*

EXPLANATION:

(A) *Incorrect.* There is no "epidural" space in the retrobulbar region.
(B) *Incorrect.* The block is not performed intracranially, so it is not likely to cause increased intracranial pressure (ICP). Increased ICP may cause respiratory derangements (Cushing's triad), but it is a late sign.
(C) *Incorrect.* There is no "oculopontine reflex." This is a distracter term that sounds similar to the oculocardiac reflex that causes bradycardia.
(D) *Incorrect.* Intraarterial injection of local anesthetic causes seizures.
(E) *Correct.* High levels of local anesthetic in the CSF can cause unconsciousness and apnea.

This question tests knowledge of the potential complications of retrobulbar blockade for eye surgery. Retrobulbar blocks are performed blindly. The needle is advanced into the orbit without visualizing the structures that are encountered along the way or where, exactly, the needle is placed. Local anesthetic may be injected into any structure: vein, artery, nerve, or the eye itself. The most likely complication in this patient is inadvertent brain stem anesthesia from subarachnoid injection. The best answer is E.

REFERENCE:

Barash PG, Cullen BF, Stoelting RK. Clinical Anesthesia, 4th ed. Philadelphia, Lippincott Williams & Wilkins, 2001, pp. 977–979.
Morgan GE, Mikhail MS, Murray MJ. Clinical Anesthesiology, 3d ed. New York, McGraw-Hill, 2002, p. 766.

BOOK B:

Answer E

Cardiovascular

QUESTION 55

QUESTION (Choose single best answer):

A 40-year-old man is undergoing open reduction and internal fixation of a fractured femur. During anesthesia with fentanyl, enflurane, and oxygen, his heart rate decreases to 20 beats per minute, and 6 premature ventricular contractions per minute are noted. No pulse is detected. The most appropriate next step is to

(A) Administer atropine.
(B) Administer epinephrine.
(C) Administer lidocaine.
(D) Apply a transthoracic pacemaker.
(E) Start cardiopulmonary resuscitation.

CORRECT ANSWER: E

SUMMARY:

Enflurane, as well as isoflurane and halothane, depresses the sinoatrial (SA) node rate and prolongs conduction through the atrioventricular (AV) node, which can result in junctional rhythms or slow sinus rates with escape beats. Regardless of the type of anesthetic used, a patient without a detectable pulse has insufficient tissue perfusion, and cardiopulmonary resuscitation (CPR) should be initiated immediately. This patient shows electrical activity on the monitor but no detectable pulse. This clinical presentation is described as pulseless electrical activity (PEA). The most common causes of PEA are known as the "five H's and five T's"—hypovolemia, hypoxia, hydrogen ion acidosis, hyper/hypokalemia, and hypothermia and tablets (overdose), tamponade, tension pneumothorax, coronary thrombosis, and pulmonary thrombosis. After initiating supportive measures for the patient with PEA, the root cause should be identified and treated.

EXPLANATION:

(A) **Incorrect.** Atropine may increase the electrical rate but not pressure. Without a pulse, there will not be any mechanism to circulate the drug.
(B) **Incorrect.** Epinephrine has both chronotropic and vasopressor properties. Without a pulse, there will not be any mechanism to circulate the drug.
(C) **Incorrect.** Lidocaine has some antiarrythmic properties, but like all local anesthetics, it decreases depolarization rates and has negative inotropic properties.[1] Lidocaine typically is used for premature ventricular beats, stable ventricular tachycardia, and refractory ventricular fibrillation/pulseless ventricular tachycardia. However, without a pulse, there will not be any mechanism to circulate the drug.

(D) *Incorrect.* A transthoracic pacemaker will take precious time to institute and will only increase rate, not provide for a blood pressure. The American Heart Association describes transthoracic pacing as a "disappointing" treatment for PEA.

(E) *Correct.* CPR is the most appropriate next step in a patient without a pulse.

REASONING:

The patient with PEA may need all the interventions listed in the choices to survive. However, without a discernible pulse pressure, medication administered may not be distributed to the sites of action. The primary survey for a patient with PEA involves chest compressions, the secondary survey has the rescuer administering drugs and assessing for pseudo-PEA (blood flow present but too low to be felt by palpation), and finally, treating for reversible causes.

REFERENCES:

1. Miller RD, Miller ED, Reves JG, et al. Anesthesia, 5th ed. New York, Churchill Livingstone, 2000, p. 512.
2. Advanced Cardiac Life Support. Dallas, American Heart Association, 2003, pp. 36, 83, 99.
3. Morgan GE, Mikhail MS, Murray MJ. Clinical Anesthesiology, 3d ed. New York, McGraw-Hill, 2002, p. 363.

BOOK B:

Answer D

Cardiovascular

QUESTION 56

QUESTION (Choose single best answer):

A 35-year-old woman with systemic lupus erythematosus is admitted to the critical care unit following sudden onset of severe chest pain. Examination shows tachycardia, hypotension, pulmonary edema, and a blowing systolic murmur in the left parasternal region. The most appropriate management is

(A) Aerosol administration of terbutaline.
(B) Intravenous infusion of phenylephrine and nitroglycerin.
(C) Intravenous infusion of esmolol.
(D) Intravenous infusion of epinephrine and nitroprusside.
(E) Volume loading with lactated Ringer's solution.

CORRECT ANSWER: D

SUMMARY:

Systemic lupus erythematosus (SLE) can have various cardiac manifestations, including pericarditis, myocarditis, coronary artery disease, dysrhythmias, and valvular disease.[1] Over 50 percent of patients with SLE have been shown to have valvular abnormalities on echocardiographic studies. These are commonly noninfectious vegetations known as Libman-Sacks endocarditis *and affect the mitral and aortic valves.[1] Pathology of the valves includes thickening and fibrosis that eventually may cause retraction of the valves and result in insufficiency or stenosis. The clinical constellation described is one of acute mitral insufficiency. Mitral regurgitation causes volume overload of the left ventricle, resulting in decreased cardiac output and elevated left atrial pressure (LAP). This is manifested clinically by tachycardia, hypotension, and pulmonary edema.[2]*

EXPLANATION:

(A) *Incorrect.* Aerosolized terbutaline is a beta-adrenergic agonist used to treat asthma. This does not address the patient's clinical problem.

(B) *Incorrect.* Intravenous infusion of phenylephrine may increase blood pressure, but it also will increase systemic vascular resistance and therefore worsen mitral regurgitation.[2] Nitroglycerin might help to vasodilate the coronary arteries but also may dilate venous capacitance vessels, resulting in decreased ventricular preload.[2]

(C) **Incorrect.** Intravenous infusion of esmolol is contraindicated because a goal of management is to maintain a normal to slightly elevated heart rate. This serves to decrease time for regurgitation in the cardiac cycle and improve cardiac output.[2]

(D) **Correct.** Intravenous infusion of epinephrine may improve contractility and chronotropy. Nitroprusside may decrease systemic vascular resistance, promoting forward flow and decreasing the regurgitant flow.[2]

(E) **Incorrect.** Volume loading with lactated Ringer's solution is contraindicated because the patient's problem is not inadequate preload but an inability of the left ventricle to maintain forward flow. Volume loading will further volume overload the left ventricle and increase the regurgitant volume.[2]

REASONING:

This question tests knowledge of the pathophysiology of acute mitral regurgitation. Choice A can be eliminated immediately by knowing that the problem is not pulmonary but cardiac in origin. The next step is to determine that the signs and symptoms suggest valvular regurgitation. This is especially challenging because the symptoms could be consistent with aortic insufficiency (AI) as well. Knowing that the murmur of AI is primarily diastolic would help to differentiate between these two etiologies. Fortunately, goals in management are similar for both mitral and aortic regurgitation: maintaining normal to elevated heart rate, gentle vasodilation, maintaining cardiac output, and avoiding fluid overloading.[2] Thus choices B, C, and E also may be ruled out. D is the best answer.

REFERENCES:

1. Braunwald D, Zipes P. Heart Disease, 6th ed. Philadelphia, Saunders, 2001, pp. 2204–2206.
2. Miller RD, Miller ED, Reves JG, et al. Anesthesia, 5th ed. New York, Churchill Livingstone, 2000, pp. 1768–1770.
3. Morgan GE, Mikhail MS, Murray MJ. Clinical Anesthesiology, 3d ed. New York, McGraw-Hill, 2002, pp. 412–414, 419–420.

BOOK B:

QUESTION 57

Answer A

Pharmacology

QUESTION (Choose single best answer):

The following table shows the pharmacokinetic effects of a new neuromuscular blocker.

	Normal	Renal Failure
Volume of distribution	15 L	21 L
Clearance	200 mL/min	100 mL/min

In a patient with renal failure, which of the following will result in a response to this drug most similar to that of a normal individual?

(A) Increased loading dose
(B) The same maintenance dose
(C) Decreased maintenance dose interval
(D) Avoidance of continuous infusion
(E) Increased dose of anticholinesterase for reversal

CORRECT ANSWER: A

SUMMARY:

The volume of distribution (V_d) is the apparent volume in which a drug is distributed. It is determined by a drug's lipid solubility, amount of protein binding, and organ perfusion. A large V_d implies extensive spread and tissue uptake of a drug so that a smaller fraction is available at the effector site. In a patient with a large V_d, as in renal failure, a larger dose may be required initially to achieve the same therapeutic level. The clearance is the rate of a drug's elimination either by metabolism or excretion and, along with redistribution, helps to terminate the drug's effect. Administering the same maintenance dose given to a normal patient or using continuous infusion when a drug's clearance is compromised by renal failure can result in undesirable prolonged drug effects. Decreasing the maintenance dose interval is a possible option but may result in periods of subtherapeutic drug levels. The volume of distribution of the anticholinesterase drug neostigmine is not affected significantly by renal failure, and the loading dose would not need to be increased.[1]

EXPLANATION:

(A) **Correct.** A larger volume of distribution (V_d) means that a larger loading dose is necessary to achieve the same drug plasma concentration. We assume that the response in the question is the time to onset of neuromuscular blockade.

(B) **Incorrect.** This will result in drug accumulation.

(C) **Incorrect.** This will result in drug accumulation.

(D) **Incorrect.** This is a somewhat vaguely worded choice. If the continuous infusion were adjusted to clearance (half the rate), this would not be a problem. We are not given this information and assume that the constant infusion is at the same rate as for a healthy patient. This would result in drug accumulation.

(E) **Incorrect.** The pharmacokinetics of neostigmine have been studied in patients with renal failure using a two-compartment model. The volume of distribution is not affected significantly, and the loading dose of neostigmine would not need to be increased.[1]

REASONING:

This question tests knowledge of pharmacokinetics and the concept of volume of distribution. A decreased renal clearance does not preclude use of a continuous infusion as long as the maintenance dose or dosing interval or both are decreased. There is considerable ambiguity regarding what "response" is being measured and the proposed dose of the continuous infusion. An increased loading dose and an increased dosing interval or a reduced infusion rate would be the most complete answer to this question. Considering these limitations, A seems like the best answer.

REFERENCES:

1. Cronnelly R, Stanski DR, Miller RD, et al. Renal function and the pharmacokinetics of neostigmine in anesthetized man. Anesthesiology 51(3):222–226, 1979.

2. Barash PG, Cullen BF, Stoelting RK. Clinical Anesthesia, 4th ed. Philadelphia, Lippincott Williams & Wilkins, 2001, pp. 249–254.

3. Morgan GE, Mikhail MS, Murray MJ. Clinical Anesthesiology, 3d ed. New York, McGraw-Hill, 2002, p. 153.

Answer A

Physiology

QUESTION (Choose single best answer)

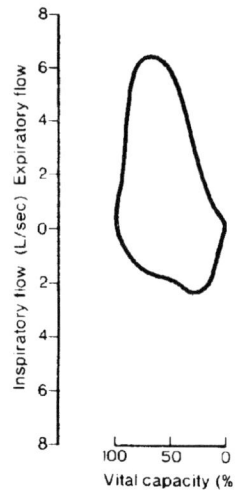

The flow-volume loop shown above is most likely from a patient with which of the following?

(A) Bilateral vocal cord paralysis
(B) Chronic bronchitis
(C) Tracheal stenosis 6 months after a previous tracheostomy
(D) Tumor of the lower trachea
(E) Normal respiratory status

CORRECT ANSWER: A

SUMMARY:

Flow-volume loops can be used to differentiate different types of obstructive and restrictive pulmonary diseases. The subject is asked to inhale fully to total lung capacity, then to exhale completely, and finally, to inhale maximally back to total lung capacity. The flow generated is plotted against the volume inspired/expired, forming the flow-volume loop. Obstructive pulmonary diseases result in decreased flows, whereas restrictive diseases result in decreased volumes. The loop also can distinguish between variable intrathoracic and extrathoracic obstruction because of decreases in expiratory and inspiratory flows, respectively. Finally, fixed large airway obstruction will result in decreases in inspiratory and expiratory flows.

EXPLANATION:

(A) **Correct.** Bilateral vocal cord paralysis is an example of variable extrathoracic obstruction. The *inspiratory* loop is flattened because negative pressure of forced inspiration causes airway collapse resulting in reduced flow. In addition, the ratio of expiratory over inspiratory flow at mid-vital capacity is usually greater than 2.0.[1]
(B) **Incorrect.** Chronic bronchitis is an example of diffuse airway obstruction. The flow-volume loop would show abnormally *decreased* flow ("scooped out") on end *expiration.*[1]
(C) **Incorrect.** Tracheal stenosis from tracheostomy is an example of a fixed obstruction. The flow-volume loop would show a plateau during both the inspiratory and expiratory effort-dependent portions of the curve because the airway diameter does

not change owing to the obstruction. The ratio of the expiratory over i[?]
flow at mid-vital capacity usually would be around 1.0.[1]

(D) *Incorrect.* Tumor of the lower trachea is an example of a variable int[?]
obstruction. The flow-volume loop would show a plateau during the *ex*[?]
phase because negative inspiratory pressure would not be present to ke[?]
way open.[1]

(E) *Incorrect.* This is not an example of normal respiratory status because[?]
tory flow would be much greater than the inspiratory flow. In a normal[?]
volume loop, the ratio of expiratory over inspiratory flow at mid-vital c[?]
usually around 1.0.[1]

REASONING:

This question tests knowledge of the flow-volume loop and how different path[?]
generate different loops. The reader should be able to recognize that the flow-[?]
shown demonstrates decreased inspiratory flow with relatively normal expi[?]
i.e., the mid-vital capacity ratio of expiratory flow to inspiratory flow is 6/2[?]
consistent with variable extrathoracic obstruction (choice A). The other cho[?]
amples of pathologic states that would have distinctly different flow-volume[?]

REFERENCE:

1. Miller RD, Miller ED, Reves JG, et al. Anesthesia, 5th ed. New York, Churchill[?]
2000, pp. 893–895.
2. Morgan GE, Mikhail MS, Murray MJ. Clinical Anesthesiology, 3d ed. New York, M[?]
2002, pp. 242–243.

BOOK B: QUESTION 59

Answer C

Cardiovascular

QUESTION (Choose single best answer):

A 66-year-old patient with aortic stenosis is scheduled for aortic valve replac[?]
amination shows blood pressure of 110/60 mm Hg and sinus rhythm at a rate [?]
per minute. Pulmonary artery occlusion pressure (PAOP) is 20 mm Hg with a[?]
a wave on the tracing. Which of the following is the most appropriate manage[?]

(A) Increasing myocardial contractility
(B) Maintaining PAOP below 20 mm Hg
(C) Maintaining sinus rhythm
(D) Promoting mild tachycardia
(E) Decreasing peripheral resistance

CORRECT ANSWER: C

SUMMARY:

The pathophysiology of aortic stenosis involves the gradual development of ob[?]
to flow through the aortic valve. This leads to increased systolic left ventricular p[?]
left ventricular hypertrophy (LVH), impaired diastolic function, and eventually,[?]
mise of systolic function of the left ventricle. Well-timed atrial contractions bec[?]
portant for left ventricular filling and help to offset the decreased ventricular co[?]
from LVH. The classic presentation of the symptomatic patient with aortic stenos[?]
pnea on exertion, angina, and syncope.

EXPLANATION:

(A) *Incorrect.* The left ventricle is already operating maximally or has lost the[?]
to increase contractility. Increased contractility will increase oxygen deman[?]
ther stressing the heart.

3

(B) **Incorrect.** The high wedge pressure is a reflection of the stiff ventricle. The PAOP should be maintained at a high level to ensure adequate left ventricular filling and cardiac output.

(C) **Correct.** Patients with aortic stenosis often depend on well-timed atrial contractions to augment left ventricular filling.

(D) **Incorrect.** Tachycardia leaves less time in diastole for left ventricular filling and increases oxygen demand.

(E) **Incorrect.** Afterload reduction does little to help offset the fixed afterload increase from the stenotic aortic valve and can lead to low diastolic pressures that can impair coronary artery perfusion.

REASONING:

The patient with symptomatic aortic valve stenosis has a dismal prognosis without valve replacement. Inappropriate anesthetic management also can worsen the prognosis. Preload must be optimized to fill a noncomplaint left ventricle. Afterload is relatively fixed. Decreases in afterload do little to offset this fixed afterload increase and can lead to coronary hypoperfusion and myocardial ischemia. The heart rate can be neither too high nor too low. The left atrium can contribute as much as 40 percent of left ventricular filling. Loss of this contribution from atrial fibrillation can decrease cardiac output dramatically, leading to hypotension and decreased coronary perfusion. Subsequent myocardial ischemia further worsens myocardial function, quickly degenerating into a vicious cycle that is difficult to correct.

REFERENCE:

Barash PG, Cullen BF, Stoelting RK. Clinical Anesthesia, 4th ed. Philadelphia, Lippincott Williams & Wilkins, 2001, pp. 894–895.

Morgan GE, Mikhail MS, Murray MJ. Clinical Anesthesiology, 3d ed. New York, McGraw-Hill, 2002, pp. 416–418.

OK B:

swer D

inical Anesthesia

QUESTION 60

QUESTION (Choose single best answer):

During rapid-sequence induction prior to an emergency surgical procedure, a 20-year-old patient vomits gastric contents containing particulate matter. An endotracheal tube is easily inserted, and ventilation with pure oxygen is initiated. Despite the presence of bilateral breath sounds, SpO_2 is 90 percent. Which of the following is the most appropriate next step?

(A) Administration of broad-spectrum antibiotics
(B) Intravenous administration of high-dose methylprednisolone
(C) Bronchial lavage with normal saline solution
(D) Bronchoscopy to remove particulate matter
(E) Cancellation of the surgical procedure

CORRECT ANSWER: D

SUMMARY:

The treatment of aspiration of gastric contents is controversial. Intubation with supportive management is the mainstay of therapy in the symptomatic patient. Pharmacologic treatment is not indicated during the initial approach to aspiration. Large particles may be amenable to removal by bronchoscopy, especially if they are of a size to obstruct airways. Otherwise, it is best to leave them alone. Any attempt at lavage or removal may push the gastric contents further down the respiratory tree.

EXPLANATION:

(A) *Incorrect.* Indiscriminate use of antibiotics may select for a more virulent strain, and many patients never develop an infection if left untreated. Targeted antibiotic therapy may benefit a patient with documented cultures or a patient with bowel obstruction.

(B) *Incorrect.* Steroids have not been shown conclusively to benefit patients with aspiration.

(C) *Incorrect.* Lavage may disperse gastric contents further throughout the lungs, enlarging the area of injury.

(D) *Correct.* Large particles may be suctioned out via bronchoscopy, particulary if they are obstructing the airways.

(E) *Incorrect.* This is an emergency procedure. Presumably the reader would not begin an elective case without fasting the patient a minimum of 6 hours after a light meal (toast and clear liquids).[1] An elective case complicated by an aspiration of this magnitude should be canceled.

REASONING:

Aspiration of gastric contents can lead to aspiration pneumonitis (chemical-induced lung injury also known as *Mendelson's syndrome*) and/or pneumonia (bacterial infection). It is generally believed that aspiration of greater than 25 mL of gastric fluid with a pH of less than 2.5 can cause pulmonary pathology.[1] Signs and symptoms may include bronchospasm, coughing, pulmonary infiltration, and hypoxemia. Acute respiratory distress syndrome and even death may occur in serious cases. However, the incidence of aspiration under general anesthesia is low (0.03 percent in adults and 0.04 percent in pediatric patients) but highest in patients undergoing emergency procedures. Most patients who aspirate (64 percent of adults and 63 percent of children) are asymptomatic and do not require supportive care. Others may require supplemental oxygen, mechanical ventilation, and/or specific target therapy (e.g., bronchoscopic removal of particulate matter). Premedication with sodium citrate (to increase gastric pH), metoclopramide (to increase lower esophageal sphincter tone and gastric emptying), and rapid-sequence induction with Sellick's maneuver to secure the airway all help to decrease the likelihood and/or complications of aspiration during induction of anesthesia.

REFERENCES:

1. Barash PG, Cullen BF, Stoelting RK. Clinical Anesthesia, 4th ed. Philadelphia, Lippincott Williams & Wilkins, 2001, pp. 557, 610.

2. Marik PE. Aspiration pneumonitis and aspiration pneumonia. N Engl J Med 344(9):665–671, 2001.

3. Warner MA, Warner ME, Weber JG. Clinical significance of pulmonary aspiration during the perioperative period. Anesthesiology 78(1):56–62, 1993.

4. Warner MA, Warner ME, Warner DO, et al. Perioperative pulmonary aspiration in infants and children. Anesthesiology 90(1):66–71, 1999.

5. Morgan GE, Mikhail MS, Murray MJ. Clinical Anesthesiology, 3d ed. New York, McGraw-Hill, 2002, p. 252.

BOOK B:

QUESTION 61 (OPTIONAL)

Answer B

Equipment/Physics

QUESTION (Choose single best answer):

A radial artery catheter is to be used for blood pressure measurement during a sitting craniotomy. When zeroing the transducer, which of the following describes the best levels for placement of the transducer and opening of the system to air?

	Transducer	Opening to Air
(A)	Head	Wrist
(B)	Head	Head
(C)	Head	Heart
(D)	Heart	Heart
(E)	Heart	Wrist

SUMMARY:

Pressure transducer accuracy depends on proper zeroing and leveling of the transducer. These two distinct and separate steps often are performed simultaneously by the anesthesiologist. Zeroing the transducer involves turning the stopcock most proximal to the transducer toward the arterial line tubing connected to the patient. This effectively eliminates any contact between the pressure transducer and the patient. The pressure transducer is now exposed solely to atmospheric pressure, and the "zero" button on the anesthesia monitor is selected. This maneuver establishes the current atmospheric pressure as a zero reference point. When the stopcock is returned to its original position, connection with the patient is reestablished, and the arterial waveform measures pressure relative to the zero reference point. Leveling the transducer involves moving the transducer to the top of the fluid column of the chamber or vessel you wish to monitor.[1] In the supine position, the midchest midaxillary plane estimates the level of the heart and is used to measure systemic arterial pressures.[1] During a sitting craniotomy, the clinician is most concerned with the cerebral perfusion pressure, for which the level of the ear is used to approximate the pressure in the circle of Willis. Leveling of the transducer does not significantly affect the zero reference point initially established by opening the transducer to air. For instance, atmospheric pressure does not change significantly between the wrist and the head in the sitting position. Using the relationship

$$log_{10} \text{ P} \approx 5 - \frac{height}{15,500}$$

where P is pressure, we can calculate that atmospheric pressure decreases 0.00129 percent with a 1-m increase from sea level.[2] This change is not clinically significant. Therefore, the transducer can be opened to air at any point and does not need to be rezeroed when the transducer is releveled. (See also Question 17, Book B.)

EXPLANATION:

(A) *Incorrect.* The transducer is at the correct level. Atmospheric pressure does not change appreciably from the wrist to the head (<0.00129 percent). Opening the transducer to air at the wrist still would provide an accurate zero reference point. This choice is only incorrect because it is not the "theoretically" best location. This difference is clinically insignificant.

(B) *Correct.* The transducer is at the correct level. Theoretically, the zero reference point (opening the transducer to air) is most accurately measured here, but the difference is not clinically significant.

(C) *Incorrect.* The transducer is at the correct level. Atmospheric pressure does not change appreciably from the heart to the head

(D) *Incorrect.* The transducer should be leveled at the head during a sitting craniotomy so that it provides a better estimate of cerebral perfusion pressure to the brain.[1]

(E) *Incorrect.* See above.

REASONING:

This is a challenging question because it implies that rezeroing (opening the transducer to air) is necessary when a transducer is releveled. This is not the case. Atmospheric pressure does not vary significantly between the wrist, heart, and head. Zeroing (opening the transducer to air) at any of these locations would provide an accurate atmospheric zero reference point. Leveling of the transducer to the top of the fluid column of a specific chamber or vessel simply establishes the arterial pressure at that location. The pressure difference between the head and the wrist is simply the hydrostatic pressure of the fluid column between the two sites (7.46 mm Hg decrease in pressure for every 10 cm increase in height, assuming 1.34 cm H_2O = 1 mm Hg). Choices A, B, and C all will provide clinically accurate zero reference points. On an actual examination, we would select choice B only because it is theoretically the "best" location for zeroing and leveling. This difference, however, is not clinically significant.

REFERENCES:

1. Miller RD, Miller ED, Reves JG, et al. Anesthesia, 5th ed. New York, Churchill Livingstone, 2000, pp. 1136–1137.
2. Environmental Test Methods and Engineering Guidelines. US Department of Defence Military Standard 810E. Washington, DC, US Government Printing Office, 1989.
3. Morgan GE, Mikhail MS, Murray MJ. Clinical Anesthesiology, 3d ed. New York, McGraw-Hill, 2002, pp. 94–95.

BOOK B:

QUESTION 62

Answer B

Equipment/Physics

QUESTION (Choose single best answer):

The gauge pressure on a cylinder of nitrous oxide

(A) Varies with the size of the cylinder.
(B) Is the same for full and half-full cylinders.
(C) Is the same as that of a full cylinder of oxygen if both are full.
(D) Is independent of the temperature of the cylinder.
(E) Reliably indicates the amount of nitrous oxide in the cylinder.

CORRECT ANSWER: B

SUMMARY:

Nitrous oxide is an inorganic, colorless, compressible, and odorless inhaled anesthetic agent that is a gas at room temperature but can be stored as a liquid while under pressure. These unique properties account for the characteristic of the gas in compressed tanks. Oxygen cylinder pressure readings reflect the quantity of gas left in the tank. In contrast, nitrous oxide will have the same cylinder pressure (745 psi) until the liquid N_2O is exhausted. As N_2O is depleted, the liquid vaporizes at the same rate as it is being consumed from the tank until there is no liquid left. The only accurate method to estimate the amount of N_2O in a cylinder is to weigh the tank and subtract the tare weight (weight of the empty tank).

EXPLANATION:

(A) *Incorrect.* The pressure of a tank of N_2O will read 745 psi regardless of the tank size because liquid N_2O is vaporized at the same rate at which it is consumed (at normal ambient temperature and assuming that the cylinder is not completely devoid of liquid N_2O).

(B) *Correct.* The pressure in a cylinder of N_2O will be the same until the tank is nearly empty (about 400 L of N_2O) and no more liquid is available to vaporize as the gas is being consumed. This is so because the rate at which the liquid converts to the gaseous phase is the same as the rate of gas consumption from the cylinder until there is no liquid left to convert.

(C) *Incorrect.* A full cylinder of oxygen has a pressure of 1800 to 2200 psi at 20°C. The pressure of a cylinder of N_2O at the same temperature is 745 psi.

(D) *Incorrect.* N_2O is a compressible gas. Increases in temperature cause transformation of some liquid to the gaseous phase, but this is not usually accompanied by a significant increase in pressure. Large increases in temperature may overcome the compressibility of the gas and result in increased cylinder pressures.

345

(E) **Incorrect.** Only the weight of the tank can reliably indicate the amount of N_2O remaining because the pressure will be constant until only 400 L of N_2O is left in the tank and liquid N_2O is depleted (the point where the tank pressure will begin to fall).

REASONING:

This question tests knowledge of the properties of compressed anesthetic gases in cylinders. Choice A can be eliminated because the size of a cylinder has nothing to do with the vapor pressure of a gas. Choice C is clearly incorrect based on the standard tank pressures for N_2O and O_2. Choice D is incorrect with respect to large increases in temperature (although small temperature changes do not result in significant increases in pressure). The magnitude of temperature change is not a specified, making choice D a poor one. The best answer is B.

REFERENCE:

Barash PG, Cullen BF, Stoelting RK. Clinical Anesthesia, 4th ed. Philadelphia, Lippincott Williams & Wilkins, 2001, p. 568.

Morgan GE, Mikhail MS, Murray MJ. Clinical Anesthesiology, 3d ed. New York, McGraw-Hill, 2002, pp.17–18.

BOOK B:

Answer E

Neuroanesthesia

QUESTION 63

QUESTION (Choose single best answer):

Immediately after sustaining severe head injury, a 20-year-old man has a blood pressure of 150/90 mm Hg and an intracranial pressure (ICP) of 35 mm Hg. After 1 hour of thiopental infusion, blood pressure is 105/60 mm Hg, ICP is 20 mm Hg, central venous pressure (CVP) is 5 mm Hg, and temperature is 36°C. The electroencephalogram (EEG) shows slow-wave activity. The most appropriate next step is administration of

(A) Additional thiopental.
(B) A corticosteroid.
(C) Furosemide.
(D) Nimodipine.
(E) Phenylephrine.

CORRECT ANSWER: E

SUMMARY:

Barbiturates have been used in the management of patients with increased ICP because they are potent cerebral vasoconstrictors and decrease the cerebral blood volume contribution to ICP.[1] A potential side effect of barbiturates use is hypotension owing to myocardial depression. If hypotension is sufficiently profound, cerebral perfusion pressure (CPP) may no longer be maintained. This may manifest as EEG changes. It is important to note that CPP = mean arterial pressure (MAP) – ICP. Efforts should focus on increasing MAP to improve the cerebral perfusion pressure. Immediate treatment should include vasopressors such as phenylephrine or dopamine and colloid fluid resuscitation if the patient is volume depleted.[1]

EXPLANATION:

(A) **Incorrect.** Additional thiopental most likely would worsen the hypotension.
(B) **Incorrect.** Although corticosteroids may have a role in reducing vasogenic edema, their routine use in head trauma is controversial. Steroids alone will not improve the main problem of hypotension.

(C) *Incorrect.* Loop diuretics are effective in decreasing ICP but may take up to 30 minutes to show a clinical effect and can worsen hypotension in patients who are already volume depleted.

(D) *Incorrect.* Nimodipine is a useful drug in preventing and treating vasospasm that can occur after subarachnoid hemorrhage. It does not decrease ICP and can produce hypotension.

(E) *Correct.* Hypotension is a potential side effect of barbiturate therapy and can be particularly profound in patients who are volume depleted.[1] In addition to replacing intravascular volume with colloid, vasopressors such as phenylephrine can be useful in maintaining cerebral perfusion.

REASONING:

The key to this question is identifying the main problem. Although the patient still has increased ICP of 20 mm Hg, this is less that than the initial presentation. The presence of new EEG changes in the setting of hypotension would indicate inadequate cerebral perfusion. The initial goal of therapy should be to increase blood pressure using vasopressors and colloid. Drugs that can cause hypotension should be avoided. The best answer is E.

REFERENCE:

1. Stoelting RK, Miller RD. Basics of Anesthesia, 4th ed. New York, Churchill Livingstone, 2000, pp. 445–447.
2. Morgan GE, Mikhail MS, Murray MJ. Clinical Anesthesiology, 3d ed. New York, McGraw-Hill, 2002, pp. 568–569, 575–578, 797–798.

BOOK B: **QUESTION 64**

Answer E

Cardiovascular

QUESTION (Choose single best answer):

Following induction of anesthesia with sufentanil and pancuronium, a patient with left main coronary artery disease has a decrease in blood pressure from 110/70 to 60/40 mm Hg. There is no change in heart rate or electrocardiogram (ECG). The most appropriate management of the hypotension is administration of

(A) Calcium chloride.
(B) Ephedrine.
(C) Epinephrine.
(D) Isoproterenol.
(E) Phenylephrine.

CORRECT ANSWER: E

SUMMARY:

Patients with left main disease can have severe three-vessel disease and are at risk of myocardial ischemia jeopardizing their entire left ventricle. It is important to resolve any myocardial supply-demand imbalance immediately by treating any hypotension, tachycardia, or hypertension. Phenylephrine increases diastolic blood pressure without the concomitant increase in heart rate associated with ephedrine, epinephrine, and isoproterenol. Calcium chloride would not be the most appropriate treatment for this severe hypotension.

EXPLANATION:

(A) *Incorrect.* Calcium chloride would not be the most effective or appropriate treatment for this severe hypotension. Calcium also increases myocardial contractility and increases myocardial oxygen demand.

(B) *Incorrect.* Ephedrine would increase the heart rate, leading to increased myocardial oxygen demand.

(C) *Incorrect.* Epinephrine would increase myocardial oxygen demand and worsen the myocardial oxygen supply-demand imbalance.

(D) *Incorrect.* Isoproterenol would increase the myocardial oxygen demand and worsen the myocardial oxygen supply-demand imbalance.

(E) *Correct.* Phenylephrine is a pure alpha-adrenergic agonist and would increase coronary perfusion pressure without significantly increasing myocardial oxygen demand.

REASONING:

It is important to minimize myocardial oxygen demand in patients with impaired oxygen supply to the heart (i.e., coronary artery disease). The key is optimizing myocardial O_2 supply while minimizing or avoiding increased demand. Phenylephrine will elevate the diastolic blood pressure and improve oxygen delivery while minimizing oxygen demand by avoiding tachycardia, hypertension, and increased wall tension or chamber size.

REFERENCE:

Hensley F, Martin DE, Gravlee FP. Practical Approach to Cardiac Anesthesia, 3d ed. Philadelphia, Lippincott Williams & Wilkins, 2002, pp. 280–282.

Morgan GE, Mikhail MS, Murray MJ. Clinical Anesthesiology, 3d ed. New York, McGraw-Hill, 2002, pp. 395–405, particularly p. 401.

BOOK B: **QUESTION 65**

Answer D

Pharamacology

QUESTION (Choose single best answer):

In a 35-year-old patient, which of the following is associated with an increased duration of clinical narcosis following infusion of a total dose of 10 mg/kg thiopental over 3 hours?

(A) Alcoholism in remission
(B) Asthma
(C) Fever
(D) Obesity
(E) Use of appetite suppressants

CORRECT ANSWER: D

SUMMARY:

Thiopental is a barbiturate used for induction of anesthesia. Its sedative-hypnotic effects are a result of activation of gamma-aminobutryic acid (GABA) inhibitory neurotransmitters.[1] The rapid onset of an induction dose is due to rapid equilibration of blood levels with highly perfused brain tissue. The quick offset results from redistribution to moderately perfused lean tissue such as muscle. Poorly perfused organs such as adipose tissue take up thiopental much more slowly. This accounts for the prolonged duration of effect if a large induction dose is given or a continuous infusion is administered. The induction dose of thiopental should be based on lean body mass rather than actual body weight.[1]

EXPLANATION:

(A) *Incorrect.* Chronic alcohol intake does not change the thiopental anesthetic requirement, pharmacokinetics, or pharmacodynamics. Swerdlow and colleagues also examined the pharmacokinetics and pharmacodynamics of thiopental in alcoholics after 1 month of abstinence. Again, no differences were found.[2]

(B) *Incorrect.* While there is a greater incidence of wheezing in asthmatic patients receiving thiopental compared with propofol for induction,[1] there is no evidence that asthma affects the pharmacokinetics of thiopental.

(C) *Incorrect.* Fever can increase heart rate and metabolic rate. There is no evidence that it will increase the duration of narcosis with thiopental.

(D) *Correct.* If thiopental is given as a large dose or is delivered by infusion over a period of time, termination of effect is prolonged because clearance will depend more on uptake into adipose tissue than on lean tissue that has reached equilibrium with the blood compartment.[3] This is in contrast to the rapid redistribution to brain and lean tissue that explains the termination of effect of an induction dose.

(E) *Incorrect.* Appetite suppressants include drugs with different mechanisms of action, including serotonin reuptake inhibitors such as fenfluramine and phenteramine, serotonin, norepinephrine reuptake inhibitors such as sibutramine, and amphetamines. While these drugs have various side effects such as primary pulmonary hypertension for fenfluramine, they do not include increased narcosis with thiopental.[1,4]

REASONING:

This question tests knowledge of the pharmacokinetics and pharmacodynamics of thiopental. Choice A can be easily ruled out based on either the common misconception that chronic alcoholics require a greater dose of barbiturates for induction or knowledge of the fact that there is no difference between alcoholics and nonalcoholics. The pulmonary system is not involved in the metabolism of thiopental, so choice B can be ruled out. Choices C and E both increase metabolic rate, which logically might increase metabolism of drugs. There is no evidence that either has any effect on thiopental, so both can be eliminated. Finally, obesity increases the potential adipose reservoir in which thiopental can accumulate when infused over 3 hours. Thus D is the best answer.

REFERENCES:

1. Stoelting RK, Dierdorf SF. Anesthesia and Co-Existing Disease, 4th ed. New York, Churchill Livingstone, 2002, pp. 201–202, 443.

2. Swerdlow BN, Holley FO, Maitre PO, Stanski DR. Chronic alcohol intake does not change thiopental anesthetic requirement, pharmacokinetics, or pharmacodynamics. Anesthesiology 72:455–461, 1990.

3. Miller RD, Miller ED, Reves JG, et al. Anesthesia, 5th ed. New York, Churchill Livingstone, 2000, pp. 209–227.

4. Hardman JG, Limbird LE, Gilman AG. Goodman and Gilman's The Pharmacologic Basis of Therapeutics, 10th ed. New York, McGraw-Hill, 2001, p. 241.

5. Morgan GE, Mikhail MS, Murray MJ. Clinical Anesthesiology, 3d ed. New York, McGraw-Hill, 2002, pp. 156–159.

BOOK B: QUESTION 66

Answer D

Clinical Anesthesia

QUESTION (Choose single best answer):

A previously healthy 60-kg, 17-year-old boy is undergoing emergency surgery for a gunshot wound involving the iliac vein. Ventilation is controlled with a tidal volume of 700 mL/breath, rate of 10/min, and peak inspiratory pressure of 30 cm H_2O. Body temperature is normal. The most likely cause of an end-tidal carbon dioxide partial pressure of 16 mm Hg is

(A) Endobronchial intubation.
(B) Excessive expiratory time.
(C) Excessive tidal volume.
(D) Low cardiac output.
(E) Pulmonary aspiration.

SUMMARY:

An ETco2 of 16 mm Hg is abnormally low. Causes of low ETco2 include an increased A–a CO2 gradient or mechanical/measurement artifacts. Causes of artifacts include a partial or complete circuit disconnection, esophageal intubation, improper aspiration rate of the sidestream capnography line, and water precipitation in the sampling tubing. An increased A–a CO2 gradient can be due to any significant increase in alveolar dead space (ventilation without perfusion) such as low cardiac output or pulmonary embolism.

EXPLANATION:

(A) *Incorrect.* Endobronchial intubation results in increased pulmonary shunting (perfusion without ventilation) that should not significantly increase dead space (ventilation without perfusion) or change end-tidal CO_2.

(B) *Incorrect.* A prolonged expiratory time would not be expected to decrease ET_{CO_2}. Decreased minute ventilation may occur as a result of decreased inspiratory time, but that would increase end-tidal CO_2 rather than decrease it.

(C) *Incorrect.* The tidal volume in a patient with normal lung function during mechanical ventilation as part of a routine general anesthetic is kept between 8 and 11 mL/kg to avoid atelectasis. A 700-mL tidal volume is acceptable in this 60-kg patient and does not explain such a low ET_{CO_2}.

(D) *Correct.* The A–a CO_2 gradient is increased in a low cardiac output state because decreased pulmonary perfusion increases alveolar dead space (ventilated, nonperfused alveoli). A lower end-tidal CO_2 is expected.

(E) *Incorrect.* Pulmonary aspiration results in impaired alveolar gas exchange and ventilation. This may lead to increased pulmonary shunting (perfusion without ventilation) and does not increase dead space or significantly affect the A–a CO_2 gradient.

REASONING:

This question tests knowledge of A–a CO_2 gradient and associated etiologies for decreased measured ET_{CO_2}. It is important to note that increased alveolar dead space is the primary etiology for a widened A–a CO_2 gradient, although other artifacts also can lead to incorrect ET_{CO_2} measurement. D is the best answer.

REFERENCE:

Barash PG, Cullen BF, Stoelting RK. Clinical Anesthesia, 4th ed. Philadelphia, Lippincott Williams & Wilkins, 2001, pp. 802–803.
Morgan GE, Mikhail MS, Murray MJ. Clinical Anesthesiology, 3d ed. New York, McGraw-Hill, 2002, pp. 111–112.

BOOK B:

Answer A

Equipment/Physics

QUESTION 67

QUESTION (Choose single best answer):

Which of the following statements concerning anesthetic management for MRIs is true?

(A) ECG wires are associated with patient burns.
(B) Mechanical ventilation of the lungs is not feasible.
(C) Monitors with ferromagnetic components may be used.
(D) Oxygen analysis of inspired gas is inaccurate.
(E) Pulse oximetry is not reliable near the MR scanner.

CORRECT ANSWER: A

SUMMARY:

Anesthesia for patients undergoing magnetic resonance imaging (MRI) examinations poses significant problems and threats to patient safety. First and foremost, all ferromagnetic objects must be removed from the patient because the scanner acts as a powerful magnet to attract these objects. Patients with pacemakers, prosthetic joints, and surgical clips must not undergo MRI. In addition, all external metal objects (credit cards, watches, jewelry, pens, etc.) must be removed from the patient. ECG wires with metal leads and pulse oximeters with wire cables can cause patient burns. The wires can attract high radiofrequency energy and transmit that energy to the patient in the form of heat. MRI does not interfere with the monitoring of inspired oxygen or with the ability to measure oxygen saturation adequately by pulse oximetry. Special O_2 cylinders and ventilators are available to enable mechanical ventilation of the lungs in the MRI suite.

EXPLANATION:

(A) **Correct.** Regular ECG wires have been associated with patient burns because they attract energy in the form of radiofrequency waves and may transmit that energy in the form of heat.

(B) **Incorrect.** Mechanical ventilation of the lungs is possible with a nonmetal endotracheal tube and an aluminum oxygen cylinder. Special MRI-compatible mechanical ventilators are also available.

(C) **Incorrect.** The ferromagnetic components of patient monitors are attracted by the MRI magnet and pose a safety hazard to the patient and MRI staff.

(D) **Incorrect.** MRI scanners do not interfere with the analysis of oxygen in inspired air.

(E) **Incorrect.** Pulse oximetry is reliable in the MRI suite because it uses spectrophotometric measurement of transmitted light to determine oxygen saturation. It is not affected by magnetic energy.

REASONING:

This question tests knowledge of anesthesia safety in the MRI scanner. Choices B and E can be eliminated because these options imply that MRI scans are not safe for patients requiring airway and oxygenation monitoring. This is certainly not the case because intubated patients are commonly taken to the MRI suite. Pulse oximetry is mandatory in the MRI suite because adequate oxygenation otherwise cannot be assessed adequately while patients are in the scanner. Choice C cannot be true because MRI uses powerful magnetic fields to create images of different tissues, and these magnetic fields attract metallic objects. Choice D is false because electromagnetic energy does not interfere with the process used to analyze inspired oxygen (electrochemical gas analysis). This leaves A as the best answer.

REFERENCE:

Barash PG, Cullen BF, Stoelting RK. Clinical Anesthesia, 4th ed. Philadelphia, Lippincott Williams & Wilkins, 2001, pp. 1332–1333.

Morgan GE, Mikhail MS, Murray MJ. Clinical Anesthesiology, 3d ed. New York, McGraw-Hill, 2002, pp. 123–124.

BOOK B: **QUESTION 68**

Answer C

Physiology

QUESTION (Choose single best answer):

Intraocular pressure is

(A) Decreased by glycopyrrolate.
(B) Increased by hyperventilation.
(C) Decreased by halothane.
(D) Increased by nondepolarizing muscle relaxants.
(E) Increased by phenylephrine eye drops.

CORRECT ANSWER: C

SUMMARY:

The ocular globe is exquisitely sensitive to volume and intraocular pressure (IOP). An increase in arterial pressure, Pa_{CO_2}, or central venous pressure (CVP) and topical anticholinesterase agents effectively raise IOP by increasing aqueous volume or decreasing its drainage. IOP also increases with coughing and the Trendelenburg and prone positions, laryngoscopy, and decreased Pa_{O_2}. In contrast, most inhalational and intravenous anesthetic agents lower IOP, with the exception of succinylcholine, which raises it. The effect of ketamine on IOP remains controversial.

EXPLANATION:

(A) *Incorrect.* Glycopyrrolate and atropine are used often to attenuate the oculocardiac reflex during eye surgeries. They have been shown to have no significant effect on IOP when used as premedications and even reduce IOP during a general anesthesia.[1,2]

(B) *Incorrect.* Hyperventilation decreases Pa_{CO_2} and thus decreases IOP.

(C) *Correct.* Inhalational anesthetics, including halothane, reduce IOP in a dose-related fashion.

(D) *Incorrect.* With the exception of succinylcholine, neuromuscular blocking drugs directly decrease IOP by muscle relaxation. This effect may be attenuated if the resulting apnea elevates Pa_{CO_2} sufficiently to raise IOP.[3]

(E) *Incorrect.* Capillary decongestion caused by the topical application of phenylephrine improves aqueous drainage from the eye, thereby decreasing IOP.[3] Phenylephrine eye drops should be administered with caution because they can exhibit significant systemic absorption and lead to hypertension.

REASONING:

This question tests knowledge of determinants of intraocular pressure (IOP) and the drugs that may influence changes in IOP. The reader should ensure that the side effects of common drugs used for eye surgery are reviewed carefully. Some examples include phenylephrine (can lead to systemic hypertension), sulfur hexafluoride (can increase IOP in the presence of N_2O for up to 10 days), and echothiophate (can inhibit pseudocholinesterase activity for 3 to 14 days).[3] The best answer is C.

REFERENCES:

1. Cozanitis DA, Dundee JW, Buchanan TA, Archer DB. Atropine versus glycopyrrolate: A study of intraocular pressure and pupil size in man. Anaesthesia 34(3):236–238, 1979.

2. Salem MG, Ahearn RS. The effects of atropine and glycopyrrolate on intra-ocular pressure in anaesthetised elderly patients. Anaesthesia 39(8):809–812, 1984.

3. Barash PG, Cullen BF, Stoelting RK. Clinical Anesthesia, 4th ed. Philadelphia, Lippincott Williams & Wilkins, 2001, pp. 286, 487, 972–973.

4. Morgan GE, Mikhail MS, Murray MJ. Clinical Anesthesiology, 3d ed. New York, McGraw-Hill, 2002, pp. 761–763, Tables 38-1 and 38–3.

BOOK B: **QUESTION 69**

Answer B

Physiology

QUESTION (Choose single best answer):

Compared with adult hemoglobin, which of the following is a characteristic of fetal hemoglobin?

(A) It has a greater oxygen-carrying capacity.
(B) It has a lower P_{50}.
(C) It is more likely to cause an artifactual increase in Sp_{O_2}.
(D) It is more likely to sickle.
(E) It unloads oxygen more readily at the tissues.

CORRECT ANSWER: B

SUMMARY:

Fetal hemoglobin (hemoglobin F) is composed of two alpha subunits and two gamma sub-units. It is characterized by a lower P_{50} and greater affinity for oxygen compared with adult hemoglobin.[1] Since hemoglobin F unloads oxygen less readily at the tissue level, neonates must maintain peripheral oxygen delivery with higher cardiac outputs and higher hemoglobin concentrations.[1] By age 3 months, infants develop physiologic anemia as their fetal hemoglobin is replaced with adult hemoglobin.

EXPLANATION:

(A) **Incorrect.** Although fetal hemoglobin has a greater affinity for oxygen, it does not have a greater oxygen-carrying capacity compared with adult hemoglobin. Each hemoglobin molecule can bind up to 4 molecules of oxygen.

(B) **Correct.** The P_{50} for normal adult hemoglobin is 26 mm Hg. Fetal hemoglobin has a lower P_{50} of approximately 19 mm Hg.[1]

(C) **Incorrect.** Fetal hemoglobin can produce an artifactual decrease in SpO_2 owing to decreased unloading of oxygen in the periphery.

(D) **Incorrect.** Large amounts of hemoglobin F actually can help to prevent sickling in patients with sickle cell anemia.

(E) **Incorrect.** The hemoglobin-oxygen dissociation curve for fetal hemoglobin is shifted to the left in comparison with adult hemoglobin. As a result, hemoglobin F unloads oxygen less readily at the tissues.

REASONING:

This question tests knowledge of fetal hemoglobin and the hemoglobin-oxygen dissociation curve. The left shift of the oxygen dissociation curve for hemoglobin F has an important role in fetal life because a high oxygen affinity facilitates transfer of maternal oxygen across the placenta. The single best answer is B.

REFERENCE:

1. Stoelting RK, Miller RD. Basics of Anesthesia, 4th ed. New York, Churchill Livingstone, 2000, p. 364.
2. Morgan GE, Mikhail MS, Murray MJ. Clinical Anesthesiology, 3d ed. New York, McGraw-Hill, 2002, pp. 501, 640, Fig. 22-23 (p. 502), The Effects of Changes in Acid-Base Status, Body Temperature, and 2,3-DPG on the Hemoglobin-Oxygen Dissociation Curve.

BOOK B: **QUESTION 70**

Answer A

Clinical Anesthesia

QUESTION (Choose single best answer):

Which of the following is most effective in decontaminating an anesthesia machine that was splattered with human immunodeficiency virus (HIV)–contaminated blood?

(A) Bleach
(B) Deionized water
(C) Ethylene oxide
(D) Hydrogen peroxide
(E) Isopropyl alcohol

CORRECT ANSWER: A

SUMMARY:

Vectors implicated in HIV transmission include blood products, body fluids, and tissues. Although the risk of environmentally mediated HIV transmission is negligible, it is theo-

retically possible. Fortunately, HIV is easily inactivated or killed from surfaces. Multiple reports recommend first cleaning a surface contaminated with HIV to reduce the organic load prior to attempted disinfection. Bleach, 70% isopropyl alcohol, ultraviolet (UV) light, and aldehyde preparations are among the possible options. The cheapest and most convenient remains a 1:10 or 1:100 dilution of household bleach.[1]

EXPLANATION:

(A) *Correct.* Sodium hypochlorite (bleach) has been proven to be effective in intactivating HIV virus when used in appropriate concentration and in the presence of a low amount of serum. Cleaning a surface prior to disinfection with bleach is recommended to reduce the organic load. In cases where prior cleaning is impossible, care must be taken to use a higher bleach concentration (a minimum of 10,000 ppm available chlorine).[2]

(B) *Incorrect.* Water is deionized when all anions and cations are removed. No disinfectant property exists.

(C) *Incorrect.* Ethylene oxide is a colorless flammable gas used in steam sterilization such as an autoclave and is not a practical agent for decontamination of an anesthesia machine.

(D) *Incorrect.* Hydrogen peroxide is a poor antiseptic that reacts with the enzyme catalase to yield water and oxygen.

(E) *Incorrect.* Isopropyl alcohol 70% has been shown to rapidly deactivate high titers of HIV in suspension but only partially inactivated virus dried onto a surface.[3] Alcohol also quickly evaporates when sprayed and is an unreliable chemical disinfectant for surfaces contaminated with HIV virus.

REASONING:

This question tests knowledge of best practices for chemical disinfection of HIV surface contamination. Choice B is incorrect because it has no disinfectant property, whereas choice D is a poor antiseptic. Choice C can be eliminated because it is an inappropriate method for decontamination of an anesthesia machine. Choices A or E are both plausible answers. However, alcohol evaporates quickly from surfaces and only partially inactivates the virus. A is the best answer.

REFERENCES:

1. Crutcher JM, Lamm SH, Hall TA. Procedures to protect health-care workers from HIV infection: Category I (health-care) workers. Am Ind Hyg Assoc J 52(2):A100–103, 1991.
2. Van Bueren J, Simpson RA, Salman H, et al. Inactivation of HIV-1 by chemical disinfectants: Sodium hypochlorite. Epidemiol Infect 115(3):567–579, 1995.
3. Van Bueren J, Larkin DP, Simpson RA. Inactivation of human immunodeficiency virus type 1 by alcohols. J Hosp Infect 28(2):137–148, 1994.

BOOK B:

QUESTION 71

Answer B

Pharmacology

QUESTION (Choose single best answer):

Which of the following is greater in an obese patient than in a nonobese patient of equal height?

(A) Milliliters of local anesthetic required for epidural block
(B) Milligrams of succinylcholine required for intubation
(C) Clearance of diazepam
(D) Clearance of fentanyl
(E) Oxygen consumption per body surface area

CORRECT ANSWER: B

SUMMARY:

Pharmacokinetics in obese patients are difficult to predict. High fat stores, larger volumes of distribution, increased cardiac output and glomerular filtration rate, and other derangements of obesity all can have variable effects on drug distribution, binding, metabolism, and elimination. In general, water-soluble drugs will have smaller volumes of distribution compared with lipid-soluble drugs. The reader should carefully review the factors affecting drug pharmacokinetics and pharmacodynamics in obesity.[1] In general, the most prudent approach is to dose drugs based on ideal body weight. Dosing according to actual body weight can lead to gross overdosing. An increased dose of succinylcholine (1.2 mg/kg for lean body weight to 1.5 mg/kg for ideal weight) usually is recommended to achieve optimal intubating conditions.[1] The obese patient should receive 10 to 20 percent less local anesthetic volume for neuraxial anesthesia. Oxygen consumption increases directly with increasing weight.

EXPLANATION:

(A) *Incorrect.* Obese patients require a smaller volume (75 to 80 percent of normal) of local anesthetic agent for epidural analgesia.[1] This is probably due to a smaller epidural space resulting from increased fat and engorged epidural veins.

(B) *Correct.* Obese patients have higher pseudocholinesterase levels and require a higher dose of succinylcholine to achieve equivalent levels at the neuromuscular junction.[1]

(C) *Incorrect.* Diazepam is lipophilic, so it has a large volume of distribution and a longer elimination half-life. However, clearance of the drug does not appear to be affected by obesity.

(D) *Incorrect.* Fentanyl pharmacokinetics are not significantly altered by obesity when it is administered based on actual body weight.[1]

(E) *Incorrect.* Oxygen consumption is higher for the obese. However, it is roughly equal at rest when adjusted for body surface area.

REASONING:

This question is challenging given the many and often conflicting effects of obesity on pharmacokinetics and pharmacodynamics. Choice A is clearly incorrect. Lipophilic drugs (e.g., diazepam and thiopental) do take longer to remove from the body (elimination) owing to increased stores in the fat, but removal from the blood (clearance) is the same in obese and nonobese patients. Obese patients have higher basal metabolic rates and increased demand for oxygen, but this is directly related to size. B is the best answer.

REFERENCE:

1. Barash PG, Cullen BF, Stoelting RK. Clinical Anesthesia, 4th ed. Philadelphia, Lippincott Williams & Wilkins, 2001, pp. 1037–1038, 1041, Table 37-1.
2. Morgan GE, Mikhail MS, Murray MJ. Clinical Anesthesiology, 3d ed. New York, McGraw-Hill, 2002, pp. 748–749.

BOOK B:

Answer D

Pharmacology

QUESTION 72

QUESTION (Choose single best answer):

The best premedication regimen for a known active narcotic addict would include

(A) Secobarbital.
(B) Diazepam.
(C) Nalbuphine.
(D) Morphine.
(E) Droperidol.

CORRECT ANSWER: D

SUMMARY:

Opiate withdrawal from acute drug cessation is an important preoperative concern for patients with narcotic addiction or dependency. Opiate withdrawal can present with multiple signs and symptoms, including tachycardia, hypertension, mydriasis, gooseflesh, diaphoresis, rhinorrhea, diarrhea, agitation, anxiety, mood lability, and drug-seeking behaviors.[1] The incidence of withdrawal symptoms peaks 1 to 3 days after acute cessation of opiates such as morphine, heroin, or meperidine.[1] Anesthesiologists should attempt to maintain opioid medications at their usual level to prevent acute opiate withdrawal.[2] Administration of opioid antagonist agents such as naloxone should be avoided.[2]

EXPLANATION:

(A) *Incorrect.* Secobarbital is a barbiturate that can cause mild stimulation at low doses and can lead to sedation and unconsciousness with higher doses. It acts at the gamma-aminobutyric acid (GABA) receptor and would not be useful for withdrawal prophylaxis in an opioid addict.

(B) *Incorrect.* Diazepam is a benzodiazepine that also acts at the GABA receptor. It would not be useful for withdrawal prophylaxis in an opioid addict.

(C) *Incorrect.* Nalbuphine is an opioid agonist-antagonist and can precipitate acute opioid withdrawal.

(D) *Correct.* Morphine is an opioid agonist agent that is suitable for maintenance of a patient's usual narcotic dose and provides prophylaxis against opioid withdrawal symptoms.

(E) *Incorrect.* Droperidol is a dopamine antagonist that acts centrally to interfere with serotonin, norepinephrine, and GABA transmissions. It would not be useful for withdrawal prophylaxis in an opioid addict.

REASONING:

This question tests knowledge of preoperative management of patients with opiate addiction. The best premedication regimen to prevent acute opiate withdrawal in these patients is administration of an opiate agonist medication such as morphine or methadone. Barbiturates, benzodiazepines, and butyrophenones such as droperidol do not act at the opioid receptor and would not be useful for opioid withdrawal prophylaxis. Mixed opioid agonist-antagonist agents such as nalbupine or buprenorphine also should be avoid because their antagonist properties have the potential to precipitate acute withdrawal. Morphine is the only option that is a pure opioid agonist. D is the best answer.

REFERENCES:

1. Noble J, Ii H, Greene W, et al. Textbook of Primary Care Medicine, 3d ed. St Louis, Mosby, 2001, p. 447.

2. Barash PG, Cullen BF, Stoelting RK. Clinical Anesthesia, 4th ed. Philadelphia, Lippincott Williams & Wilkins, 2001, p. 562.

3. Morgan GE, Mikhail MS, Murray MJ. Clinical Anesthesiology, 3d ed. New York, McGraw-Hill, 2002, p. 594.

Answer D

Cardiovascular

QUESTION (Choose single best answer):

During cardiopulmonary bypass (CPB) at a nasopharyngeal temperature of 28°C and a hematocrit of 20 percent, temperature-corrected Pa_{CO_2} is 50 mm Hg and uncorrected Pa_{CO_2} is 60 mm Hg. The most appropriate management is to

(A) Administer additional opioid.
(B) Administer packed red blood cells to increase the hematocrit to 25 percent.
(C) Further decrease the patient's temperature.
(D) Increase fresh gas flow to the oxygenator.
(E) Institute mechanical ventilation.

CORRECT ANSWER: D

SUMMARY:

Acid-base management during hypothermic cardiopulmonary bypass (CPB) (i.e., alpha-stat versus pH-stat) is controversial.[1] pH-stat acid-base management uses temperature-corrected blood gases to guide management, whereas alpha-stat management uses temperature-uncorrected blood gas analysis. In a normal patient, ventilation is controlled by varying the delivered minute ventilation. Ventilation and perfusion can be controlled separately during CPB. Perfusion is controlled by varying flow rates and ventilation is controlled by varying total gas flow through the oxygenator. Regardless of which method of acid-base management is employed during hypothermic CPB, Pa_{CO_2} is controlled by varying total gas flows. Hypercarbia should be treated by increasing the total gas flow through the oxygenator.

EXPLANATION:

(A) *Incorrect.* Additional opioid will not affect hypercarbia during CPB. If sympathetic stimulation is suspected, opioid may be given, but the ventilation still needs to be increased.
(B) *Incorrect.* A hematocrit of 20 percent is well tolerated under hypothermic conditions. Low hematocrit decreases blood viscosity and improves the rheology of the microcirculation. Administration of packed red blood cells would not help to correct the underlying respiratory acidosis.
(C) *Incorrect.* The magnitude of hypothermia used during CPB is determined by type of surgery and the duration and magnitude of flows during bypass. Hypothermia will not help to correct the significant respiratory acidosis.
(D) *Correct.* Increasing the fresh gas flow to the oxygenator will increase ventilation and help to correct the respiratory acidosis.
(E) *Incorrect.* The pulmonary circulation is isolated during CPB. There is no benefit to ventilating lungs that are not perfused. Mechanical ventilation would not correct the respiratory acidosis.

REASONING:

This question tests knowledge of acid-base management during hypothermic cardiopulmonary bypass. Discussions of the interpretation of blood gas analysis in hypothermic patients are often difficult to understand because many readers find certain concepts confusing. It is important to understand that the partial pressure of a gas in a liquid is defined as the partial pressure of that gas which would be present in a gas mixture in equilibrium with the liquid. Therefore, Pa_{CO_2} is a measure of the partial pressure of CO_2 in a gas mixture in equilibrium with blood. It is not a direct measure of the CO_2 content in the blood itself.

Interpretation of blood gas results during hypothermia is difficult because the solubility of CO_2 in solution increases, as does CO_2 binding to hemoglobin.[2] As a result, a larger amount of CO_2 gas will dissolve into blood as temperature decreases. In a closed system (i.e., sealed heparinized blood gas syringe), the total amount of CO_2 must remain the same. When temperature decreases, CO_2 solubility and hemoglobin binding increase, causing additional CO_2 gas to dissolve into blood. Because this is a closed system, the partial pressure of CO_2 must decrease as the concentration in solution increases. This explains why the Pa_{CO_2} decreases as temperature decreases. (Note that although more CO_2 is dissolved in blood at lower temperatures, the molecular interaction between water and CO_2 is decreased with hypothermia, and therefore, formation of H^+ is minimal.)

Because blood samples are heated to 37°C prior to measuring gas tensions, they will overestimate the true arterial CO_2 gas tension in a hypothermic patient.[1] Temperature-corrected values can be generated to estimate the true arterial CO_2 gas tension and pH at the patient's actual temperature. Management of acid-base status during hypothermic CPB can be achieved through either pH-stat or alpha-stat management. pH-stat management uses temperature-corrected values to guide management, whereas alpha-stat uses temperature-uncorrected measurements. The goal in both is the same: to maintain a normal arterial Pa_{CO_2} of 40 mm Hg and a pH of 7.40. In this question we are given a temperature-corrected Pa_{CO_2} value of 50 mm Hg and a temperature-uncorrected value of 60 mm Hg. Regardless of management technique, the hypercarbia should be treated by increasing "ventilation." Accordingly, fresh gas flow to the oxygenator should be increased. D is the best answer.

REFERENCES:

1. Miller RD, Miller ED, Reves JG, et al. Anesthesia, 5th ed. New York, Churchill Livingstone, 2000, pp. 1409–1410.
2. Kofstad J. Blood gases and hypothermia: Some theoretical and practical considerations. Scand J Clin Lab Invest 56(suppl 224):21–26, 1996.
3. Hensley WJ, Loblay RH, Tiller DJ. Fluid, Electrolyte and Acid-Base Disturbances: A Practical Guide for Interns. New York, Wiley, 1976, p. 488.
4. Kaplan JA. Cardiac Anesthesia, 4th ed. Philadelphia, Saunders, 1999, pp. 1069–1070.
5. Morgan GE, Mikhail MS, Murray MJ. Clinical Anesthesiology, 3d ed. New York, McGraw-Hill, 2002, p. 436.

BOOK B:

QUESTION 74

Answer B

Physiology

QUESTION (Choose single best answer):

Two days after coronary artery bypass grafting, a 62-year-old man remains sedated, tracheally intubated, and mechanically ventilated with full neuromuscular block. Over the next 3 hours, Pa_{O_2} decreases from 90 to 70 mm Hg at an FI_{O_2} of 0.7, peak inspiratory pressure (PIP) measured proximally in the ventilatory circuit increases from 40 to 66 cm H_2O, and plateau pressure remains unchanged at 30 cm H_2O. Which of the following is the most likely cause of these changes?

(A) Adult respiratory distress syndrome (ARDS)
(B) Bronchial mucus plugging
(C) Left ventricular failure
(D) Lobar pneumonia
(E) Tension pneumothorax

CORRECT ANSWER: B

SUMMARY:

Peak inspiratory pressure (PIP) measures dynamic lung compliance. Plateau pressure (PP) is measured at end inspiration (zero gas flow) and reflects static lung compliance.

Both PIP and PP are increased when tidal volume is increased or lung compliance is decreased. Increased PIP with unchanged PP is seen with increased inspiratory gas flow or increased airway resistance (e.g., bronchospasm, mucus plugging, airway compression, etc.).

EXPLANATION:

(A) **Incorrect.** ARDS results in increased PIP and PP owing to decreased lung compliance.

(B) **Correct.** Increased PIP with unchanged PP is seen with increased inspiratory gas flow and increased airway resistance (e.g., bronchospasm, mucus plugging, kinked endotracheal tube, foreign-body aspiration, airway compression, and endotracheal tube cuff herniation).

(C) **Incorrect.** Left ventricular failure leading to pulmonary edema would result in decreased lung compliance and a corresponding increase in PIP and PP.

(D) **Incorrect.** Lobar pneumonia would lead to decreased lung compliance and a corresponding increase in PIP and PP.

(E) **Incorrect.** Both PIP and PP would be expected to rise with a tension pneumothorax.

REASONING:

This question tests knowledge of the differences between PIP and PP and corresponding differences in dynamic versus static lung compliance. PIP is the highest pressure generated in the breathing circuit during inspiration and reflects dynamic compliance. PP is measured during inspiratory pause and reflects static lung compliance. Normally, PIP is equal to or slightly more than PP. If PIP and PP are both increased, this suggests a decrease in lung compliance or increased tidal volumes (Trendelenburg position, pleural effusion, ascites, tension pneumothorax, endobronchial intubation, abdominal packing, retractors, insufflation, alveolar diseases such as ARDS, PNA, or pulmonary edema). Alternatively, an increase in airway resistance or inspiratory gas flow likely has occurred if PIP is increased but PP is unchanged. The best answer is B.

REFERENCE:

Barash PG, Cullen BF, Stoelting RK. Clinical Anesthesia, 4th ed. Philadelphia, Lippincott Williams & Wilkins, 2001, pp. 794–795.

Morgan GE, Mikhail MS, Murray MJ. Clinical Anesthesiology, 3d ed. New York, McGraw-Hill, 2002, p. 47.

BOOK B:

QUESTION 75

Answer A

OB/Regional

QUESTION (Choose single best answer):

A combined epidural and general anesthetic is used for aortofemoral bypass surgery. Just prior to extubation, the patient received morphine 5 mg through the epidural catheter. Eleven hours later, he is unresponsive while breathing 40% oxygen from a face mask. Respiratory rate is 6 breaths per minute and SpO_2 is 92% percent. Arterial blood gas analysis shows a PaO_2 of 80 mm Hg, a $PaCO_2$ of 84 mm Hg, and a pH of 7.16. Which of the following statements concerning this patient is true?

(A) Hypercarbia is contributing to the decreased level of consciousness.

(B) Naloxone is ineffective for reversing the respiratory depression.

(C) The oxygen saturation is higher than expected because of the pH.

(D) The risk for respiratory depression would have been lower with subarachnoid administration of 0.5 mg morphine.

(E) Residual local anesthetic is contributing to the respiratory depression.

CORRECT ANSWER: A

SUMMARY:

Epidural opiates are effective agents for postoperative pain relief. Morphine given in doses up to 10 mg has an onset of 1 to 2 hours and a duration of 12 to 24 hours.[1] Side effects are dose-dependent and include pruritus, nausea and vomiting, urinary retention, and respiratory depression. All can be ameliorated by administration of naloxone, which also will decrease the analgesic properties. It is important to remember that these side effects can occur at any point in the duration of the action, and delayed respiratory depression can occur. Because of the dose-dependent nature of side effects and limited analgesic efficacy with increased doses, the recommended dose of epidural morphine is approximately 5 mg.[1]

EXPLANATION:

(A) **Correct.** Increased $PaCO_2$ is associated with agitation, sedation, and even coma. These mental status changes are thought to be due to intracranial hypertension secondary to increased cerebral blood flow and severe intracellular acidosis.

(B) **Incorrect.** Naloxone *is* effective for reversing respiratory depression from epidural morphine.[1]

(C) **Incorrect.** Based on the oxyhemoglobin dissociation curve, an oxygen saturation of 90 percent corresponds to a PaO_2 of 60 mm Hg. This patient has a PaO_2 of 80 mm Hg, and the oxygen saturation is 92 percent, which is slightly lower than would be expected.

(D) **Incorrect.** The risk of respiratory depression is higher with intrathecal narcotics than with epidural narcotics.[1]

(E) **Incorrect.** Local anesthetics do not cause respiratory depression.[1]

REASONING:

This patient is experiencing delayed respiratory depression from epidural narcotics resulting in alveolar hypoventilation. He has a pure respiratory acidosis and impaired level of consciousness with relatively normal oxygenation. Choice C is incorrect because the saturation is not higher than expected. Choice B is incorrect because naloxone can reverse respiratory depression, and choice E is incorrect because local anesthetics are not associated with respiratory depression. This makes A the best answer.

REFERENCES:

1. Barash PG, Cullen BF, Stoelting RK. Clinical Anesthesia, 4th ed. Philadelphia, Lippincott Williams & Wilkins, 2001, pp. 1417–1418.
2. Miller RD, Miller ED, Reves JG, et al. Anesthesia, 5th ed. New York, Churchill Livingstone, 2000, pp. 2330–2333.
3. Morgan GE, Mikhail MS, Murray MJ. Clinical Anesthesiology, 3d ed. New York, McGraw-Hill, 2002, pp. 501–502, 650–652.

BOOK B:

QUESTION 76

Answer B

Physiology

QUESTION (Choose single best answer):

A rapid, shallow ventilatory pattern is most energy efficient for a patient who

(A) Has a low ratio of forced expiratory volume in 1 second to vital capacity (FEV_1/VC).
(B) Has a high ratio of tidal volume to vital capacity and diminished vital capacity.
(C) Has increased pulmonary compliance.
(D) Is using the accessory muscles of respiration.
(E) Has increased airway resistance.

SUMMARY:

Patients with restrictive lung disease have decreased pulmonary compliance and characteristically exhibit a rapid, shallow breathing pattern that decreases the work of breathing. All lung volumes typically are reduced on spirometry, with vital capacity affected to a greater extent than tidal volume. The FEV_1/FVC ratio remains normal because both are decreased proportionally.

EXPLANATION:

(A) *Incorrect.* A low ratio of FEV_1 to vital capacity is characteristic of *obstructive* lung disease. Patients with obstructive lung disease do not benefit from a rapid, shallow ventilatory pattern.

(B) *Correct.* All lung volumes are decreased in restrictive lung disease.[2] However, vital capacity is affected to a greater extent than tidal volume.

(C) *Incorrect.* A rapid, shallow breathing pattern is most energy efficient for patients with restrictive lung disease who have *decreased* pulmonary compliance.[1]

(D) *Incorrect.* Patients using accessory muscles of respiration may be in respiratory distress. A rapid, shallow breathing pattern in these patients is not energy efficient and can represent impending respiratory failure.

(E) *Incorrect.* Patients with increased airway resistance benefit from a slower ventilatory pattern with emphasis on prolonged expiratory time. Obstructive lung disease is characterized by decreased flows, whereas patients with restrictive lung disease have decreased volumes.[2]

REASONING:

This question emphasizes the differences between obstructive and restrictive lung disease. The characteristic features of restrictive lung disease result from reduced lung compliance: smaller lung volumes and a rapid, shallow breathing pattern. Choice B may not be obvious at first, but it makes sense that vital capacity should be affected more than tidal volume during normal breathing because inspiratory reserve will be severely impaired by decreased lung compliance.

REFERENCES:

1. Stoelting RK, Miller RD. Basics of Anesthesia, 4th ed. New York, Churchill Livingstone, 2000, p. 275.
2. Barash PG, Cullen BF, Stoelting RK. Clinical Anesthesia, 4th ed. Philadelphia, Lippincott Williams & Wilkins, 2001, pp. 762, 764
3. Morgan GE, Mikhail MS, Murray MJ. Clinical Anesthesiology, 3d ed. New York, McGraw-Hill, 2002, pp. 489, 512, 518.

BOOK B:

QUESTION 77

Answer E

Clinical Anesthesia

QUESTION (Choose single best answer):

A 70-year-old patient has absence of the left radial pulse 1 month after repair of an aortic aneurysm. Arterial pressure was monitored perioperatively with a 20-gauge left radial artery catheter. Which of the following statements concerning this complication is true?

(A) A preoperative Allen's test would have predicted this complication.
(B) Stellate ganglion block should be performed.
(C) This complication would have been less likely with an 18-gauge catheter.
(D) This patient has poor collateral circulation in the hand.
(E) The pulse likely will return.

CORRECT ANSWER: E

SUMMARY:

The radial artery is used most often for continuous blood pressure monitoring because the location is accessible and there is usually good collateral circulation in the hand. This is often assessed with the Allen test. The test is thought to be unreliable owing to documented instances of ischemic injury despite normal Allen's tests. Successful and uncomplicated arterial catheterizations also have been documented despite abnormal Allen's tests.[1] In addition to thromboses, complications can include median nerve dysfunction, hematoma, infection, blood or air emboli, hand ischemia, skin necrosis, pseudoaneurysm, and arteriovenous fistula formation.[2] Avoidance of large catheters, longer duration of catheterization, and use of polypropelene-tapered catheters can help to decrease the incidence of complications.

EXPLANATION:

(A) *Incorrect.* The Allen's test does not reliably predict adverse outcomes from radial artery catheterization. Moreover, radial artery cannulations have been performed safely despite abnormal Allen's tests.[1]

(B) *Incorrect.* Stellate ganglion block is used to treat head, neck, arm, and upper chest pain. It also can be used after accidental intraarterial injection of thiopental.[2] But there is no evidence that such a block is indicated.

(C) *Incorrect.* Complications would be *more* likely with an 18-gauge catheter. The larger the catheter, the greater is the risk of thrombosis.[3]

(D) *Incorrect.* The fact that the radial artery is occluded does not necessarily mean that there is poor collateral circulation of the hand. The ulnar artery may be normal, patent, and supplying adequate blood to the rest of the hand even with the radial artery occluded. The patient described in this question has absence of radial pulse, not ischemia of the entire hand.

(E) *Correct.* In a study of 1700 patients who had radial artery cannulation, 25 percent had evidence of radial artery occlusion after decannulation. However, there were no ischemic complications.[1] Blood flow usually normalizes in 3 to 70 days.[2]

REASONING:

This question tests knowledge of the indications, placement technique, potential complications, and their treatment for radial arterial catheters. Knowing that the Allen's test is unreliable should allow choice A to be eliminated. Stellate ganglion block may help dilate the artery, but there is no evidence that this should be performed, so choice B can be ruled out. Choice C can be eliminated because catheter size is related to the incidence of complications. Absent radial pulse does not mean that there is poor circulation of that hand, so choice D can be eliminated. Finally, even though it may take time, recanulation of the artery usually occurs, making E the best answer.

REFERENCES:

1. Miller RD, Miller ED, Reves JG, et al. Anesthesia, 5th ed. New York, Churchill Livingstone, 2000, pp. 1124–1131.

2. Barash PG, Cullen BF, Stoelting RK. Clinical Anesthesia, 4th ed. Philadelphia, Lippincott Williams & Wilkins, 2001, pp. 673–674, 1240.

3. Benumof JL. Clinical Procedures in Anesthesia and Intensive Care. Philadelphia, Lippincott, 1992, pp. 383–384.

4. Morgan GE, Mikhail MS, Murray MJ. Clinical Anesthesiology, 3d ed. New York, McGraw-Hill, 2002, pp. 91–93, 332–333.

Answer A

OB/Regional

QUESTION (Choose single best answer):

Five minutes after intrathecal administration of tetracaine 12 mg in hyperbaric solution, a 60-year-old man has a weak hand grasp. Respirations are normal, heart rate has decreased from 80 to 45 beats per minute, and blood pressure has decreased from 150/80 to 90/50 mm Hg. The most appropriate management at this time is

(A) Administration of atropine.
(B) Administration of ephedrine.
(C) Administration of phenylephrine.
(D) Placement of the patient in the head-down position.
(E) Observation.

CORRECT ANSWER: A

SUMMARY:

With neuraxial anesthesia, the most readily anesthetized fibers are the small sympathetic nerves, followed by the unmyelinated and then the myelinated fibers associated with pain and touch, and finally, the myelinated motor neurons. When patients with spinal or epidural anesthesia exhibit decreased hand strength, the block is at least to the high thoracic and low cervical levels because the motor innervation to the hand is derived from C5–T1. This situation will result in significant decreases in blood pressure and heart rate owing to blockade of the sympathetic vasomotor fibers at T5–L1 and cardioaccelerator fibers at T1–4. Hypotension and bradycardia leading to full arrest are possible in this situation, especially in patients with high vagal tone.[1] The anesthesiologist must be prepared to treat the patient with fluids and medications such as atropine, ephedrine, and possibly epinephrine in order to increase cardiac output and systemic perfusion.[1]

EXPLANATION:

(A) *Correct.* The blockade of the cardioaccelerator fibers is causing severe bradycardia. When combined with the decreased vasomotor tone associated with sympathectomy, cardiac arrest is possible. Atropine is the medication of choice for this patient.

(B) *Incorrect.* Ephedrine is an indirect-acting alpha- and beta-agonist. It may be a second-line agent for treating this patient after atropine.[1]

(C) *Incorrect.* Phenylephrine is a direct alpha-agonist that will provide vasoconstriction, possibly resulting in a reflex bradycardia that would not be optimal in this patient.

(D) *Incorrect.* The solution is hyperbaric, which means that its spread in the intrathecal space depends on gravity. Placing this patient in the head-down position potentially could cause the block to move even higher.

(E) *Incorrect.* This patient does require careful observation for signs that his block is compromising respiratory function, but not in the absence of treating his current problems.

REASONING:

This question is testing what you should do *first*. The high level of neuraxial blockade is evidenced by the decreased grip strength in the hands. The cardiovascular effects of the spinal are manifested by decreased heart rate and blood pressure. In the setting of spinal (or epidural) anesthesia, bradycardia combined with the decreased venous return to the heart from the sympathectomy can lead to complete cardiac arrest. The first course of action should be to increase the heart rate. The drug of choice for this is atropine, followed by ephedrine and/or epinephrine if it is not effective.[1] A is the best answer.

REFERENCE:

1. Pollard JB. Cardiac arrest during spinal anesthesia: Common mechanisms and strategies for prevention. Anesth Analg 92:252–256, 2001.
2. Morgan GE, Mikhail MS, Murray MJ. Clinical Anesthesiology, 3d ed. New York, McGraw-Hill, 2002, pp. 258–260, 277.

BOOK B:

Answer B

Equipment/Physics

QUESTION 79

QUESTION (Choose single best answer):

A burn is found at the site of the electrocautery pad. Which of the following is most likely?

(A) The electrosurgical unit was in the bipolar mode.
(B) The electrocautery pad became partially detached.
(C) The electrosurgical unit ground wire was severed.
(D) The line-isolation monitor alarmed.
(E) The patient became grounded.

CORRECT ANSWER: B

SUMMARY:

The great majority of patient burns in the operating room are caused by incorrect or inadequate placement of the electrocautery pad on the patient. Electrocautery devices send ultrahigh-frequency current from the machine to the tip of the cauterizing electrode. The current has a high density at the electrocautery tip and is able to exert coagulation and cutting at the tissue level. The current enters the patient at the cautery tip and exits through the electrocautery pad. The pad should be placed on skin that is devoid of bony protuberances and should cover a large surface area. It is the large surface area of the electrocautery pad that prevents concentration of electrical current in a small area that would cause a burn. Inadequate surface-area coverage or placement over a bony protuberance that attracts current in high density can lead to unintended thermal injury in the operating room.

EXPLANATION:

(A) *Incorrect.* The bipolar mode of the electrocautery unit returns current through an adjacent return electrode in close proximity to the cautery tip. This confines the current flow to a few millimeters and eliminates the need for an electrocautery pad.
(B) *Correct.* Inadequate surface-area contact between the electrocautery pad and the patient can concentrate electric current on the exit limb of the circuit and lead to a patient burn at the site of the electrocautery pad.
(C) *Incorrect.* If an electrosurgical ground unit wire becomes severed, the isolation transformer (installed in most operating rooms in the United States) would protect the patient from electric shock. Because isolation transformers create a second ungrounded circuit loop, patient contact with a single live wire will not cause a shock or burn because no electric circuit is completed.
(D) *Incorrect.* The line-isolation monitor (LIM) alarm indicates that a single fault between a power line and ground has occurred. Because most operating rooms have isolation transformers, two faults have to occur in order for electric shock to occur. The most likely cause of thermal injury in this patient is a partially detached electrocautery pad. This event would not cause the LIM to alarm.
(E) *Incorrect.* If the patient becomes grounded in a modern operating room setting, an isolation transformer would prevent electric shock or burns by isolating the patient from completing an electric circuit.

REASONING:

This question tests knowledge of electrical safety in the operating room and causes of inadvertent thermal injury from electrocautery. Choice A can be eliminated because bipolar mode does not use an electrocautery pad. Choices C, D, and E are associated with electric shock and not burns or diathermy. B therefore is the best choice because it relates to burn injuries, and the mechanism involved clearly increases the risk for thermal injury (a smaller surface area of electric current causing a burn).

REFERENCE:

Barash PG, Cullen BF, Stoelting RK. Clinical Anesthesia, 4th ed. Philadelphia, Lippincott Williams & Wilkins, 2001, pp. 159–160.
Morgan GE, Mikhail MS, Murray MJ. Clinical Anesthesiology, 3d ed. New York, McGraw-Hill, 2002, pp. 23–25, Figs. 2-7, 2-8, and 2-10.

BOOK B:

QUESTION 80

Answer C

Equipment/Physics

QUESTION (Choose single best answer):

Which property of oxygen is detected by the fail-safe device on the anesthesia machine?

(A) Concentration
(B) Flow
(C) Pressure
(D) Partial pressure
(E) Reserve volume

CORRECT ANSWER: C

SUMMARY:

The fail-safe device on an anesthesia machine helps to prevents delivery of a hypoxic mixture of gas to patients. The device measures the pressure of oxygen across a valve near the oxygen flowmeter. Should the pressure of oxygen fall below 25 psig (normal is approximately 50 psig), the fail-safe valve will shut off automatically or proportionally decrease flow of all other gases.[1] When this occurs, an alarm will sound. The fail-safe mechanism does not protect against all causes of hypoxic gas mixtures such as insufficient O_2 concentration in the oxygen supply, inadvertent switching of the gas pipeline supplies, or hypoxic proportioning of gases at the flowmeter assembly (in the absence of a flow-proportioning system).

EXPLANATION:

(A) *Incorrect.* The fail-safe mechanism does not measure concentration of O_2. It measures the pressure in the oxygen pipeline across the valve.
(B) *Incorrect.* The flow of gases does not determine whether the gas mixture is hypoxic. Low flow can occur at 100% concentration of O_2, and there would be no need to shut off the delivery of other gases in this situation.
(C) *Correct.* The device measures the pressure of O_2 across the fail-safe valve. When it falls below 25 psig, it will shut off or proportionally decrease flow of all other gases, and an alarm will sound.
(D) *Incorrect.* The fail-safe valve measures the pressure of O_2 across a valve near the O_2 flowmeter, not the partial pressure of oxygen.
(E) *Incorrect.* The fail-safe device does not measure the reserve volume of oxygen in either the cylinders or the central supply.

REASONING:

This question tests knowledge of the fail-safe valve in an anesthesia machine. Choice A can be eliminated because the fail-safe valve does not measure the concentration of oxygen in the pipeline. Choice B potentially could be normal even when a gas mixture is hypoxic (i.e., if the flow of other gases is very high), so B is not a good answer. Choice E does not make sense because the fail-safe device is in the machine itself and not at the level of the oxygen tank or central supply of oxygen (where volume would have to be measured). This leaves choices C and D. The concentration of inspired oxygen is measured by an oxygen sensor in the inspiratory limb. The partial pressure of expired oxygen is measured by the gas analyzer. The pressure of oxygen (in psig) is measured by the fail-safe device. The best answer is C.

REFERENCE:

1. Barash PG, Cullen BF, Stoelting RK. Clinical Anesthesia, 4th ed. Philadelphia, Lippincott Williams & Wilkins, 2001, pp. 567, 668.
2. Morgan GE, Mikhail MS, Murray MJ. Clinical Anesthesiology, 3d ed. New York, McGraw-Hill, 2002, pp. 42–43.

BOOK B:

Answer A

OB/Regional

QUESTION 81

QUESTION (Choose single best answer):

Which of the following nerves should be blocked for an operation at the medial aspect of the lower leg?

(A) Femoral
(B) Sciatic
(C) Obturator
(D) Common peroneal
(E) Tibial

CORRECT ANSWER: A

SUMMARY:

Lower extremity nerve blocks are effective at providing both intraoperative and postoperative analgesia to patients undergoing surgery of the thigh, knee, or ankle. Blocking the femoral nerve at a level approximately 2 cm below the inguinal ligament (just lateral to the arterial pulse) will provide analgesia to the medial and anterior aspects of the thigh, as well as to the patellar region. The saphenous nerve comes off the posterior branch of the femoral nerve and supplies the medial portion of the lower leg to the level of the maleolus. Blocking the femoral nerve also will block areas of the lower extremity innervated by the saphenous nerve. Femoral nerve blockade is useful for surgeries of the anterior and medial aspects of the lower leg. For surgeries below the knee, femoral nerve blocks often are combined with sciatic and/or lateral femoral cutaneous nerve blocks to increase the lateral and posterior distributions of analgesia.

EXPLANATION:

(A) **Correct.** The femoral nerve supplies the anterior and medial aspects of the thigh and leg below the knee. It also supplies the knee joint and the ligaments within the joint. Blocking the femoral nerve is the single best regional technique for surgeries of the medial aspect of the lower leg. Combining femoral and sciatic nerve block is best for surgeries below the knee.

(B) **Incorrect.** The sciatic nerve supplies the posterior aspect of the thigh and gluteal region. Its branches supply the lateral aspect of the lower leg and the dorsolateral aspect of the foot. Sciatic nerve blocks by themselves will not provide analgesia for the medial aspect of the lower leg.

(C) **Incorrect.** The obturator nerve innervates the hip, the deep adductor muscles, and the lower aspect of the inner thigh. Obturator nerve block is indicated as a supplement to femoral, sciatic, and lateral femoral cutaneous nerve blocks. Alone it does not provide adequate surgical analgesia for procedures of the lower limb. The most common use of the obturator nerve block is in diagnosis of painful conditions of the hip or relief of adductor muscle spasms.

(D) **Incorrect.** The common peroneal nerve supplies the lateral (not medial) aspect of the lower leg.

(E) **Incorrect.** The tibial nerve supplies the lateral aspect of the ankle and the plantar surface of the foot.

REASONING:

This question tests knowledge of the nerve supply to the lower limb and differences in innervation to the medial and lateral aspects of the lower leg. Choices C and E can be eliminated because they do not supply the lower leg at all. Choice D can be eliminated if the reader knows that the peroneal nerve runs on the lateral aspect of the leg (derived from the sciatic nerve branches). This leaves choices A and B (femoral and sciatic). The sciatic nerve runs posteriorly, and branches wrap around to supply the lateral aspect of the leg. Thus the femoral nerve, choice A, is the best answer.

REFERENCE:

Cousins MJ, Bridenbaugh PO. Neural Blockade in Clinical Anesthesia and Management of Pain, 3d ed. Philadelphia, Lippincott, 1997, pp. 382–384.

Morgan GE, Mikhail MS, Murray MJ. Clinical Anesthesiology, 3d ed. New York, McGraw-Hill, 2002, pp. 298–305.

BOOK B: **QUESTION 82**

Answer B

Equipment/Physics

QUESTION (Choose single best answer):

Which of the following is most effective in preventing intraoperative hypothermia in adults?

(A) Heating and humidifying inspired gases
(B) Maintaining a warm operating room
(C) Using a circulating warm-water mattress
(D) Using reflective coverings
(E) Warming intravenous fluids

CORRECT ANSWER: B

SUMMARY:

Intraoperative hypothermia is a common complication in patients undergoing surgery. Heat loss occurs primarily through radiation, conduction, and convection from the patient's skin and open body cavities to surrounding ambient air and surfaces in contact with skin. Convection is by far the most important mechanism of heat loss.[1] Methods to prevent intraoperative hypothermia include administration of warm intravenous fluids, use of warmed and humidified inspired gases, maintaining a warm operating room environment, use of forced-air warming blankets (Bair Huggers), use of circulating warm-water mattresses, use of resistive heating pads, and use of reflective coverings. Of these, maintaining a warm operating room environment and forced-air warming (addressing convective heat loss) are the most efficient methods. Circulating warm-water mattresses and warming intravenous fluids are somewhat effective, whereas warm inspired gases and reflective coverings have been shown to be relatively ineffective at preventing hypothermia. Newer methods employing resistive heating techniques have been shown to be as effective as forced-air warming.

EXPLANATION:

(A) *Incorrect.* Heating and humidification of inspired gases are a relatively ineffective method of preventing intraoperative hypothermia.

(B) *Correct.* Conductive heat loss will not occur if the operating room environment is warmer than the patient's core temperature. However, this is difficult to accomplish while surgeons work under heavily gowned conditions. For this reason, other methods of preventing hypothermia must be employed.

(C) *Incorrect.* Circulating warm-air mattresses are used commonly in the pediatric operating room suite and are effective at providing conductive heat transfer. However, only the side of the body in contact with the mattress is treated, and therefore, this method is not as effective as maintaining high ambient air temperatures.

(D) *Incorrect.* Use of reflective coverings is relatively ineffective at preventing hypothermia.[2,3]

(E) *Incorrect.* Warming intravenous fluids is relatively ineffective at preventing hypothermia by itself because the total body surface area addressed by the intravascular system is small compared with skin.

REASONING:

This question is challenging because it requires comparing several different warming methods and fails to provide the most commonly used method (forced-air warming) as an answer option. Common sense can help to eliminate choices that are not used commonly in the operating room suite (choice A and D). The most efficient methods to prevent heat loss involve transfer of heat to the patient over a large surface area. Methods that provide contact between warm fluid or air with skin have the greatest surface-area exposure and therefore would be the best answers. Choice E can be eliminated by realizing that the total surface area of the intravascular system is relatively small compared with skin and that warming is limited by the total amount of intravenous fluid administered. This leaves choices B and C. B is the best answer because it involves contact with the largest surface area.

REFERENCES:

1. Buggy DJ, Crossley AWA. Thermoregulation, mild perioperative hypothermia and post-anaesthetic shivering. Br J Anaesth 84(5):615–628, 2000.
2. Bennett J, Ramachandra V, Webster J, Carli F. Prevention of hypothermia during hip surgery: Effect of passive compared with active skin surface warming. Br J Anaesth 73(2):180–183, 1994.
3. Ng SF, Oo CS, Loh KH, et al. A comparative study of three warming interventions to determine the most effective in maintaining perioperative normothermia. Anesth Analg 96(1):171–176, 2003.
4. Morgan GE, Mikhail MS, Murray MJ. Clinical Anesthesiology, 3d ed. New York, McGraw-Hill, 2002, pp. 117–120.

Answer C

Equipment/Physics

QUESTION (Choose single best answer):

Which of the following shaded areas most accurately represents the dead space of a properly functioning circle system?

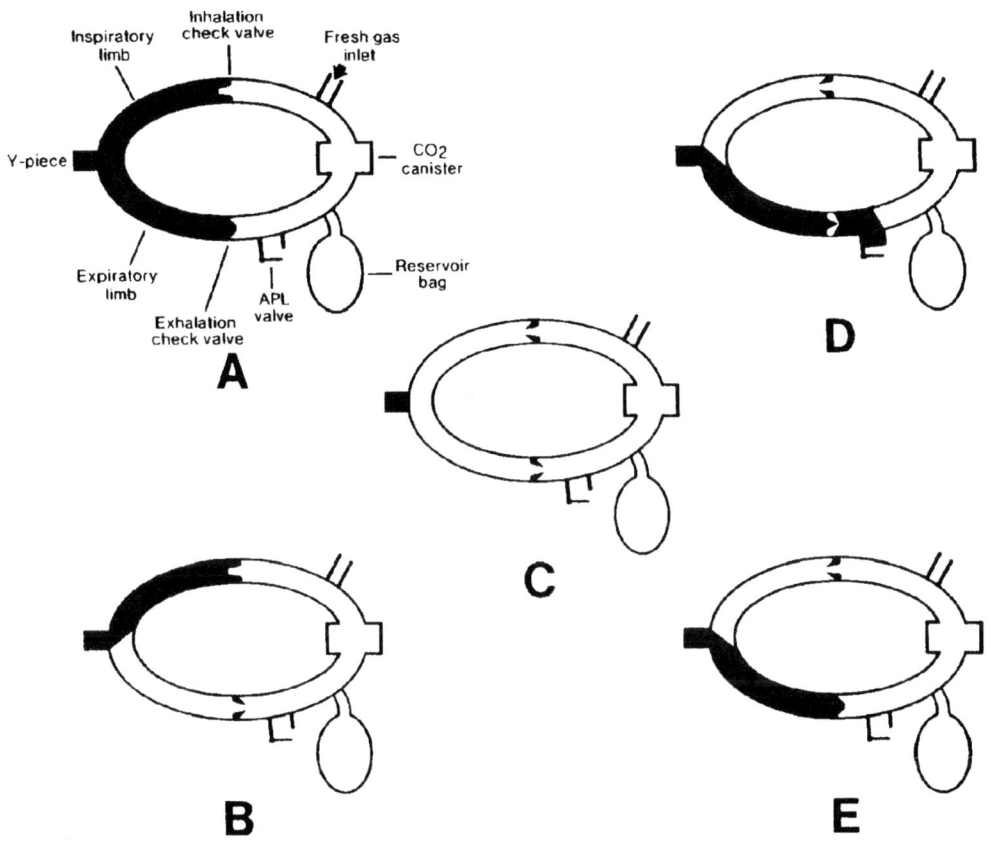

CORRECT ANSWER: C

SUMMARY:

The circle system used on most modern anesthesia machines was developed in an attempt to address the inefficiencies of the Mapleson and Bain circuits. Most important, the circle system overcomes the problem of rebreathing exhaled gases. In the circle system, the expiratory and inspiratory limbs are separated proximal to the Y-piece, and a unidirectional valve is employed in both limbs. This allows fresh gases to enter the system and exhaled gases to exit the system in separate limbs proximal to the Y-piece. The area of the circle system distal to the Y-piece is the only dead space of the circle system because it is the only place where inspired and exhaled gases are mixed. Areas of the circuit proximal to the Y-piece do not represent dead space.

EXPLANATION:

(A) *Incorrect.* The areas in the inspiratory and expiratory limbs that are proximal to the Y-piece do not represent dead space (see items B and E below).

(B) *Incorrect.* Because inspired gas only moves unidirectionally (toward the patient), the area between the inspiratory valve and the Y-piece is not dead space.

(C) *Correct.* Only the area distal to the Y-piece is dead space in the circle system. This is so because there is no mixing of inspired and expired gases proximal to the Y-piece.

(D) *Incorrect.* Neither the exhaled gas between the Y-piece and the expiratory valve nor that between the expiratory valve and the APL valve is dead space because no remixing of inspired and expired gas occurs.

(E) *Incorrect.* Since exhaled gases do not move backward across the expiratory valve, the area between the Y-piece and the expiratory valve is not dead space.

REASONING:

This question tests knowledge of dead space in the circle system. *Dead space* as it relates to breathing systems is defined as the part of tidal volume that does not participate in alveolar ventilation. Careful examination of the diagrams in this question should reveal that the volumes of gas in the inspiratory and expiratory limbs participate in alveolar ventilation during some part of their transit. Only the area in diagram C distal to the Y-piece contains mixed inspiratory and expiratory gases that does not undergo alveolar ventilation. Therefore, C is the best answer.

REFERENCE:

Barash PG, Cullen BF, Stoelting RK. Clinical Anesthesia, 4th ed. Philadelphia, Lippincott Williams & Wilkins, 2001, p. 581.

Morgan GE, Mikhail MS, Murray MJ. Clinical Anesthesiology, 3d ed. New York, McGraw-Hill, 2002, pp. 32–37.

BOOK B:

QUESTION 84

Answer B

Pharmacology

QUESTION (Choose single best answer):

The effect of succinylcholine is terminated at postsynaptic effector cells by

(A) Binding and uptake by effector cells.
(B) Diffusion into capillaries.
(C) Hydrolysis by junctional cholinesterase.
(D) Hydrolysis by pseudocholinesterase.
(E) Spontaneous degradation to succinylmonocholine.

CORRECT ANSWER: B

SUMMARY:

Succinylcholine is a rapidly acting depolarizing muscle relaxant that binds to receptors in the neuromuscular junction (NMJ) and mimics the action of acetylcholine. Succinylcholine works by inducing a long period of depolarization at the postsynaptic receptor such that acetylcholine cannot bind and cause muscle contraction. Succinylcholine undergoes rapid hydrolysis in the circulation by plasma cholinesterases. Its primary clinical effect occurs when drug that is not degraded in plasma reaches and binds to receptors at the level of the NMJ. Once bound, there is little available cholinesterase in the NMJ to terminate drug effect. Drug bound to postsynaptic NMJ receptors undergoes diffusion from the NMJ into the extracellular fluid. Degradation of succinylcholine occurs both at the level of the plasma (rapid hydrolysis) and at postsynaptic receptor cells (slow diffusion). This question specifically asks for the mechanism at postsynaptic cells.

EXPLANATION:

(A) *Incorrect.* The action of succinylcholine is terminated by hydrolysis at the level of the plasma and NMJ and by diffusion of unbound drug from the NMJ into capillaries. Binding of succinylcholine at effector cells would result in depolarizing blockade, not drug termination.

(B) **Correct.** Once succinylcholine is bound to receptor cells, termination of action occurs by diffusion into capillaries. This reduces the amount of available succinylcholine in the NMJ but does not terminate drug action once bound.

(C) **Incorrect.** Cholinesterases are not present in sufficiently large quantities in the NMJ to contribute to termination of action at the level of the postsynaptic receptors.

(D) **Incorrect.** Hydrolysis by pseudocholinesterases occurs in plasma with respect to unbound drug, not to drug already bound to NMJ receptors.

(E) **Incorrect.** Although succinylmonocholine is a major metabolite of succinylcholine, this metabolite is produced primarily in the circulation after hydrolysis, not at the level of the postsynaptic effector cells.

REASONING:

This question tests knowledge of the three sites at which succinylcholine is metabolized. Choice A can be eliminated because uptake and binding at effector cells likely would produce drug action, not termination. Choices D and E describe degradation of unbound drug in plasma, not at effector cells. Choice C is not a good choice because cholinesterases are not present in sufficient quantities in the NMJ. The vast amount of succinylcholine that reaches the NMJ and binds to receptors is removed via diffusion into extracellular fluid and capillaries. B is the best answer.

REFERENCE:

Stoelting RK. Pharmacology and Physiology in Anesthetic Practice, 3d ed. Philadelphia, Lippincott-Williams & Wilkins, 1998, pp. 189–190.
Morgan GE, Mikhail MS, Murray MJ. Clinical Anesthesiology, 3d ed. New York, McGraw-Hill, 2002, p. 183.

BOOK B:

Answer D

OB/Regional

QUESTION 85 (OPTIONAL)

QUESTION (Choose single best answer):

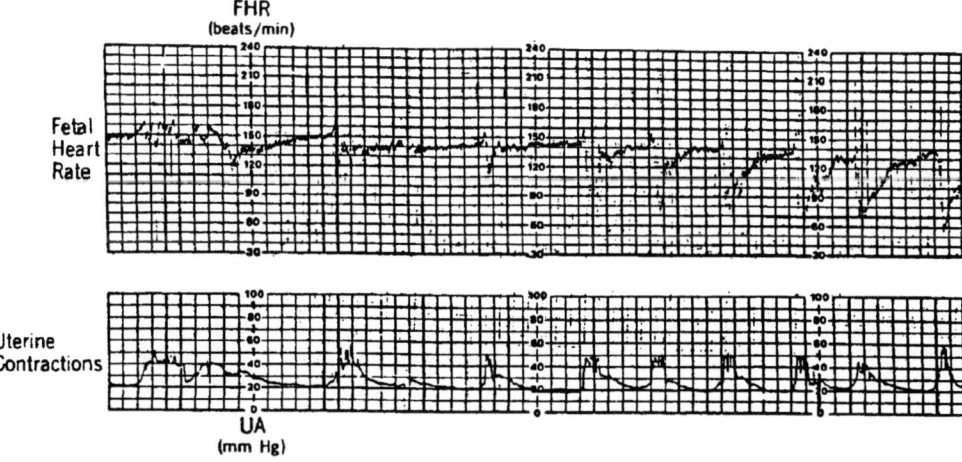

The fetal heart rate and uterine contraction tracings shown above are most consistent with

(A) Fetal acidosis.
(B) Fetal cerebral hemorrhage.
(C) Fetal head compression.
(D) Fetal hypoxia.
(E) Uteroplacental insufficiency.

CORRECT ANSWER: D

SUMMARY:

It is essential for the anesthesiologist to possess an understanding of fetal heart rate monitoring because it is a useful tool for measuring fetal oxygenation and well-being. The fetal heart rate tracing should be measured in conjunction with uterine contractions. U-shaped decelerations that predictably occur with contractions are referred to as "early" or "late" depending on when they occur. Early decelerations have their onset with the contraction, nadir at the peak, and return to baseline by the end of the contraction. These decelerations are a reassuring pattern associated with fetal head compression. Late decelerations begin after the onset of the contraction, nadir after the peak, and return to baseline after the contraction. This pattern is associated with uteroplacental insufficiency and is commonly a nonreassuring pattern depending on the fetal baseline heart rate and variablilty. Variable decelerations have an abrupt onset and variable association with contractions, and the change from baseline is greater than with other types of decelerations. This pattern tends to be nonreassuring and is associated with acute interruptions in umbilical cord blood flow. Over time, fetal hypoxia can develop with both variable and late patterns owing to a decreased ability of the fetus to compensate for the interruptions in blood flow.

EXPLANATION:

(A) *Incorrect.* While lactic acidosis can develop over time in a compromised fetus, there is not a predictable pattern associated with fetal acidosis.

(B) *Incorrect.* There is currently no reliable method to detect fetal cerebral hemorrhage from the fetal heart rate tracing.

(C) *Incorrect.* Fetal head compression is associated with early decelerations. While the onset of this patient's decelerations occurs with contractions and the nadir is close to the peak in a couple of the decelerations, the lowest heart rate is much lower than what is usually associated with early decelerations, and the return to baseline is long after the contraction is over.

(D) *Correct.* The fetus is exhibiting variable decelerations in the second stage of labor (one can see that the patient is pushing based on the up and down pattern with the uterine contractions). This is a common pattern in this stage of labor.[1] However, the slow return to baseline as the labor progresses indicates a decreased ability to tolerate the acute decreases in umbilical cord blood flow, and the decelerations become more profound and the return to baseline becomes slower. This is a pattern associated with fetal hypoxia.[1]

(E) *Incorrect.* Uteroplacental insufficiency is associated with late decelerations, which are not seen in this tracing.

REASONING:

This is a difficult question because the fetal heart rate tracing is not straightforward. Choice B can be eliminated immediately because there is not a pattern associated with cerebral hemorrhage. The next step is to determine what types of decelerations are displayed. Since they have an abrupt onset and low nadir, they are variables. Why not early or late? It is possible that the first few decelerations are early, but the overwhelming pattern is one with acute decelerations, gradually getting lower, and a return to baseline that is getting slower. This pattern is associated with variable decelerations, and the slow return to baseline over time is associated with hypoxia.[1] Knowing this, one can eliminate choices C and E. We know that the baby is compromised, but we would not know it was acidotic without performing a blood gas analysis. Choice A can be eliminated. The best answer is D. The reader should not be discouraged by the difficulty of this question. We were only able to interpret this tracing correctly after extensive research and consultation with senior maternal-fetal medicine specialists at Stanford.

REFERENCES:

1. Gibb D, Arulkumaran S. Fetal Monitoring in Practice, 2d ed. Oxford, UK, Butterworth Heinemann, 1997, pp. 45–70, 130–131.
2. Freeman RK, Garite TJ, Nageotte MP. Fetal Heart Rate Monitoring, 2d ed. Baltimore, Williams & Wilkins, 1991, pp. 13–17, 71–83.
3. Hughes SC, Levinson G, Rosen MA. Shnider and Levinson's Anesthesia for Obstetrics, 4th ed. Philadelphia, Lippincott Williams & Wilkins, 2002, pp. 3–8.
4. Morgan GE, Mikhail MS, Murray MJ. Clinical Anesthesiology, 3d ed. New York, McGraw-Hill, 2002, pp. 840–842, Fig. 43-3, Periodic Changes in Fetal Heart Rate Related to Uterine Contractions.

BOOK B:

None of the choices are correct.

Basic Science

QUESTION 86 (OPTIONAL)

QUESTION (Choose single best answer):

The cardiovascular effects of an inhalational anesthetic are evaluated in 10 normal volunteers in the awake resting state and after 15 minutes of constant inspired concentration. Results were analyzed by t test for paired data and are presented below as mean ± standard deviation.

	Mean Arterial Pressure (mm Hg)	Heart Rate (bpm)	Cardiac Output (L/min)
Awake	94±5	82±2	4.2±0.5
Anesthetized	83±9	90±2*	3.9±0.7

*$p < .05$.

Based on these data, which of the following conclusions is most valid?

(A) A decrease in cardiac output would have been evident if more subjects were included in the study.
(B) The anesthetic decreases mean arterial pressure.
(C) The anesthetic does not cause cardiac depression.
(D) The anesthetic is unsafe for patients with coronary artery disease.
(E) The is a 95 to 100 percent chance that the anesthetic increases heart rate.

CORRECT ANSWER: None of the choices are correct.

SUMMARY:

Anesthesiologists should have a basic understanding of epidemiology and statistics in order to interpret the quality of evidence presented in scientific journals. Anesthetic practice should be guided by evidence-based principles that are supported by high-quality research. This question describes a crossover study in which the patient serves as his or her own control. Measurements first were performed awake and then repeated while the patient was anesthetized. The outcome measures (mean arterial pressure, heart rate, and cardiac output) are all continuous variables and can be described by their average value (mean) and standard deviation (a measure of variance from the mean). The correct statistical test for analyzing continuous variables in a crossover study is the paired t *test because it accounts for the decreased sample variance when a subject is used as his or her own control. A* p *value indicates the probability of committing a type I error, i.e., the chance that we reject the null hypothesis, H_0, when it is actually true. In this case, the H_0 would state: "There is no significant change in heart rate when a patient is anesthetized." The* p *< .05 for the heart rate variable indicates that this H_0 can be rejected with a 5 percent chance of committing a type I error. Restated, we can be at least 95 percent certain that anesthia increases heart rate.*

EXPLANATION:

(A) *Incorrect.* This study did not show a statistically significant difference in cardiac output when the patient was anesthetized. Negative findings should prompt the reader to question the power of the study to resolve the difference it observed. Statistical power is the probability of concluding that there was a difference when a difference truly exists. In other words, power reflects our confidence that we could detect a difference in cardiac output if there were truly a difference. The computed post hoc power for this study is approximately 20 percent.[1] Thus we are only 20 percent confident that we could detect a difference in cardiac output if a difference truly exists. Therefore, it is possible that we may find a difference if a larger cohort of patients were studied. However, we cannot conclude with certainty that this would be the case.

(B) *Incorrect.* The difference on this measure did not reach statistical significance ($p < .05$), and we cannot reject the H_0.

(C) *Incorrect.* We cannot make a conclusion on this measure because this study did not evaluate "cardiac depression." We presume that cardiac depression means negative inotropy, although this is not specified.

(D) *Incorrect.* We cannot make this conclusion based on the current study design. The cohort used in this study did not have coronary artery disease. In addition, the outcome measure "anesthetic is unsafe" would need to be defined more clearly (e.g., incidence of perioperative myocardial infarction, drop in MAP greater than 20 mm Hg with induction, etc.).

(E) *Incorrect.* The difference on this measure did reach statistical significance ($p < .05$), and we can reject the H_0 with 95 percent certainty. Therefore, we can say that the anesthetic increases heart rate with at least 95 percent certainty. Please note, however, that this is not the same as saying, "There is a 95 to 100 percent chance that the anesthetic increases heart rate." In truth, the anesthetic either increases heart rate or it does not. This is truth, and it is fixed. Therefore, there is not a 95 percent chance that the anesthetic increases heart rate; it simply does or it does not. Scientific methods and statistical analysis allow us to report that we can be 95 percent certain that we captured the truth. In addition, it should be noted that nothing can be proven to have a 100 percent certainty of being correct.

REASONING:

This question tests knowledge of basic epidemiology and statistics for interpretation of experimental evidence. Choice D can be eliminated immediately because patients with coronary artery disease were not studied in this experiment. Choice A can be eliminated even though the study did not have adequate power to resolve the observed difference in cardiac output. We cannot know with certainty that a difference would be found if a larger cohort were studied. Choice B can be eliminated because we did not achieve statistical significance ($p < .05$) on this measure. Choice C can be eliminated because "cardiac depression" was not measured in this study. The only outcome measure that was statistically significant was an increase in heart rate. Choice E is not correct because the anesthetic cannot have a "chance" of increasing heart rate—it either does or does not. We can report that we have a 95 percent certainty that it increases heart rate, but we can never claim that we have 100 percent certainty in resolving the truth. On an actual examination, we would choose choice E because it best reflects the intent of the question. However, none of the answers are correct.

REFERENCE:

1. Norman GR, Streiner DL. Biostatistics: The Bare Essentials. Ontario, BC Decker, 2000, Chap. 7, pp. 62–68.
2. Morgan GE, Mikhail MS, Murray MJ. Clinical Anesthesiology, 3d ed. New York, McGraw-Hill, 2002, pp. 137–145.

Answer D

Clinical Anesthesia

QUESTION (Choose single best answer):

A patient with alcoholic cirrhosis, ascites, and gastrointestinal bleeding receives 4 units of red blood cells prior to anesthesia with isoflurane in oxygen for emergency exploratory laparotomy. After the peritoneum is opened and the fluid is drained, blood pressure decreases to 60/40 mm Hg and SpO$_2$ decreases to 90 percent. The most likely cause of the hypoxemia is

(A) Acute myocardial ischemia.
(B) Decreased 2,3-diphosphoglycerate in transfused blood.
(C) Increased intrapulmonary shunting.
(D) Relative hypovolemia.
(E) Venous air embolism.

CORRECT ANSWER: D

SUMMARY:

Liver cirrhosis is characterized by a hyperdynamic circulatory state with arteriovenous shunting present in both the systemic and pulmonary systems. Low blood viscosity owing to chronic anemia and hypoalbuminemia further contributes to this hyperdynamic state of high cardiac output and low peripheral vascular resistance. Ascites fluid increases intraabdominal pressure on the diaphragm and creates a restrictive pulmonary physiology. Hypoxemia results from a combination of pulmonary arteriovenous (AV) communications and $\dot{V}/\dot{Q}$ mismatch. Although the circulatory and ventilatory systems generally are compensated, infection, blood loss, rapid volume shifts, and cardiac dysfunction can quickly upset this fragile balance and lead to circulatory collapse.

EXPLANATION:

(A) *Incorrect.* Myocaridal infarction can cause hypotension and hypoxemia. However, in this patient, the symptoms presented during decompression of the peritoneum on opening the abdomen. The most likely clinical explanation is that the rapid fluid drainage caused an intravascular volume shift to the extravascular space, creating a relative hypovolemia. Decreased venous return to the heart lowers pulmonary perfusion and increases alveolar dead space, which results in hypoxemia.

(B) *Incorrect.* Transfused packed red blood cells are depleted of 2,3-DPG and cause a leftward shift of the oxyhemoglobin dissociation curve, impeding unloading of oxygen from hemoglobin. The transfusion was given prior to anesthesia, and the SpO$_2$ was apparently normal prior to induction. The timing of the symptoms makes this an unlikely cause of hypoxemia in this patient.

(C) *Incorrect.* Increased intrapulmonary shunting would exacerbate hypoxia. However, the abdominal decompression is expected to relieve the pressure on the diaphragm and improve pulmonary gas exchange instead of making it worse.

(D) *Correct.* Intraabdominal bleeding can be extensive in a patient with liver failure and presumed coagulopathy. Although bleeding may have been slowed temporarily by a tamponade effect, hypovolemia can be unmasked rapidly once the peritoneum is opened and bleeding resumes.

(E) *Incorrect.* Venous air embolism is a rare complication that is unlikely in this patient.

REASONING:

This question tests knowledge of the pathophysiology of alcoholic cirrhosis and liver failure. The clinical scenario of hypotension and hypoxemia can happen in the setting of myocardial infarction, VAE, and hypovolemia. The most likely cause in this patient is relative hypovolemia, choice D.

REFERENCE:

Barash PG, Cullen BF, Stoelting RK. Clinical Anesthesia, 4th ed. Philadelphia, Lippincott Williams & Wilkins, 2001, pp. 1256–1258.

Morgan GE, Mikhail MS, Murray MJ. Clinical Anesthesiology, 3d ed. New York, McGraw-Hill, 2002, pp. 726–728.

BOOK B:

QUESTION 88

Answer D

Neuroanesthesia

QUESTION (Choose single best answer):

Which of the following statements concerning barbiturate protection from cerebral ischemia is true?

(A) It may be achieved with dosages low enough to avoid cardiovascular effects.
(B) It is linearly dose-related.
(C) It improves neurologic outcome following cardiac arrest.
(D) It is most useful in patients with focal ischemia.
(E) It is unrelated to electroencephalographic (EEG) activity.

CORRECT ANSWER: D

SUMMARY:

Barbiturates can maximally reduce the cerebral metabolic requirement for oxygen ($CMRO_2$) at doses high enough to induce an isoelectric EEG.[1] In addition, barbiturates can cause inverse steal by vasoconstricting blood vessels in areas of healthy brain and shunting blood to ischemic brain tissue, reduce calcium influx, block sodium channels, and inhibit free-radical formation. Cerebral protection by barbiturates is limited to focal ischemic events. They do not confer any significant benefit following global ischemia owing to cardiac arrest.

EXPLANATION:

(A) *Incorrect.* Barbiturates induce burst suppression on the EEG after a large bolus of 15 to 40 mg/kg. This often requires administration of vasopressors to avoid significant hypotension.
(B) *Incorrect.* The cerebral protective effect of barbiturates plateaus with the onset of burst suppression. Higher doses result in an increased incidence of side effects without additional benefits.
(C) *Incorrect.* There is no clear evidence that any anesthetic agent is effective in protecting the brain from global ischemic events such as cardiac arrest.
(D) *Correct.* Electrical silence induced by barbiturates provides some cerebral protection in patients who suffer focal ischemic events.
(E) *Incorrect.* The cerebral protective effect of barbiturates is directly related to the onset of burst suppression. Maximal reduction in $CMRO_2$ is achieved when the EEG is isoelectric.[1]

REASONING:

This question tests knowledge of barbiturate protection from cerebral ischemia. Choice A can be eliminated because large bolus doses of barbiturates can require administration of vasopressor medications to treat or prevent hypotension. Choice E can be eliminated because cerebral protection often involves modulation of $CMRO_2$ and EEG activity. Choice C can be eliminated because no study has shown conclusively that barbiturates improve neurologic outcome following cardiac arrest. D is be the best answer.[2]

REFERENCES:

1. Stoelting RK, Dierdorf SF. Anesthesia and Co-Existing Diseases, 3d ed. New York, Churchill Livingstone, 1993, p. 63.

2. Barash PG, Cullen BF, Stoelting RK. Clinical Anesthesia, 4th ed. Philadelphia, Lippincott Williams & Wilkins, 2001, p. 707.

3. Morgan GE, Mikhail MS, Murray MJ. Clinical Anesthesiology, 3d ed. New York, McGraw-Hill, 2002, pp. 156–159, 561–562.

BOOK B:

Answer D

Clinical Anesthesia

QUESTION 89

QUESTION (Choose single best answer):

A 77-year-old woman is still intubated and breathing spontaneously following a total hip replacement. The muscle relaxant has been reversed. Tidal volume is 400 mL, end-tidal carbon dioxide tension is 45 mm Hg, and SpO_2 is 98 percent at an FIO_2 of 1.0. On transfer from the operating table to the gurney, her heart rate increases from 65 to 100 beats per minute, and her blood pressure decreases from 130/80 to 80/50 mm Hg. End-tidal carbon dioxide tension ($ETCO_2$) is 30 mm Hg, and SpO_2 is 94 percent. The most likely diagnosis is

(A) Anaphylactic reaction.
(B) Bronchospasm.
(C) Myocardial infarction.
(D) Pulmonary embolism.
(E) Unreplaced blood loss.

CORRECT ANSWER: D

SUMMARY:

Three potentially life-threatening complications associated with total hip replacement (THR) are cement implantation syndrome, thromboembolism, and intraoperative hemorrhage. Cement implantation syndrome typically occurs at the time of insertion of the joint prosthesis and presents with systemic hypotension, hypoxia, and pulmonary hypertension. The etiology is now thought to be related to medullary fat embolization rather than to intrinsic cement toxicity.[1,2] Methyl methacrylate is an acrylic cement compound used to fuse the joint prosthesis to bone in arthroplastic procedures. The cement produces an exothermic reaction that can lyse blood cells and bone marrow.[3] Conversion of methyl methacrylate to methacrylate acid and absorption of its volatile monomer also may contribute to toxicity.[3] Deep venous thrombosis is the most frequent postoperative complication associated with lower extremity joint replacement, with a reported prevalence as high as 80 percent.[4] Clinically significant pulmonary embolism occurs in 2 to 10 percent of these patients. The incidence of fatal pulmonary embolism after hip arthroplasty is 1 to 2 percent.[5]

EXPLANATION:

(A) ***Incorrect.*** Anaphylactic reaction to the cement or anesthetic can occur, but it is a rare complication. Hypersensitivity reactions to methyl methacrylate cement typically occur in dental workers after chronic exposure. Anaphylactic reactions often are correlated temporally with a specific exposure. This patient's sudden hypotension in the absence of an inciting exposure makes this choice less likely.

(B) ***Incorrect.*** Bronchospasm is characterized by increased expiratory effort and polyphonic expiratory wheezes that usually are accompanied by coughing, shortness of breath, or complaints of chest tightness. We are not given any other information to suspect this finding.

(C) ***Incorrect.*** A sudden acute myocardial infarction leading to hemodynamic compromise and collapse could explain the observed findings, but it is not the most likely diagnosis in this patient.

(D) **Correct.** Patients undergoing hip replacement surgery have a high incidence of developing deep venous thrombosis (DVT). They also have an increased risk of developing clinically significant and/or fatal pulmonary embolism. Pulmonary embolism acutely increases pulmonary vascular resistance, causing a localized or generalized reflex bronchoconstriction to areas affected by the embolic event. The result is an increase in pulmonary shunting and hypoxemia. Tachycardia, elevated central venous pressure (CVP), and hypotension also may occur owing to progressive right ventricular failure.

(E) **Incorrect.** Only hypovolemia owing to rapid blood loss could explain these acute cardiovascular changes. We have no reason to suspect it in this patient.

REASONING:

This question tests knowledge of common complications following hip replacement surgery. It is important to understand that these patients are at increased perioperative risk for developing clinically significant and/or fatal pulmonary embolism from DVT. Cement implantation syndrome also places these patients at increased risk of hypotension, hypoxia, and pulmonary embolism during femoral reaming and joint placement. The temporal association of the patient's hypotension with transfer from the operating table makes dislodgment of a DVT and subsequent pulmonary embolism the most likely diagnosis. D is the best answer.

REFERENCES:

1. Byrick RJ. Cement implantation syndrome: A time-limited embolic phenomenon. Can J Anaesth 44:107–111, 1997.
2. Orsini EC, Byrick RJ, Mullen JBM, et al. Cardiopulmonary function and pulmonary microemboli during arthroplasty using cemented or noncemented components: The role of intramedullary pressure. J Bone Joint Surg 69A:822–832, 1987.
3. Barash PG, Cullen BF, Stoelting RK. Clinical Anesthesia, 4th ed. Philadelphia, Lippincott Williams & Wilkins, 2001, p. 1117.
4. Anderson FS Jr, Wheeler HB, Goldberg RJ, et al. A population-based perspective of the hospital incidence and case-fatality rates of deep vein thrombosis and pulmonary embolism: A community-wide survey. J Vasc Surg 151:933–938, 1991.
5. Lieberman JR. Venous thromboembolism after total hip arthroplasty. In Callaghan JJ, Rosenberg AG, Rubash HE, eds. The Adult Hip. Philadelphia, Lippincott-Raven, 1998, pp. 633–646.
6. Morgan GE, Mikhail MS, Murray MJ. Clinical Anesthesiology, 3d ed. New York, McGraw-Hill, 2002, pp. 520, 786.

BOOK B: **QUESTION 90**

Answer D

Pain

QUESTION (Choose single best answer):

A 40-year-old woman has continuous nondermatomal burning pain of the distal foot 4 weeks after sustaining a metatarsal fracture. On examination, the foot is mildly swollen, tender, and cool. Which of the following statements concerning this condition is true?

(A) A radiograph of the distal bones of the painful foot will show severe osteoporosis.
(B) A technetium scan of the distal joints of the painful foot will show decreased uptake.
(C) Early use of the opioid analgesia will prevent progression of the symptoms.
(D) Intravenous phentolamine will relieve the pain.
(E) The chance of spontaneous recovery within 8 weeks is greater than 80 percent.

CORRECT ANSWER: D

SUMMARY:

This question describes the syndrome of reflex sympathetic dystrophy now know as complex regional pain syndrome type I *(CRPS). During the acute phase, a technetium bone scan will show increased uptake, and the x-ray will be normal. Opioids have no effect on the course of the disease. If the pain is sympathetically maintained, blockade with the alpha-blocker phentolamine may relieve it.[1] The chance of recovery has been reported to be high if treatment is initiated within a month of symptom onset.*

EXPLANATION:

(A) *Incorrect.* The condition has only occurred for 4 weeks, during which time only minimal changes would be expected. No specific test is available for CRPS. Plain radiographs can show patchy osteoporosis as early as 2 weeks after the onset of CRPS. As the disease progresses, the bones may have a ground glass appearance, and cortical erosions may be present.

(B) *Incorrect.* As stated above, the classic finding would be increased uptake on technetium scan. A technetium scan of the affected joints has been studied for CRPS. It has been reported to be sensitive but not specific. Classic findings include increased periarticular uptake, although the reverse sometimes can be seen.[2]

(C) *Incorrect.* Opioids do not prevent progression of the disease and are controversial in the treatment of this disease because they often are not effective.

(D) *Correct.* Intravenous phentolamine will relieve the pain. This effect is dose-dependent and correlates with relief provided by local anesthetic sympathetic block.

(E) *Incorrect.* Aggressive treatment with physical therapy and sympathetic blockade is required to achieve a high rate of recovery.

REASONING:

This question tests knowledge of the diagnosis and treatment of CRPS. The diagnosis requires the presence of regional pain and sensory changes following a noxious event (either a serious or trivial injury). Furthermore, the pain is associated with findings such as abnormal skin color, temperature change, abnormal sudomotor activity, or edema. The combination of these findings exceeds their expected magnitude in response to known physical damage during and following the inciting event. These changes occur in the absence of other concomitant conditions that might account for the findings. Two types of CRPS have been recognized. Type I corresponds to reflex sympathetic dystrophy (RSD) and occurs without a definable nerve lesion. Type II, formerly called *causalgia,* refers to cases where a definable nerve lesion is present.[3] A hallmark of these conditions is the presence of sympathetically maintained pain that can be relieved by regional sympathetic block, intravenous regional block, or infusion of the alpha-adrenergic blocker phentolamine. Aggressive early intervention is needed to produce a high rate of recovery.

REFERENCES:

1. Arner S. Intravenous phentolamine test: Diagnostic and prognostic use in reflex sympathetic dystrophy. Pain 46(1):17–22, 1991.

2. Rho R, Brewer RP, Lamer TJ, Wilson PR. Complex regional pain syndrome. Mayo Clin Proc 77(2):174–180, 2002.

3. Stanton-Hicks M, Jänig W, Hassenbusch S, et al. Reflex sympathetic dystrophy: Changing concepts and taxonomy. Pain 63:127–133, 1995.

4. Morgan GE, Mikhail MS, Murray MJ. Clinical Anesthesiology, 3d ed. New York, McGraw-Hill, 2002, pp. 308–309.

Answer D

Clinical Anesthesia

QUESTION (Choose single best answer):

Evaluation of a postoperative neurologic deficit discloses an inability to oppose the thumb and little finger, weakness of abduction of the thumb, and loss of flexion of the distal phalanx of the index finger. This problem is most likely related to

(A) Paresthesia occurring during an interscalene brachial plexus block.
(B) Attempted radial artery cannulation at the wrist.
(C) Inadequate padding under the elbow.
(D) Attempted venipuncture in the antecubital fossa.
(E) Abduction of the upper humerus against an "ether screen."

CORRECT ANSWER: D

SUMMARY:

The median nerve lies next to the medial cubital and basilic veins in the antecubital fossa and may be traumatized by attempts at cannulation (arterial or venous) or by the extravasation of intravenous medications such as thiopental.[1,2] This nerve is rarely injured by improper positioning (e.g., extreme dorsiflexion at the wrist). A median nerve injury will result in an inability to oppose the thumb and little finger, weakness of thumb abduction, loss of flexion of the distal phalanx of the index finger, and decreased sensation over the palmar surface of the thumb, index finger, and lateral half of the middle finger.[2]

EXPLANATION:

(A) *Incorrect.* An interscalene brachial plexus block affects the C5–T1 dermatomes and is useful for surgery on the shoulder, arm, and forearm. Paresthesias elicited during the performance of this block will not result in an isolated median nerve palsy.
(B) *Incorrect.* Radial artery cannulation has been associated with hematomas, thrombosis, air embolization, and infection, and would be more likely to harm the radial nerve.
(C) *Incorrect.* Inadequate padding under the elbow may result in an ulnar neuropathy, the most common perioperative peripheral nerve injury. This nerve is injured most frequently when the forearm is flexed or pronated. There is usually elbow pain and impairment of flexion at the proximal finger joints and abduction/adduction of the fingers. Risk factors for ulnar neuropathies include male gender, a hospital stay greater than 2 weeks, and a very large or very thin body habitus.
(D) *Correct.* Attempts at venipuncture in the cubital fossa may result in a median nerve palsy, as described above.
(E) *Incorrect.* Compression of the upper lateral humerus predisposes to a radial nerve injury leading to wrist drop, inability to extend at the metacarpophalangeal joints, and weak abduction of the thumb.

REASONING:

This question tests knowledge of neuroanatomy and innervation to the upper extremity and hand. Choice D is clearly correct because the question describes a neurologic deficit consistent with a median nerve injury, given the distribution of the injury. It is also important to understand that trauma from attempted venipuncture is the most likely mechanism of injury in this patient. D is the best answer.

REFERENCES:

1. Gravenstein N, Kirby RR. Complications in Anesthesiology, 2d ed. Philadelphia, Lippincott-Raven, 1996, pp. 372–375.
2. Stoelting RK, Miller RD. Basics of Anesthesia, 4th ed. New York, Churchill Livingstone, 2000, p. 206.
3. Morgan GE, Mikhail MS, Murray MJ. Clinical Anesthesiology, 3d ed. New York, McGraw-Hill, 2002, pp. 93, 295, 288–289, 296ff, 893, 897ff, 899t.

QUESTION (Choose single best answer):

Arterial oxyhemoglobin desaturation develops more rapidly following apnea in a pregnant patient at term than in a nonpregnant patient with a large intraabdominal tumor. Which of the following findings in pregnancy is the most likely cause?

(A) Higher cardiac output.
(B) Higher oxygen consumption.
(C) Larger anatomic dead space.
(D) Smaller blood volume.
(E) Smaller functional residual capacity.

CORRECT ANSWER: B

SUMMARY:

Many physiologic changes occur during pregnancy. Changes affecting the cardiorespiratory system include increased blood volume by 35 percent, increased plasma volume by 45 percent, increased cardiac output by 40 percent, increased oxygen consumption by up to 50 percent, increased tidal volume by 40 percent, increased minute ventilation by 50 percent, and decreased functional residual capacity (FRC) by 20 percent. Under normal circumstances, increased minute ventilation and tidal volume compensate for the increased oxygen consumption. However, when parturients become apenic, the increased oxygen consumption combined with the smaller FRC causes rapid arterial oxyhemoglobin desaturation, even when compared with a patient with a large intraabdominal tumor of comparable size to the gravid uterus.

EXPLANATION:

(A) *Incorrect.* Parturients have an increase in cardiac output by up to 40 percent at term. This serves to increase oxygen delivery to the tissues and does not contribute to arterial desaturation.

(B) *Correct.*

$$\text{Apneic time} = (\text{FRC} \times \text{F}_{IO_2})/\dot{V}_{O_2}$$

where apneic time is the period of time from the beginning of apnea until arterial oxyhemoglobin desaturation occurs, FRC is the functional residual capacity, F_{IO_2} is the alveolar oxygen concentration, and $\dot{V}_{O_2}$ is the rate of oxygen consumption. $\dot{V}_{O_2}$ increases by 20 to 50 percent in pregnancy mainly owing to fetal consumption. Patients who have a large intraabdominal tumor do not have an increased $\dot{V}_{O_2}$ and therefore do not desaturate as quickly as a parturient.

(C) *Incorrect.* Anatomic dead space is not changed in parturients.[1]

(D) *Incorrect.* Parturients have a 35 percent increase in blood volume at term.

(E) *Incorrect.* FRC is decreased by 20 percent in parturients.

REASONING:

This question requires knowledge of the major cardiopulmonary physiologic changes in pregnancy. These include decreased FRC, increased oxygen consumption, increased cardiac output, and increased blood volume. These facts eliminate choice D. Anatomic dead space is a parameter that does not change in pregnancy, which eliminates answer C. While a patient with a large intraabdominal tumor will have a decreased FRC and possibly an increased cardiac output depending on the vascularity of the tumor, these patients do not have a significant source of oxygen consumption such as a growing fetus, which eliminates answers A and E. B is the best answer.

REFERENCE:

1. Hughes SC, Levinson G, Rosen MA. Shnider and Levinson's Anesthesia for Obstetrics, 4th ed. Philadelphia, Lippincott Williams & Wilkins, 2002, pp. 3–8.
2. Morgan GE, Mikhail MS, Murray MJ. Clinical Anesthesiology, 3d ed. New York, McGraw-Hill, 2002, pp. 805–806, Table 42-1, Average Maximum Physiologic Changes Associated with Pregnancy.

BOOK B: **QUESTION 93**

Answer D

Neuroanesthesia

QUESTION (Choose single best answer):

Which of the following best describes the relationship between cerebral perfusion pressure and cerebral blood flow in a patient with untreated chronic hypertension?

(A) It is constant at mean blood pressures between 50 and 150 mm Hg.
(B) It is linear for all blood pressures.
(C) The flow-versus-pressure curve is hyperbolic.
(D) The flow-versus-pressure curve is shifted to the right.
(E) The flow-versus-pressure curve is shifted to the left.

CORRECT ANSWER: D

SUMMARY:

The relationship between cerebral perfusion pressure (CPP) and cerebral blood flow (CBF) is determined by cerebral autoregulation. This physiologic relationship regulates cerebral vascular tone to maintain constant CBF between mean arterial pressures of 50 and 150 mm Hg in normotensive patients.[1] Flow becomes pressure-dependent above or below these limits. In patients with chronic hypertension, the entire curve shifts rightward. Thus higher CPPs are required to maintain CBF in patients with untreated chronic hypertension. The clinical implication is that hypertensive patients are more likely to experience cerebral hypoperfusion at "normal" blood pressure ranges. Intraoperative blood pressure management in these patients should account for this rightward shift in the cerebral autoregulation curve to ensure adequate cerebral perfusion.

EXPLANATION:

(A) *Incorrect.* This relationship is true for normotensive patients. Patients with untreated chronic hypertension may require higher mean blood pressures to ensure constant CBF.
(B) *Incorrect.* Flow increases and decreases linearly with pressure only at the extremes of pressure.
(C) *Incorrect.* The basic shape of the curve is similar for normotensive and hypertensive patients.
(D) *Correct.* Patients with untreated chronic hypertension may need higher CPPs to ensure constant CBF. This causes the flow-versus-pressure curve to shift to the right.
(E) *Incorrect.* The flow-versus-pressure curve is shifted to the right, not the left.

REASONING:

This question tests knowledge of cerebral autoregulation of blood flow and the flow-versus-pressure curve that describes that relationship. The cerebral vasculature modulates vascular resistance to maintain a constant flow within a certain range of CPPs. CBF becomes pressure-dependent outside this range. Untreated chronic hypertension modifies this relationship, shifting the flow-versus-pressure curve to the right. The best answer is D.

REFERENCE:

1. Barash PG, Cullen BF, Stoelting RK. Clinical Anesthesia, 4th ed. Philadelphia, Lippincott Williams & Wilkins, 2001, p. 746, Fig. 28-5.
2. Morgan GE, Mikhail MS, Murray MJ. Clinical Anesthesiology, 3d ed. New York, McGraw-Hill, 2002, pp. 553–554.

Answer B

Equipment/Physics

QUESTION (Choose single best answer):

The accuracy of oxyhemoglobin saturation determined by digital pulse oximetry is affected significantly by each of the following *except*

(A) Movement of the patient.
(B) Isovolemic hemodilution to a hematocrit of 23 percent.
(C) Position of the operating room light.
(D) Intravenous administration of methylene blue.
(E) Infusion of phenylephrine.

CORRECT ANSWER: B

SUMMARY:

Pulse oximetry is a noninvasive technique that uses a combination of plethysmography and oximetry to estimate SpO$_2$, the oxyhemoglobin saturation of arterial blood. These monitors transmit light in the red (660 nm) and infrared (940 nm) wavelengths, which are absorbed by deoxyhemoglobin and oxyhemoglobin, respectively.[1] The light at these wavelengths passes through perfused tissue (i.e., finger, ear, etc.) and is measured by a photodetector. The ratio of light detected at these two wavelengths is used to determine the SpO$_2$. An algorithm corrects for light absorbed by nonpulsatile tissue. Low perfusion caused by peripheral vasoconstriction, increased vascular resistance, low cardiac output, hypovolemia, or hypothermia can degrade the light signal and cause inaccurate measurement. Excessive ambient light, dyshemoglobins, nail polish, patient motion, dyes such as methylene blue, and poor sensor positioning also can result in an inaccurate SpO$_2$ reading.[1]

EXPLANATION:

(A) *Incorrect.* Patient motion may interfere with plethysmography, making it difficult for the pulse oximeter to isolate arterial pulsations and to correct for light absorption by nonpulsatile venous tissue.
(B) *Correct.* Isovolemic hemodilution to a hematocrit of 23 percent will not reduce perfusion and should not affect the accuracy of pulse oximetry.
(C) *Incorrect.* An operating room light may provide excessive ambient light, interfering with detection of red and infrared light absorption.
(D) *Incorrect.* Methylene blue will produce a transient false decrease in SpO$_2$.
(E) *Incorrect.* Infusion of phenylephrine, an alpha$_1$-adrenergic agonist, will cause peripheral vasoconstriction that may result in a loss of signal.

REASONING:

This question test knowledge of pulse oximetry. Choices A, C, and D are clearly incorrect. The key to answering this question is understanding that a phenylephrine infusion may cause peripheral vasoconstriction that may decrease tissue perfusion at the monitoring site leading to inaccurate SpO$_2$ readings. Choice B describes an isovolemic state with normal tissue perfusion. This will not affect the accuracy of SpO$_2$ readings. B is the best answer.

REFERENCE:

1. Barash PG, Cullen BF, Stoelting RK. Clinical Anesthesia, 4th ed. Philadelphia, Lippincott Williams & Wilkins, 2001, pp. 670–671.
2. Morgan GE, Mikhail MS, Murray MJ. Clinical Anesthesiology, 3d ed. New York, McGraw-Hill, 2002, pp. 108–110, 216.

QUESTION (Choose single best answer):

The use of droperidol as a preanesthetic medication has been associated with each of the following *except*

(A) Acute anxiety.
(B) Anterograde amnesia.
(C) Hypotension.
(D) Extrapyramidal signs.
(E) Catalepsy.

CORRECT ANSWER: B

SUMMARY:

Droperidol is a derivative of haloperidol and is the first butyrophenone designed with the intent to produce an "artificial hibernation" without significant circulatory or respiratory depression.[1] Droperidol interferes with dopamine, serotonin, norepinephrine, and gamma-aminobutyric acid (GABA) receptors in the central nervous system. This results in sedative and antiemetic effects, in addition to side effects such as hypotension, extrapyramidal effects, and catalepsy. Droperidol also has been reported to cause neuroleptic malignant syndrome. Droperidol use has decreased recently owing to a Food and Drug Administration (FDA) black box warning linking the drug to prolonged QT intervals and resulting torsades de points ventricular dysrhythmias. This FDA warning has prompted reconsideration of the perioperative risks associated with droperidol administration.[2]

EXPLANATION:

(A) *Incorrect.* Used as a preanesthetic medication, droperidol may cause patients to appear sedate, but on further examination, they will admit to feeling dysphoric and restless and may even refuse surgery.[1]
(B) *Correct.* At usual premedication doses, droperidol does not cause unconsciousness, analgesia, or amnesia.
(C) *Incorrect.* Droperidol has alpha-adrenergic blocking effects that can cause hypotension. Droperidol is also contraindicated in patients with pheochromocytoma because it can cause release of catecholamines from the adrenal medulla, resulting in severe hypertension.
(D) *Incorrect.* Use of droperidol can cause extrapyramidal reactions such as oculogyric crisis, torticollis, and agitation owing to antidopaminergic effects. These symptoms may be treated with diphenhydramine. Droperidol also can antagonize the effects of levodopa and should be avoided in patients with Parkinson's disease.
(E) *Incorrect.* Droperidol can cause a cataleptic immobility manifested by a trance-like state with mobile but stiff extremities.[1]

REASONING:

This question tests understanding of the pharmacology of droperidol. Knowing that droperidol is a butyrophenone, which are fluorinated derivatives of phenothiazines, the reader should be able to rule out choices A, D, and E. These are known side effects of phenothiazines. Hypotension is a known cardiovascular effect of droperidol, so choice C also can be eliminated. This leaves choice B. Although there has been a report of the amnestic effects of droperidol in the literature,[3] anterograde amnesia is usually not a property commonly associated with droperidol.

REFERENCES:

1. Miller RD, Miller ED, Reves JG, et al. Anesthesia, 5th ed. New York, Churchill Livingstone, 2000, pp. 256–259.

2. Shafer SL. Safety of patients reason for FDA black box warning on droperidol. Anesth Analg 98(2):551–552, 2004 (author reply p. 552).

3. Wille RT, Barnett JL, Chey WD, et al. Routine droperidol premedication improves sedation for ERCP. Gastrointest Endosc 52(3):362–366, 2000.

4. Morgan GE, Mikhail MS, Murray MJ. Clinical Anesthesiology, 3d ed. New York, McGraw-Hill, 2002, pp. 174–175.

BOOK B:

Answer E

Physiology

QUESTION 96

QUESTION (Choose single best answer):

Each of the following changes is expected with deliberate hypothermia *except*

(A) Decreased unloading of oxygen from hemoglobin.
(B) A 5 percent decrease in MAC for each 1°C decrease in temperature.
(C) Increased arterial oxygen and carbon dioxide contents.
(D) A 50 percent decrease in cerebral metabolic rate at 28°C.
(E) Spike and dome EEG activity at temperatures below 30°C.

CORRECT ANSWER: E

SUMMARY:

Hypothermia will shift the oxyhemoglobin dissociation curve to the left, increasing the affinity of hemoglobin for oxygen and making it less available to the tissues. A 1°C reduction in temperature will result in about a 5 percent decrease in MAC[1] and a 6 percent drop in the cerebral metabolic requirement for oxygen ($CMRO_2$).[2] Hypothermia will increase the solubility of gases in blood, so dissolved arterial oxygen and carbon dioxide content will increase. Spike and dome electroencephalographic (EEG) activity is related to specific epileptic states and not to hypothermia, which would tend to slow and then suppress brain waves.

EXPLANATION:

(A) *Incorrect.* There is decreased unloading of oxygen to the tissues with hypothermia.

(B) *Incorrect.* There is a 5 percent decrease in MAC for each 1°C drop in temperature.

(C) *Incorrect.* The solubility of gases increases with hypothermia. However, while the content of dissolved O_2 and CO_2 in arterial blood will increase, their partial pressures, the PO_2 and PCO_2, will decrease. (*See also Question 73, Book B.*) Arterial blood with a PCO_2 of 40 mm Hg and a pH of 7.4, when cooled to 25°C, will have a PCO_2 of 23 mm Hg and a pH of 7.60. Correction of the respiratory alkalosis in a hypothermic patient will result in severe acidosis on rewarming.

(D) *Incorrect.* A temperature of 28°C (a 9°C reduction in normal body temperature) will result in an approximately 50 percent reduction in $CMRO_2$.

(E) *Correct.* Hypothermia is associated with EEG slowing, burst suppression, and then an isoelectric pattern with the progressive suppression of neuronal activity.

REASONING:

This question tests knowledge of physiologic consequence of hypothermia. The key to answering this type of question is recognizing the single wrong answer, i.e., that hypothermia is associated with EEG slowing, burst suppression, and isoelectric activity. A spike and dome EEG pattern does not occur with hypothermia but has been reported during anesthesia with enflurane.[3] The best answer is E.

REFERENCES:

1. Sessler DI. Hypothermia, mild (core temperature 34–36°C). In Roizen MF, Fleischer LA, eds. Essence of Anesthesia Practice, 2d ed. Philadelphia, Saunders, 2002, p. 189.
2. Miller RD, Miller ED, Reves JG, et al. Anesthesia, 5th ed. New York, Churchill Livingstone, 2000, pp. 697–698.
3. Neigh JL, Garman JK, Harp JR. The electroencephalographic pattern during anesthesia with ethrane: Effects of depth of anesthesia, PaCO_2, and nitrous oxide. Anesthesiology 35(5):482–487, 1971.
4. Schubert A. Symposium article: Side effects of mild hypothermia. J Neurosurg Anesthesiol 7(2):141, 1995.
5. Morgan GE, Mikhail MS, Murray MJ. Clinical Anesthesiology, 3d ed. New York, McGraw-Hill, 2002, pp. 136, 446–447, 453, 502ff.

BOOK B:

Answer E

Pharmacology

QUESTION 97

QUESTION (Choose single best answer):

Each of the following drugs is a cause of central anticholinergic syndrome *except*

(A) Amitriptyline.
(B) Atropine.
(C) Diphenhydramine.
(D) Promethazine.
(E) Ranitidine.

CORRECT ANSWER: E

SUMMARY:

Central anticholinergic syndrome (CAS) occurs with the administration of medications that have centrally acting antimuscarinic properties. CNS symptoms range from stupor to delirium. Medications associated with CAS include antihistamines, tricyclic antidepressants, topical cycloplegic eyedrops, gastrointestinal antispasmodics, synthetic opioids, and antipsychotics.[1] The CNS effects are related to the degree to which these drugs cross the blood-brain barrier and antagonize muscarinic acetylcholine receptors in the brain. While all the medications listed as choices fall into the preceding classes, ranitidine only has weak penetration into the CNS and would be unlikely to cause CAS. CAS is treated with administration of physostigmine, a lipid-soluble tertiary amine cholinesterase inhibitor that can effectively cross the blood-brain barrier.

EXPLANATION:

(A) *Incorrect.* Amitryptyline is a tricyclic antidepressant that works by blocking reuptake of norepinephrine and serotonin. Amytryptyline has high antimuscarinic activity and tends to be the most sedating tricyclic antidepressant. It also can potentiate other centrally acting anticholinergic agents and contribute to postoperative delirium.

(B) *Incorrect.* CAS is also known as *atropine toxicity.*[1] Atropine is a tertiary amine and belladonna alkaloid that readily crosses the blood-brain barrier. It can cause mild postoperative memory loss at the usual dose and delirium and CNS excitation at toxic doses.

(C) *Incorrect.* Diphenhydramine is an ethanolamine and H_1-receptor antagonist that readily crosses the blood-brain barrier. Its antimuscarinic and antiserotoninergic activities confer hypnotic and antiemetic properties.

(D) *Incorrect.* Promethazine, like diphenhydramine, diphendyrinate, and chlorpheniramine, is an H_1-receptor blocker with sedative and antiemetic properties that has been implicated in CAS.

(E) **Correct.** H_2-receptor blockers such as cimetidine have been associated with
lethargy, hallucinations, and seizures, especially in elderly patients. However, ranitidine, famotidine, and nizatidine penetrate the blood-brain barrier poorly and have
minimal CNS effects.

REASONING:

This question tests knowledge of drugs that cause central anticholinergic syndrome. The
reader should ensure that these drugs are reviewed carefully.[1] All the medications listed
in this question fall into classes of drugs that have antimuscarinic effects. However, choice
E is the only medication that does not have CNS effects because it does not cross the
blood-brain barrier.

REFERENCE:

1. Barash PG, Cullen BF, Stoelting RK. Clinical Anesthesia, 4th ed. Philadelphia, Lippincott
Williams & Wilkins, 2001, pp. 288–289, 289, Table 12-12.
2. Morgan GE, Mikhail MS, Murray MJ. Clinical Anesthesiology, 3d ed. New York, McGraw-Hill,
2002, pp. 209–211, 243–245, 337t, 591.

BOOK B:

Answer E

Pharmacology

QUESTION 98

QUESTION (Choose single best answer):

A 24-year-old woman requires anesthesia for emergency repair of open fractures of the
tibia and fibula. She used cocaine 2 hours ago. Blood pressure is 170/110 mm Hg. Each
of the following is useful in managing the hypertension *except*

(A) Hydralazine.
(B) Labetalol.
(C) Nitroprusside.
(D) Phentolamine.
(E) Propanolol.

CORRECT ANSWER: E

SUMMARY:

*Cocaine is an ester local anesthetic. It is unique among local anesthetics in that it in-
hibits the reuptake of norepinephrine in adrenergic nerve terminals and potentiates the
effects of adrenergic stimulation. Norepinephrine is a potent agonist to alpha$_1$ and alpha$_2$
receptors and somewhat less of an agonist to beta$_1$ receptors.[1] The patient in this question is hypertensive. Both alpha-blockade and beta-blockade are necessary when treating cocaine-induced hypertension. Sole beta-blockade therapy could result in lethal hypertension owing to unopposed alpha-adrenergic tone. Cocaine-induced hypertension can
be potentiated by other sympathomimetic agents such as epinephrine and phenylephrine,
as well as by tricyclic antidepressants and monoamine oxidase inhibitors.*

EXPLANATION:

(A) **Incorrect.** Hydralazine is a direct-acting vasodilator that would decrease systemic
vascular resistance. It would be useful in treating the hypertension.
(B) **Incorrect.** Labetolol blocks alpha$_1$, beta$_1$, and beta$_2$ receptors at a ratio of 1:7
alpha-to-beta blockade. Unlike hydralazine, labetolol lowers overall peripheral
vascular resistance without reflex tachycardia because of its combined effect.
(C) **Incorrect.** Nitroprusside relaxes both arterial and venous smooth muscle. It primarily reduces preload. It could be used to treat the hypertension.

387

(D) **Incorrect.** Phentolamine lowers blood pressure by competitively blocking alpha receptors nonselectively. Reflex tachycardia and postural hypotension limit its utility in this patient.

(E) **Correct.** Propranolol is a nonselective beta-blocker that lowers blood pressure by decreasing myocardial contractility and decreasing heart rate. This would lead to unopposed alpha effects and exacerbate this patient's hypertension. This drug should not be administered in the setting of cocaine-induced hypertension.

REASONING:

This question tests knowledge of the pathophysiology and treatment of acute cocaine intoxication. All the choices can be used to treat hypertension, but certain drugs should not be administered in the setting of acute cocaine intoxication. The high levels of circulating norepinephrine possess alpha- and beta-adrenergic agonist properties. Therapy should be directed at blocking both receptor sites. Choice D may lead to reflex tachycardia and postural hypotension. However, choice E is clearly the most incorrect choice because it will worsen the patient's malignant hypertension. The complications of pure beta-blockade during acute cocaine intoxication are well known.[1] E is the best answer.

REFERENCE:

1. Barash PG, Cullen BF, Stoelting RK. Clinical Anesthesia, 4th ed. Philadelphia, Lippincott Williams & Wilkins, 2001, pp. 277 (Table 12-13), 975.

2. Morgan GE, Mikhail MS, Murray MJ. Clinical Anesthesiology, 3d ed. New York, McGraw-Hill, 2002, pp. 239, 591.

BOOK B:

Answer B

Clinical Anesthesia

QUESTION 99

QUESTION (Choose single best answer):

Carbon monoxide poisoning with a carboxyhemoglobin concentration of 20 percent is characterized by each of the following *except*

(A) Decreased oxygen-carrying capacity of hemoglobin.
(B) Decreased PaO_2.
(C) Shift of the oxyhemoglobin dissociation curve to the left.
(D) Normal minute volume of ventilation.
(E) Headache and nausea.

CORRECT ANSWER: B

SUMMARY:

Carbon monoxide combines with hemoglobin to form carboxyhemoglobin, interfering with oxygen binding and resulting in a leftward shift in the oxyhemoglobin dissociation curve.[1] Carbon monoxide poisoning occurs when carboxyhemoglobin concentrations exceed 15 percent in the blood. Levels approaching 20 percent or more cause altered mental status, headaches, nausea, vomiting, and eventually coma and shock. Carboxyhemoglobin levels greater than 40 to 60 percent can be fatal. Carbon monoxide poisoning does not affect the arterial oxygen tension. Normal carboxyhemoglobin levels are 1.5 percent in nonsmokers and up to 15 percent in chronic smokers.

EXPLANATION:

(A) **Incorrect.** Carbon monoxide has a 200-fold greater affinity for hemoglobin than oxygen. When carboxyhemoglobin is formed, it shifts the oxyhemoglobin dissociation curve leftward, reducing the oxyhemoglobin concentration and impairing the delivery and release of oxygen to tissues.[1]

(B) **Correct.** Carbon monoxide poisoning decreases oxygen-hemoglobin saturation, but PaO_2 and skin color may remain normal.

(C) **Incorrect.** Carbon monoxide toxicity interferes with the unloading of oxygen at the tissues, shifting the oxyhemoglobin curve to the left.

(D) **Incorrect.** Carbon monoxide toxicity can occur without lung injury. The PaO_2 should be normal if lung injury has not occurred.[1] The carotid bodies are sensitive to PaO_2, not the O_2 content of the blood. CO_2 elimination and the ventilatory response to $PaCO_2$ and PaO_2 remain unchanged. Minute ventilation should be normal in the absence of lung injury.

(E) **Incorrect.** Severity of carbon monoxide poisoning depends on the amount of carboxyhemoglobin present, the patient's tissue oxygen demands, and hemoglobin concentration. Mild carbon monoxide poisoning results in headache, dizziness, and confusion, whereas severe poisoning can result in death.

REASONING:

This question tests knowledge of the pathophysiology of carbon monoxide poisoning. Choice D is somewhat correct. Carbon monoxide poisoning accompanied by lung injury will reduced the arterial oxygen tension and will result in tachypnea.[1] However, we cannot assume that this patient has concurrent lung injury. B is the single best answer.

REFERENCE:

1. Barash PG, Cullen BF, Stoelting RK. Clinical Anesthesia, 4th ed. Philadelphia, Lippincott Williams & Wilkins, 2001, p. 1275.
2. Morgan GE, Mikhail MS, Murray MJ. Clinical Anesthesiology, 3d ed. New York, McGraw-Hill, 2002, pp. 801–802.

BOOK B: QUESTION 100

Answer E

Pharmacology

QUESTION (Choose single best answer):

A 40-year-old woman receives alfentanil 75 μg/kg followed by an infusion of 1.5 μg/kg per minute for a 1-hour cholecystectomy and cholangiogram. This regimen could be associated with each of the following *except*

(A) Muscle rigidity.
(B) Increased biliary tract pressure.
(C) Inadequate anesthesia.
(D) Postoperative respiratory depression.
(E) Two to 4 hours postoperative analgesia.

CORRECT ANSWER: E

SUMMARY:

Alfentanil is a synthetic opioid that is characterized by a very rapid onset and brief duration of action. Approximately 90 percent of the drug is in a lipid-soluble nonionized form at physiologic pH owing to a low pK_a of 6.8.[1] The typical loading dose of alfentanil is 8 to 100 μg/kg, with maintenance infusion rates of 0.5 to 3 μg/kg per minute. Side effects of alfentanil are similar to those of other opioids and include nausea and vomiting, chest wall rigidity, respiratory depression, increased biliary pressure, and decreased peristalsis.

EXPLANATION:

(A) **Incorrect.** All opioids potentially can cause muscle rigidity following rapid bolus administration. Chest wall rigidity occurs more commonly with alfentanil, sufentanil, and fentanyl.

(B) *Incorrect.* Opioids such as alfentanil can cause spasm of the sphincter of Oddi. This can produce a rise in biliary tract pressure and result in symptoms of biliary colic.

(C) *Incorrect.* Although opioids can produce intense analgesia and sedation, they do not reliably provide amnesia and can result in inadequate anesthesia when used alone. One also must assume that alfentanil is the sole anesthetic agent being administered to this patient.

(D) *Incorrect.* Opioids shift the CO_2 response curve to the right, resulting in higher resting $PaCO_2$, decreased ventilatory response to CO_2, and higher apneic threshold. These effects can persist for up to 2 hours into the postoperative period.[1] Opioid-induced respiratory depression is increased in the elderly and in combination with other sedatives.[2]

(E) *Correct.* The context-sensitive half-time for alfentanil is approximately 60 minutes for infusions of up to 10 hours. The terminal half-life of alfentanil is 84 to 90 minutes.[1]

REASONING:

This question tests knowledge of the unique pharmacology of alfentanil. Its rapid onset and minimal accumulation make it an ideal opioid for continuous intravenous infusion. Choices A through D are true for all opioids including alfentanil. However, it is not associated with significant postoperative analgesia after discontinuation, making choice E incorrect. E is the best answer.

REFERENCES:

1. Barash PG, Cullen BF, Stoelting RK. Clinical Anesthesia, 4th ed. Philadelphia, Lippincott Williams & Wilkins, 2001, pp. 346–347.

2. Stoelting RK, Miller RD. Basics of Anesthesia, 4th ed. New York, Churchill Livingstone, 2000, p. 71, Table 6-4.

3. Morgan GE, Mikhail MS, Murray MJ. Clinical Anesthesiology, 3d ed. New York, McGraw-Hill, 2002, pp. 167–169; Table 8-6 (p. 168), Uses and Doses of Common Opioids, Fig. 8-7 (p. 167).

BOOK B:

Answer B

Neuroanesthesia

QUESTION 101

QUESTION (Choose single best answer)

Monitoring sensory evoked potentials may be useful in detecting functional derangement of each of the following *except*

(A) Cranial nerve pathways during posterior fossa operations.
(B) Motor pathways during anterior cervical diskectomy.
(C) Dorsal column pathways during operations for spinal tumors.
(D) Visual pathways during operations on the sphenoid wing.
(E) Cortical pathways during carotid artery operations.

CORRECT ANSWER: B

SUMMARY:

Sensory evoked potential monitoring is a noninvasive method to assess neurologic function. For example, an electric current is delivered to the tibial nerve. If the neural pathway is intact, an evoked potential will be transmitted to the contralateral sensory cortex. There are three types of sensory evoked potentials (SEPs) in clinical use: somatosensory evoked potentials (SSEPs), visual evoked potentials (VEPs), and brain stem auditory evoked potential (BAEPs). It is important to note that intact sensory evoked potentials do not ensure normal motor function.

EXPLANATION:

(A) **Incorrect.** Cranial nerves (e.g., optic nerve) carry sensory information. These pathways are monitored by SEPs.

(B) **Correct.** SEPs evaluate dorsal spinal column pathways, whereas motor evoked potentials (MEPs) evaluate ventral spinal cord function. Because of this differing anatomy, normal SEPs do not ensure normal motor function.

(C) **Incorrect.** Dorsal column pathways carry sensory information. These pathways are monitored by SEPs.

(D) **Incorrect.** Visual pathways carry sensory information. These pathways are monitored by SEPs.

(E) **Incorrect.** Cortical pathways carry sensory information. These pathways are monitored by SEPs.

REASONING:

SEPs are influenced by anesthetics and drugs in a dose-dependent fashion. SEPs are altered by hypothermia, volatile anesthetics, and multiple intravenous anesthetic agents, including benzodiazepines and barbiturates. The reader should review these pharmacologic effects on SEPs carefully.[1] Of the SEPs listed above, BAEPs are the most resistant to anesthetics. Functional derangement is suggested by an increase in latency and a decrease in amplitude in the evoked potential.[1] SEPs evaluate ascending sensory pathways, whereas MEPs are useful in assessing descending motor pathways. Choice B should stand out because it states "motor pathways." The others refer to sensory pathways. B is the single best answer.

REFERENCE:

1. Barash PG, Cullen BF, Stoelting RK. Clinical Anesthesia, 4th ed. Philadelphia, Lippincott Williams & Wilkins, 2001, pp. 754–756, Table 28-8.
2. Morgan GE, Mikhail MS, Murray MJ. Clinical Anesthesiology, 3d ed. New York, McGraw-Hill, 2002, pp. 115–116.

BOOK B:

Answer E

OB/Regional

QUESTION 102

QUESTION (Choose single best answer):

Which of the following drugs is *least* likely to cross the placenta?

(A) Lidocaine
(B) Meperidine
(C) Midazolam
(D) Thiopental
(E) Vecuronium

CORRECT ANSWER: E

SUMMARY:

Assuming constant uterine artery blood flow, transfer of free drug (non–protein-bound) from the maternal to fetal circulation can be described by the Fick equation

$$\frac{\Delta q}{\Delta t} = \frac{KA(C_m - C_f)}{X}$$

where $\Delta q/\Delta t$ represents rate of transfer of the drug, A is the surface area of the membrane, C_m is the maternal drug concentration, C_f is the fetal drug concentration, X is the thickness of the membrane, and K is a diffusion constant determined by drug properties such as molecular weight, lipid solubility, degree of ionization, and spatial configuration. Since the surface area and membrane thickness of the placenta will remain constant, non–

ionized, lipid-soluble, non–protein-bound drugs will cross the placenta more readily. Examples of lipid-soluble agents that readily cross the placenta and enter the fetal circulation include thiopental, benzodiazepines, and opiates. Highly water-soluble agents such as muscle relaxants do not cross the placenta in significant amounts. This is why babies delivered by cesarean section from mothers who have been given muscle relaxants do not exhibit neuromuscular blockade. (See also Question 51, Book B.)

EXPLANATION:

(A) *Incorrect.* Lidocaine has little maternal protein binding and therefore crosses the placenta.

(B) *Incorrect.* Meperidine is a lipid-soluble opiate and has been shown to cross the placenta.

(C) *Incorrect.* Midazolam is a benzodiazepine, and all benzodiazepines are lipid-soluble and cross the placenta. Midazolam is water soluble at a pH of less than 6.0 but lipid soluble at a pH greater than 6.0. This allows it to readily cross the placenta at physiologic pH.

(D) *Incorrect.* Thiopental is the most commonly used induction agent in obstetric anesthesia. It is highly lipid soluble and readily crosses the placenta, reaching fetal circulation within 30 seconds of an intravenous dose.[1] Interestingly, the incidence of neonatal depression is minimal in babies whose mothers are given less than 4 mg/kg.

(E) *Correct.* Vecuronium is a nondepolarizing muscle relaxant. This class of drugs is highly water soluble, and therefore, such drugs do not cross the placenta in significant amounts.

REASONING:

This question tests knowledge of the pharmacology of anesthetic drugs across the placenta. The first thing to note about this question is the format. It asks which drug is the *least* likely to cross the placenta. This means that there must be something very different about one of the drugs in the list. Keeping in mind that ionized, water-soluble, protein-bound drugs will not cross the placenta, one can eliminate midazolam, meperidine, and thiopental owing to their lipid solubility. Lidocaine can be eliminated because it has little protein binding. Alternatively, one can answer the question by knowing that the drug on the list that is the most water soluble, vecuronium, will cross the placenta the least. E is the best answer.

REFERENCE:

1. Hughes SC, Levinson G, Rosen MA. Shnider and Levinson's Anesthesia for Obstetrics, 4th ed. Philadelphia, Lippincott Williams & Wilkins, 2002, p. 217.
2. Morgan GE, Mikhail MS, Murray MJ. Clinical Anesthesiology, 3d ed. New York, McGraw-Hill, 2002, pp. 160–167, 810–811.

BOOK B:

QUESTION 103

Answer D

Physiology

QUESTION (K-type):

Characteristics of a depolarizing neuromuscular block include

(1) Tetanic fade at 50 Hz for 5 seconds.
(2) Decreased train-of-four ratio.
(3) Posttetanic facilitation.
(4) Decreased twitch height.

CORRECT ANSWER: D (4 only is correct)

SUMMARY:

Depolarizing neuromuscular blockers such as succinylcholine bind to acetylcholine receptors and generate continuous motor end plate depolarization. This prevents the reopening of prejunctional sodium channels, resulting in muscle relaxation. Phase I depolarizing neuromuscular blockade elicited by the usual intubating doses of succinylcholine exhibits constant but decreased twitch height responses (i.e., no fade) to train-of-four, tetanic, and double-burst peripheral nerve stimulation. Furthermore, posttetanic potentiation is also absent in depolarizing blockade.

EXPLANATION:

(1) *Incorrect.* There would be a constant but reduced-height evoked response to a 5-second 50-Hz tetanic stimulus in a depolarizing block.

(2) *Incorrect.* The height of all four twitches in a train-of-four stimulus (0.2-ms 2-Hz twitches over 2 seconds) would be diminished but equal.

(3) *Incorrect.* Posttetanic potentiation or the ability of a tetanic stimulus to increase the height of a subsequent twitch response is characteristic of a nondepolarizing or phase II blockade.

(4) *Correct.* A typical depolarizing blockade would result in a decreased twitch height without fade.

REASONING:

This question tests knowledge of twitch response in depolarizing neuromuscular blockade. Choice 3 is clearly incorrect because posttetanic facilitation is seen only in nondepolarizing or a phase II depolarizing block. We should assume that this question refers to a phase I depolarizing block that is achieved with the usual dose of succinylcholine. Phase II blockade can be seen after prolonged exposure to succinylcholine.[1] This rules out answers A, B, and E. Choice 2 is incorrect because the train-of-four ratio in a phase I depolarizing block would have a shortened twitch height but the same ratio from the first to the fourth twitch. D is the best answer.

REFERENCE:

1. Barash PG, Cullen BF, Stoelting RK. Clinical Anesthesia, 4th ed. Philadelphia, Lippincott Williams & Wilkins, 2001, p. 422.

2. Morgan GE, Mikhail MS, Murray MJ. Clinical Anesthesiology, 3d ed. New York, McGraw-Hill, 2002, pp. 181–183, 182ff.

BOOK B: QUESTION 104

Answer A

OB/Regional

QUESTION (K-type):

Before awake nasal intubation in a patient who has been NPO, areas to be anesthetized are supplied by which of the following nerves?

(1) Glossopharyngeal
(2) Superior laryngeal
(3) Recurrent laryngeal
(4) Hypoglossal

CORRECT ANSWER: A (1, 2, and 3 are correct)

SUMMARY:

Anesthetizing the naso-, oro-, and hypopharynx and larynx will facilitate an awake nasal intubation. Branches of the trigeminal nerve provide sensation to the mucous membranes of the nose and anterior tongue. The glossopharyngeal nerve provides sensation to the back of the tongue, pharynx, tonsils, and soft palate. The vagus nerve, which branches into the superior laryngeal nerve and the recurrent laryngeal nerve, provides sensory innervation to the hypopharynx and larynx.

EXPLANATION:

(1) ***Correct.*** The glossopharyngeal nerve, cranial nerve (CN) IX, provides sensory innervation to the posterior third of the tongue with branches to the soft palate and oropharynx. This nerve may be blocked by the application of aerosolized lidocaine or by bilateral injection of local anesthetic at the base of the ipsilateral anterior tonsillar pillar.

(2) ***Correct.*** The superior laryngeal nerve, which is a branch of the vagus nerve (CN X), provides sensory innervation to the lower pharynx and the larynx above the vocal cords. This nerve can be blocked in between the greater cornu of the hyoid bone and the superior cornu of the thyroid cartilage or by instillation of topical lidocaine by transtracheal injection through the cricothyroid ligament.

(3) ***Correct.*** The recurrent laryngeal nerve, another branch of the vagus nerve, provides sensation to the vocal cords and the larynx.

(4) ***Incorrect.*** The hypoglossal nerve (CN XII) is the motor nerve of the tongue and does not need to anesthetized prior to an awake nasal intubation.

REASONING:

This question tests knowledge of the innervation of the larynx and nasopharynx. Recognizing that the hypoglossal nerve is purely a motor nerve rules out choice 4 and answers C, D, and E. Therefore, choices 1 and 3 must be correct. The superior laryngeal nerve typically is blocked in an awake nasal or oral fiberoptic intubation, so choice 2 also must be correct. The best answer is A.

REFERENCE:

Barash PG, Cullen BF, Stoelting RK. Clinical Anesthesia, 4th ed. Philadelphia, Lippincott Williams & Wilkins, 2001, pp. 288–289, 289.

Morgan GE, Mikhail MS, Murray MJ. Clinical Anesthesiology, 3d ed. New York, McGraw-Hill, 2002, pp. 59–62, 62t, 83.

BOOK B:

QUESTION 105

Answer A

Pain

QUESTION (K-type):

A 40-year-old patient is referred to a pain clinic for evaluation of right upper quadrant pain 6 months after cholecystectomy performed through a subcostal incision. Which of the following procedures would provide diagnostic information?

(1) Intercostal nerve blocks
(2) Celiac plexus block
(3) Differential spinal block
(4) Lumbar sympathetic block

CORRECT ANSWER: A (1, 2, and 3 are correct)

SUMMARY:

Intercostal nerve blocks inhibit nociceptive signals of somatic origin on the body wall but not visceral nociceptive signals. Celiac plexus blocks inhibit transmission of visceral nociceptive signals from all the abdominal viscera but will not block somatic nociception. Differential spinal blockade helps to distinguish between psychogenic, somatic, sympathetic, and central pain states. Thus these three tests can be used to help to determine the anatomic location and mechanism of the patient's pain. Lumbar sympathetic block is used for diagnosis and treatment of pain and vascular insufficiency in the lower extremity.

EXPLANATION:

(1) **Correct.** Intercostal nerve blocks act on the ventral rami of spinal nerves and result in blockade of sensation from the abdominal wall. A visceral origin of the pain would be excluded if this block produced pain relief for the patient.

(2) **Correct.** Celiac plexus blockade (CPB) will interrupt the transmission of sensation by the visceral afferents that run along with sympathetic efferent nerves through the celiac plexus. CPB will block nociception from virtually all the abdominal viscera except the left side of the colon and the pelvic viscera. Pain relief following CPB would exclude a musculoskeletal cause of the pain.

(3) **Correct.** Differential spinal blockade is predicated on the differential sensitivity of nerve fibers to local anesthetic and could be used to provide further diagnosis information regarding this patient's pain.[1] Classically, four different intrathecal sequential injections are given.

Saline. Pain relief suggests a placebo responder or psychogenic pain.
Procaine 0.25%. Pain relief suggests a sympathetic mechanism to the pain.
Procaine 0.5%. Pain relief suggests a somatic origin or organic pain.
Procaine 1% or 5%. Lack of pain relief suggests a central nervous system (CNS) mechanism for the pain.

(4) **Incorrect.** Lumbar sympathetic block inhibits the transmission of sympathetic efferent signals to the lower extremity and blocks visceral afferent information from the lower extremity. It would have very little utility in the assessment of right upper quadrant pain.

REASONING:

This question tests knowledge of diagnostic nerve blockade in patients with chronic pain. Choices 1 and 2 (intercostal and celiac plexus block) more clearly provide diagnostic information than differential spinal blockade. However, once choices 1 and 2 are known to be correct, choice 3 must be correct, and the only question remaining is whether choice 4 is correct. As outlined above, choice 4 (lumbar sympathetic block) is used for lower extremity sympathetic block and is not likely to be useful in a patient with abdominal pain. Therefore, A is the best answer.

REFERENCE:

1. Benzon H, Raja S, et al. Essentials of Pain Medicine and Regional Anesthesia. New York, Elsevier, 1999, p. 84.
2. Morgan GE, Mikhail MS, Murray MJ. Clinical Anesthesiology, 3d ed. New York, McGraw-Hill, 2002, pp. 295–298, Table 18-8.

BOOK B:

QUESTION 106

Answer D

Pain

QUESTION (K-type):

Compared with intermittent injections of intramuscular opioids for postoperative pain relief, patient-controlled analgesia is associated with

(1) A lower incidence of nausea and vomiting.
(2) An increased risk for ventilatory depression.
(3) A greater variability in opioid pharmacokinetics.
(4) A lower total opioid requirement.

CORRECT ANSWER: D (4 only is correct)

SUMMARY:

Patient-controlled analgesia (PCA) involves the use of computerized infusion pumps to deliver analgesic medication in response to patient demand (i.e., pushing a button). A background maintenance infusion can be programmed and often is used in conjunction with PCA-delivered bolus dosing.[1] With bolus dosing, a certain dose of analgesic is delivered when the button is pushed, assuming that the maximum dose or lockout interval has not been reached. PCA has many advantages when compared with intramuscular opioid administration. PCA use is associated with a lower total opioid requirement, superior analgesia, less sleep disturbance, and less sedation and concomitant ventilatory depression. Intramuscular opioids are associated with marked variability in opioid pharmacokinetics. PCA is not necessarily associated with a lower incidence of nausea and vomiting.

EXPLANATION:

(1) *Incorrect.* PCA does not reliably lower the incidence of nausea and vomiting.
(2) *Incorrect.* The PCA is less likely to produce the sedation and concomitant ventilatory depression that results from unpredictable absorption of intramuscular boluses.
(3) *Incorrect.* PCA use is associated with less variability in opioid pharmacokinetics.
(4) *Correct.* PCA has been associated with a lower total opioid requirement and less variability in pharmacokinetics than intramuscular opioid administration.

REASONING:

This question tests knowledge of patient-controlled analgesia. It is important to understand that its use results in less overall opioid consumption. Therefore, choice 4 is correct, and answers A and B can be eliminated. The principal criticism of the intramuscular use of opioids has been the erratic absorption that often results. Therefore, choice 3 is incorrect, and answer E can be eliminated. PCA decreases the risk of ventilatory depression compared with intramuscular administration of opioids. Answer C can be eliminated, leaving D as the best answer.

REFERENCE:

1. Barash PG, Cullen BF, Stoelting RK. Clinical Anesthesia, 4th ed. Philadelphia, Lippincott Williams & Wilkins, 2001, p. 1416.
2. Morgan GE, Mikhail MS, Murray MJ. Clinical Anesthesiology, 3d ed. New York, McGraw-Hill, 2002, pp. 304–305.

BOOK B:

QUESTION 107

Answer E

Pharmacology

QUESTION (K-type):

Adverse reactions to protamine include

(1) Markedly increased pulmonary vascular resistance.
(2) Anaphylaxis.
(3) Decreased systemic vascular resistance.
(4) Noncardiogenic pulmonary edema.

CORRECT ANSWER: E (All are correct)

SUMMARY:

Protamine is a polycationic protein isolated from salmon sperm that is used to bind and neutralize heparin, a highly negatively charged polysaccharide. These heparin-protamine complexes are then cleared by the reticuloendothelial system. Adverse reactions to protamine include anaphylactic as well as anaphylactoid reactions characterized by a decrease in systemic vascular resistance. Rapid administration of protamine also has been associated with the sudden onset of profound pulmonary hypertension and systemic hypotension. Noncardiogenic pulmonary edema (NCPE) is a rare complication of protamine administration that is associated with a mortality rate that can approach 30 percent.[1]

EXPLANATION:

(1) **Correct.** Markedly increased pulmonary vascular resistance is a sudden, potentially devastating, and yet short-lived complication of protamine administration. It occurs in approximately 1 percent of patients. The deposition of protamine-heparin complexes mediates pulmonary vasoconstriction through the release of thromboxane and C5a anaphylatoxin.[2] This reaction is accompanied by an elevation in central venous pressure (CVP) and systemic hypotension. Protamine usually has minimal effects when is administered slowly (i.e., up to 50 mg over 10 minutes).

(2) **Correct.** Anaphylaxis may occur with protamine administration. The risk is higher in patients who have been sensitized previously to protamine from cardiac catheterizations, cardiac surgeries, dialysis, or neutral protamine Hagedorn (NPH) or protamine zinc insulin therapy. This reaction is characterized by increased airway resistance, cutaneous flushing, systemic hypotension, and decreased systemic vascular resistance.[2]

(3) **Correct.** Decreased systemic vascular resistance may accompany an anaphylactic or pulmonary hypertensive response to protamine.

(4) **Correct.** Administration of protamine is associated with NCPE.[1] The mechanism is unclear but may involve C3a and C5a anaphylatoxins that mediate histamine release from mast cells and leukocytes.[1] It is a rare adverse event with a prevalence rate of only 0.2 percent of patients on cardiopulmonary bypass. The mortality can approach 30 percent.[3]

REASONING:

This question tests knowledge of the adverse reactions associated with administration of protamine sulfate. Choices 1 and 2 are well-known complications of intravenously administered protamine. Choice 3 is associated with both these complications. Choice 4 is a rare complication of rapid protamine administration that is associated with mortality of up to 30 percent. E is the best answer.

REFERENCES:

1. Brooks JC. Noncardiogenic pulmonary edema immediately following rapid protamine administration. Ann Pharmacother 33(9):927–930, 1999.

2. Barash PG, Cullen BF, Stoelting RK. Clinical Anesthesia, 4th ed. Philadelphia, Lippincott Williams & Wilkins, 2001, pp. 916, 1299, 1306.

3. Holland CL, Singh AK, McMaster PRB, Fang W. Adverse reactions to protamine sulfate following cardiac surgery. Clin Cardiol 7:157–162, 1984.

4. Morgan GE, Mikhail MS, Murray MJ. Clinical Anesthesiology, 3d ed. New York, McGraw-Hill, 2002, pp. 434, 457–458.

BOOK B:

Answer B

Physiology

QUESTION 108

QUESTION (K-type):

Causes of the hypoxemia that occurs in patients with advanced cirrhosis include

(1) Decreased total lung capacity.
(2) Decreased cardiac output.
(3) Right-to-left pulmonary shunting.
(4) Decreased 2,3-diphosphoglycerate concentration in erythrocytes.

CORRECT ANSWER: B (1 and 3 are correct)

SUMMARY:

Patients with hepatic cirrhosis are prone to hypoxemia for several reasons. Some of these reasons include (1) hypoventilation owing to decreased lung volumes and increased intraabdominal pressures from ascites, (2) right-to-left pulmonary shunts, (3) $\dot{V}/\dot{Q}$ abnormalities from impaired hypoxic vasoconstriction, and (4) decreased pulmonary diffusing capacity from increased extracellular fluid. A rightward shift of the oxyhemoglobin dissociation curve owing to increased 2,3-diphosphoglycerate can also occur.[1]

EXPLANATION:

(1) *Correct.* The presence of ascites in the abdomen causes mechanically induced restriction of the diaphragm, which reduces all lung volumes and all lung capacities. This can lead to hypoventilation, atelectasis, and hypoxemia.[1]

(2) *Incorrect.* End-stage liver disease is characterized by a hyperdynamic state that includes an increased cardiac output and low peripheral vascular resistance in the setting of normal heart rates and filling pressures.

(3) *Correct.* Right-to-left shunting across the lungs is seen in advanced cirrhotics owing to portopulmonary-pulmonary communications, spider angiomas in the lungs, and the secretion of vasodilatory substances such as glucagons, vasoactive intestinal protein (VIP), and ferritin. These vasodilatory substances are thought to impair hypoxic vasoconstriction and contribute to ventilation-perfusion abnormalities.

(4) *Incorrect.* Because of the propensity toward hypoxemia, advanced cirrhotics must compensate by unloading oxygen more readily than normal individuals. This is accomplished by a rightward shift in the oxyhemoglobin dissociation curve. Factors that cause a rightward shift in the oxyhemoglobin curve include acidosis, hyperthermia, and an increase in 2,3-diphosoglycerate concentration.

REASONING:

This question tests knowledge of pulmonary physiology contributing to hypoxemia in the setting of hepatic failure. The reader should carefully review factors that contribute to hypoxemia in patients with hepatic cirrhosis.[1] It is helpful to remember the physiologic mechanisms that help to compensate for hypoxemia. A rightward shift of the oxyhemoglobin dissociation curve decreases the affinity of hemoglobin for oxygen. This facilitates unloading of oxygen from hemoglobin and the delivery of oxygen to end organs. A decrease in 2,3-diphosphoglycerate would cause a leftward shift of the oxyhemoglobin curve, so choice 4 is wrong. The best answer is B.

REFERENCE:

1. Barash PG, Cullen BF, Stoelting RK. Clinical Anesthesia, 4th ed. Philadelphia, Lippincott Williams & Wilkins, 2001, pp. 1085–1087, Table 39-5.
2. Morgan GE, Mikhail MS, Murray MJ. Clinical Anesthesiology, 3d ed. New York, McGraw-Hill, 2002, pp. 502, 726–728, 945.

BOOK B:

Answer A

Clinical Anesthesia

QUESTION 109

QUESTION (K-type):

In a patient who is breathing room air spontaneously at the conclusion of a nitrous oxide (70%)–opioid anesthetic, causes of hypoxemia include

(1) Decreased functional residual capacity.
(2) Dilution of alveolar oxygen by outpouring of nitrous oxide.
(3) Opioid-induced respiratory depression.
(4) Increased physiologic dead space.

CORRECT ANSWER: A (1, 2, and 3 are correct)

SUMMARY:

All patients undergoing general anesthesia are at risk for hypoxemia during emergence. The combined effects of residual potent inhalational anesthetic agent and opioid medications attenuate the ventilatory response to hypoxemia and hypercarbia.[1] Restrictive changes in pulmonary function after surgery result in a decreased functional residual capacity (FRC).[1] A decreased FRC can contribute to atelectasis and shunting that can lead to hypoxemia. Rapid elimination of nitrous oxide from the lungs at the end of surgery can dilute alveolar O_2 and CO_2, leading to diffusion hypoxia.[2]

EXPLANATION:

(1) **Correct.** The most important predictor of the degree of restrictive lung physiology and postoperative pulmonary complications is the site of the surgical wound. Non-laparoscopic abdominal surgeries can lead to a 40 to 50 percent decrease in FRC from preoperative levels. Intracranial, peripheral, and ENT surgeries may only have a 15 to 20 percent decrease.[1]

(2) **Correct.** At the end of a general anesthetic, significant hypoxemia can result from the rapid elimination of nitrous oxide, which can dilute oxygen and CO_2 in the alveoli. Administering 100% oxygen at the conclusion of a general anesthetic can easily prevent this diffusion hypoxia.[2]

(3) **Correct.** Opioid medications attenuate the ventilatory response to hypoxia and hypercarbia. The carbon dioxide–ventilatory response curve is shifted to the right.[1] The typical ventilatory pattern is a decreased respiratory rate with increased tidal volumes.[1]

(4) **Incorrect.** Physiologic dead space is composed of anatomic and alveolar dead space. Anatomic dead space involves the parts of the respiratory tree that do not exchange gas; it includes the oropharynx and extends to the terminal and respiratory bronchioles. Factors that alter anatomic dead space are tracheal intubation, tracheostomy, the ventilator Y-piece, and excessive ventilator tubing. Alveolar dead space arises from areas of the lung that are ventilated but not perfused. Alveolar dead space would increase in any disease state that decreases the overall perfusion to the lungs. At the conclusion of a general anesthetic, there is collapse of alveoli (atelectasis) resulting in increased shunting (perfused and unventilated alveoli). Dead space ventilation, however, is not increased.

REASONING:

This question tests knowledge of the changes in respiratory physiology associated with surgery and anesthesia. The key phrase in this question is "spontaneously breathing room air at the conclusion of nitrous oxide (70%)–opioid anesthetic." We assume that the patient is supine. Decreased FRC is a well-known complication of surgery and anesthesia. Diffusion hypoxia also can occur during emergence and in the immediate postoperative period owing to rapid dilution of alveolar oxygen with nitrous oxide (diffusion hypoxia). Furthermore, at the conclusion of a general anesthesia, the reader should expect increased shunting (areas that are perfused but not ventilated), not increased dead space. The best answer is A.

REFERENCES:

1. Barash PG, Cullen BF, Stoelting RK. Clinical Anesthesia, 4th ed. Philadelphia, Lippincott Williams & Wilkins, 2001, pp. 799–800 (Table 29-4), 809, 814.
2. Fink BR. Diffusion anoxia. Anesthesiology 6(4):511–519, 1955.
3. Morgan GE, Mikhail MS, Murray MJ. Clinical Anesthesiology, 3d ed. New York, McGraw-Hill, 2002, pp. 945, 133.

Answer A

Pharmacology

QUESTION (K-type):

Compared with an induction dose of midazolam, an induction dose of thiopental causes a greater decrease in

(1) Blood pressure.
(2) Cerebral blood flow.
(3) Cerebral metabolic rate.
(4) Cortical electroencephalographic (EEG) activity.

CORRECT ANSWER: A (1, 2, and 3 are correct)

SUMMARY:

Midazolam and thiopental are both intravenous anesthetics useful for induction of anesthesia that exert their clinical CNS effects by interacting with gamma-aminobutyric acid (GABA) receptors. When used for induction, benzodiazepines produce minimal cardiovascular depression. Barbiturates reduce $CMRo_2$, cerebral blood flow (CBF), and intracranial pressure (ICP) to a greater extent than benzodiazepines. Thiopental can produce electrical silence on the EEG. Unlike midazolam, this effect is not apparent at typical induction doses.

EXPLANATION:

(1) **Correct.** Induction doses of thiopental can produce hypotension from peripheral vasodilation and tachycardia owing to vagolysis. Hypovolemic patients are more prone to the cardiovascular effects of this drug. In contrast, midazolam and other benzodiazepines have minimal effects on blood pressure.
(2) **Correct.** Benzodiazepines decrease CBF to a lesser extent than barbiturates. Barbiturates are potent cerebral vasoconstrictors and reduce CBF in a dose-dependent fashion.
(3) **Correct.** Midazolam has a ceiling on its effect on $CMRo_2$ corresponding to its EEG effect.[1] Thiopental reduces $CMRo_2$ uniformly throughout the brain to a greater extent than midazolam.
(4) **Incorrect.** Thiopental can produce burst suppression on EEG, whereas midazolam is not able to produce similar EEG effects.[2] However, this difference is not apparent at typical induction doses.

REASONING:

This answer to this question is controversial because commonly used textbooks disagree. Barbiturates exert a greater effect on blood pressure, CBF, and $CMRo_2$ than benzodiazepines at typical induction doses. Choice 4 is also somewhat vague. At 3 mg/kg of thiopental, one probably would only see activation of the EEG, which also would be seen with midazolam. However, at 5 mg/kg, the biphasic EEG pattern of thiopental would be evident with EEG slowing, whereas midazolam still would show only EEG activation. If choice 4 were worded "dose-dependent cortical EEG inhibition," then it would be correct. However, because of the vague wording, A is the best answer.

REFERENCES:

1. Barash PG, Cullen BF, Stoelting RK. Clinical Anesthesia, 4th ed. Philadelphia, Lippincott Williams & Wilkins, 2001, pp. 317, 319.
2. Stoelting RK, Miller RD. Basics of Anesthesia, 4th ed. New York, Churchill Livingstone, 2000, p. 68.
3. Morgan GE, Mikhail MS, Murray MJ. Clinical Anesthesiology, 3d ed. New York, McGraw-Hill, 2002, pp. 158, 161, 164, Table 8-8 (p. 171), Summary of Nonvolatile Anesthetic Effects on Organ Systems, Table 25-1 (p. 558), Comparative Effects of Anesthetic Agents on Cerebral Physiology, 559–560.

Answer E

Equipment/Physics

QUESTION (K-type):

The FI_{O_2} achieved by nasal prongs with oxygen flowing at 8 L/min depends on

(1) Tidal volume.
(2) Respiratory frequency.
(3) Inspiratory flow rate.
(4) Volume of the nasopharynx.

CORRECT ANSWER: E (All are correct)

SUMMARY:

Two types of equipment can provide supplemental oxygen: low-flow (variable performance) or high-flow (fixed performance) equipment.[1] Low-flow or variable-performance equipment includes nasal cannulas, nasal masks, nonreservoir oxygen masks, and reservoir masks. Fixed-performance equipment includes anesthesia bag/bag-mask valve systems, air entrainment venturi masks, and air entrainment nebulizers. Fixed-performance delivery systems provide a consistent and predictable delivered FI_{O_2} but require flow rates three to four times the patients minute ventilation. Variable-performance equipment supplies oxygen at a lower flow, and these devices are appropriate for patients with stable breathing patterns.

EXPLANATION:

(1) *Correct.* Inspired oxygen will be diluted by various amounts of entrained room air as ventilatory demand changes. Oxygen fills the nasopharynx during exhalation. However, during inspiration, both oxygen and air are drawn into the respiratory system. The fractional concentration of inspired oxygen therefore is lowered.
(2) *Correct.* With rapid respiration rates, inspired gas flows will exceed oxygen supply because nasal prongs deliver oxygen at fixed flows. The respiratory frequency affects the fractional concentration of inspired oxygen when nasal prongs are used.
(3) *Correct.* The FI_{O_2} decreases with decreased oxygen flow rates.
(4) *Correct.* The nasopharynx acts as an oxygen reservoir when nasal prongs are used.

REASONING:

This question tests knowledge of anesthetic equipment and respiratory physiology. Low-flow oxygen delivery devices such as nasal prongs are used commonly in the perioperative care of surgical patients. The approximate values of delivered FI_{O_2} for these devices should be reviewed by the reader.[1] In patients with normal, stable breathing patterns, nasal prongs can achieve an FI_{O_2} of 0.24 to 0.44 (1 to 6 L/min), oxygen mask 0.40 to 0.60 (5 to 8 L/min), and a mask with reservoir bag 0.6 to 0.80 or more (6 to 10 L/min). All the options are correct, and E is the best answer.

REFERENCE:

1. Miller RD, Miller ED, Reves JG, et al. Anesthesia, 5th ed. New York, Churchill Livingstone, 2000, pp. 2404–2406, Table 72-1.
2. Morgan GE, Mikhail MS, Murray MJ. Clinical Anesthesiology, 3d ed. New York, McGraw-Hill, 2002, p. 955.

Answer C

Pharmacology

QUESTION (K-type):

The administration of mannitol 1 g/kg over 15 minutes produces an acute increase in

(1) Serum potassium concentration.
(2) Central venous pressure.
(3) Systemic vascular resistance.
(4) Serum osmolality.

CORRECT ANSWER: C (2 and 4 are correct)

SUMMARY:

Mannitol is an osmotic diuretic that typically is used in anesthesia for decreasing brain volume and intracranial pressure (ICP) during neurosurgical procedures.[1] It also increases renal blood flow and scavenges free radicals and has been used to provide putative renal protection during aortic cross-clamping.[2] Acutely, mannitol increases the plasma osmolality, causing an extracellular shift of water and expanding the intravascular volume. While mannitol has been demonstrated to increase serum potassium concentration, this does not occur until higher doses are used.

EXPLANATION:

(1) *Incorrect.* Increased serum potassium levels are seen when 2 g/kg of mannitol are used.[3]
(2) *Correct.* Mannitol administration is associated with an increase in intravascular volume. This will increase the central venous pressure. Increased intravascular volume can precipitate acute congestive heart failure in patients with limited cardiac reserve.
(3) *Incorrect.* A transient decrease in mean arterial pressure (MAP) after administration of mannitol owing to decreased systemic vascular resistance is not uncommon. The phenomenon has been studied in animal models, but the exact mechanism is unclear.[4,5]
(4) *Correct.* Mannitol is a hypertonic solution. It will increase the serum osmolality.

REASONING:

This is a somewhat challenging question that tests knowledge of the acute effects of mannitol adminstration. Mannitol is an osmotic diuretic that should be administered slowly ($\geq$10 minutes) to prevent a transient increase in ICP in patients with intracranial hypertension.[1] Caution also should be used in patients with impaired cardiac function because the increased preload associated with rapid mannitol administration can precipitate left ventricular failure and acute congestive heart failure (CHF). When mannitol is used in typical clinical doses, it actually will cause a slight decrease in the serum potassium concentration. However, at higher doses (2 g/kg), it will increase serum potassium.[3] This question limits the amount of mannitol to 1 g/kg. The best answer is C.

REFERENCES:

1. Barash PG, Cullen BF, Stoelting RK. Clinical Anesthesia, 4th ed. Philadelphia, Lippincott Williams & Wilkins, 2001, p. 762.
2. Miller RD, Miller ED, Reves JG, et al. Anesthesia, 5th ed. New York, Churchill Livingstone, 2000, p. 686.
3. Manninen PH, Lam AM, Gelb AW, Brown SC. The effect of high dose mannitol on serum and urine electrolytes and osmolality in neurosurgical patients. Can J Anaesth 34(5):442–446, 1987.

4. Cote CJ, Greenhow DE, Marshall BE. The hypotensive response to rapid intravenous adminis-tration of hypertonic solutions in man and in the rabbit. Anesthesiology 50(1):30–35, 1979.

5. Stiff JL, Munch DF, Bromberger-Barnea B. Hypotension and respiratory distress caused by rapid infusion of mannitol or hypertonic saline. Anesth Analg 58(1):42–48, 1979.

6. Morgan GE, Mikhail MS, Murray MJ. Clinical Anesthesiology, 3d ed. New York, McGraw-Hill, 2002, p. 674.

BOOK B:

Answer C

Pediatrics

QUESTION 113

QUESTION (K-type):

Compared with a term infant, an infant born at 32 weeks' gestation who receives anes-thesia at 2 months of age is at increased risk for

(1) Pulmonary oxygen toxicity.
(2) Postoperative apnea.
(3) Renal failure.
(4) Retrolental fibroplasia.

CORRECT ANSWER: C (2 and 4 are correct)

SUMMARY:

Premature infants are at increased risk for retrolental fibroplasia and postoperative ap-nea. Anesthesiologists caring for infants younger than 44 weeks postconceptional age should attempt to maintain normal neonatal Pao_2 between 60 and 80 mm Hg intraoper-atively to prevent retinopathy. Infants younger than 50 weeks postconceptional age are not good candidates for elective or outpatient surgery and should be admitted at least 12 hours postoperatively for apnea monitoring.

EXPLANATION:

(1) *Incorrect.* High alveolar oxygen tensions for prolonged periods of time may gen-erate oxygen free radicals. Bronchopulmonary dysplasia is a chronic disorder that presents with pulmonary dysfunction in the first year of life.[1]

(2) *Correct.* Premature infants are at increased risk for postoperative apnea up to 60 weeks of postconceptional age. Other risk factors for postoperative apnea include anemia (hematocrit < 30 percent), hypothermia, infection, and CNS disease.

(3) *Incorrect.* Prematurity alone is not a risk factor for renal failure.

(4) *Correct.* Retrolental fibroplasia, also known as *retinopathy of prematurity*, is a disease associated with hyperoxia in infants younger than 44 weeks postconcep-tional age. Normal Pao_2 in the neonate is between 60 and 80 mm Hg. Maintaining the Pao_2 at less than 140 mm Hg generally is considered safe.

REASONING:

This questions highlights the special diseases particular to premature neonates: retrolen-tal fibroplasia and apnea of prematurity. Choices 1 and 3 can be eliminated because oxy-gen toxicity and renal failure are not problems that are specific to premature neonates. The best answer is C.

REFERENCE:

1. Stoelting RK, Miller RD. Basics of Anesthesia, 4th ed. New York, Churchill Livingstone, 2000, p. 371.

2. Morgan GE, Mikhail MS, Murray MJ. Clinical Anesthesiology, 3d ed. New York, McGraw-Hill, 2002, pp. 864, 959.

QUESTION 114

QUESTION (K-type):

Advantages of performing spinal anesthesia via the lateral approach include

(1) Larger opening for needle insertion than for the midline approach.
(2) Avoidance of the calcified interspinous ligament in the elderly.
(3) Less flexion of the spine required than for the midline approach.
(4) Less likelihood of peridural vein puncture than for the midline approach.

CORRECT ANSWER: A (1, 2, and 3 are correct)

SUMMARY:

Spinal anesthesia may be performed by the midline or lateral paramedian approach. The midline technique is done in the sitting or lateral position and is facilitated by the patient flexing his or her back. The spinous processes are palpated, and the needle is placed in the middle of the interspinous space. As the needle is advanced, the layers encountered are skin, subcutaneous tissue, supraspinous ligament, interspinous ligament, ligamentum flavum, epidural space, dura, and finally, the subarachnoid space. The paramedian approach is helpful in patients who have calcified ligaments or may be uncooperative with flexion of the spine. Owing to the sharp angle of the thoracic spinous processes, the paramedian technique may be useful when performing a thoracic epidural. The needle is inserted 1 cm lateral to the lower border of the desired interspace and angled 45 degrees cephalad and approximately 15 degrees medial.[1] In contrast to the midline approach, the first significant resistance encountered is ligamentum flavum. It is also important to note that the incidence of venous puncture is higher with the paramedian approach because veins travel anterior and lateral in the epidural space.[1]

EXPLANATION:

(1) **Correct.** The opening into the spinal canal is larger laterally rather than via the midline approach.
(2) **Correct.** Elderly patients often have calcified interspinous ligaments that can make the midline approach difficult.
(3) **Correct.** Flexion of the spine facilitates the midline approach by making the intervertebral spaces larger and has limited effect when one uses the paramedian approach.
(4) **Incorrect.** The epidural and spinal veins traverse laterally in the spinal canal and therefore are more likely to be punctured with the lateral paramedian approach.

REASONING:

This question tests knowledge of vertebral anatomy. The paramedian technique is used by many practitioners when the interspinous ligaments are calcified or the patient is uncooperative or unable to flex the spine to facilitate the midline technique. Choices 1, 2, and 3 are all advantages of the technique. Choice 4 can be eliminated because of the fact that the veins are located laterally in the spinal column. A is the correct answer.

REFERENCE:

1. Barash PG, Cullen BF, Stoelting RK. Clinical Anesthesia, 4th ed. Philadelphia, Lippincott Williams & Wilkins, 2001, pp. 646, 651.
2. Morgan GE, Mikhail MS, Murray MJ. Clinical Anesthesiology, 3d ed. New York, McGraw-Hill, 2002, pp. 263–266.

QUESTION (K-type):

In meralgia paresthetica

(1) There is pain in the anterolateral aspect of the thigh.
(2) The obturator nerve is involved.
(3) Obesity is an associated factor.
(4) Neurolytic alcohol block is the treatment of choice.

CORRECT ANSWER: B (1 and 3 are correct)

SUMMARY:

Meralgia paresthetica is an entrapment neuropathy involving the lateral femoral cutaneous nerve. The site of entrapment is the anterior iliac spine under the inguinal ligament. There is usually pain, paresthesias, or numbness in the anterolateral thigh distal to this site. Meralgia paresthetica can be diagnosed with nerve conduction studies, electromyography, or blockade of this nerve with local anesthetic, which also provides temporary pain relief. The treatment of choice is symptomatic management with nonsteroidal anti-inflammatory drugs (NSAIDs) or corticosteroid injections. Intractable symptoms may require surgery.

EXPLANATION:

(1) *Correct.* The lateral femoral cutaneous nerve provides sensation to the anterolateral thigh, and meralgia paresthetica typically involves pain in this area.
(2) *Incorrect.* Entrapment of the obturator nerve usually occurs in the obturator canal, which results in pain in the upper medial thigh.
(3) *Correct.* Obesity increases the likelihood of nerve entrapment and is an associated factor.
(4) *Incorrect.* Neurolytic alcohol blocks cause temporary nonselective destruction of nerve fibers and ganglia. They are used as treatments of last resort for severe intractable cancer pain. NSAIDs and rest are the treatments of choice in meralgia paresthetica.

REASONING:

This question tests knowledge of the pathophysiology of meralgia paresthetica. Choice 2 is obviously incorrect because this syndrome involves the lateral femoral cutaneous nerve. This rules out answers A, C, and E. Since choice 1 is correct, answer D is incorrect, and B is the only possible answer.

REFERENCE:

Barash PG, Cullen BF, Stoelting RK. Clinical Anesthesia, 4th ed. Philadelphia, Lippincott Williams & Wilkins, 2001, p. 737.
Morgan GE, Mikhail MS, Murray MJ. Clinical Anesthesiology, 3d ed. New York, McGraw-Hill, 2002, pp. 336, 351, 351t, figures inside back cover.

Answer E

Neuroanesthesia

QUESTION (K-type):

In patients undergoing transsphenoidal hypophysectomy for acromegaly, anesthesia is complicated by

(1) Decreased subglottic diameter.
(2) Temporomandibular joint dysfunction.
(3) Glucose intolerance.
(4) Diabetes insipidus.

CORRECT ANSWER: E (All are correct)

SUMMARY:

Acromegaly is an endocrine disorder that involves oversecretion of growth hormone. It has an overall population prevalence of 50 to 70 cases per million with an annual incidence rate of only 3 to 4 cases per million people.[1] It is a multisystem disease that affects the viscera, skeletal muscles, and soft and connective tissues. Diabetes, hypertension, heart disease, and sleep apnea are physical manifestations of acromegaly that are particularly concerning to the anesthesiologist.[2] A difficult airway should be anticipated in patients with acromegaly. Enlargement of the tongue and epiglottis, as well as the increased length of the mandible, predisposes to difficult upper airway management and endotracheal intubation. Moreover, the recurrent laryngeal nerve may be paralyzed owing to the excessive stretching caused by overgrowth of cartilaginous structures. A decrease in subglottic diameter also should be anticipated if the patient complains of dyspnea on exertion. Excessive growth hormone affects carbohydrate metabolism and may lead to glucose intolerance. Because of connective tissue overgrowth, these patients also may have temporomandibular joint dysfunction. An important complication of transsphenoidal hypophysectomy is increased risk of pituitary hypofunction. Postoperative diabetes insipidus can occur in up to 40 percent of patients.

EXPLANATION:

(1) *Correct.* Stridor on examination is suggestive of tissue overgrowth in the subglottic region.
(2) *Correct.* Acromegaly causes an overgrowth of connective tissue that would affect all joints, including the temporomandibular joint.
(3) *Correct.* Alteration in carbohydrate metabolism caused by excessive growth hormone may predispose these patients to develop diabetes mellitus. Insulin therapy may be required in severe cases.
(4) *Correct.* While not a complication of acromegaly, diabetes insipidus (DI) may develop as a complication of the surgical procedure. DI typically is seen during the first 12 hours postoperatively and lasts for 2 to 4 days.[3] It is characterized by polyuria (2 to 15 L/day), hyponatremia, and decreased urine osmolality and specific gravity.[3]

REASONING:

This question tests knowledge of the anesthetic complications associated with acromegaly. It is a multisystemic disease that can manifest all the findings presented in choices 1, 2, and 3. DI is a complication associated with the surgical procedure, transsphenoidal hypophysectomy. All the choices are correct, and the best answer is E.

REFERENCES:

1. Melmed S. Acromegaly. N Engl J Med 322(14):966–977, 1990.
2. Seidman PA, Kofke WA, Policare R, Young M. Anaesthetic complications of acromegaly. Br J Anaesth 84(2):179–182, 2000.
3. Barash PG, Cullen BF, Stoelting RK. Clinical Anesthesia, 4th ed. Philadelphia, Lippincott Williams & Wilkins, 2001, p. 769.
4. Stoelting R, Dierdorf S. Anesthesia and Co-Existing Disease, 4th ed. New York, Churchill Livingstone, 2002, pp. 437–438.
5. Morgan GE, Mikhail MS, Murray MJ. Clinical Anesthesiology, 3d ed. New York, McGraw-Hill, 2002, p. 581.

BOOK B:	QUESTION 117

Answer B

Pediatrics

QUESTION (K-type):

The infant airway differs from that of the adult in which of the following ways?

(1) The larynx is more cephalad.
(2) The vocal cords are perpendicular to the plane of the trachea.
(3) The cricoid cartilage is the narrowest part of the airway.
(4) The larynx is more anterior.

CORRECT ANSWER: B (1 and 3 correct)

SUMMARY:

Several features differentiate the infant airway from the adult airway and may contribute to difficult tracheal intubation: a more cephalad larynx, a long and stiff epiglottis, a short trachea and neck, and a proportionately larger head and tongue. The larynx in infants actually is not anterior compared with adults, contrary to common perception.[1]

EXPLANATION:

(1) **Correct.** The larynx is found at the level of C4 in infants and C6 in adults.
(2) **Incorrect.** In the adult larynx, the vocal cords are more perpendicular to the tracheal plane. The vocal cords in infants are angled in relation to the tracheal plane.[2]
(3) **Correct.** The narrowest portion of the infant airway is the cricoid ring.
(4) **Incorrect.** The larynx is more cephalad but not more anterior in infants compared with adults.[1] Sometimes overextension of the infant head can displace the larynx anteriorly during endotracheal intubation.[3]

REASONING:

This commonly tested question asks for comparisons between pediatric and adult airways. This may be a controversial question owing to choice 4 because textbooks disagree on this point. However, choice 2 is definitely not correct, making B the best answer.

REFERENCES:

1. Cote CJ. A Practice of Anesthesia for Infants and Children, 3d ed. Philadelphia, Saunders, 2001, pp. 81–82.
2. Barash PG, Cullen BF, Stoelting RK. Clinical Anesthesia, 4th ed. Philadelphia, Lippincott Williams & Wilkins, 2001, p. 596, Table 23-1.
3. Gregory GA. Pediatric Anesthesia, 4th ed. New York, Churchill Livingstone, 2002, p. 224.
4. Morgan GE, Mikhail MS, Murray MJ. Clinical Anesthesiology, 3d ed. New York, McGraw-Hill, 2002, pp. 850–851, Table 44-1 (p. 851), Characteristics of Neonates and Infants that Differentiate Them from Adult Patients.

Answer D

OB/Regional

QUESTION (K-type):

The duration of an epidural block can be increased clinically by

(1) Use of a local anesthetic with low protein binding.
(2) Use of a local anesthetic with a low pK_a.
(3) Addition of sodium bicarbonate to the local anesthetic.
(4) Increasing the total dose of the local anesthetic.

CORRECT ANSWER: D (4 only is correct)

SUMMARY:

The duration of epidural or spinal anesthesia depends on the properties of the local anesthetic used and the total drug concentration administered.[1] Drugs that have high protein binding such as etidocaine and bupivicaine have a longer duration than those with less protein binding such as lidocaine. The addition of sodium bicarbonate to lidocaine can hasten onset by increasing the pH of the solution, whereas adding epinephrine to a local anesthetic increases the duration by causing local vasoconstriction and decreased tissue uptake.

EXPLANATION:

(1) *Incorrect.* Local anesthetics with high protein binding will have longer duration.
(2) *Incorrect.* All local anesthetics are weak bases and have pK_a values greater than physiologic pH. Those with comparably lower pH have a faster onset owing to a higher concentration of drug in the nonionized form, but this property does not correlate with duration.
(3) *Incorrect.* The addition of sodium bicarbonate to local anesthetic increases the pH of the solution. This increases the nonionized free-base form of local anesthetics, which hastens the onset of the drug but does not prolong the duration.[2]
(4) *Correct.* Higher total doses of local anesthetic correlate with prolonged duration.[1] However, one must take into consideration other properties of the agent used and determine the toxic dose prior to attempting to increase the duration of an epidural based on total dose alone.

REASONING:

This question tests knowledge of the pharmacokinetics of local anesthetics. It is common practice to add sodium bicarbonate to a local anesthetic solution to hasten onset of analgesia. However, this does not increase the duration of action. Other additives such as epinephrine are added for this purpose. This eliminates choice 3, and thus choice 1 can be eliminated as well, even if the reader is unsure of the relationship between protein binding and duration. Choice 2 is incorrect because of the fact that the pK_a relates to *onset* rather than duration. Thus D the best answer.

REFERENCES:

1. Barash PG, Cullen BF, Stoelting RK. Clinical Anesthesia, 4th ed. Philadelphia, Lippincott Williams & Wilkins, 2001, pp. 455–456.
2. Hughes SC, Levinson G, Rosen MA. Shnider and Levinson's Anesthesia for Obstetrics, 4th ed. Philadelphia, Lippincott Williams & Wilkins, 2002, p. 87.
3. Morgan GE, Mikhail MS, Murray MJ. Clinical Anesthesiology, 3d ed. New York, McGraw-Hill, 2002, pp. 234–238, Table 14-1, Physiochemical Properties of Local Anesthetics.

Answer D

OB/Regional

QUESTION (K-type):

Prior to vaginal delivery at term, a primiparous woman receives epidural anesthesia administered through a catheter inserted at L2–3. The following day she has left footdrop and sensory loss over the left outer calf. Causes of these complications include

(1) Compression of the obturator nerve by excessive thigh flexion.
(2) Compression of the lumbosacral trunk by the fetal head.
(3) Nerve root injury by the epidural needle.
(4) Compression of the common peroneal nerve by the stirrup.

CORRECT ANSWER: D (4 only is correct)

SUMMARY:

Peripartum nerve injuries can occur after vaginal delivery with or without neuraxial analgesia. It is important to distinguish peripheral from central nerve injuries by recognizing the distribution of lower extremity peripheral nerves and dermatomes of the lumbar and sacral nerve roots. Examples of nerve distributions are obturator—medial upper thigh, lateral femoral cutaneous—lateral upper thigh; saphenous—medial lower leg; and common peroneal—lateral lower leg and medial foot. The inguinal region corresponds to the L1 dermatome, whereas L4 is the knee and L5 is the lateral lower leg and medial foot. Epidural anesthesia can contribute to peripheral nerve injuries by allowing a patient to tolerate a position that compromises the nerve and otherwise would be painful.[1] Examples include femoral neuropathy from prolonged extreme lithotomy position during the second stage of labor or common peroneal neuropathy from excessive pressure on the lateral lower leg owing to stirrups.

EXPLANATION:

(1) *Incorrect.* Obturator nerve injury would cause sensory loss over the medial upper leg.
(2) *Incorrect.* Compression of the lumbosacral trunk by the fetal head would result in sensory loss over the inguinal region, upper thigh, knee, and medial foot.
(3) *Incorrect.* The epidural was placed at L2–3. If a nerve root is injured at this level, the sensory loss would occur over the upper thigh.
(4) *Correct.* The foot drop and distribution of the sensory loss correspond with the common peroneal nerve, which can be compressed by stirrups. It is important to note that this also can happen to patients placed in the lithotomy position in the operating room, and the reader must monitor carefully for compression over this nerve.

REASONING:

The key to correctly answering this question is knowledge of the dermatomal distribution of the nerve roots and the sensory distribution of the peripheral nerves in the leg. These should be reviewed carefully by the reader.[2] The only possible answer that corresponds to the correct anatomic position is choice 4, making the correct answer D.

REFERENCES:

1. Hughes SC, Levinson G, Rosen MA. Shnider and Levinson's Anesthesia for Obstetrics, 4th ed. Philadelphia, Lippincott Williams & Wilkins, 2002, p. 410.
2. Barash PG, Cullen BF, Stoelting RK. Clinical Anesthesia, 4th ed. Philadelphia, Lippincott Williams & Wilkins, 2001, pp. 736–737.
3. Morgan GE, Mikhail MS, Murray MJ. Clinical Anesthesiology, 3d ed. New York, McGraw-Hill, 2002, pp. 303, 893.

Answer D

Pediatrics

QUESTION (K-type):

A 2-year-old boy with tetralogy of Fallot is scheduled for repair of bilateral inguinal hernias. True statements concerning this child include

(1) Oxygen saturation will improve with crying.
(2) Cyanosis will increase with use of halothane.
(3) Resistance to pulmonary outflow will be fixed.
(4) An increased red cell mass will compensate for right-to-left shunt.

CORRECT ANSWER: D (4 only is correct)

SUMMARY:

Tetralogy of Fallot is composed of a ventricular septal defect, overriding aorta, right ventricular outflow tract (RVOT) obstruction, and right ventricular hypertrophy. It is the most common congenital cardiac anomaly that results in right-to-left shunting and cyanosis.[1] RVOT obstruction is dynamic and increases with sympathetic stimulation. The management of patients with uncorrected tetralogy of Fallot should include maintenance of intravascular volume and hematocrit and avoidance of low systemic vascular resistance and high pulmonary vascular resistance.

EXPLANATION:

(1) *Incorrect.* Crying actually can trigger hypercyanotic episodes or "tet spells."[1] Infundibular spasm increases the magnitude of right-to-left shunting and worsens cyanosis.
(2) *Incorrect.* Volatile anesthetics are indicated in anesthetizing children with tetralogy of Fallot because they relax RVOT dynamic obstruction by decreasing myocardial contractility. It is true that decreased systemic vascular resistance (SVR) can lead to an increase in right-to-left shunting.[1] However, halothane has very little impact on SVR and can be administered safely to these children.
(3) *Incorrect.* In most patients, RVOT obstruction is due to hypertrophy of infundibular muscle. The resistance to pulmonary outflow is dynamic and can be increased by sympathetic tone.
(4) *Correct.* Patients with tetralogy of Fallot tend to have higher hematocrits in order to compensate for their chronic right-to-left shunt.

REASONING:

This question tests knowledge of the pathophysiology and anesthetic management of tetralogy of Fallot. A similar question is virtually guaranteed to be asked on the reader's board examination. Fortunately, this question is fairly straightforward. It is important to understand that the management of patients with right-to-left shunts always depends on balancing pulmonary vascular resistance (PVR) and SVR. The best answer is D.

REFERENCE:

1. Stoelting RK, Miller RD. Basics of Anesthesia, 4th ed. New York, Churchill Livingstone, 2000, pp. 258–259.
2. Morgan GE, Mikhail MS, Murray MJ. Clinical Anesthesiology, 3d ed. New York, McGraw-Hill, 2002, pp. 425–26.

Answer D

Neuroanesthesia
clipping: anesthetic
management

QUESTION (K-type):

A previously healthy 28-year-old woman who had a subarachnoid hemorrhage 2 days ago is scheduled for a craniotomy and clipping of an anterior communicating artery aneurysm. She is awake, oriented, and neurologically intact. True statements concerning anesthetic management include

(1) The arterial pressure should be maintained above the preoperative values during induction.
(2) Hyperventilation to a $PaCO_2$ of 25 to 30 mm Hg should be initiated prior to endotracheal intubation.
(3) Mannitol should be given immediately following induction.
(4) The mean arterial pressure (MAP) should be decreased to 50 mm Hg if necessary for surgical exposure.

CORRECT ANSWER: D (4 only is correct)

SUMMARY:

Appropriate anesthetic management of a patient undergoing cerebral aneurysm clipping includes avoiding increases in transmural pressure that can lead to aneurysm rupture, maintaining cerebral perfusion pressure, and facilitating surgical exposure.[1] Transmural pressure is defined as MAP − intracranial pressure (ICP). Increases in MAP during induction or decreases in ICP prior to opening of the dura can lead to aneurysm rupture. Hyperventilation may decrease ICP dramatically, increasing the transmural pressure and the likelihood of aneurysm rupture. It also may compromise cerebral blood flow (CBF) and should be avoided in patients with vasospasm.

EXPLANATION:

(1) **Incorrect.** MAP should be maintained at preoperative values during induction. Hypertension during induction will increase transmural pressure and potentially cause aneurysm rupture.[1]
(2) **Incorrect.** Extreme hyperventilation prior to intubation may increase the risk of aneurysm rupture by reducing ICP and increasing transmural pressure. In addition, patients who have suffered a subarachnoid hemorrhage are at risk for cerebral vasospasm and require maintenance of CBF.
(3) **Incorrect.** Administration of mannitol following opening of the dura is a technique employed to induce brain relaxation and facilitate surgical dissection. An osmotic diuretic given immediately following induction offers no advantage and may worsen dehydration in patients following a subarachnoid hemorrage.[1]
(4) **Correct.** Deliberate hypotension may be used to facilitate exposure during surgical dissection as long as the benefit outweighs the risk. Patients with cardiovascular disease, renal insufficiency, or other end-organ disease may not be good candidates for deliberate hypotension.[1] An alternative technique induces regional instead of global hypotension by placement of a temporary clip on a major artery feeding the aneurysm.[2]

REASONING:

This question tests knowledge of anesthetic management in patients with cerebral aneurysms. It is important to understand that transmural pressure across the wall of the aneurysm = MAP − ICP. Goals during induction include avoiding sudden increases in MAP or decreases in ICP. Hyperventilation, osmotic diuresis, and deliberate hypotension are all techniques used to facilitate surgical exposure once the dura is open.

REFERENCES:

1. Barash PG, Cullen BF, Stoelting RK. Clinical Anesthesia, 4th ed. Philadelphia, Lippincott Williams & Wilkins, 2001, p. 728.
2. Stoelting RK, Miller RD. Basics of Anesthesia, 4th ed. New York, Churchill Livingstone, 2000, p. 328.
3. Morgan GE, Mikhail MS, Murray MJ. Clinical Anesthesiology, 3d ed. New York, McGraw-Hill, 2002, pp. 578–579.

BOOK B:

Answer C

Clinical Anesthesia

QUESTION 122

QUESTION (K-type):

A 45-year-old man is scheduled for elective antrectomy and vagotomy. He has drunk a 6-pack of beer daily for 20 years. Laboratory evaluation shows the following findings:

	Patient	Normal
AST (SGOT) (units/L)	75	0–45
ALT (SGPT) (units/L)	56	0–45
LDH (units/L)	300	50–250
Alkaline phosphatase (units/L)	120	25–115
Bilirubin (mg/dL)	1.2	0.1–1.2

Based on these laboratory findings, anticipated problems in anesthetic management include

(1) Increased risk for halothane hepatotoxicioty.
(2) Coagulation disorders.
(3) Large peripheral arteriovenous shunts.
(4) Increased anesthetic requirements.

CORRECT ANSWER: C (2 and 4 are correct)

SUMMARY:

Impaired synthetic liver function and elevated liver enzyme tests are to be expected in the setting of chronic alcohol abuse. Ten to fifteen years of chronic alcohol consumption can lead to cirrhosis and subsequent liver failure. Extensive hepatocellular injury results in numerous physiologic consequences than can include portal hypertension and coagulopathy. This patient has mildly elevated liver enzyme values suggestive of either alcoholic hepatitis or alcoholic cirrhosis. It is difficult to assess the extent of liver dysfunction in the absence of a physical examination or other markers of synthetic liver function such as INR or albumin. However, given the duration of alcohol abuse, we can anticipate increased anesthetic requirements (owing to induction of P450) as well as potential coagulation disorders (due to impaired hepatic synthesis of clotting factors).

EXPLANATION:

(1) *Incorrect.* Halothane hepatitis is a rare occurrence (1 in 22,000 to 35,000 cases). Risk factors include middle age, adults, females, obesity, and multiple prior exposures at short intervals. There are two proposed mechanisms leading to halothane-induced hepatotoxicity. According to hepatic oxygen-deprivation theory, hepatocellular injury is due to halothane-induced reduction in oxygen supply to the hepatocytes. Another theory proposes that immunologic response to halothane toxic metabolites leads to hepatocyte injury. At present, there is no compelling evidence associating halothane with exacerbation of preexisting liver disease. However, avoidance probably is warranted to minimize clinical uncertainty if worsening liver function occurs in the postoperative period.

(2) **Correct.** Coagulation disorder is seen commonly in patients with cirrhosis. Prothrombin time (PT) is a sensitive indicator of hepatic synthetic function. A persistently elevated international normalization ratio (INR) of 1.5 or greater despite administration of vitamin K is suggestive of hepatic synthetic dysfunction.

(3) **Incorrect.** Intrapulmonary shunts, not large peripheral arteriovenous shunts, can be expected in hepatic cirrhosis.

(4) **Correct.** Chronic alcohol abuse increases anesthetic requirements, whereas acute alcoholic intoxication decreases anesthetic requirements.

REASONING:

As mentioned above, these laboratory findings are suggestive of either alcoholic hepatitis or alcoholic cirrhosis. In clinical practice we would obtain further medical history, perform a physical examination, and obtain appropriate laboratory studies to determine the extent of liver damage. The key word in this question is *anticipated*. Without more specific information, it would be prudent to anticipate potential liver dysfunction and the associated implications for anesthetic management. In addition, knowing the risk factors of halothane-induced hepatotoxicity is also expected. C is the best answer.

REFERENCES:

Miller RD, Miller ED, Reves JG, et al. Anesthesia, 5th ed. New York, Churchill Livingstone, 2000, pp. 657–658.

Stoelting R, Dierdorf S. Anesthesia and Co-Existing Disease, 4th ed. New York, Churchill Livingstone, 2002, p. 307.

Morgan GE, Mikhail MS, Murray MJ. Clinical Anesthesiology, 3d ed. New York, McGraw-Hill, 2002, pp. 139–140.

BOOK B: **QUESTION 123**

Answer C

Cardiovascular

QUESTION (K-type)

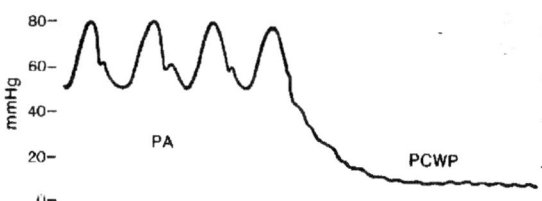

Causes of the pulmonary artery pressure and pulmonary artery occlusion pressure waveforms shown above include

(1) Catheter overwedging.
(2) Protamine reaction.
(3) Acute mitral regurgitation.
(4) Primary pulmonary hypertension.

CORRECT ANSWER: C (2 and 4 are correct)

SUMMARY:

Flow-directed pulmonary artery catheters (PACs) can be used to provide estimates of left ventricular end-diastolic pressures.[1] Flotation of the catheter into the pulmonary artery allows the pulmonary arterial (PA) pressure waveform to be transduced. When the balloon at the tip of the catheter is inflated and "wedged" into the distal PA circulation, a pulmonary catheter wedge pressure (PCWP) waveform can be recorded. The PCWP (also sometimes referred to as the pulmonary artery occlusion pressure [PAOP]) provides an estimate of left ventricular end-diastolic pressure (LVEDP), assuming that the path from the catheter tip to the left ventricle is unobstructed and ventricular compliance is normal. Ideally, the pulmonary artery diastolic pressure will approximate the PCWP. This PAC tracing is abnormal. It indicates very high PA pressures (normal PA pressures 10 to 25 mm Hg/5 to 15 mm Hg) with a normal PCWP. This relationship is seen in any disease state that increases pulmonary vascular resistance, such as primary pulmonary hypertension or protamine reaction. A protamine reaction can cause acute pulmonary vasoconstriction. (See also Question 107, Book B.)

EXPLANATION:

(1) *Incorrect.* An overwedged catheter would produce a ramplike trace with loss of pulsatile flow. The PA pressures would be normal.

(2) *Correct.* See below.

(3) *Incorrect.* Acute mitral regurgitation (MR) would produce prominent *v* waves on the PA tracing. The predictive value of prominent V waves for acute MR has been confirmed.[2]

(4) *Correct.* Elevated PA systolic and diastolic pressure (80/45 mm Hg) with normal wedge pressure (15 mm Hg) is seen in any condition that can produce elevated pulmonary vascular resistance, such as cor pulmonale, pulmonary embolism, and collagen-vascular disease. This results in right ventricular hypertrophy (RVH) and elevated right ventricular and pulmonary artery pressures over time. A similar presentation can be seen with protamine reaction secondary to thromboxane release producing pulmonary vasoconstriction.

REASONING:

This question tests knowledge of the interpretation of a PAC tracing and the effects of pulmonary hypertension on PAP and PCWP. The reader should review the criteria for placement and interpretation of PAC monitoring and its limitations carefully.[1] Choices 1 and 3 can be ruled out based on this knowledge. D is the best answer.

REFERENCES:

1. Barash PG, Cullen BF, Stoelting RK. Clinical Anesthesia, 4th ed. Philadelphia, Lippincott Williams & Wilkins, 2001, pp. 657–679.

2. Snyder RW 2d, Glamann DB, Lange RA, et al. Predictive value of prominent pulmonary arterial wedge v waves in assessing the presence and severity of mitral regurgitation. Am J Cardiol 73(8):568–570, 1994.

3. Stoelting RK, Dierdorf SF. Anesthesia and Co-Existing Diseases, 3d ed. New York, Churchill Livingstone, 1993, pp. 103–106.

4. Morgan GE, Mikhail MS, Murray MJ. Clinical Anesthesiology, 3d ed. New York, McGraw-Hill, 2002, pp. 457–458.

BOOK B:

QUESTION 124

Answer D

Pediatrics

QUESTION (K-type):

Electrolyte profiles consistent with pyloric stenosis in a 6-week-old infant include

	Na$^+$ (mEq/L)	K$^+$ (mEq/L)	Cl$^-$ (mEq/L)	HCO$_3^-$ (mEq/L)
(1)	145	3.5	108	24
(2)	145	2.5	85	15
(3)	160	5.5	120	36
(4)	128	2.5	85	32

SUMMARY:

Pyloric stenosis owing to hypertrophy of the pyloric smooth muscle classically presents with persistent nonbilious vomiting. Infants with this disease typically present with dehydration and depletion of sodium, potassium, and chloride, resulting in hypochloremic metabolic alkalosis. Pyloric stenosis is a medical emergency, but surgery should be delayed until fluids and electrolytes have been replaced.[1] Long-standing metabolic alkalosis can lead to respiratory depression postoperatively owing to persistent cerebrospinal fluid (CSF) alkalosis.

EXPLANATION:

(1) **Incorrect.** This set of electrolytes is in the near-normal range.
(2) **Incorrect.** The sodium should be low and bicarbonate high in pyloric stenosis.
(3) **Incorrect.** The sodium, potassium, and chloride should be low in pyloric stenosis.
(4) **Correct.** This set of electrolytes is most consistent with pyloric stenosis: low sodium, potassium, and chloride and high bicarbonate.

REASONING:

This question tests knowledge of the electrolyte abnormalities associated with pyloric stenosis. These abnormalities are due to chronic vomiting. Since gastric fluid contains hydrochloric acid, vomiting results in hypochloremic metabolic alkalosis. Even if the reader is unsure about sodium or potassium levels, choice 4 is the only one with low chloride and high bicarbonate. D is the best answer.

REFERENCE:

1. Stoelting RK, Miller RD. Basics of Anesthesia, 4th ed. New York, Churchill Livingstone, 2000, pp. 374–375.
2. Morgan GE, Mikhail MS, Murray MJ. Clinical Anesthesiology, 3d ed. New York, McGraw-Hill, 2002, pp. 866–867.

BOOK B: **QUESTION 125**

Answer B

Regional Anesthesia

QUESTION (K-type):

True statements concerning regional anesthesia with peripheral nerve blocks for an operation on a knee using a tourniquet include

(1) The inguinal perivascular block includes the obturator nerve.
(2) Paresthesias are required during sciatic block.
(3) The lateral femoral cutaneous nerve must be blocked.
(4) Block of the lumbar plexus in the psoas compartment provides adequate anesthesia.

SUMMARY:

Operations on the knee using a tourniquet require anesthesia of the anterior, medial, lateral, and posterior aspects of the thigh. These areas are innervated by the femoral, obturator, lateral femoral cutaneous, and posterior cutaneous nerves of the thigh, respectively. These are the nerves that must be blocked. Inguinal perivascular block and block of the lumbar plexus in the psoas compartment both aim to block the femoral, obturator, and lateral femoral cutaneous nerves, but not the posterior cutaneous nerve of the thigh.

EXPLANATION:

(1) **Correct.** An inguinal perivascular block aims to have local anesthetic spread proximally along the facial compartment containing the femoral nerve to include the obturator and lateral femoral cutaneous nerves.

(2) **Incorrect.** A sciatic block may be accomplished without paresthesias.

(3) **Correct.** The lateral thigh must be anesthetized with blockade of the lateral femoral cutaneous nerve, particularly if a tourniquet is to be used.

(4) **Incorrect.** Blockade of the lumbar plexus will not block the posterior cutaneous nerve of the thigh and thus will be inadequate for knee surgery using a tourniquet.

REASONING:

This question tests knowledge of the innervation of the lower leg and thigh. The reader hopefully will note by now the frequency with which innervation to the lower extremity is tested. (*See also Questions 37, Book A; 81, Book B; 115, Book B; 119, Book B; and 134, Book B.*) The importance of this topic for careful review by the reader cannot be overstated. It is important to note the use of the tourniquet in order to identify the entire area of anesthesia required for surgery. B is the best answer.

REFERENCE:

Cousins M, Bridenbaugh P. Neural Blockade in Clinical Anesthesia and Management of Pain, 3d ed. Philadelphia, Saunders, 1998, pp. 373–380.

Morgan GE, Mikhail MS, Murray MJ. Clinical Anesthesiology, 3d ed. New York, McGraw-Hill, 2002, pp. 262–266.

BOOK B:

Answer E

OB/Regional

QUESTION 126

QUESTION (K-type):

Proximal spread of a local anesthetic solution placed in the axillary perivascular space is promoted by

(1) Increased volume of the local anesthetic agent.
(2) Digital pressure distal to the injection site.
(3) Cephalad direction of the needle.
(4) Adduction of the shoulder after the injection.

CORRECT ANSWER: E (All are correct)

SUMMARY:

Factors affecting spread of local anesthetic during placement of axillary blocks are important because proximal spread of local anesthetic leads to more complete and reliable blockade. Interventions that promote proximal spread of local anesthetic include the following: increased volume of local anesthetic, digital pressure distal to the injection site, cephalad direction of the needle, and adduction of the shoulder after the injection.

EXPLANATION:

(1) **Correct.** Large-volume injection promotes spread in all directions.

(2) **Correct.** Factors leading to inadequate axillary block include the septation of the axillary perivascular space and the proximal departure of the musculocutaneous nerve from the axillary sheath. Proximal spread of the local anesthetic helps to overcome both these problems and achieves a more effective block. Digital pressure distal to the site of injection has been advocated to encourage spread proximally rather than distally.

(3) *Correct.* Cephalad direction of the needle has been advocated for promoting proximal spread but may incur a small risk of pneumothorax.

(4) *Correct.* Multiple authors note that overabduction of the arm during placement of the block may cause forward displacement of the humeral head leading to an attenuated axillary pulse. Similarly, adduction of the shoulder after injection can reduce the pressure caused by forward displacement of the humeral head that may reduce proximal spread of local anesthetic.

REASONING:

This question tests knowledge of the placement of an axillary block. Factors that affect proximal spread of local anesthetic in the sheath include the volume of anesthetic used, digital pressure distal to the injection, cephalad direction of the needle, and adduction of the shoulder after the injection. All choices are correct, and therefore, the best answer is E.

REFERENCES:

Barash PG, Cullen BF, Stoelting RK. Clinical Anesthesia, 4th ed. Philadelphia, Lippincott Williams & Wilkins, 2001, pp. 726–727.

Cousins M, Bridenbaugh P. Neural Blockade in Clinical Anesthesia and Management of Pain, 3d ed. Philadelphia, Saunders, 1998, pp. 359–361.

Morgan GE, Mikhail MS, Murray MJ. Clinical Anesthesiology, 3d ed. New York, McGraw-Hill, 2002, pp. 254–256.

BOOK B: **QUESTION 127**

Answer D

Pain

QUESTION (K-type):

Indications for neurolytic celiac plexus ablation include pain due to carcinoma of the

(1) Sigmoid colon.
(2) Kidney.
(3) Ovary.
(4) Pancreas.

CORRECT ANSWER: D (4 only is correct)

SUMMARY:

Celiac plexus neurolysis is indicated for pain control in upper abdominal and retroperitoneal malignancy. It is generally thought to be helpful for pain originating in the distal esophagus, stomach, duodenum, small intestines, and ascending and proximal transverse colon. Organs supplied by the celiac artery that receive contributions from the celiac plexus include the liver, biliary system, spleen, and pancreas. Textbooks differ on whether the visceral afferents from the kidney course through the celiac plexus. Review of the literature available on Medline from 1966 to 2003 resulted in no reports of celiac plexus blockade for renal cell carcinoma. Carcinoma of the sigmoid colon, ovaries, and other pelvic viscera may be treated with hypogastric plexus blocks.

EXPLANATION:

(1) *Incorrect.* Celiac plexus block will relieve intestinal pain related to the mid-transverse colon and higher but does not cover the sigmoid colon, which may be covered with other blocks such as a superior hypogastric plexus block.

(2) *Incorrect.* While texts differ on whether visceral afferent fibers from the kidneys travel through the celiac plexus, cancer of the kidney is clearly not an indication for a neurolytic celiac plexus block. No cases of such treatment could be found in an extensive Medline search.

(3) **Incorrect.** Ovaries are thought to be innervated by fibers originating lower than the celiac plexus.

(4) **Correct.** There is extensive literature supporting use of neurolytic celiac plexus block for pancreatic cancer, with reported success rates generally between 80 and 90 percent, often resulting in cessation of opioid use.

REASONING:

This question tests knowledge of the celiac plexus block. A hallmark of celiac plexus blockade is that it does not cover the sigmoid colon. Therefore, choice 1 is incorrect, and answers A, B, and E can be eliminated. Differentiating between answers C and D requires only a determination of whether pain due to carcinoma of the kidney is an indication for neurolytic celiac plexus block. There is no literature in the Medline database to support this indication. D is the best answer.

REFERENCES:

Benzon H, Raja S, et al. Essentials of Pain Medicine and Regional Anesthesia. New York, Elsevier 1999, p. 323.

Cousins M, Bridenbaugh P. Neural Blockade in Clinical Anesthesia and Management of Pain. 3d ed. Philadelphia, Saunders, 1998, pp. 463–465.

Nikiforov S, Cronin A, Murray B, Hall V. Subcutaneous paravertebral block for renal colic. Anesthesiology 94:531–532, 2001.

Waldman S. Atlas of Interventional Pain Management, 2d ed. Philadelphia, Saunders, 2004, pp. 265–271.

Morgan GE, Mikhail MS, Murray MJ. Clinical Anesthesiology, 3d ed. New York, McGraw-Hill, 2002, pp. 295–296.

BOOK B:

QUESTION 128

Answer A

Pharmacology

QUESTION (K-type):

Compared with a 20-year-old patient, an 80-year-old patient will

(1) Have similar electroencephalographic (EEG) sensitivity to the same blood concentrations of thiopental.
(2) Require lower induction doses (mg/kg) of thiopental.
(3) Have increased sensitivity to volatile anesthetics.
(4) Require lower doses (mg/kg) of succinylcholine.

CORRECT ANSWER: A (1, 2, and 3 are correct)

SUMMARY:

Pharmacokinetic and pharmacodynamic changes occur with age. These changes alter dosing and duration of anesthetics. In general, the geriatric patient has decreased total-body water owing to decreased muscle mass and increased body fat. This results in a decreased volume of distribution for water-soluble drugs, whereas an increased volume of distribution is seen with more lipid-soluble drugs. Plasma concentrations of drugs parallel these changes in volume of distribution. Hepatic and renal function generally is decreased in the elderly patients, leading to impaired elimination and clearance that can result in a prolonged drug effect.

EXPLANATION:

(1) **Correct.** A study by Homer and Stanski demonstrated through pharmacodynamic modeling that EEG brain sensitivity to thiopental does not change with age.[1]
(2) **Correct.** An octegarian will achieve higher plasma levels of thiopental compared with a 20-year old if given the same dose. This is due to the slower redistribution

of the drug to peripheral compartments. A typical octegarian requires less than half the induction dose of thiopental required by a 20-year-old patient.

(3) **Correct.** The MAC for inhalational agents is reduced for the geriatric patient. In general, a 4 percent reduction per decade is seen in MAC for those over age 40.

(4) *Incorrect.* There is no evidence to suggest an alteration in the action of succinylcholine in the elderly.[2]

REASONING:

This question tests knowledge of pharmacokinetic and pharmacodynamic changes that occur with age. It is important to note that the main pharmacodynamic effect of age is reduced anesthetic requirements (i.e., decreased MAC). Careful titration of anesthetic agents can help to prevent inadvertent overdosing. Elimination and clearance of certain drugs also can be impaired, leading to prolonged duration of action. It is important to note with choice 1 that the age-independent effect on EEG brain sensitivity is specific to thiopental. Propofol is a more commonly used induction agent today. Studies have shown that elderly patients are more sensitive to the hypnotic and EEG effects of propofol than are younger patients.[3] Choice 4 is incorrect because response to succinylcholine is unaltered with age. The best answer is A.

REFERENCES:

1. Homer TD, Stanski DR. The effect of increasing age on thiopental disposition and anesthetic requirement. Anesthesiology 62(6):714–724, 1985.
2. Cope TM, Hunter JM. Selecting neuromuscular-blocking drugs for elderly patients. Drugs Aging 20(2):125–140, 2003.
3. Schnider TW, Minto CF, Shafer SL, et al. The influence of age on propofol pharmacodynamics. Anesthesiology 90(6):1502–1516, 1999.
4. Morgan GE, Mikhail MS, Murray MJ. Clinical Anesthesiology, 3d ed. New York, McGraw-Hill, 2002, pp. 875–881, 157–158.

BOOK B:

QUESTION 129 (OPTIONAL)

Answer D

Clinical Anesthesia

QUESTION (K-type):

Induction of anesthesia with usual drug dosages and concentrations may lead to cardiovascular signs of overdose in patients with hypothyroidism because of expected decreases in

(1) Respiratory quotient.
(2) Minute volume of breathing.
(3) Circulating blood volume.
(4) Cardiac output.

CORRECT ANSWER: D (3 and 4 are correct)

SUMMARY:

A diagnosis of hypothyroidism is made based on the presence of low free T$_4$ levels. It is important to remember that thyroid hormone increases fat and carbohydrate metabolism, thus affecting growth and metabolic rates. A lack of thyroid hormone results in a decreased metabolic rate, thereby decreasing the rate of oxygen consumption and carbon dioxide production. This decrease in carbon dioxide production indirectly decreases minute ventilation. The cardiovascular and respiratory systems generally are depressed. Cardiac output, stroke volume, myocardial contractility, and heart rate are decreased, whereas ventilatory responses to hypoxia and hypercarbia are depressed. Other possible manifestations include slow mental function, slow movement, dry skin, arthralgias, carpal tunnel syndrome, periorbital edema, intolerance to cold, impaired clearance of free water with or without hyponatremia, and slow gastric emptying.[1]

EXPLANATION:

(1) **Incorrect.** The respiratory quotient is the ratio of carbon dioxide production to oxygen consumption. This ratio typically reflects the body's principal energy source—carbohydrates, lipids, and proteins. The normal respiratory quotient is 0.8. The quotient rises to 1 if carbohydrate metabolism is predominant and down to 0.7 if fat metabolism increases.[1] Studies have shown that the respiratory quotient decreases when thyroid hormone levels are elevated.[2] A change in respiratory quotient would not predispose to cardiovascular signs of induction agent overdose.

(2) **Incorrect.** Patients with hypothyroid have decreased minute ventilation, likely related to decreased metabolic rate and carbon dioxide production.[3] However, decreased minute ventilation would not predispose to cardiovascular signs of induction agent overdose.

(3) **Correct.** Hypothyroid patients are more likely to develop hypotension from anesthetic agents owing to decreased cardiac output (from decreased stroke volume and heart rate), blunted baroreceptor reflexes, and a diminished intravascular volume.[4] This results in a narrowed pulse pressure, prolonged circulation time, and decreased tissue perfusion.[4]

(4) **Correct.** Hypothyroid patients do have depressed myocardial contractility, heart rate, and stroke volume and, therefore, decreased cardiac output. A decreased cardiac output would contribute to cardiovascular signs of induction agent overdose.

REASONING:

This question tests knowledge of the pathophysiology and anesthetic implications of hypothyroidism. It is fairly easy to exclude choices 1 and 2 because they would not be expected to contribute to cardiovascular signs of induction agent overdose (i.e., hypotension). Choices 3 and 4 are both correct. However, a K-type question does not offer this combination as a selection. On an actual examination, we would select D (4 only is correct) because depression of cardiac output is a well-known association of hypothyroidism, and choice 3 cannot be selected individually.

REFERENCES:

1. Miller RD, Miller ED, Reves JG, et al. Anesthesia, 5th ed. New York, Churchill Livingstone, 2000, pp. 599, 929.
2. Clement K, Viguerie N, Diehn M, et al. In vivo regulation of human skeletal muscle gene expression by thyroid hormone. Genome Res 12(2):281–291, 2002.
3. Zwillich CW, Pierson DJ, Hofeldt F, et al. Ventilatory control in myxedema and hypothyroidism. N Engl J Med 292(13):662–665, 1975.
4. Williams RH, Larsen PR, Kronenberg HM, et al. Williams' Textbook of Endocrinology, 10th ed. Philadelphia, Saunders, 2002, p. 425.
5. Morgan GE, Mikhail MS, Murray MJ. Clinical Anesthesiology, 3d ed. New York, McGraw-Hill, 2002, pp. 741–742, 476–467.

BOOK B:

Answer D

Pharmacology

QUESTION 130

QUESTION (K-type):

The duration of the anticoagulant effect of heparin is

(1) Independent of body temperature.
(2) Determined primarily by renal excretion.
(3) Prolonged two to three times with hypoalbuminemia.
(4) Dose-dependent.

CORRECT ANSWER: D (4 only is correct)

Heparin is a polyanionic glycosaminoglycan that acts as an anticoagulant by binding to the serine protease antithrombin III (AT-III) and increasing its activity 1000-fold. AT-III irreversibly binds and inhibits the activated clotting factors thrombin and factors Xa, XIa, XIIa, and XIIIa. Most of the anticoagulant effect is derived from the inhibition of thrombin and factor Xa. The in vivo half-life of heparin varies among individuals and is dose- and temperature-dependent. Heparin does not bind albumin, and its activity is unaffected by hypoalbuminemia. Heparin is eliminated primarily by the reticuloendothelial system. A small percentage is excreted unchanged by the kidneys.[1]

EXPLANATION:

(1) *Incorrect.* The rate of clearance of heparin from the plasma decreases in proportion to the degree of hypothermia.[2]
(2) *Incorrect.* Heparin is degraded and cleared primarily by the reticuloendothelial system. A small amount of undegraded heparin appears in the urine. The half-life of heparin may be increased mildly in patients with end-stage renal disease.
(3) *Incorrect.* Heparin does not bind albumin and is unaffected by low-albumin states. Plasma proteins vitronectin and platelet factor 4 bind heparin and competitively inhibit heparin binding to AT-III. These heparin-binding proteins account for the variation in heparin dosing among individuals to reach a therapeutic ACT.[1]
(4) *Correct.* The anticoagulant effect of heparin is directly dose-dependent. The approximate half-lives for 100, 400, and 800 units/kg of intraveneous heparin administered at normal body temperature are 60, 180, and 300 minutes, respectively.[1]

REASONING:

This question tests knowledge of the pharmacology of heparin. It is important to understand the mechanism of heparin's action on the coagulation system. Choice 4 is obviously correct, ruling out answers A and B. Since choice 2 is incorrect, D is the best answer.

REFERENCES:

1. Hardman JG, Gilman AG, Limbird LE. Goodman & Gilman's The Pharmacological Basis of Therapeutics, 9th ed. New York, McGraw-Hill, 1996, pp. 1343–1346.
2. Barash PG, Cullen BF, Stoelting RK. Clinical Anesthesia, 4th ed. Philadelphia, Lippincott Williams & Wilkins, 2001, pp. 222, 228, 905.
3. Morgan GE, Mikhail MS, Murray MJ. Clinical Anesthesiology, 3d ed. New York, McGraw-Hill, 2002, pp. 351t, 449–450.

BOOK B: **QUESTION 131**

Answer B

Clinical Anesthesia

QUESTION (K-type):

During general endotracheal anesthesia, early signs of an acute asthma attack include

(1) Alteration of the expiratory plateau on capnography.
(2) Increased Pa_{CO_2}.
(3) Increased peak airway pressure.
(4) Hypoxemia.

CORRECT ANSWER: B (1 and 3 are correct)

SUMMARY:

Early signs of acute intraoperative bronchospasm usually manifest as increased peak inspiratory pressures, decreased exhaled tidal volumes, an up-sloping capnograph, and wheezing. The severity of the obstruction is inversely correlated with the rate of rise of the carbon dioxide capnograph. During an acute attack, the total lung capacity (TLC), residual volume, and functional residual capacity (FRC) are all increased. Hypoxemia occurs later as the number of alveolar units with low ventilation-perfusion ratios increases. Other signs of a severe asthma attack include pulsus paradoxus and right-sided heart strain (right bundle-branch block, right-axis deviation, and ST-segment changes).

EXPLANATION:

(1) **Correct.** A slowly rising waveform or a sloping waveform on the capnograph occurs during an acute asthma attack.
(2) **Incorrect.** Carbon dioxide is readily diffusible. As such, a rise in the partial pressure of arterial carbon dioxide will not be an early sign.
(3) **Correct.** Bronchoconstriction will result in increased peak airway pressure but unchanged plateau pressure.
(4) **Incorrect.** Assuming that the patient is mechanically ventilated, hypoxemia will not be an early sign of an acute asthma attack.

REASONING:

This question tests knowledge of the early signs of an acute asthma attack. All the choices listed will occur in a spontaneously breathing patient. However, this event occurs during general endotracheal anesthesia. We assume that mechanical ventilation is involved. Furthermore, this question asks about *early* signs of an acute asthma attack. Choices 1 and 3 are correct; therefore, the best answer is B.

REFERENCE:

Miller RD, Miller ED, Reves JG, et al. Anesthesia, 5th ed. New York, Churchill Livingstone, 2000, pp. 2410, 2436–2437.
Morgan GE, Mikhail MS, Murray MJ. Clinical Anesthesiology, 3d ed. New York, McGraw-Hill, 2002, pp. 513–516.

BOOK B:

QUESTION 132

Answer B

OB/Regional

QUESTION (K-type):

At the placental interface, the efficiency of oxygen transport to the fetus is enhanced by

(1) Movement of the maternal oxyhemoglobin dissociation curve to the right.
(2) Diffusion of carbon dioxide from fetal blood.
(3) Movement of the fetal oxyhemoglobin dissociation curve to the left.
(4) Maternal hyperventilation.

CORRECT ANSWER: B (1 and 3 are correct)

SUMMARY:

Because the fetus is unable to store oxygen, placental transfer of respiratory gases is critically important. Oxygen transfer depends on maternal and fetal placental blood flow and maternal and fetal oxygen tension. The oxyhemoglobin dissociation curve in the mother is shifted to the right, thereby decreasing affinity and increasing unloading of oxygen to the fetus. Conversely, the fetal oxyhemoglobin dissociation curve is shifted to the left, resulting in increased oxygen affinity. This physiologic state facilitates oxygen transfer to the fetus. Any maternal condition that decreases oxygen tension or shifts the maternal oxyhemoglobin dissociation curve to the left (maternal hyperventilation and alkalosis) will decrease oxygen delivery to the fetus, potentially resulting in fetal asphyxia.

EXPLANATION:

(1) **Correct.** As stated above, the maternal oxyhemoglobin curve is shifted to the right.
(2) **Incorrect.** Carbon dioxide readily diffuses from the fetus into the maternal circulation and does not appear to affect fetal oxygenation.[1]
(3) **Correct.** The fetal oxyhemoglobin curve is shifted to the left.
(4) **Incorrect.** While the maternal Pa_{CO_2} decreases slightly during pregnancy, there is little acid-base disturbance owing to renal compensation. However, maternal hyperventilation resulting in hypocarbia and alkalosis causes decreased uterine blood flow and a shift of the oxyhemoglobin curve to the left, both of which impair oxygen delivery to the fetus.[1]

REASONING:

The reader should review the conditions that result in changes in the oxyhemoglobin dissociation curve carefully.[2] One of these is conditions is pregnancy. The goal of the fetus is to take the nutrients and oxygen it needs for survival, and the maternal physiology changes to accomplish this goal. The maternal curve shifts to the right, and the fetal curve shifts to the left. Knowing that alkalosis will shift the curve to the left eliminates choice 4 and answers D and E. Carbon dioxide and oxygen diffuse across the placenta independently, which eliminates choice 2 and answer A. B is the best answer.

REFERENCES:

1. Hughes SC, Levinson G, Rosen MA. Shnider and Levinson's Anesthesia for Obstetrics, 4th ed. Philadelphia, Lippincott Williams & Wilkins, 2002, pp. 3, 26, 36.
2. Barash PG, Cullen BF, Stoelting RK. Clinical Anesthesia, 4th ed. Philadelphia, Lippincott Williams & Wilkins, 2001, p. 670, Fig. 25-2.
3. Morgan GE, Mikhail MS, Murray MJ. Clinical Anesthesiology, 3d ed. New York, McGraw-Hill, 2002, pp. 808–811, 501–502, Fig. 22-23 (p. 502), The Effects of Changes in Acid-Base Status, Body Temperature, and 2,3-DPG Concentration on the Hemoglobin-Oxygen Dissociation Curve.

BOOK B:

QUESTION 133

Answer C

Physiology

QUESTION (K-type):

During a carbon dioxide challenge test in a healthy patient, the Pa_{CO_2} increases to 60 mm Hg. Expected effects include

(1) Decreased pulmonary vascular resistance.
(2) Increased cardiac output.
(3) Renovascular dilatation.
(4) Sympathetic stimulation.

CORRECT ANSWER: C (2 and 4 are correct)

SUMMARY:

Hypercapnia has multiple systemic effects. Hypercapnia activates the sympathetic system, which typically results in increased cardiac output, increased arterial blood pressure, and increased propensity toward dysrhythmias. As the arterial partial pressure of carbon dioxide increases, cerebral blood flow increases proportionally. Partial pressures of carbon dioxide greater than 80 mm Hg lead to unconsciousness as the cerebral pH becomes more acidotic. Furthermore, hypercapnia is a strong respiratory stimulant. Minute ventilation increases up to 3 L/min for each 1 mm Hg increase in Pa_{CO_2} in awake subjects.

EXPLANATION:

(1) **Incorrect.** Hypoxia, hypercapnia, and acidosis are vasoconstrictors of the pulmonary vasculature.

(2) *Correct.* Although carbon dioxide is a myocardial depressant, it causes a reflex stimulation of the sympathetic system that masks these effects.[1] Cardiac output and blood pressure are increased with hypercarbia.[1]

(3) *Incorrect.* Sympathetic stimulation releases adrenergic substances such as norepinephrine that cause renal vasoconstriction.[2]

(4) *Correct.* Hypercapnia is associated with a reflex simulation of the sympathetic system.

REASONING:

This question tests knowledge of the cardiovascular effects of hypercapnia. The term *carbon dioxide challenge test* is a red herring. This relatively obscure test has been reported in the literature as a diagnostic tool for panic disorders but is not used in anesthesia.[3] Fortunately, this question simply asks for the physiologic response to hypercapnia. Choices 2 and 4 are correct; therefore, the best answer is C.

REFERENCES:

1. Miller RD, Miller ED, Reves JG, et al. Anesthesia, 5th ed. New York, Churchill Livingstone, 2000, pp. 613–614, Table 15-5.

2. Sharkey RA, Mulloy EM, O'Neill SJ. Acute effects of hypoxaemia, hyperoxaemia and hypercapnia on renal blood flow in normal and renal transplant subjects. Eur Respir J 12(3):653–657, 1998.

3. Valença A, Nardi A, Nascimento I, et al. Carbon dioxide test as an additional clinical measure of treatment response in panic disorder. Arq Neuropsiquiatr 60(2B):358–361, 2002.

4. Morgan GE, Mikhail MS, Murray MJ. Clinical Anesthesiology, 3d ed. New York, McGraw-Hill, 2002, pp. 38–39, 671, 493.

BOOK B: QUESTION 134

Answer B

OB/Regional

QUESTION (K-type):

Which of the following peripheral nerves must be blocked for removal of a glass splinter from the plantar surface of the heel?

(1) Tibial
(2) Saphenous
(3) Sural
(4) Superficial peroneal

CORRECT ANSWER: B (1 and 3 are correct)

SUMMARY:

The posterior tibial nerve provides sensory innervation to the medial and anterolateral sole of the foot and most of the heel. It is a continuation of the tibal nerve, entering the foot posterior to the medial malleolus, where it branches into the lateral and medial plantar nerves. The rest of the heel is innervated by the sural nerve, which provides sensation to the lateral foot. None of the other three nerves that supply cutaneous sensation to the foot—the superficial peroneal nerve, the deep peroneal nerve, and the saphenous nerve—innervates the heel.

EXPLANATION:

(1) *Correct.* The tibial nerve is the major nerve to the plantar surface of the foot and provides sensation to all but the lateral heel. The posterior tibial nerve may be blocked posterior to the medial malleolus behind the posterior tibial artery.

(2) **Incorrect.** The saphenous nerve, which is a continuation of the femoral nerve and the only nerve to the foot that is not an offshoot of the sciatic nerve system, is responsible for sensation to the anteromedial foot. It is found most consistently anterior to the medial malleolus.

(3) **Correct.** The sural nerve, which branches off from the tibial nerve, supplies sensation to the lateral heel. It may be blocked by deep subcutaneous fan infiltration of local anesthetic between the Achilles tendon and the lateral malleolus.

(4) **Incorrect.** The superficial peroneal nerve, which branches from the common peroneal nerve, enters the foot lateral to extensor digitorum longus at the medial malleolus and provides cutaneous sensation to the dorsum of foot and to the five toes.

REASONING:

The key to answering this question is understanding the anatomy of the ankle block. The sensation to the plantar surface of the foot is mostly supplied by the posterior tibial nerve, with a small area of the lateral heel innervated by the sural nerve and a small area of the anteromedial foot by the saphenous nerve. The superficial and deep peroneal nerves innervate only the dorsal foot.

REFERENCE:

Barash PG, Cullen BF, Stoelting RK. Clinical Anesthesia, 4th ed. Philadelphia, Lippincott Williams & Wilkins, 2001, pp. 740–741.

Morgan GE, Mikhail MS, Murray MJ. Clinical Anesthesiology, 3d ed. New York, McGraw-Hill, 2002, p. 303.

BOOK B: QUESTION 135

Answer E

Clinical Anesthesia

QUESTION (K-type):

A 26-year-old woman is to undergo emergency laparotomy for a ruptured appendix. She has been taking propylthiouracil and an oral beta-adrenergic blocker for 2 days for acute hyperthyroidism. Appropriate perioperative therapy includes administration of

(1) Potassium iodide.
(2) Hydrocortisone.
(3) Propranolol.
(4) Propylthiouracil.

CORRECT ANSWER: E (All are correct)

SUMMARY:

Any hyperthyroid patient should be made euthyroid prior to any elective surgery. The goal of medical treatment in hyperthyroidism is threefold: (1) inhibition of hormone synthesis with drugs such as propylthiouracil, (2) prevention of hormone release with iodide salts, and (3) prevention of the symptoms of adrenergic activity with beta-blockade. When surgery cannot be postponed, the main goal of an anesthetic is to maintain hemodynamic stability and control the blood pressure with beta-blockade. Perioperative hyperthyroid medications should be continued. All the medications are appropriate in the treatment of acute hyperthyroidism.[1]

EXPLANATION:

(1) **Correct.** Potassium or sodium iodide can be administered perioperatively to prevent hormone release. Iodide ions are actively transported into the thyroid gland and immediately oxidized to iodine. It is iodine that combines with tyrosine to

form the two thyroid hormones, triiodothryonine (T_3) and thyroxine (T_4). The presence of iodine in the thyroid gland autoregulates thyroid hormone synthesis.

(2) **Correct.** Corticosteroids block conversion of T_4 to T_3 and are useful in the treatment of hyperthyroidism.

(3) **Correct.** In acute hyperthyroidism, patients have a hyperdynamic circulation that results in tachycardia, tachydysrhythmias, and increased cardiac output. This increased activity of the sympathetic system can be attenuated with beta-blockers. Propranolol has an added advantage of decreasing peripheral conversion of T_4 to the active T_3 form.[2]

(4) **Correct.** Propylthiouracil, carbimazole, and methimazole are drugs that are used to treat hyperthyroidism by inhibiting hormone synthesis.

REASONING:

This question tests knowledge of perioperative management of hyperthyroidsm. The key to this question is knowledge of the medical therapies that can be used to help achieve euthyroidism acutely for a hyperthyroid patient presenting for emergent surgery.

REFERENCES:

1. Barash PG, Cullen BF, Stoelting RK. Clinical Anesthesia, 4th ed. Philadelphia, Lippincott Williams & Wilkins, 2001, p. 1121.
2. Wiersinga WM. Propranolol and thyroid hormone metabolism. Thyroid 1(3):273–277, 1991.
3. Stoelting RK, Miller RD. Basics of Anesthesia, 4th ed. New York, Churchill Livingstone, 2000, pp. 411–417.
4. Morgan GE, Mikhail MS, Murray MJ. Clinical Anesthesiology, 3d ed. New York, McGraw-Hill, 2002, pp. 741–743.

BOOK B:

QUESTION 136

Answer B

Pharmacology

QUESTION (K-type):

A previously healthy 55-year-old patient is spontaneously breathing oxygen, nitrous oxide, and halothane during a minor surgical procedure. The end-tidal halothane concentration measured by mass spectrometry is 0.7 percent, end-tidal nitrous oxide concentration is 50 percent, and end-tidal carbon dioxide concentration is 9 percent. Findings consistent with these concentrations include

(1) Tachycardia.
(2) Decreased requirement for halothane.
(3) Premature ventricular contractions.
(4) Serum bicarbonate concentration of 35 mEq/L.

CORRECT ANSWER: B (1 and 3 correct)

SUMMARY:

The key to this question is recognizing that the patient is significantly hypercarbic, most likely from attenuation of the ventilatory response to hypercarbia related to anesthesia.[1] One MAC of halothane decreases the ventilatory response to carbon dioxide by approximately 50 percent.[1] End-tidal carbon dioxide concentrations typically are not reported as a percent of expired gases, and many readers may not realize that the normal ET_{CO_2} is 5 percent. Conversion of 9 percent CO_2 to millimeters of mercury requires knowing the atmospheric pressure, which we assume is the sea-level pressure (760 mm Hg). Thus 0.09 × 760 mm Hg = 68 mm Hg. Physiologic signs of hypercarbia include tachycardia, hypertension, arrythmias, and pulmonary hypertension. Renal compensation for acute respiratory acidosis is limited, and HCO_3^- increases only about 1 mEq/L for each 10 mm Hg increase in Pa_{CO_2} above 40 mm Hg. Here, the expected HCO_3^- would be 24 + (68 − 40)/10 = 26.8 mEq/L.

426

EXPLANATION:

(1) **Correct.** Tachycardia is a well-known complication associated with hypercarbia.
(2) **Incorrect.** Hypercarbia does not affect MAC and would not decrease the halothane requirements.[1]
(3) **Correct.** Arrythmias are also associated with hypercarbia.
(4) **Incorrect.** Renal compensation for an acute respiratory acidosis is limited and would not explain a serum bicarbonate concentration of 35 mEq/L.

REASONING:

This is a somewhat challenging question that tests knowledge of hypercarbia and the associated cardiovascular complications. It is important to note that there are many causes of hypercapnia: increased production (fever, malignant hyperthermia, hyperthyroid, etc.), decreased excretion (hypoventilation, partial airway obstruction, etc.), and increased delivery to the lungs (increased cardiac output, right-to-left shunting). In the absence of any known pathology, we presume that this patient's hypercarbia is due to hypoventilation stemming from attenuation of the ventilatory response to hypercarbia related to anesthesia. The key to the question is to first recognize the patient has an elevated $ETCO_2$ by converting from percent composition of expired gas to partial pressure in millimeters of mercury. It is also important to note that some texts list hypercarbia of greater than 90 mm Hg as a factor that can decrease MAC. In this patient, the hypercarbia still would be insufficient to decrease MAC by these standards. The best answer is B.

REFERENCE:

1. Barash PG, Cullen BF, Stoelting RK. Clinical Anesthesia, 4th ed. Philadelphia, Lippincott Williams & Wilkins, 2001, pp. 389–399, Fig. 15-25.

BOOK B: **QUESTION 137**

Answer C

Clinical Anesthesia

QUESTION (K-type):

A 48-year-old man who is undergoing a right upper lobectomy for cancer has a PaO_2 of 67 mm Hg while his left lung is being ventilated at 10 mL/kg at a rate of 10 breaths per minute. Measures to increase PaO_2 include

(1) Hyperventilation to a $PaCO_2$ of 30 mm Hg.
(2) Insufflation of the right lung with continuous positive airway pressure (CPAP).
(3) Application of positive end-expiratory pressure of 15 cm H_2O to the left lung.
(4) Partial occlusion of right pulmonary blood flow.

CORRECT ANSWER: C (2 and 4 correct)

SUMMARY:

Hypoxemia is a known risk of one-lung ventilation. Effective measures to increase the PaO_2 include the following: (1) 5 to 10 cm H_2O of CPAP to the collapsed lung, (2) periodic inflation of the collapsed lung, and (3) clamping of the ipsilateral pulmonary artery to decrease shunting of blood to the unventilated lung.

EXPLANATION:

(1) **Incorrect.** It is important to avoid hyperventilation because hypocapnia increases pulmonary vascular resistance (PVR) in the dependent lung and inhibits hypoxic pulmonary vasoconstriction (HPV) in the nondependent lung. This leads to increased shunting and decreased PaO_2 that will worsen the hypoxemia.[1]

(2) **Correct.** Application of 5 to 10 cm H_2O of CPAP to the collapsed lung is employed commonly to improve oxygenation.

(3) **Incorrect.** Application of 10 cm H_2O of PEEP has the potential to improve oxygenation by increasing FRC and improving the $\dot{V}/\dot{Q}$ relationship in the dependent lung. Most studies, however, have shown little benefit to this technique. This is probably due to the increased lung volumes compressing small interalveolar vessels and increasing PVR, diverting blood to the nonventilated lung, and worsening the shunt.[1] The 15 cm H_2O of PEEP that is suggested also seems somewhat high.

(4) **Correct.** Ligation or clamping of the ipsilateral pulmonary artery will decrease shunting.

REASONING:

This question tests knowledge of the management of one-lung ventilation during anesthesia. It is important to review the proper placement and evaluation of a double-lumen endotracheal tube and to understand the intraoperative management of one-lung ventilation because these are commonly tested topics.[1] Choices 2 and 4 were selected because these measures clearly are effective in improving oxygenation during one-lung ventilation. Choice 1 is clearly wrong because it actually can lead to a decreased Pa_{O_2} by worsening shunting.[1] Choice 3 is somewhat difficult to eliminate because PEEP to the ventilated lung is used commonly by some anesthesiologists to attempt to improve Pa_{O_2}. However, the current literature does not support this practice, and the amount of PEEP suggested seems somewhat high. The best answer therefore is C.

REFERENCE:

1. Barash PG, Cullen BF, Stoelting RK. Clinical Anesthesia, 4th ed. Philadelphia, Lippincott Williams & Wilkins, 2001, pp. 824–826, 829, 831–833.
2. Morgan GE, Mikhail MS, Murray MJ. Clinical Anesthesiology, 3d ed. New York, McGraw-Hill, 2002, p. 539.

BOOK B:

Answer C

OB/Regional

QUESTION 138

QUESTION (K-type):

Uterine contractility is decreased by

(1) Epidural lidocaine.
(2) Terbutaline.
(3) Ketamine anesthesia.
(4) Halothane.

CORRECT ANSWER: C (2 and 4 are correct)

SUMMARY:

Agents that decrease uterine tone are used to treat preterm labor and uterine hypertonus or to facilitate removal of a retained placenta. The uterus contracts owing to a rise in myometrial cell calcium concentration that occurs in response to an enzyme cascade set in motion by circulating hormones or other mediators.[1] Uterine beta$_2$-receptor activation results in an increase in cAMP, decreasing intracellular calcium and inhibiting the myosin light chain kinase.[2] Beta-agonists such as terbutaline and ritrodine act via this mechanism. Magnesium sulfate and calcium channel blockers such as nifedipine relax the uterus by decreasing intracellular calcium.[2] Nitroglycerin causes nitric oxide–mediated uterine relaxation.[2] Halogenated anesthetic agents also provide uterine relaxation, although their mechanism is less well understood.

EXPLANATION:

(1) **Incorrect.** Epidural lidocaine has not been shown to inhibit uterine contractility.[2]

(2) **Correct.** Terbutaline is a beta-agonist with beta$_1$ and beta$_2$ activity. It results in uterine relaxation via its beta$_2$ effects.

(3) **Incorrect.** Ketamine has been shown to increase uterine contractions, especially in the second trimester.[2] When given closer to delivery (i.e., at cesarean section), ketamine has little effect on uterine tone.[2]

(4) **Correct.** Halothane and all other volatile agents cause a dose-dependent decrease in uterine tone.

REASONING:

This question tests knowledge of the pharmacologic effects of various anesthetics on uterine tone. Choices 2 and 4 are agents used commonly to provide uterine relaxation in obstetric practice and therefore are correct. The reader must determine if the remaining two choices are correct in order to differentiate between answers E and C. Epidural lidocaine does not decrease uterine contractility, which eliminates both choices 1 and 3 (alternatively, if the reader knows that ketamine does not provide uterine relaxation, choice 1 could be eliminated). The best answer is C.

REFERENCES:

1. Chestnut DH. Obstetric Anesthesia Principles and Practice, 2d ed. St Louis, Mosby, 1999, pp. 668–670.

2. Hughes SC, Levinson G, Rosen MA. Shnider and Levinson's Anesthesia for Obstetrics, 4th ed. Philadelphia, Lippincott Williams & Wilkins, 2002, pp. 44–45, 324–326.

3. Morgan GE, Mikhail MS, Murray MJ. Clinical Anesthesiology, 3d ed. New York, McGraw-Hill, 2002, p. 837.

BOOK B: **QUESTION 139**

Answer B

Neuroanesthesia

QUESTION (K-type):

During induction of anesthesia for removal of a large intracranial tumor, effects of adding 1 MAC of isoflurane at normocarbia include

(1) Decreased cerebral metabolic rate.
(2) Attenuated cerebrovascular response to Pa$_{CO_2}$.
(3) Increased intracranial pressure (ICP).
(4) Abolished cerebral autoregulation.

CORRECT ANSWER: B (1 and 3 are correct)

SUMMARY:

All volatile anesthetics produce a dose-dependent decrease in cerebral metabolic rate (CMR) and impairment of cerebral autoregulation of blood flow. The cerebral vasculature, however, maintains its responsiveness to carbon dioxide with all volatile anesthetics. The vasodilating potency of various inhalational anesthetics is approximately halothane >> enflurane > isoflurane = sevoflurane = desflurane.[1]

EXPLANATION:

(1) **Correct.** All volatile anesthetic agents cause a reduction in CMR.[1]

(2) **Incorrect.** Cerebrovascular responsiveness to Pa$_{CO_2}$ is well maintained during anesthesia with all the volatile anesthetic agents.[1]

(3) **Correct.** All volatile anesthetic agents cause a dose-dependent increase in cerebral vasodilation.[1] Unless other measures are employed (i.e., simultaneous hyperventilation, etc.), cerebral vessels will dilate and increase ICP.

(4) **Incorrect.** 1 MAC of isoflurane will not abolish autoregulation.[1]

This question tests knowledge of the effects of volatile anesthetics on cerebral autoregulation of blood flow. It is important to remember that all intravenous anesthetic agents tend to cause parallel changes in cerebral blood flow (CBF) and CMR. In contrast, volatile anesthetics decrease CMR but generally increase CBF to some extent. The net magnitude of this increase may be a combination of decreased CBF in response to decreased CMR and the direct vasodilating property of these agents.[1] B is the best answer.

REFERENCE:

1. Miller RD, Miller ED, Reves JG, et al. Anesthesia, 5th ed. New York, Churchill Livingstone, 2000, pp. 707–709, 1989.
2. Morgan GE, Mikhail MS, Murray MJ. Clinical Anesthesiology, 3d ed. New York, McGraw-Hill, 2002, pp. 557–558.

BOOK B:

Answer A

Physiology

QUESTION 140

QUESTION (K-type):

Intraoperative events that may cause an increased arterial to end-tidal carbon dioxide tension difference include

(1) Pulmonary embolus.
(2) Induced hypotension.
(3) Application of positive end-expiratory pressure.
(4) Atelectasis.

CORRECT ANSWER: A (1, 2, and 3 are correct)

SUMMARY:

End-tidal carbon dioxide tension (PET_{CO_2}) is used clinically as an estimate of arterial carbon dioxide tension (Pa_{CO_2}). The normal gradient between Pa_{CO_2} and PET_{CO_2} is 5 mm Hg. This gradient is due to the dilution of alveolar gas with carbon dioxide–free gas from alveolar dead space. Increases in the Pa_{CO_2}–PET_{CO_2} gradient are seen with decreases in lung perfusion or increases in alveolar dead space. Significant decreases in lung perfusion will increase this gradient, as seen with air embolism, decreased cardiac output, or decreased blood pressure. Furthermore, increases in alveolar dead space also will increase this gradient. Positive end-expiratory pressure (PEEP) actually can increase alveolar dead space by overdistending bronchi and alveoli. Other factors that increase dead space include increasing age, positive-pressure ventilation, and chronic obstructive pulmonary disease (COPD).

EXPLANATION:

(1) **Correct.** Pulmonary embolus increases alveolar dead space (ventilated and unperfused alveoli), which increases dilution of alveolar gas.
(2) **Correct.** Induced hypotension increases alveolar dead space.
(3) **Correct.** Application of excessive PEEP also can increase alveolar dead space.
(4) **Incorrect.** Atelectasis or collapse of alveoli decreases dead space and therefore would decrease arterial to end-tidal carbon dioxide tension differences.

REASONING:

This question tests knowledge of the etiology of increased alveolar dead space. Fortunately, the question is made significantly easier by the fact that choice 4 is the only answer that does not increase alveolar dead space (it increases shunting instead). Choices 1, 2, and 3 are correct. Therefore, the best answer is A.

REFERENCE:

Barash PG, Cullen BF, Stoelting RK. Clinical Anesthesia, 4th ed. Philadelphia, Lippincott Williams & Wilkins, 2001, pp. 802, 1388.

Morgan GE, Mikhail MS, Murray MJ. Clinical Anesthesiology, 3d ed. New York, McGraw-Hill, 2002, pp. 501, 111–112.

BOOK B:

Answer C

OB/Regional

QUESTION 141

QUESTION (K-type):

Factors that decrease beat-to-beat variability of the fetal heart rate include

(1) Epidural administration of lidocaine.
(2) Maternal hypotension.
(3) Intravenous administration of ephedrine.
(4) Intravenous adminstration of glycopyrrolate.

CORRECT ANSWER: C (2 and 4 are correct)

SUMMARY:

Fetal heart rate monitoring is the most widely available method for assessing fetal status during pregnancy and labor. The most important parameter is beat-to-beat variability. Variability is measured clinically by visual recognition of a "wavy baseline" that normally has an amplitude range of 5 to 25 beats per minute. It represents an intact pathway between the fetal central nervous system, vagus nerve, and cardiac conduction system. Minimal variability alone usually is unrelated to fetal academia. However, loss of varaiability in association with tachycardia or decelerations is the most sensitive indicator of metabolic acidosis. Conditions associated with decreased variability include fetal sleep state, congenital neurologic or cardiac abnormalities, severe asphyxia, extreme prematurity, and idiopathic causes. Drugs known to decrease variability include opiates, general anesthesia, barbiturates, diazepam, phenothiazines, and parasympatholytics such as atropine.

EXPLANATION:

(1) **Incorrect.** Epidural lidocaine has not been shown to change beat-to-beat variability.
(2) **Correct.** Persistent maternal hypotension can lead to decreased oxygen delivery to the fetus. This can result in asphyxia and lead to decreased beat-to-beat variability.
(3) **Incorrect.** Ephedrine is an indirect- and direct-acting sympathomimetic drug and docs not affcct bcat-to-bcat variability.
(4) **Correct.** Parasympatholytic drugs such as atropine and glycopyrolate change the fetal autonomic responses, resulting in tachycardia and decreased beat-to-beat variability.[1]

REASONING:

A compromised fetus has decreased beat-to-beat variability. Maternal hypotension leads to decreased oxygen delivery, so choice 2 is correct. With a K-type question, choice 4 must be correct, and now one must determine if choices 1 or 3 are correct. In the absence of hypotension, epidural lidocaine does not cause fetal depression or decreased oxygen delivery. Choice 1 therefore is incorrect. Thus the best answer is C.

REFERENCE:

1. Freeman RK, Garite TJ, Nageotte MP. Fetal Heart Rate Monitoring, 2d ed. Baltimore, Williams & Wilkins, 1991, pp. 13–17, 71–83.
2. Morgan GE, Mikhail MS, Murray MJ. Clinical Anesthesiology, 3d ed. New York, McGraw-Hill, 2002, pp. 840–843.

Answer C

Pain

QUESTION (K-type):

Neural fibers that transmit pain include

(1) B fibers.
(2) C fibers.
(3) Aα fibers.
(4) Aδ fibers.

CORRECT ANSWER: C (2 and 4 are correct)

SUMMARY:

Pain information is transmitted within the nervous system by either small unmyelinated C fibers (i.e., C polymodal nociceptors) or myelinated Aδ fibers (i.e., high-threshold mechanoreceptors). Aδ fibers are associated with sharp, well-localized pain with smaller receptive fields.[1] C fibers are associated with dull, aching and poorly localized pain with large receptive fields.[1] Aα fibers are large myelinated motor neurons, and B fibers are preganglionic myelinated sympathetic fibers.

EXPLANATION:

(1) ***Incorrect.*** B fibers are preganglionic myelinated sympathetic fibers. They do not carry pain information.
(2) ***Correct.*** C fibers are unmyelinated nerves that carry pain, warm and cold temperature, and touch sensation. These small fibers (0.4 to 1.2 mm) also have a slow conduction speed (0.2 to 2 m/s).
(3) ***Incorrect.*** Aα fibers carry motor, proprioception, and touch information. These large-diameter fibers (12 to 20 mm) have fast conduction speeds (70 to 120 m/s). They do not carry pain information.
(4) ***Correct.*** Aδ fibers carry pain, cold temperature, and touch information. These fibers are 2 to 4 mm in diameter and have conduction speeds ranging from 12 to 30 m/s.

REASONING:

This question tests knowledge of nerve fiber anatomy. It is important for the reader to review neurophysiology related to pain nociception and the associated central mechanisms that can modulate responses to pain.[1] The best answer is C.

REFERENCES:

1. Miller RD, Miller ED, Reves JG, et al. Anesthesia, 5th ed. New York, Churchill Livingstone, 2000, pp. 2352–2353.
2. Waldman SD. Interventional Pain Management, 2d ed. Philadelphia, Saunders, 2001, pp. 11–13.
3. Morgan GE, Mikhail MS, Murray MJ. Clinical Anesthesiology, 3d ed. New York, McGraw-Hill, 2002, pp. 218, 276–283.

Answer A

Basic Science

QUESTION (K-type):

Gas flow through an endotracheal tube is

(1) Directly related to the change in pressure along the length of the tube.
(2) Inversely related to the viscosity of the gas.
(3) Inversely related to the length of the tube.
(4) Directly related to the square of the radius of the tube.

CORRECT ANSWER: A (1, 2, and 3 are correct)

SUMMARY:

The flow of gas through the upper airway and bronchial tree is a mixture of laminar and turbulent flow. Laminar flow describes concentric cylinders of gas flowing at varying velocities within a tube, with highest-velocity flow in the center and decreasing outward. Turbulent flow involves random movement of gas down the airway and usually occurs at high gas flows at branching points or sharp angles in the airway[1]. The type of flow (i.e., laminar versus turbulent) can be predicted by the Reynolds number. A low Reynolds number (<1000) is associated with laminar flow, and high values (>1500) produce turbulent flow.

Gas flow through a straight, unbranched tube can be described by laminar flow.[1] The relationship between determinants of laminar flow through an endotracheal tube can be described by Hagen-Poiseuille's law

$$R = \frac{8 \times length \times viscosity}{\pi \times radius^4} = \frac{P_B - P_A}{flow}$$

where R is resistance, P_B is barometric pressure, and P_A is alveolar gas pressure.[1] Solving for flow, the equation becomes

$$Flow = (P_A - P_B) \times \frac{\pi \times radius^4}{8 \times length \times viscosity}$$

EXPLANATION:

(1) **Correct.** Laminar flow is directly related to pressure along the length of the tube.
(2) **Correct.** Laminar flow is inversely related to the viscosity of the gas.
(3) **Correct.** Laminar flow is inversely related to the length of the tube.
(4) **Incorrect.** Laminar flow is related to the fourth power of the radius of the tube.

REASONING:

This question tests knowledge of the biophysics of airflow within an endotracheal tube. The differences between laminar flow and turbulent flow should be reviewed. This question is challenging because airflow in the airways is both laminar and turbulent. We have assumed that airflow through an endotracheal tube is laminar, but the flow also can be turbulent.[2] Indeed, the Hagen-Poiseulle law discussed above assumes laminar flow. These estimates of flow generally are higher than actual measurements taken under in vivo conditions.[3] Factors that contribute to this discrepancy include turbulent flow from sharp-angled connectors and the fact that an endotracheal tube becomes curved when it is placed in vivo to adapt to the upper airway anatomy. Indeed, authors have found that endotracheal tubes with 4.0- to 7.0-mm inside diameters show both laminar and turbulent flows in the normal range of gas flows used clinically.[2] Laminar flow through a curved endotracheal tube is best described by the Ito formula.[4] Turbulent flow through a curved endotracheal tube is described by the Blasius formula.[5] Technically, this question is unanswerable unless we are provided a Reynold's number that is consistent with laminar flow. However, on an actual examination, we would select A because none of the selections is consistent with a description of turbulent flow.

REFERENCES:

1. Barash PG, Cullen BF, Stoelting RK. Clinical Anesthesia, 4th ed. Philadelphia, Lippincott Williams & Wilkins, 2001, p. 795.
2. Jarreau PH, Louis B, Dassieu G, et al. Estimation of inspiratory pressure drop in neonatal and pediatric endotracheal tubes. J Appl Physiol 87(1):36–46, 1999.
3. O'Grady K, Doyle DJ, Irish J, Gullane P. Biophysics of airflow within the airway: a review. J Otolaryngol 26(2):123–128, 1997.

4. Ito H. Laminar flow in curved pipes. Z Angev Math Mech 49:653–663, 1969.

5. Schlighting H. Boundary-Layer Theory. New York, McGraw-Hill, 1979.

6. Morgan GE, Mikhail MS, Murray MJ. Clinical Anesthesiology, 3d ed. New York, McGraw-Hill, 2002, pp. 485–486.

BOOK B:

Answer C

Pharmacology

QUESTION 144

QUESTION (K-type):

Hetastarch

(1) Produces a hypercoagulable state.
(2) Complicates blood cross-matching.
(3) Is contraindicated in patients with diabetes mellitus.
(4) Is metabolized by amylase.

CORRECT ANSWER: C (2 and 4 are correct).

SUMMARY:

Hetastarch, or hydroxyethyl starch, is a synthetic colloid. Hemodilution of more than 30 percent with hetastarch has been shown to affect platelet function and fibrin formation, leading to a hypocoagulable state.[1] These effects likely are dose-dependent and usually occur when the maximum daily dose for volume expansion has exceeded (20 mL/kg). Hetastarch also complicates blood cross-matching. Larger molecules require amylase to be broken down. Hetastarch does not significantly affect blood glucose levels and is not contraindicated in diabetics.

EXPLANATION:

(1) *Incorrect.* Hetastarch causes hypocoagulation via a dilution of coagulation factors, as well as platelet dysfunction and, ultimately, decreased fibrin formation. Hetastarch coats the surface of platelets, reducing the availability of the functional receptor for fibrinogen on the platelet surface.[2]

(2) *Correct.* Increased rouleaux formation of hetastarch-containing blood samples has been shown to cause difficulties in the interpretation of typing and antibody screening of blood samples by blood bank personnel.[3]

(3) *Incorrect.* Studies of diabetic and nondiabetic rats have shown that hetastarch does not cause or aggravate hyperglycemia.[4] These findings may be applicable to humans.

(4) *Correct.* Hetastarch with small molecular weight can be eliminated directly by the kidneys, whereas larger ones first must be degraded by amylase.

REASONING:

This question tests knowledge of the complications associated with volume expansion using hetastarch. The most important facts to remember are that hetastarch can impair coagulation at excessive doses (>20 mL/kg per day) and can interfere with blood antibody testing. The best answer is C.

REFERENCES:

1. Blanloeil Y, Trossaert M, Rigal JC, Rozec B. [Effects of plasma substitutes on hemostasis.] Ann Fr Anesth Reanim 21(8):648–667, 2002.

2. Franz A, Braunlich P, Gamsjager T, et al. The effects of hydroxyethyl starches of varying molecular weight on platelet function. Anesth Analg 92(6):1402–1407, 2001.

3. Daniels MJ, Strauss RG, Smith-Floss AM. Effects of hydroxyethyl starch on erythrocyte typing and blood cross-matching. Transfusion 22(3):226–228, 1982.

4. Hofer RE, Lanier WL. Effect of hydroxylethyl starch solutions on blood glucose concentrations in diabetic and nondiabetic rats. Crit Care Med 20(2):211–215, 1992.

5. Barash PG, Cullen BF, Stoelting RK. Clinical Anesthesia, 4th ed. Philadelphia, Lippincott Williams &Wilkins, 2001, p. 176.

6. Mishler JM. Pharmacological effects produced by the acute and chronic administration of hydroxyethyl starch. J Clin Apheresis 2(1):52–62, 1984.

7. Morgan GE, Mikhail MS, Murray MJ. Clinical Anesthesiology, 3d ed. New York, McGraw-Hill, 2002, p. 630.

BOOK B:

QUESTION 145 (OPTIONAL)

Answer A

Physiology

QUESTION (K-type):

During pelvic laparoscopy under epidural anesthesia, the patient is placed in the Trendelenburg position, and the abdomen is distended by insufflation of carbon dioxide. Anticipated responses include

(1) Hyperpnea to maintain normal minute ventilation.
(2) Pain despite sensory block to T4.
(3) Decreased venous return and cardiac output.
(4) Metabolic acidosis from absorption of carbon dioxide.

CORRECT ANSWER: A (1, 2, and 3 are correct)

SUMMARY:

Laparoscopic surgery is made possible by the creation of a pneumoperitoneum using insufflation of carbon dioxide gas. This pneumoperitoneum has many important physiologic and metabolic consequences. First, carbon dioxide is absorbed by the abdominal vasculature because it is highly soluble. This can lead to higher arterial carbon dioxide levels and a resulting respiratory acidosis. The increase in intraabdominal pressure (IAP) from the pneumoperitoneum results in cephalad displacement of the diaphragm, leading to decreased lung compliance and increased peak inspiratory pressures. The Trendelenburg position also contributes to the resulting atelectasis, decreased functional residual capacity (FRC), and increased ventilation-perfusion mismatch that leads to impaired arterial oxygenation. Expected cardiovascular consequences of pneumoperitoneum with high insufflation pressures include decreased preload and cardiac output. While laparoscopic surgery is performed most commonly under general anesthesia, other anesthetics have been employed, such as local anesthesia with monitored anesthesia care or neuroaxial blockade. A patient undergoing laparoscopic surgery using an epidural or spinal technique requires a high level of blockade to facilitate complete muscle relaxation and the prevention of diaphragmatic irritation.

EXPLANATION:

(1) **Possibly correct.** Increased IAP from pneumoperitoneum and Trendelenburg position contributes to decreased tidal volumes. Hyperpnea can help to maintain normal minute ventilation. However, increased Pa_{CO_2} from insufflation with CO_2 gas will increase the ventilatory drive. An *increased* minute ventilation is expected.

(2) **Correct.** A T2 level is needed to optimize muscle relaxation and to prevent diaphragmatic irritation. Diaphragmatic irritation sometimes can present as referred shoulder pain.

(3) **Correct.** Insufflation is associated with a transient increase in venous return followed by an impedance of flow.[1] Cardiac output decreases proportionately with IAP. One study found a 30 percent reduction in cardiac index (CI) after insufflation to 15 mm Hg.[2]

(4) **Incorrect.** Carbon dioxide is highly absorbable via the peritoneal vasculature and can result in a respiratory acidosis, not metabolic acidosis.

435

REASONING:

This question tests knowledge of the physiologic changes associated with laparoscopy and pneumoperitoneum. It is somewhat challenging because choice 1 is not entirely correct. Decreased tidal volumes requiring hyperpnea to maintain normal minute ventilation might be anticipated as a consequence of increased IAP and Trendelenburg positioning. However, it is not entirely clear that normal minute ventilation should be anticipated because increased $PaCO_2$ from the pneumoperitoneum should increase the ventilatory drive and minute ventilation. Most readers would find choices 2 and 3 correct, providing additional confidence that choice 1 is also correct. Therefore, A is the best answer.

REFERENCES:

1. Barash PG, Cullen BF, Stoelting RK. Clinical Anesthesia, 4th ed. Philadelphia, Lippincott Williams & Wilkins, 2001, pp. 1058–1061.
2. Westerband A, Van De Water J, Amzallag M, et al. Cardiovascular changes during laparoscopic cholecystectomy. Surg Gynecol Obstet 175(6):535–538, 1992.
3. Morgan GE, Mikhail MS, Murray MJ. Clinical Anesthesiology, 3d ed. New York, McGraw-Hill, 2002, pp. 522–524.

BOOK B:

Answer A

Cardiovascular

QUESTION 146

QUESTION (K-type):

When triggered by the R wave, the intraaortic balloon pump (IABP) is likely to be ineffective with

(1) Prolonged use of electrocautery.
(2) Development of rapid atrial fibrillation.
(3) Sudden onset of aortic regurgitation.
(4) Sudden onset of mitral regurgitation.

CORRECT ANSWER: A (1, 2, and 3 are correct)

SUMMARY:

An intraaortic balloon pump is a mechanical device that is used to provide temporary assistance to a heart with impaired function. It is usually inserted in the femoral artery and placed with the tip distal to the subclavian artery. A 25-cm balloon is used to provide synchronized counterpulsation to decrease afterload and augment diastolic perfusion of the myocardium.[1] The IABP is timed to deflate just prior to systole and to inflate during diastole. The deflation just prior to systole increases forward flow from the heart and decreases myocardial oxygen consumption through afterload reduction. Inflation of the balloon during diastole improves coronary perfusion by increasing diastolic blood pressure, therefore increasing myocardial oxygen delivery. Improper timing of counterpulsations can be caused by electrocradiographic (ECG) artifact, rapid heart rates, and cardiac dysrhythmias and renders the IABP ineffective.

EXPLANATION:

(1) ***Correct.*** Prolonged use of electrocautery would distort the ECG and result in improper timing of the IABP.
(2) ***Correct.*** Rapid atrial fibrillation also would distort the ECG and result in improper timing of the IABP.
(3) ***Correct.*** The use of an IABP would exacerbate acute aortic regurgitation because inflation of the balloon during diastole would worsen the regurgitant fraction into the left ventricle.
(4) ***Incorrect.*** The management of mitral regurgitation includes improving forward flow, which is what occurs when the IABP deflates during systole.

REASONING:

This question tests knowledge related to the function of intraaortic ballon pumps. The reader should understand that the IABP is used to provide temporary assistance to a failing heart and is contraindicated in patients with irreversible cardiac disease who are not candidates for transplantation or patients who have severe aortic insufficiency. The indications and contraindications for IABP should be reviewed.[1] The principle of IABP is synchronized counterpulsation to assist forward flow with afterload reduction and to augment diastolic coronary perfusion. The best answer is A.

REFERENCE:

1. Barash PG, Cullen BF, Stoelting RK. Clinical Anesthesia, 4th ed. Philadelphia, Lippincott Williams & Wilkins, 2001, pp. 915–916, Table 32-27.
2. Morgan GE, Mikhail MS, Murray MJ. Clinical Anesthesiology, 3d ed. New York, McGraw-Hill, 2002, pp. 456–457.

BOOK B:

Answer B

Cardiovascular

QUESTION 147

QUESTION (K-type):

An asymptomatic 40-year-old woman with a systolic click and a late systolic murmur is scheduled for total abdominal hysterectomy. Anesthetic considerations include

(1) Prophylactic antibiotics are recommended.
(2) Intraoperative fluid restriction is indicated.
(3) The patient is predisposed to tachyarrhythmias.
(4) Myocardial depressant inhalational agents are contraindicated.

CORRECT ANSWER: B (1 and 3 are correct)

SUMMARY:

Mitral valve prolapse (MVP) is the most common valvular disorder of the heart and occurs in 5 to 17 percent of otherwise healthy individuals.[1] Most patients are asymptomatic but can present with palpitations, syncope, shortness of breath, and atypical chest pain. There is a higher incidence in females. The only clinical finding may be a midsystolic click, with or without the late systolic murmur of mitral regurgitation. Anesthetic considerations include antibiotic prophylaxis against endocarditis, maintaining adequate preload, and prevention of sympathetic stimulation, which can accentuate left ventricular emptying and worsen the severity of mitral valve prolapse. These patients are also at risk for dysrhythmias. Supraventricular arrhythmias occur in more that 50 percent of patients, and ventricular arrhythmias occur in 45 percent of these patients.[1]

EXPLANATION:

(1) **Correct.** Patients with mitral valve prolapse benefit from antibiotics as prophylaxis against endocarditis.
(2) **Incorrect.** These patients need to have adequate preload and benefit from fluid loading.
(3) **Correct.** Patients with MVP are at increased risk of supraventricular, ventricular, and bradyarrhythmias, and this may explain the observed sudden cardiac death in some of these patients.[1]
(4) **Incorrect.** There is no contraindication to inhalational agents. Good depth of anesthesia can help to prevent a sympathetic response to surgical stimulus and the tachyarrythmias associated with increased sympathetic stimulation in these patients. Myocardial depression by inhalational agents is not a specific concern for these patients. Increased myocardial contractility actually can exacerbate the severity of MVP by facilitating left ventricular emptying.

REASONING;

This question tests knowledge of the mechanism of mitral regurgitation (MR) in MVP and the anesthetic implications and pathophysiology associated with MVP. The important anesthetic implications for patients with MVP are to ensure maintenance of normovolemia and avoid factors that increase left ventricular empting (i.e., sympathetic stimulation, increased myocardial contractility, tachycardia, prolonged afterload reduction). The best answer is B.

REFERENCE:

1. Miller RD, Miller ED, Reves JG, et al. Anesthesia, 5th ed. New York, Churchill Livingstone, 2000, pp. 956–957.
2. Morgan GE, Mikhail MS, Murray MJ. Clinical Anesthesiology, 3d ed. New York, McGraw-Hill, 2002, pp. 414–416.

BOOK B:

Answer B

OB/Regional

QUESTION 148

QUESTION (K-type):

A 24-year-old woman who is receiving magnesium sulfate for severe preeclampsia requires emergency cesarean delivery. True statements concerning succinylcholine-induced muscle relaxation in this patient include

(1) It will be potentiated by the magnesium sulfate.
(2) Fasciculations will be absent following succinylcholine administration.
(3) It will be prolonged.
(4) It can be antagonized by calcium chloride.

CORRECT ANSWER: B (1 and 3 are correct)

SUMMARY:

Magnesium sulfate is used in obstetrics for seizure prophylaxis in patients with preeclampsia and for tocolysis in those with preterm labor. It acts at the cellular level, decreasing nerve transmission and uterine activity and antagonizing the effects of calcium on smooth muscle cells. Profound muscular weakness results from decreased release of acetylcholine and sensitivity of the motor end plate to acetylcholine. Patients receiving magnesium treatment who require neuromuscular blockade for cesarean section or other surgical procedures have increased sensitivity to depolarizing and nondepolarizing neuromuscular blockade. Other side effects of magnesium include pulmonary edema, altered sensorium, respiratory paralysis, impaired cardiac conduction, and even death.

EXPLANATION:

(1) **Correct.** Patients receiving magnesium have increased sensitivity to nondepolarizing and depolarizing neuromuscular blocking drugs owing to decreased neuromuscular transmission at the motor end plate and excitability of the muscle membrane.[1] However, studies in preeclamptic and normal patients receiving magnesium demonstrate that the initial intubating dose required should not be changed in the presence of magnesium.[1]

(2) **Incorrect.** The incidence of succinylcholine-induced fasiculations is decreased in parturients. However, fasiculations are not eliminated completely, even in the presence of magnesium.[2]

(3) **Correct.** Prolongation of succinlycholine in patients receiving magnesium is due to development of a phase II block and is most common with repeated doses of succinlycholine or continuous infusion of magnesium.[1]

(4) **Incorrect.** Calcium antagonizes the effects of magnesium but has not been shown to antagonize the effects of succinylcholine.

REASONING:

This question is difficult because it addresses controversial topics in clinical obstetric anesthesia, many of which have been studied in animals but not humans. The important point to remember is that magnesium alters neuromuscular transmission, prolonging the effects of depolarizing and nondepolarizing muscle relaxants. This makes choices 1 and 3 correct. As a general rule, it is best to avoid statements such as those in choice 2 ("will be absent"), and indeed, this statement is incorrect. Choice 4 is incorrect because calcium only antagonizes magnesium. The best answer is B.

REFERENCES:

1. Hughes SC, Levinson G, Rosen MA. Shnider and Levinson's Anesthesia for Obstetrics, 4th ed. Philadelphia, Lippincott Williams & Wilkins, 2002, pp. 305, 331.
2. Stacey MRW, Barclay K, Asai T, Vaughn RS. Effects of magnesium sulphate on suxamethonium-induced complications during rapid-sequence induction of anaesthesia. Anaesthesia 50:933–936, 1995.
3. Morgan GE, Mikhail MS, Murray MJ. Clinical Anesthesiology, 3d ed. New York, McGraw-Hill, 2002, pp. 813, 838.

BOOK B:

QUESTION 149 (OPTIONAL)

Answer D

Neuroanesthesia

QUESTION (K-type)

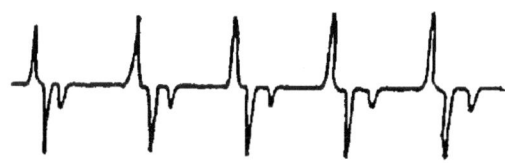

During posterior fossa surgery in the sitting position,

(1) A single-lumen central venous catheter should display the electrocardiogram (ECG) shown above.
(2) Pulmonary artery occlusion pressures greater than 10 mm Hg prevent paradoxical air embolism.
(3) If venous air embolism occurs, pulmonary artery pressure increases before precordial Doppler sounds change.
(4) If venous air embolism occurs, aspiration of air from the distal lumen of a pulmonary artery catheter is less effective than aspiration from a multiorificed central venous catheter.

CORRECT ANSWER: D (4 only is correct)

SUMMARY:

Venous air embolism (VAE) is a concern whenever the operative site is above the level of the heart, such as the sitting position during a craniotomy. Central lines are placed during craniotomies for infusion of vasoactive substances and the ability to aspirate air in the event of a VAE. If a VAE is suspected, treatment may include irrigating the operative site and/or applying wax to bone margins, lowering the head of the bed below the level of the heart, increasing central filling pressures with administration of intravenous fluid, and aspirating the entrained air through a right atrial catheter. The optimal position of the catheter is at the junction of the superior vena cava (SVC) and the right atrium

(RA). Multiorifice catheters are superior to single-orifice catheters for aspiration of VAE. Pulmonary artery catheters are not as useful for aspirating entrained air owing to their smaller lumen and slower rate of blood return.

EXPLANATION:

(1) ***Incorrect.*** The proper placement of a central venous catheter for aspiration of VAE during craniotomy in the sitting position is at the SVC-RA junction. An intravenous electrocardiographic (IV-ECG) technique can been employed to position a central venous catheter properly.[1,2] This technique involves transducing the ECG lead (II or V) from the tip of the catheter. As the catheter is advanced, the P wave becomes peaked as it advances toward the heart. A biphasic P wave is seen as the catheter passes the sinoatrial (SA) node. The ideal position for the central line is at the junction of the SVC and RA. This occurs just prior to the peaked P wave (P-atriale). The ECG in the question appears to be transduced from lead V and is not biphasic nor P-atriale. The catheter is likely advanced far past the atrium and needs to be withdrawn.

(2) ***Incorrect.*** Paradoxical air embolism can occur in patients with patent foramen ovale when the right atrial pressure is greater than the left atrial pressure. An intraatrial pressure of 10 cm H_2O or greater may lead to paradoxical air embolism.

(3) ***Incorrrect.*** The most sensitive indicator of intracardiac air is TEE, followed by Doppler. Other findings characteristic of VAE occur later. Changes in end-tidal nitrogen concentrations occur before the decrease in PET_{CO_2} and increased pulmonary artery pressures. The classic "mill wheel" murmur is a late sign of VAE.

(4) ***Correct.*** Right atrial multiorifice catheters allow for larger volumes of intracardiac air to be aspirated as opposed to the distal lumen of a pulmonary artery catheter.[2]

REASONING:

This question tests knowledge of intraoperative management of VAE and the IV-ECG technique for central venous catheter placement. The question is made challenging by the ECG tracing, which is difficult to interpret. Even with a good understanding of the IV-ECG technique, it is difficult on first examination to determine if the P wave is peaked (P-atriale) or biphasic. Indeed, even detailed discussions with electrophysiology specialists at Stanford failed to yield a definitive answer. When our experts compared the tracing with sample tracings from Cottrell,[2] they concluded that the P wave was not biphasic and that the tracing likely was transduced from lead V because the QRS complex and T wave deflected downward. If the P wave were P-atriale, it would be deflected in the same direction as the QRS complex and T wave. Since the P wave is deflected in the opposite direction, we must conclude that the catheter has passed the midatrial position and that choice 1 is incorrect. Choice 4 is certainly true, and since choice 3 is incorrect, one would only have to decide if the choice 2 is correct. Thankfully, it is not, and the reader does not even need to evaluate choice 1. The correct answer is D.

REFERENCES:

1. Chu KS, Hsu JH, Wang SS, et al. Accurate central venous port-A catheter placement: Intravenous electrocardiography and surface landmark techniques compared by using transesophageal echocardiography. Anesth Analg 98(4):910–914, 2004.

2. Cottrell JE, Smith DS. Anesthesia and Neurosurgery. St Louis, Mosby, 2001, pp. 342–344, Fig. 17-1.

3. Stoelting RK, Dierdorf SF. Anesthesia and Co-Existing Disease, 4th ed. New York, Churchill Livingstone, 2002, pp. 243–245.

4. Morgan GE, Mikhail MS, Murray MJ. Clinical Anesthesiology, 3d ed. New York, McGraw-Hill, 2002, pp. 574–575.

Answer C

Clinical Anesthesia

QUESTION (K-type):

A patient undergoing strabismus repair develops acute bradycardia during traction on an eye muscle. This response is

(1) Mediated by a facial nerve afferent.
(2) Also manifested by ventricular ectopy.
(3) Prevented by preanesthetic intramuscular administration of atropine.
(4) Treated by stopping the surgical stimulus.

CORRECT ANSWER: C (2 and 4 correct)

SUMMARY:

The oculocardiac reflex occurs with traction on extraocular muscles or when pressure is applied to the ocular globe. Such stimulus can elicit cardiac dysrhythmias. This reflex is seen commonly in pediatric patients undergoing strabismus surgery but can occur in all patient populations undergoing a variety of ophthalmologic procedures such as enucleation, cataract extraction, retinal detachment repair, and even placement of a retrobulbar block. The first step in managing cardiac dysrthymias associated with this reflex is to temporarily cease the inciting stimulus.

EXPLANATION:

(1) *Incorrect.* The afferent pathway is the trigeminal nerve, and the efferent pathway is the vagus.
(2) *Correct.* The oculocardiac reflex can elicit a wide variety of cardiac dysrhythmias, including bradycardia, ventricular ectopy, ventricular fibrillation, and sinus arrest.
(3) *Incorrect.* Intramuscular premedication with anticholinergic medications is not as effective as intravenous administration in the prevention of the oculocardiac reflex. The possibility of eliciting a response cannot be eliminated completely by premedication.
(4) *Correct.* Intraoperative management of the oculocardiac reflex includes supportive care, cessation of surgical stimulus, administration of anticholinergic medications, and infiltration of the rectus muscles with local anesthetics.

REASONING:

This question tests knowledge of the etiology and treatment of the oculocardiac reflex. A key point to answering this question correctly is understanding that while bradycardia is seen often with the oculocardiac reflex, other dysrthymias are possible. Appropriate management of the reflex includes immediate removal of the inciting stimulus and treatment with anticholinergic agents, if necessary.

REFERENCE:

Miller RD, Miller ED, Reves JG, et al. Anesthesia, 5th ed. New York, Churchill Livingstone, 2000, p. 2181.
Morgan GE, Mikhail MS, Murray MJ. Clinical Anesthesiology, 3d ed. New York, McGraw-Hill, 2002, p. 763.

Answer E

Clinical Anesthesia

QUESTION (K-type):

In a patient treated with propranolol and phenoxybenzamine prior to resection of a solitary pheochromocytoma, factors contributing to postoperative hypotension include

(1) Residual alpha-adrenergic block.
(2) Heart failure.
(3) Residual beta-adrenergic block.
(4) Adrenal insufficiency.

CORRECT ANSWER: E (all are correct)

SUMMARY:

Pheochromocytomas are norepinephrine- and epinephrine-secreting tumors of chromaffin tissues. Chronic catecholamine excess causes downregulation of adrenergic receptors, which is thought to be a protective response to avoid catecholamine toxicity. Cardiovascular manifestations of pheochromocytoma include increased peripheral vascular resistance and systemic hypertension from $alpha_1$ stimulation. An increase in ventricular ectopy and automaticity also can be seen from $beta_1$ stimulation. These patients are placed on $alpha_1$-antagonists and beta-blockers prior to resection. Patients should never be placed solely on beta-blockade because this can lead to unopposed alpha-adrenergic tone, life-threatening hypertension associated with increases in afterload, and may precipitate heart failure. Hypotension, not hypertension, is the primary problem after tumor resection. Postresection hypotension usually is due to hypovolemia, the sudden drop in catecholamine levels, and persistent adrenergic blockade. Fluid resuscitation and possible adrenergic support with norepinephrine, epinephrine, or phenylephrine may be necessary.

EXPLANATION:

(1) ***Correct.*** Residual alpha-adrenergic blockade can result in postoperative hypotension.
(2) ***Correct.*** Prolonged exposure to catecholamines can result in catecholamine-induced cardiomyopathy. The increased peripheral vascular resistance can lead to ventricular hypertrophy and congestive heart failure because of the increased myocardial workload.
(3) ***Correct.*** Residual beta-blockade also can result in postoperative hypotension.
(4) ***Correct.*** Adrenal insufficiency can occur even with solitary pheochromocytoma resection because some have been shown to produce adrenocorticotropic hormone (ACTH). Of course, with bilateral resection, adrenal insufficiency is expected, which is why many surgeons try to leave a piece of normal adrenal tissue to avoid the lifelong need for replacement.

REASONING:

This question tests knowledge of the pathophysiology and anesthetic implications of pheochromocytoma. Choices 1 and 3 are well-known etiologies of postoperative hypotension after pheochromocytoma resection. Choice 2 also was selected because plasma catecholamine levels stay persistently elevated for 1 to 3 days postoperatively. Therefore, an increase in myocardial workload still can occur and predispose to congestive heart failure (CHF). Adrenal insufficiency after resection of a solitary pheochromocytoma can occur. Thus the best answer is E.

REFERENCE:

Miller RD, Miller ED, Reves JG, et al. Anesthesia, 5th ed. New York, Churchill Livingstone, 2000, pp. 924–925.
Morgan GE, Mikhail MS, Murray MJ. Clinical Anesthesiology, 3d ed. New York, McGraw-Hill, 2002, pp. 222–223, 747–748.

Answer B

Physiology

QUESTION (K-type):

Anesthesia is induced with isoflurane and nitrous oxide in a patient with low cardiac output. Compared with a patient with normal cardiac function, which of the following will occur?

(1) Alveolar isoflurane concentration will approach the inspired concentration more rapidly.
(2) Total uptake of isoflurane will be higher during the first 11 minutes.
(3) The rate of rise of the alveolar concentration of isoflurane will be affected more than that of nitrous oxide.
(4) Induction will be slower.

CORRECT ANSWER: B (1 and 3 are correct)

SUMMARY:

Brain tissue concentration determines the clinical effect of inhalational agents. The brain tissue concentration is directly proportional to the partial pressure of the anesthetic in the brain. Brain partial pressure is approximated by alveolar partial pressure of the inhalational agent. Therefore, the clinical effect of an inhalational agent is proportional to the alveolar partial pressure. The greater the uptake of inhalational agent, the greater is the difference between inspired and alveolar concentration, and the slower is the rate of induction. The following factors affect anesthetic uptake: ventilation, anesthetic solubility in the blood, alveolar blood flow, and the partial pressure difference between alveolar gas and venous blood. The effect of changing cardiac output on rate of induction is more pronounced with soluble inhalational agents. As cardiac output decreases, less blood is perfused to the lungs, and there will be less uptake of the inhalational agent by the blood. This results in a more rapid rise in the alveolar partial pressure. Since alveolar partial pressure approximates brain tissue concentration of the inhalational agents, this results in a quicker induction in patients with low cardiac outputs as compared with those with normal cardiac outputs.

EXPLANATION:

(1) **Correct.** Alveolar isoflurane concentration approaches inspired concentration more rapidly in low cardiac output states compared with normal cardiac output states. This is so because less volatile anesthetic is taken up by the blood in low cardiac output states.
(2) **Incorrect.** Uptake of isoflurane will be less during low cardiac output states as compared with normal cardiac output states. The rate of rise of F_A/F_I (and anesthetic uptake) is not constant and typically decreases after the first 8 minutes owing to saturation of the vessel-rich group.[1] The total uptake of isoflurane may be greater during the first 11 minutes of the anesthetic, but patients with decreased cardiac output will still have less uptake during this period of time compared with patients with normal cardiac function.
(3) **Correct.** The rate of rise of the alveolar concentration of isoflurane is increased during low cardiac output states. Nitrous oxide uptake is not affected significantly by changing cardiac output because it is highly insoluble.
(4) **Incorrect.** Induction will be faster. See above.

REASONING:

The effects of volatile gas solubility and cardiac output on the speed of induction and rate of uptake is tested commonly on the written boards. The subject is not intuitive to many readers. The correct answer here can only be reached by a firm grasp of the pharmacokinetics of inhalational anesthetics. Choices 1 and 3 are correct; therefore, the answer is B.

REFERENCE:

1. Miller RD, Miller ED, Reves JG, et al. Anesthesia, 5th ed. New York, Churchill Livingstone, 2000, pp. 74–79.

2. Morgan GE, Mikhail MS, Murray MJ. Clinical Anesthesiology, 3d ed. New York, McGraw-Hill, 2002, pp.129–130.

BOOK B:

Answer C

Pediatrics

QUESTION 153 (OPTIONAL)

QUESTION (K-type):

Factors associated with postintubation croup in children include

(1) Age less than 3 months.
(2) History of recent upper respiratory infection.
(3) Use of a nasotracheal tube.
(4) Surgery of the head and neck.

CORRECT ANSWER: C (2 and 4 are correct)

SUMMARY:

Postintubation croup is a complication that most commonly affects children aged 1 to 4 years. It can present in the postoperative period, usually within 3 hours of extubation, and results from glottic or subglottic edema. Risk factors for postintubation croup include age 1 to 4 years, excessively large endotracheal tube (no leak over 25 cm H_2O), head and neck surgery, surgery longer than 1 hour, repeated movement of the endotracheal tube, and traumatic intubation.[1]

EXPLANATION:

(1) *Incorrect.* Postintubation croup occurs most commonly in children 1 to 4 years of age.
(2) *Correct.* In a large study using a prospectively collected database with 1283 children with a preoperative upper respiratory infection (URI) and over 20,000 children without a URI, children with a preoperative URI had a high relative risk of developing postoperative croup.[2]
(3) *Incorrect.* Use of a nasotracheal tube is not associated with increased risk compared with an orotracheal tube.
(4) *Correct.* Surgery of the head and neck is a risk factor for postintubation croup.

REASONING:

This question tests knowledge of postoperative respiratory complications in children. Choice 2 is very controversial. There are sources for and against recent URI being a risk factor for postintubation croup.[1] Even a major pediatric anesthesia textbook states that there is no correlation between URI and postintubation croup.[3] However, a study of over 22,000 patients by Cohen and colleagues published in 1991 (prior to this board examination) demonstrated a high relative risk of postintubation croup in patients with a URI.[2]

REFERENCES:

1. Cote CJ. A Practice of Anesthesia for Infants and Children, 3d ed. Philadelphia, Saunders, 2001, p. 93.

2. Cohen MM, Cameron CB. Should you cancel the operation when a child has an upper respiratory tract infection? Anesth Analg 72(3):282–288, 1991.

3. Gregory GA. Pediatric Anesthesia, 4th ed. New York, Churchill Livingstone, 2002, p. 242.

4. Morgan GE, Mikhail MS, Murray MJ. Clinical Anesthesiology, 3d ed. New York, McGraw-Hill, 2002, pp. 78, 850, 863.

Answer A

Pharmacology

QUESTION (K-type):

True statements concerning the effects of amrinone include

(1) Systemic vascular resistance is decreased.
(2) Intracellular levels of cyclic AMP are increased.
(3) It acts independently of beta$_1$-adrenergic receptors.
(4) Simultaneous administration of nonrepinephrine enhances ventricular dysrhythmias.

CORRECT ANSWER: A (1, 2, and 3 are correct)

SUMMARY:

Amrinone is a bipyridine-derivative phosphodiesterase inhibitor. It produces mild positive inotropism with strong vasodilatory effects. The mechanism is cAMP-mediated. Amrinone acts at the cell membrane and impedes the breakdown of cAMP. As cAMP increases, protein kinase is activated, promoting phosphorylation of the sarcoplasmic reticulum. Phosphorylation increases the slow inward movement of calcium current, increasing intracellular calcium and myocyte inotropy. In peripheral smooth muscle, increased cAMP levels cause vasodilation.

EXPLANATION:

(1) **Correct.** Amrinone causes vasodilation. Decreased systemic vascular resistance should be expected.
(2) **Correct.** Phosphodiesterase inhibitors impede the breakdown of cAMP. Increased intracellular levels of cAMP are responsible for the clinical effects of amrinone.
(3) **Correct.** Amrinone acts independently of catecholamine receptors. It is a phosphodiesterase inhibitor.
(4) **Incorrect.** Norepinephrine is a direct alpha- and beta-agonist. While administration of norepinephrine with amrinone may help to offset vasodilation, amrinone does not act synergistically with norepinephrine to increase the incidence of ventricular dysrhythmias.

REASONING:

This question tests knowledge of the pharmacology of amrinone. It is important to understand that the mechanism of phosphodiesterase inhibitors is distinct from that of other agents that act on adrenergic receptors. Drugs such as amrinone specifically inhibit phosphodiesterase III, which acts specifically on cyclic AMP. These agents are useful for positive ionotropy in the treatment of low-output cardiac disease. Important but uncommon side effects associated with amrinone include dose-related thrombocytopenia and centrilobular hepatic necrosis.[1] A is the best answer.

REFERENCE:

1. Barash PG, Cullen BF, Stoelting RK. Clinical Anesthesia, 4th ed. Philadelphia, Lippincott Williams & Wilkins, 2001, pp. 305–306.
2. Morgan GE, Mikhail MS, Murray MJ. Clinical Anesthesiology, 3d ed. New York, McGraw-Hill, 2002, pp. 456t, 457.

Answer A

Clinical Anesthesia

QUESTION (K-type):

Deflation of a leg tourniquet after 2 hours of inflation decreases

(1) Mixed venous oxygen saturation.
(2) Core temperature.
(3) Systemic vascular resistance.
(4) End-tidal carbon dioxide tension.

CORRECT ANSWER: A (1, 2, and 3 are correct)

SUMMARY:

Tourniquets are employed to minimize the blood loss in peripheral orthopedic procedures. Typically, the tourniquet is inflated to 100 mm Hg above systolic blood pressure. Deleterious effects of tourniquets are time- and pressure-dependent. Damage to nerves, skeletal muscles, and vessels has been reported with prolonged usage. Most changes are completely reversible for inflations of 1 to 2 hours.[1] The observed physiologic changes are due to washout of acid and potassium from the isolated limb. Physiologic derangements expected with tourniquet release include (1) transient metabolic acidosis, (2) increased arterial carbon dioxide tensions (1 to 8 mm Hg), (3) increased heart rate (10 to 15 percent), (4) increased serum potassium concentration (5 to 10 percent), and (5) decreased systemic vascular resistance (SVR).

EXPLANATION:

(1) **Correct.** Mixed venous oxygen tension represents the overall balance between oxygen consumption and oxygen delivery. A decreased mixed oxygen venous tension is seen during increased oxygen consumption or decreased oxygen delivery. During 2 hours of tourniquet time, a patient's limb would experience decreased blood flow. On reperfusion after tourniquet removal, recirculation of deoxygenated blood and increased uptake from the ischemic limb would result in a decreased mixed venous oxygen tension.
(2) **Correct.** Reestablishment of circulation to the ischemic limb would mix warm blood with that of a cold extremity, thus lowering core body temperature.[2]
(3) **Correct.** The transient metabolic acidosis seen with deflation of a leg tourniquet would result in a transient decrease in systemic vascular resistance. Expected cardiovascular changes also include a decrease in central venous pressure (CVP) and mean arterial pressure (MAP), with an increase in heart rate and a propensity for dysrhythmias.
(4) **Incorrect.** An increase in the end-tidal carbon dioxide tension would be expected owing to the "washout" of lactic acid from the ischemic limb.

REASONING:

This question tests knowledge of the physiologic effects of tourniquet application. Choice 4 can be eliminated immediately from consideration based on the common clinical observation of increased ETCO$_2$ after tourniquet release. One might reasonably expect core temperature to drop as a cool ischemic limb is reperfused (choice 2). Consequently, choices 1 and 3 also must be selected, leaving A as the correct answer.

REFERENCES:

1. Barash PG, Cullen BF, Stoelting RK. Clinical Anesthesia, 4th ed. Philadelphia, Lippincott Williams & Wilkins, 2001, p. 1115.
2. Estebe JP, Le Naoures A, Malledant Y, Ecoffey C. Use of a pneumatic tourniquet induces changes in central temperature. Br J Anaesth 77(6):786–788, 1996.

3. Morgan GE, Mikhail MS, Murray MJ. Clinical Anesthesiology, 3d ed. New York, McGraw-Hill, 2002, pp. 498, 500.

BOOK B:

Answer B

Pharmacology

QUESTION 156

QUESTION (K-type):

Compared with those of isoflurane, the respiratory effects of enflurane include

(1) Similar decrease in airway resistance.
(2) Greater attenuation of hypoxic pulmonary vasoconstriction.
(3) Greater increase in $Paco_2$ during spontaneous ventilation at 1 MAC.
(4) Less inhibition of hypoxic ventilatory drive at "MAC awake" concentrations.

CORRECT ANSWER: B (1 and 3 are correct)

SUMMARY:

All volatile anesthetics share similar effects on respiratory physiology. Isoflurane and enflurane cause respiratory depression, inhibit hypoxic pulmonary vasoconstriction, cause bronchodilation, and depress the ventilatory response to hypoxia and hypercarbia and inhibit mucociliary function.

EXPLANATION:

(1) **Correct.** Enflurane and isoflurane have similar effects on bronchomotor tone.
(2) **Incorrect.** All volatile anesthetics in animal models cause inhibition of the hypoxic pulmonary constriction reflex. There does not appear to be a difference between the various agents.[1]
(3) **Correct.** Enflurane causes a more profound respiratory depression at 1 MAC compared with isoflurane.[2]
(4) **Incorrect.** All volatile anesthetics cause equal depression of the hypoxic ventilatory drive even at the "MAC awake" concentration.

REASONING:

This is a difficult question because enflurane is not used in modern anesthesia. The important point to remember is that all volatile anesthetics suppress the ventilatory response to hypoxia and hypercarbia. Studies show that the ventilatory response to hypoxia is depressed 15 to 75 percent with as little as 0.1 MAC of volatile anesthetic.[3] This has important clinical implications for patients recovering from anesthesia.

REFERENCES:

1. Hirshman CA, McCullough RE, Cohen PJ, Weil JV. Depression of hypoxic ventilatory response by halothane, enflurane and isoflurane in dogs. Br J Anaesth 49(10):957–963, 1977.
2. Lindahl SG, Johannesson GP. Ventilatory CO_2 response, respiratory drive and timing in children anaesthetized with halothane, enflurane or isoflurane. Eur J Anaesthesiol 4(5):313–326, 1987.
3. Barash PG, Cullen BF, Stoelting RK. Clinical Anesthesia, 4th ed. Philadelphia, Lippincott Williams & Wilkins, 2001, pp. 387, 399–400.
4. Morgan GE, Mikhail MS, Murray MJ. Clinical Anesthesiology, 3d ed. New York, McGraw-Hill, 2002, pp. 142–143.

Answer A

Pharmacology

QUESTION (K-type):

Intravenous drugs that produce central nervous system effects by modulating gamma-aminobutyric acid (GABA) receptor activity include

(1) Midazolam.
(2) Thiopental.
(3) Flumazenil.
(4) Ketamine.

CORRECT ANSWER: A (1, 2, and 3 are correct)

SUMMARY:

GABA is an important inhibitory neurotransmitter. Many anesthetics enhance the inhibitory effects of GABA. GABA-receptor agonists enhance anesthesia, whereas GABA antagonists reverse some of these anesthetic affects. Benzodiazepines bind to a specific receptor in the CNS that facilitates GABA-receptor binding. Flumazenil is a specific benzodiazepine-receptor antagonist that reverses the CNS effects of benzodiazepines. Barbiturates suppress transmission of excitatory neurotransmitters and enhance transmission of inhibitory neurotransmitters (e.g., GABA). In addition, both propofol and etomidate act through modulating GABA-receptor activity. Ketamine is a unique intravenous anesthetic. It causes anesthesia by dissociating the thalamus through an N-methyl-D-aspartate receptor antagonism. It does not affect GABA activity.

EXPLANATION:

(1) *Correct.* Midazolam is the most commonly used benzodiazepine in anesthesia. It binds to the benzodiazepine receptor, which facilitates GABA binding to its receptor.
(2) *Correct.* Thiopental is the most commonly used barbiturate in anesthesia. Thiopental suppresses transmission of excitatory neurotransmitters and enhances transmission of inhibitory neurotransmitters (e.g., GABA).
(3) *Correct.* Flumazenil is a benzodiazepine antagonist with an indirect effect on the GABA receptor by reversing the effect of the benzodiazepines.
(4) *Incorrect.* Ketamine has no direct or indirect effects on GABA activity.

REASONING:

This question tests knowledge of the mechanism of action of common anesthetic agents. Since midazolam is the most likely correct answer, you can eliminate answers C and D. Since ketamine does not have GABA activity, answers D and E can be eliminated. Since choice 3 is linked to both A and B, the answer becomes obvious. The only challenge here is remembering that barbiturates have GABA activity. A is the best answer.

REFERENCE:

Barash PG, Cullen BF, Stoelting RK. Clinical Anesthesia, 4th ed. Philadelphia, Lippincott Williams & Wilkins, 2001, pp. 123–124, 327–344.
Morgan GE, Mikhail MS, Murray MJ. Clinical Anesthesiology, 3d ed. New York, McGraw-Hill, 2002, pp. 156, 160, 169.

Answer A

Clinical Anesthesia

QUESTION (K-type):

Findings consistent with heparin-induced thrombocytopenia include

(1) Platelet count of 25,000/mm^3.
(2) Subcutaneous route of heparin administration.
(3) Thrombosis.
(4) Onset within 4 hours of initiating heparin therapy.

CORRECT ANSWER: A (1, 2, and 3 are correct)

SUMMARY:

Heparin-induced thrombocytopenia (HIT) is defined as a decrease in platelet count shortly after starting heparin when other causes of thrombocytopenia have been ruled out. A milder form of HIT only results in mild thrombocytopenia and usually occurs within 4 days of starting heparin. This mild form is not thought to be immune-mediated. It usually resolves spontaneously despite continuing heparin. It is not associated with thrombosis and is thought to be a direct effect of heparin on platelets. A severe form of HIT usually occurs between days 4 and 14 of heparin therapy and is immune-mediated. It can result in both venous and arterial thrombosis. It is sometimes referred to as heparin-induced thrombocytopenia/thrombosis (HIT/T). Findings consistent with heparin-induced throm-bocytopenia include a 50 percent decrease in platelet count after receiving any form of heparin, including intravenous, subcutaneous, heparin flushes, and even heparin-coated catheters. Once HIT/T is suspected, all forms of heparin should be stopped. The platelet count should rise following discontinuation, but the patient continues to be at risk of thrombotic events, so anticoagulation with danaparoid or lepirudin should be started with the consultation of a hematologist.

EXPLANATION:

(1) **Correct.** A platelet count of 25,000/mm^3 is likely to represent a 50 percent decline from baseline.
(2) **Correct.** All forms of heparin administration have been associated with HIT/T.
(3) **Correct.** Thrombosis is clinical feature of HIT/T.
(4) **Incorrect.** It takes several days for HIT/T to occur.

REASONING:

This question tests knowledge of the pathophysiology of HIT/T. Since thrombosis is the most correct answer, choices C and D can be eliminated. Since it takes several days of heparin therapy to cause HIT/T, answer E can be eliminated. Since all forms of heparin cause HIT/T, the only correct answer is A.

REFERENCES:

Baglin TP. Heparin-induced thrombocytopenia thrombosis (HIT/T) sydrome. J Clin Pathol 54(4): 272–274, 2001.

Morgan GE, Mikhail MS, Murray MJ. Clinical Anesthesiology, 3d ed. New York, McGraw-Hill, 2002, p. 450.

Answer B

Clinical Anesthesia

QUESTION (K-type):

An anephric 12-year-old patient with a large pericardial effusion is to have pericardio-centesis under general anesthesia. Appropriate anesthetic management includes

(1) Maintenance of a high venous pressure.
(2) Prevention of tachycardia.
(3) Avoidance of positive end-expiratory pressure.
(4) Reduction of systemic vascular resistance.

CORRECT ANSWER: B (1 and 3 are correct)

SUMMARY:

Without evidence to the contrary, the reader should treat this patient as if he or she has tamponade physiology. Goals of management include maintenance of high sympathetic tone (which maintains a high venous pressure), relatively high heart rate, and relatively high afterload. Positive end-expiratory pressure (PEEP) will diminish preload and should be avoided.

EXPLANATION:

(1) **Correct.** Maintenance of high venous pressure is desirable to maintain filling of the heart in a patient with a large pericardial effusion. The effusion exerts pressure on the right atria, which will prevent diastolic filling unless venous pressures are maintained.
(2) **Incorrect.** Since the effusion impedes diastolic filling, stroke volume is relatively fixed, and reductions in heart rate will result in decreased cardiac output and may precipitate cardiac arrest.
(3) **Correct.** Increases in airway pressure (as with PEEP) will add to the intrathoracic pressure, impairing diastolic filling, and should be avoided.
(4) **Incorrect.** Since diastolic filling limits cardiac output in tamponade, a reduction in systemic vascular resistance will not be met with increased cardiac output, and blood pressure may fall precipitously.

REASONING:

This question tests knowledge of cardiovascular physiology in the setting of pericardial effusion/tamponade. Factors that diminish preload and cardiac output should be avoided. It is important to maintain heart rate, filling pressures, and afterload in these patients. Therefore, B is the best answer.

REFERENCE:

Barash PG, Cullen BF, Stoelting RK. Clinical Anesthesia, 4th ed. Philadelphia, Lippincott Williams & Wilkins, 2001, pp. 918–919.
Morgan GE, Mikhail MS, Murray MJ. Clinical Anesthesiology, 3d ed. New York, McGraw-Hill, 2002, pp. 399–400.

Answer D

Physiology

QUESTION (K-type):

Reliable indicators of left ventricular function in a patient with severe chronic obstructive pulmonary disease (COPD) include

(1) Left ventricular end-diastolic volume.
(2) Pulmonary artery diastolic pressure (PADP).
(3) Left atrial pressure (LAP).
(4) Cardiac index.

CORRECT ANSWER: D (4 only is correct)

SUMMARY:

COPD is characterized by pulmonary maldistribution of ventilation and perfusion giving rise to areas of intrapulmonary shunt and dead space. The evolution of this disease is chronic hypoxemia, erythrocytosis, pulmonary hypertension, and eventual right ventricular failure or cor pulmonale. Left ventricular function may be impaired secondarily, and hemodynamic parameters normally measured by Swan Ganz catheter no longer may be reliable in patients with severe COPD.

EXPLANATION:

(1) *Incorrect.* The left ventricular end-diastolic volume (LVEDV) can be approximated from the left ventricular end-diastolic pressure (LVEDP), assuming normal ventricular compliance. This relationship is no longer reliable in severe COPD owing to the interventricular interdependence between the right and left ventricles.[1] A distended right ventricle pushes on the interventricular septum, altering the left ventricular compliance and function.

(2) *Incorrect.* PADP is usually within a few millimeters of mercury of pulmonary catheter wedge pressure (PCWP) except in the setting of pulmonary hypertension (*See also Question 123, Book B.*)

(3) *Incorrect.* LAP is equivalent to LVEDP when there is no obstruction between the ventricle and atrium. Because PCWP is measured when there is no flow from the catheter tip to the left atrium, then PCWP = LAP = LVEDP. The possible presence of pulmonary hypertension in severe COPD makes wedging the catheter difficult, and PCWP can be artificially high, making LAP an unreliable indicator of LV function.

(4) *Correct.* Cardiac index is derived from the cardiac output measured via thermodilution technique. It reflects the rate of blood flow through the pulmonary artery and, by extension, cardiac output by the left ventricle.

REASONING:

This question tests knowledge of the pathophysiology of COPD and its effects on cardiovascular function. Complications of severe COPD include pulmonary hypertension and right ventricular failure that change the relationship between PCWP, LAP, LVEDP, and LVEDV. Because these parameters are no longer measured reliably, they are poor indicators of left ventricular function. Cardiac index that is calculated by thermodilution technique is least affected. Thus only choice 4 or D is correct.

REFERENCE:

[1] Marino PL. The ICU Book, 2d ed. Philadelphia, Lippincott Williams & Wilkins, 1998, p. 247.

QUESTION 161

QUESTION (K-type):

A 38-year-old woman who takes verapamil for idiopathic hypertrophic subaortic stenosis (IHSS) is anesthetized with enflurane, nitrous oxide, oxygen, and fentanyl for laparoscopic cholecystectomy. After inflation of the abdomen with carbon dioxide, her heart rate increases to 140 beats per minute, blood pressure decreases to 85/60 mm Hg, and ST-segment depression occurs. End-tidal carbon dioxide concentration is unchanged. Appropriate pharmacologic management includes intravenous administration of

(1) Phenylephrine.
(2) Nitroglycerin.
(3) Esmolol.
(4) Calcium chloride.

CORRECT ANSWER: B (1 and 3 are correct)

SUMMARY:

IHSS is a dynamic obstruction of the left ventricular outflow tract (LVOT) with the systolic anterior motion (SAM) of the anterior mitral leaflet abutting against the hpertrophic septum. Factors that worsen the LVOT obstruction are increased myocardial contractility, decreased left ventricular preload, and decreased left ventricular afterload. Decreasing the contractility with beta-blockers and increasing the afterload with alpha-agonists and preload augmentation with fluid and release of abdominal insufflation are all appropriate maneuvers.

EXPLANATION:

(1) **Correct.** Phenylephrine causes peripheral vasoconstriction, increasing central filling volumes, and helps prevent and treat LVOT obstruction in patients with IHSS.
(2) **Incorrect.** Nitroglycerine causes vasodilatation and decreases preload, worsening LVOT obstruction.
(3) **Correct.** Esmolol decreases the heart rate, allowing more time for diastolic filling, and decreases myocardial contractility. This helps to prevent and treat LVOT obstruction.
(4) **Incorrect.** Calcium chloride increases myocardial contractility and exacerbates the outlet obstruction.

REASONING:

This question tests knowledge of the pathophysiology and anesthetic implications of IHSS. It is important to understand the dynamic nature of the LVOT obstruction in patients with IHSS and factors that modulate the severity of obstruction. A full ventricle decreases obstruction. Factors that impair filling or increase emptying, such as increased myocardial contractility, peripheral vasodilation, and decreased preload, all worsen LVOT obstruction in these patients. B is the best answer.

REFERENCE:

Braunwald D, Zipes P. Heart Disease: A Textbook of Cardiovascular Medicine, 6th ed. Philadelphia, Saunders, 2001, p. 207.
Morgan GE, Mikhail MS, Murray MJ. Clinical Anesthesiology, 3d ed. New York, McGraw-Hill, 2002, p. 418.

Answer D

Pharmacology

QUESTION (K-type):

Compared with intermittent bolus administration, effects of continuous infusion of a short-acting anesthetic include

(1) Increased therapeutic index.
(2) Decreased serum concentration required.
(3) Prolonged recovery time.
(4) Decreased total amount of anesthetic required.

CORRECT ANSWER: D (4 only is correct)

SUMMARY:

Continuous infusion of medication during anesthetic administration has several advantages over intermittent bolus administration. Continuous infusions allow more predictable plasma drug concentrations and avoid peak and trough drug levels (peaks produce unwanted side effects, and troughs produce decreased clinical efficacy). Infusions provide the ability to titrate clinical effect more closely and thus give the clinician more precise hemodynamic and therapeutic control. There is some evidence to suggest that infusions decrease the total amount of drug required and may be associated with fewer postoperative side effects.[1] Continuous parenteral infusions do not have an impact on therapeutic index (this property of a drug is relatively constant regardless of route of administration). If anything, continuous infusions decrease recovery time because they allow slow titration of medication. The serum concentration associated with continuous infusions may be higher or lower than with bolus administration depending on whether the comparison is to peak or trough bolus concentrations.

EXPLANATION:

(1) *Incorrect.* Continuous parenteral infusions do not affect therapeutic index.
(2) *Incorrect.* This statement is not correct because it depends on whether you are comparing infusion concentrations with peak bolus drug concentrations or trough bolus drug concentrations.
(3) *Incorrect.* Continuous infusions are not associated with prolonged recovery times when titrated properly in healthy patients.
(4) *Correct.* Of all the choices listed, only decreased total amount of drug required is supported by clinical studies.[2]

REASONING:

This question tests knowledge of the pharmacokinetics of anesthetic infusions. Answers A, B, and E can be eliminated immediately simply by knowing that answer 1 is incorrect (the therapeutic index of a drug does not change based on the route of administration). This leaves answers C and D. Although it is tempting to say that the serum concentration would be lower with an infusion (choice 2), this is only true when the infusion concentration is compared with the peak bolus concentrations. During the trough phase of bolus injections, the infusion concentration may well be higher. Thus D is the best answer.

REFERENCES:

1. White PF. Use of continuous infusion versus intermittent bolus administration of fentanyl or ketamine during outpatient anesthesia. Anesthesiology 59:294–300, 1983.
2. White PF. Textbook of Intravenous Anesthesia. Baltimore, Williams & Wilkins, 1997, p. 603.
3. Newson C, Joshi GP, Victory R, et al. Comparison of propofol administration techniques for sedation during monitored anesthesia care. Anesth Analg 81:486–491, 1995.

4. Reves JG, et al. Continuous infusion of fentanyl and midazolam for cardiac surgery. Anesth Analg 70:S1–450, 1990.

5. Morgan GE, Mikhail MS, Murray MJ. Clinical Anesthesiology, 3d ed. New York, McGraw-Hill, 2002, pp. 887–888.

BOOK B:

Answer C

Pediatrics

QUESTION 163

QUESTION (K-type):

During abdominal closure for gastroschisis in a 1-day-old infant, airway pressure increases and oxygen saturation decreases. Breath sounds are bilateral, and endotracheal suctioning does not improve ventilation. After increasing FIO_2, appropriate management includes

(1) Deepening volatile anesthesia.
(2) Administering additional muscle relaxant.
(3) Adding positive end-expiratory pressure (PEEP).
(4) Foregoing primary abdominal closure.

CORRECT ANSWER: C (2 and 4 are correct)

SUMMARY:

Gastroschisis is a congenital anomaly characterized by an abdominal wall defect lateral to the umbilicus. It results from occlusion of the omphalomesenteric artery in utero and typically is not associated with other congenital anomalies.[1] The lack of a hernia sac predisposes neonates with this disorder to dehydration, infection, and hypothermia. Primary closure of the defect is not always possible because it can result in a dramatic decrease in pulmonary compliance and hypotension from abdominal compartment syndrome.

EXPLANATION:

(1) **Incorrect.** Deepening anesthesia will not necessary help to improve ventilation. In fact, higher concentrations of volatile anesthetic may worsen hypotension.
(2) **Correct.** Adequate muscle relaxation is necessary for decreasing abdominal wall tension when attempting primary closure.
(3) **Incorrect.** Oxygen desaturation in the setting of abdominal compartment syndrome results from an overall decrease in venous return and pulmonary blood flow. Since the problem is an increase in dead space, adding PEEP in this setting will not help.
(4) **Correct.** For many neonates, primary closure is not advisable because they will not tolerate drastic decreases in pulmonary compliance and venous return.

REASONING:

This question tests knowledge of the pathophysiology and anesthetic management of patients with gastroschisis. At first glance, choices 1 and 3 sound reasonable. However, the major problem with performing primary closure of a gastroschisis is abdominal compartment syndrome. Increased intraabdominal pressure results in poor pulmonary compliance, decreased venous return, decreased cardiac output, decreased pulmonary blood flow, and decreased lower extremity perfusion. Administering more volatile anesthetic and PEEP will not improve any of these conditions.

REFERENCE:

1. Cote CJ. A Practice of Anesthesia for Infants and Children, 3d ed. Philadelphia, Saunders, 2001, pp. 309–310.

2. Morgan GE, Mikhail MS, Murray MJ. Clinical Anesthesiology, 3d ed. New York, McGraw-Hill, 2002, p. 866.

QUESTION 164 (OPTIONAL)

Answer C

Clinical Anesthesia

QUESTION (K-type):

True statements concerning airway management in a patient with suspected injury to the cervical spine following head and chest trauma include

(1) Cricothyroidotomy is the preferred method of securing the airway.
(2) Injuries at Cl or C2 place the patient at greatest risk for neurologic injury during laryngoscopy.
(3) Cricoid pressure is contraindicated.
(4) Normal lateral, anteroposterior (AP), and open-mouth views of the cervical spine rule out spinal cord injury.

CORRECT ANSWER: C (2 only is correct)

SUMMARY:

Spinal cord injuries are common in major trauma patients, with cervical involvement constituting 50 percent of all spine injuries. The reader should assume that all trauma patients potentially have unstable spinal injuries. Extreme care must be taken at all steps when treating these patients to prevent further injury. All trauma patients are at high risk for aspiration and should be treated accordingly. The preferred method of securing the airway should be an awake fiberoptic intubation or a rapid-sequence induction with cricoid pressure and inline cervical stabilization.

EXPLANATION:

(1) *Incorrect.* This would be the preferred method only if the patient's associated injuries and clinical status would preclude an awake fiberoptic intubation or rapid-sequence intubation with inline cervical stabilization.
(2) *Correct.* This statement is correct. The atlanto-occipital and the upper cervical spine are the most at risk during intubation.[1]
(3) *Incorrect.* All trauma patients are at significant risk of aspiration, and cricoid pressure should be applied for all inductions. Care should be taken not to apply excessive pressure if a known C6–7 fracture is present.
(4) *Incorrect.* Ten percent of cervical injuries would be missed with only a three-view cervical spine series. An additional computed tomographic (CT) scan of the cervical spine would rule out spinal cord injury.[2]

REASONING:

This question is difficult because the only correct answer is choice 2. When faced with this dilemma, it is best to go with the most correct statement and eliminate the most incorrect. There is little evidence to support choice 1, so it is must incorrect. Therefore, on an actual examination, we would choose answer C. However, the reader should note that choice 4 is incorrect.

REFERENCES:

1. Barash PG, Cullen BF, Stoelting RK. Clinical Anesthesia, 3th ed. Philadelphia, Lippincott Williams & Wilkins, 1997, p. 580.
2. Barash PG, Cullen BF, Stoelting RK. Clinical Anesthesia, 4th ed. Philadelphia, Lippincott Williams & Wilkins, 2001, p. 1266.
3. Morgan GE, Mikhail MS, Murray MJ. Clinical Anesthesiology, 3d ed. New York, McGraw-Hill, 2002, pp. 793, 794.

QUESTION (K-type):

A 30-year-old man with gunshot wounds receives an emergency transfusion of 4 units of un-cross-matched O, Rh-negative blood. His blood type is AB, Rh-positive. For further intraoperative transfusions, he should receive

(1) O, Rh-negative red cells.
(2) AB, Rh-positive red cells.
(3) AB, Rh-positive plasma.
(4) O, Rh-negative plasma.

CORRECT ANSWER: B (1 and 3 are correct)

SUMMARY:

Human red blood cell membranes are estimated to contain at least 300 different antigenic determinants, and there are at least 20 separate blood group antigen systems. The ABO system is the most important blood typing system and accounts for the majority of transfusion reactions. An individual is either group A, B, AB, or O. Individuals will develop antibodies to whatever type they lack. For example, someone who is type A will have antibodies to B; someone who is type O will have antibodies to both A and B; and someone who is type AB will have no antibodies. Type O blood is considered the universal donor, and type AB is considered the universal recipient.

EXPLANATION:

(1) **Correct.** After a patient receives un-cross-matched blood (>2 units), he or she should continue to receive type O packed red blood cells (PRBCs).[1] This is so because a unit of PRBCs contains a small amount of plasma that contains antibodies to A and B antigens. If the patient were to receive type-specific blood, in this case type AB, there is a chance that the antibodies transferred to the patient in the donor type O unit could attack the type specific AB red cells, causing a hemolytic transfusion reaction.

(2) **Incorrect.** See above.

(3) **Correct.** Although the patient may have anti-A and anti-B antibodies passively transferred from the prior type O unit, there is not risk of hemolysis because A or B antigens are not present in plasma.

(4) **Incorrect.** Type AB–specific plasma can be given, and valuable type O–specific units should not be wasted.

REASONING:

This question tests knowledge of ABO compatibility and blood transfusions. Although not stated explicitly, we assume that the author is referring to packed red blood cells. O-negative whole blood should not be administered because the plasma could contain high titers of anti-A and anti-B antibodies.[1] It should be noted that the Rh status is somewhat of a red herring and does not matter in this question. In this question the patient is Rh-positive, so it does not matter if you use Rh-negative or Rh-positive units. This helps to limit the options to only the ABO group. B is the best answer.

REFERENCE:

1. Barash PG, Cullen BF, Stoelting RK. Clinical Anesthesia, 4th ed. Philadelphia, Lippincott Williams & Wilkins, 2001, p. 205.
2. Morgan GE, Mikhail MS, Murray MJ. Clinical Anesthesiology, 3d ed. New York, McGraw-Hill, 2002, p. 633.

Answer E

Pharmacology

QUESTION (K-type):

A 46-year-old man who takes clonidine for essential hypertension undergoes a 12-hour limb reimplantation under general anesthesia. Which of the following should be anticipated during the perioperative course?

(1) Decreased anesthetic requirements
(2) Postoperative hypertension
(3) Blunting of tachycardia with tracheal intubation
(4) Excessive postoperative drowsiness

CORRECT ANSWER: E (All are correct)

SUMMARY:

Clonidine is a presynaptic alpha$_2$-adrenergic agonist that inhibits norepinephrine release. It is used for the treatment of refractory hypertension. In addition to its antihypertensive effects, it decreases anesthetic and analgesic requirements and produces sedation and anxiolysis. It can be used in regional and neuroaxial anesthesia to provide prolongation of the block. Patients receiving clonidine for hypertension should continue the medication postoperatively because severe rebound hypertension can result from abrupt discontinuation.

EXPLANATION:

(1) **Correct.** Clonidine has been shown to decrease anesthetic requirements.
(2) **Correct.** Patients receiving clonidine for hypertension are at risk of developing postoperative hypertension from withdrawal of the medication. Signs of withdrawal include hypertension, tachycardia, insomnia, flushing, headache, apprehension, sweating, and tremulousness and usually occur 18 hours after discontinuing the drug.[1]
(3) **Correct.** Patients receiving clonidine may have a blunting of tachycardia from intubation from the decreased activation of the sympathetic nervous system and increased vagal tone.[1]
(4) **Correct.** Patients may experience postoperative sedation from either the direct effect of clonidine or through the accentuation of anesthesia and analgesia caused by clonidine.

REASONING:

This question tests knowledge of the pharmacology of clonidine. It is important for the reader to have a thorough understanding of the multiple pharmacologic effects of clonidine at its various sites of administration and to be aware of the hazards of acute clonidine withdrawal. All the statements are correct, and thus E is the best answer.

REFERENCE:

1. Barash PG, Cullen BF, Stoelting RK. Clinical Anesthesia, 4th ed. Philadelphia, Lippincott Williams & Wilkins, 2001, p. 317.
2. Morgan GE, Mikhail MS, Murray MJ. Clinical Anesthesiology, 3d ed. New York, McGraw-Hill, 2002, p. 217.

Answer A

Equipment/Physics

QUESTION (K-type):

Defective expiratory unidirectional valves in a circle system result in

(1) Increased dead space.
(2) Decreased F_{IO_2}.
(3) Prolonged anesthetic induction.
(4) Transformation to a non-rebreathing system.

CORRECT ANSWER: A (1, 2, and 3 are correct)

SUMMARY:

The circle system is a rebreathing circuit with inspiratory and expiratory unidirectional valves and a CO_2 absorber canister to prevent rebreathing of expired CO_2 gas. The inspiratory valve opens on inspiration and closes on expiration, and the expiratory valve has the opposite action. Unidirectional valves prevent rebreathing of expired CO_2, and limit the circuit's dead space.[1] Non-rebreathing systems such as the Mapleson circuits do not have unidirectional expiratory valves and depend on an adequate fresh gas flow to prevent rebreathing of expired CO_2. The circle system is designed to partially rebreathe expired gases in order to (1) warm and humidify inspired gases, (2) economize use of anesthetic agents, and (3) reduce environmental pollution with anesthetic gases. The non-rebreathing system is designed so that none of the exhaled gas is rebreathed in the circuit. Rebreathing of expired CO2 gas can occur with a faulty unidirectional valve on the circle system or inadequate fresh gas flow on the Mapleson circuits.

EXPLANATION:

(1) *Correct.* Unidirectional valves are important in decreasing the dead space of the anesthetic circuit. The only dead space is distal to the valves. If the expiratory valve is defective, this will add significant dead space to the breathing circuit.
(2) *Correct.* Since the expiratory valve prevents rebreathing, failure of this valve will allow the exhaled gas to mix with the inspiratory gas and lower the F_{IO_2}.
(3) *Correct.* Rebreathing exhaled gases causes the inspired gas concentration to be lower. At induction, the expired anesthetic gas concentration is less than inspired. The lower the inspired concentration of anesthetic, the slower is the induction.
(4) *Incorrect.* The circle system still has a functioning inspiratory valve and cannot be converted into a non-rebreathing system (i.e., Mapleson circuit) because fresh gas flow will not occur during expiration, a requirement for a non-rebreathing system.

REASONING:

This question tests knowledge of the circle system. Questions regarding the circle system, its advantages and disadvantages, associated dead space, and problems with its components are tested frequently. The reader should review these topics carefully.[2] The best answer is A.

REFERENCES:

1. Ehrenwerth J, Eisenkraft JB. Anesthesia Equipment: Principles and Applications. St Louis, Mosby–Year Book, 1993, p. 93.
2. Barash PG, Cullen BF, Stoelting RK. Clinical Anesthesia, 4th ed. Philadelphia, Lippincott Williams & Wilkins, 2001, pp. 567–594.
3. Morgan GE, Mikhail MS, Murray MJ. Clinical Anesthesiology, 3d ed. New York, McGraw-Hill, 2002, pp. 35–36.

Answer E

Equipment/Physics

QUESTION (K-type):

In the absence of a change in the ventilator settings, the measured exhaled tidal volume on the machine spirometer decreases when

(1) The endotracheal tube migrates into the right main stem bronchus.
(2) Fresh gas flow is decreased.
(3) A heated humidifier is added.
(4) The endotracheal tube cuff begins to leak.

CORRECT ANSWER: E (All are correct)

SUMMARY:

The tidal volume that is delivered by the anesthesia machine ventilator is measured by a device known as a spirometer. *There are various types of spirometers, and they measure the tidal volumes in different ways. They are usually placed in the expiratory limb of the circuit to measure exhaled tidal volume. Changes in measured exhaled tidal volume that are not due to changes in the ventilator settings can be caused by various factors. These factors include circuit leaks, loss of volume through breathing tube expansion, water condensation in the spirometer, and measurement inaccuracies with high or low fresh gas flows.*

EXPLANATION:

(1) **Correct.** As the endotracheal tube migrates into a mainstem bronchus, the peak inspiratory pressures will increase. A mainstem intubation creates a less compliant system and results in a decreased tidal volume.
(2) **Correct.** Some spirometers use a system not unlike a weather vane to measure the volume of exhaled gas. As the volume of gas passes through the vane, it spins and is translated into a volume of gas that represents the tidal volume. However, the measurement can be inaccurate at either low or high fresh gas flows owing to friction or inertia of the mechanical apparatus.
(3) **Correct.** The spirometers are calibrated at the factory for a specific density of gas. If the temperature of the gas changes, it will result in a change in the density of the gas. Adding a heated humidifier will change the density of the gas, creating a measurement error.[1]
(4) **Correct.** As the endotracheal tube cuff begins to leak, it will result in loss of part of the exhaled tidal volume from around the tube. Since the measurement of exhaled tidal volume occurs within the expiratory limb of the circuit, the volume that leaks around the cuff will be lost to measurement.

REASONING:

Questions about anesthesia machines and physics are challenging and usually require memorization. It is important not to panic when confronted with a difficult question. It is important to remember that all the questions do not need to be answered correctly to pass the examination. Careful review of delivery systems for inhaled anesthetics cannot be overstated.[2]

REFERENCES:

1. Feldman JM, Muller J. Tidal volume measurement errors: The impact of lung compliance and a circuit humidifier. Anesthesiology A468, 1990.
2. Barash PG, Cullen BF, Stoelting RK. Clinical Anesthesia, 4th ed. Philadelphia, Lippincott Williams & Wilkins, 2001, pp. 567–594.
3. Morgan GE, Mikhail MS, Murray MJ. Clinical Anesthesiology, 3d ed. New York, McGraw-Hill, 2002, pp. 44–45.

Answer D

Equipment/Physics

QUESTION (K-type)

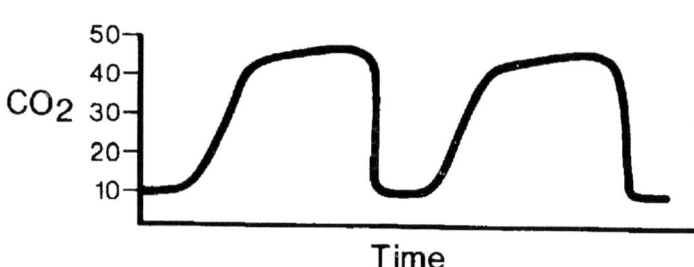

The capnographic waveform shown above was obtained during anesthesia using a semi-closed-circle system and mechanical ventilation. This waveform is consistent with

(1) Increased body temperature to 40°C.
(2) Kinking of the endotracheal tube.
(3) Inadequate minute ventilation.
(4) An incompetent expiratory value.

CORRECT ANSWER: D (4 only is correct)

SUMMARY:

Capnography is a valuable tool for the safe administration of anesthesia. It not only provides real-time confirmation of endotracheal tube placement but can also provide valuable information about various physiologic and mechanical problems in the operating room. The capnograph is divided into four parts: Phase I is the baseline trace and should be zero; phase II represents the start of exhalation with a rapid upswing in the trace; phase III represents the majority of exhalation, and the point at which it drops suddenly is phase 0, indicating the start of inhalation. The final point of phase III is described as the end-tidal CO_2. An elevation in the phase I waveform indicates rebreathing of CO_2, which could be due to an incompetent unidirectional valve or exhaustion of CO_2 absorbant.

EXPLANATION:

(1) **Incorrect.** Increased body temperature would increase the overall production of CO_2 with a resulting increase in the size of the phase II portion of the capnograph. However, the capnograph still should return to baseline despite the increased CO_2 production.
(2) **Incorrect.** Kinking of the endotracheal tube could cause an increase in airway pressure. It should not affect phase I of the capnograph.
(3) **Incorrect.** Inadequate minute ventilation will cause the end-tidal CO_2 to be elevated, but it would still return to zero in phase I of the capnograph.
(4) **Correct.** This answer is correct because an elevated phase I is associated with incompetent expiratory or inspiratory valves or exhaustion of the CO_2 absorbant, leading to rebreathing of exhaled CO_2.

REASONING:

This question tests basic knowledge of the capnogram. Fortunately, the differential diagnosis for rebreathing of CO_2, as represented by an increase from zero on the capnograph is short: incompetent valves or exhaustion of CO_2 absorber. The only correct choice is 4. D is the best answer.

REFERENCE:

Barash PG, Cullen BF, Stoelting RK. Clinical Anesthesia, 4th ed. Philadelphia, Lippincott Williams & Wilkins, 2001, pp. 668–669.
Morgan GE, Mikhail MS, Murray MJ. Clinical Anesthesiology, 3d ed. New York, McGraw-Hill, 2002, pp. 110–112.

BOOK B:

QUESTION 170

Answer A

Clinical Anesthesia

QUESTION (K-type):

A 45-year-old woman is scheduled for a cholecystectomy following an episode of acute cholecystitis. Thirty minutes after premedication with morphine and midazolam, she has nausea and acute right upper quadrant pain. Drugs that alleviate these symptoms include

(1) Glucagon.
(2) Nitroglycerin.
(3) Naloxone.
(4) Flumazenil.

CORRECT ANSWER: A (1, 2, and 3 are correct)

SUMMARY:

Choledocoduodenal sphincter (sphincter of Oddi) spasm can be induced by the administration of opioids. Smooth muscle constriction of the sphincter can cause right upper quadrant pain. The treatment options for the treatment of the spasm include naloxone, glucagon, nifedipine, and nitroglycerin.

EXPLANATION:

(1) **Correct.** Glucagon has been shown to help relax sphincter of Oddi spasm. The dose is usually 1 to 3 mg intravenously.
(2) **Correct.** Nitroglycerin also has been shown to reverse sphincter of Oddi spasm.[1,2]
(3) **Correct.** Pure opioid antagonist such as naloxone can reverse the sphincter spasm.
(4) **Incorrect.** Spincter of Oddi spasm is not caused by the administration of benzodiazepines; therefore, flumazenil will have no effect on the spasm.

REASONING:

This question tests knowledge of the etiology and treatment of cholodocoduodenal sphincter spasm. It is made more difficult because most texts list the use of naloxone and glucagon but do not make reference to the use of nitroglycerin. The correct answer includes nitroglycerin; therefore, A is the best answer.

REFERENCES:

1. Toyoyama H, Kariya N, Hase I, Toyoda Y. The use of intravenous nitroglycerin in a case of spasm of the sphincter of Oddi during laparoscopic cholecystectomy. Anesthesiology 94:708–709, 2001.
2. Velosy B, Madacsy L, Lonovics J, Csernay L. Effect of glyceryl trinitrate on the sphincter of Oddi spasm evoked by prostigmine-morphine administration. Eur J Gastroenterol Hepatol 9:1109–1112, 1997.
Morgan GE, Mikhail MS, Murray MJ. Clinical Anesthesiology, 3d ed. New York, McGraw-Hill, 2002, p. 716.

Answer E

Physiology

QUESTION (K-type):

During a blood transfusion, a patient develops sudden hypotension and oozing from the puncture sites. Laboratory studies useful in establishing the diagnosis include

(1) Serum free hemoglobin concentration.
(2) Direct antiglobulin (Coombs') test.
(3) Urine hemoglobin concentration.
(4) Serum haptoglobin concentration.

CORRECT ANSWER: E (All are correct)

SUMMARY:

Transfusion reactions are always possible when administering blood products. The most severe reaction is the acute hemolytic reaction that results from ABO incompatibility. It causes acute intravascular hemolysis and can be fatal. The signs of an acute reaction in an anesthetized patient include increased temperature, tachycardia, hypotension, hemoglobinuria, and disseminated intravascular coagulation (DIC). If a transfusion reaction is suspected, the transfusion should be stopped, and a repeat type and cross should be performed immediately. In addition, a direct Coombs test should be ordered. Additional useful labs include serum haptoglobin, urine and serum hemoglobin, complete blood count (CBC), and a DIC panel.

EXPLANATION:

(1) *Correct.* Since the principal pathologic event in an acute hemolytic reaction is intravascular hemolysis, any test that shows increased red cell destruction would be helpful in making the diagnosis. Lysed RBCs will release hemoglobin into the serum.
(2) *Correct.* This is the definitive test to confirm acute hemolytic reaction. The direct Coombs test detects antibodies bound to circulating red blood cells.
(3) *Correct.* As the free hemoglobin is cleared from the circulation, it will be excreted in the urine. This will give the urine a characteristic pink color. The patient is at risk for developing acute renal failure.
(4) *Correct.* Initially as the hemoglobin is released, it becomes bound to haptoglobin and albumin. Eventually, these sites become saturated, resulting in free hemoglobin in the blood.

REASONING:

This question tests knowledge of the pathophysiology of acute hemolytic reaction. It is an immune-mediated reaction that results in lysis of red blood cells and release of hemoglobin. All the choices are correct; therefore, the answer is E.

REFERENCE:

Barash PG, Cullen BF, Stoelting RK. Clinical Anesthesia, 4th ed. Philadelphia, Lippincott Williams & Wilkins, 2001, pp. 207–208.
Morgan GE, Mikhail MS, Murray MJ. Clinical Anesthesiology, 3d ed. New York, McGraw-Hill, 2002, p. 636.

Answer B

Pharmacology

QUESTION (K-type):

A continuous infusion of atracurium for 60 hours has been associated with

(1) Seizure activity.
(2) Histamine release.
(3) Increased anesthetic requirements.
(4) Adrenal suppression.

CORRECT ANSWER: B (1 and 3 are correct)

SUMMARY:

Atracurium is a nondepolarizing neuromuscular agent that is used often in the intensive care setting as a continuous infusion. It is degraded by non–organ-specific metabolism through both Hofmann elimination and nonspecific plasma esterases. The principal metabolite is laudanosine, which has been linked to CNS excitation and potentially seizure activity. In large- or rapid-dose administration, atracurium has been associated with histamine release.

EXPLANATION:

(1) *Correct.* The principal metabolite of atracurium is laudanosine, which has been associated with but never proven to cause seizure activity in ICU patients receiving continuous infusions.
(2) *Incorrect.* Although atracurium has been associated with histamine release, it is usually with large and rapid bolus doses of the drug. It is unlikely that a 60-hour continuous infusion of atracurium would be associated with histamine release.
(3) *Correct.* The presence of laudanosine, a by-product of long-term infusions of atracurium, has been associated with CNS stimulation and the elevation of MAC.
(4) *Incorrect.* There is no reported link between long-term infusion of atracurium and adrenal suppression.

REASONING:

This question tests knowledge of the pharmacology of atracurium. It is quite a controversial question. The "reflex" response to an atracurium question is that it releases histamine, but that would be incorrect in a long-term infusion. Based on how the question is worded (i.e., 60-hour infusion), the best answer is B.

REFERENCE:

Barash PG, Cullen BF, Stoelting RK. Clinical Anesthesia, 4th ed. Philadelphia, Lippincott Williams & Wilkins, 2001, pp. 427–428.
Morgan GE, Mikhail MS, Murray MJ. Clinical Anesthesiology, 3d ed. New York, McGraw-Hill, 2002, p. 191.

Answer A

Pharmacology

QUESTION (K-type):

The anesthetic recovery of a newborn infant is complicated by the slow return of neuromuscular function. Factors that would cause this complication include

(1) An inadequate dose of anticholinesterase.
(2) Active maternal myasthenia gravis.
(3) A core temperature of 35°C.
(4) Intraoperative administration of cefamandole.

CORRECT ANSWER: A (1, 2, and 3 are correct)

SUMMARY:

The response of neonates to nondepolarizing muscle relaxants is variable owing to their immature neuromuscular junctions, large extracellular fluid volume and resulting large volume of distribution, and immature metabolic pathways. Babies of myasthenic mothers can have transient myasthenia gravis for up to 3 weeks and will be even more sensitive to the effects of nondepolarizers. Causes of prolonged neuromuscular blockade not specific to pediatric patients include hypothermia, inadequate reversal, electrolyte abnormalities, and drug interactions.

EXPLANATION:

(1) **Correct.** An inadequate dose of anticholinesterase can result in slow return of neuromuscular function. The dose of reversal agent should be determined by response to peripheral nerve stimulation.
(2) **Correct.** Mothers with active myasthenia gravis transfer anti-Ach receptor antibodies across the placenta, causing transient neonatal myasthenia 1 to 3 weeks after birth.
(3) **Correct.** Hypothermia can prolong neuromuscular blockade by decreasing drug metabolism.
(4) **Incorrect.** Cefamandole is not used commonly in newborn infants. This issue aside, there are certain antibiotics that can interact with muscle relaxants to produce prolonged muscle paralysis, such as aminoglycosides, polymyxin, tetracycline, and clindamycin. Cefamandole is not listed as one of them.

REASONING:

This question tests knowledge of prolonged neuromuscular blockade. This problem is not specific to pediatric patients, so it is important to consider all potential causes when approaching this question. Choices 1 and 3 should be easy to identify as correct. Choice 4 can be eliminated if the reader recalls which drugs interact with muscle relaxants. Choice 2 is the only challenging option but instinctively makes sense even if the reader is not entirely sure of the answer. A is the best answer.

REFERENCE:

Barash PG, Cullen BF, Stoelting RK. Clinical Anesthesia, 4th ed. Philadelphia, Lippincott Williams & Wilkins, 2001, pp. 432–441.
Morgan GE, Mikhail MS, Murray MJ. Clinical Anesthesiology, 3d ed. New York, McGraw-Hill, 2002, pp. 185, 189, 205–206, 754, 856, Table 9-4 (p. 185), Potentiation and Resistance of Neuromuscular Blocking Agents by Other Drugs.

BOOK B:

QUESTION 174

Answer E

Pain

QUESTION (K-type):

Complications of stellate ganglion block include

(1) Elevation of the ipsilateral hemidiaphragm.
(2) Total spinal anesthesia.
(3) Seizures.
(4) Hoarseness.

CORRECT ANSWER: E (All are correct)

SUMMARY:

The stellate ganglion block is a paratracheal regional anesthetic technique that is used often in patients with head, neck, and upper extremity pain. Placement of the block involves insertion of a needle at the medial edge of the sternocleidomastoid muscle at the level of the C6 transverse process (Chassaignac's tubercle). The proximity of the insertion site to nearby structures in the neck can lead to complications related to block placement. Aberrant needle positioning in the vertebral artery when attempting stellate ganglion block can lead to an intravascular injection, resulting in seizure. Similarly, injection into the dural sleeve of a nerve root can lead to subarachnoid injection and total spinal anesthesia. Correct placement of the needle still may result in hoarseness or elevated ipsilateral hemidiaphragm with blockade of the recurrent laryngeal and phrenic nerve, respectively.

EXPLANATION:

(1) *Correct.* Ipsilateral hemidiaphragm elevation can result from inadvertent phrenic nerve blockade.
(2) *Correct.* Total spinal anesthesia can occur from inadvertent injection into the dural sleeve.
(3) *Correct.* Seizures can result from inadvertent intravascular injection into the vertebral artery.
(4) *Correct.* Hoarseness can result from inadvertent recurrent laryngeal nerve blockade.

REASONING:

This question tests knowledge of the complications associated with stellate ganglion block. Described complications include hematoma, hoarseness, phrenic nerve block, spinal block, epidural block, subdural block, pneumothorax, seizures, and contamination and infection of bone, vertebral body, and mediastinum owing to esophageal puncture. The best answer is E.

REFERENCE:

Waldman SD. Interventional Pain Management, 2d ed. Philadelphia, Saunders, 2001, pp. 367–369. Morgan GE, Mikhail MS, Murray MJ. Clinical Anesthesiology, 3d ed. New York, McGraw-Hill, 2002, p. 295.

Index